ANCIENT MEDICINE

The first edition of *Ancient Medicine* was the most complete examination of the medicine of the ancient world for a hundred years. This new edition includes the key discoveries made since the first edition, especially from important texts discovered in recent finds of papyri and manuscripts, making it the most comprehensive and up-to-date survey available.

Vivian Nutton pays particular attention to the life and work of doctors in communities, links between medicine and magic, and examines the different approaches to medicine across the ancient world. The new edition includes more on Rufus and Galen as well as augmented information on Babylonia, Hellenistic medicine and Late Antiquity.

With recently discovered texts made accessible for the first time, and providing new evidence, this broad exploration challenges currently held perspectives, and proves an invaluable resource for students of both classics and the history of medicine.

Vivian Nutton, FBA, is Professor Emeritus of the History of Medicine at University College London, and an honorary Professor in both Classics and History at the University of Warwick. He has published extensively on all aspects of medicine before the seventeenth century and, in particular, on Galen and the Renaissance.

SCIENCES OF ANTIQUITY
Series editor: Liba Taub
*Director, The Whipple Museum of the History of Science,
University of Cambridge*

Sciences of Antiquity is a series designed to cover the subject matter of what we call science. The volumes discuss how the ancients saw, interpreted and handled the natural world, from the elements to the most complex of living things. Their discussions on these matters formed a resource for those who later worked on the same topics, including scientists. The intention of this series is to show what it was in the aims, expectations, problems and circumstances of the ancient writers that formed the nature of what they wrote. A consequent purpose is to provide historians with an understanding of the materials out of which later writers, rather than passively receiving and transmitting ancient 'ideas', constructed their own world-view.

TIME IN ANTIQUITY
Robert Hannah

ANCIENT ASTROLOGY
Tamsyn Barton

ANCIENT NATURAL HISTORY
Roger French

COSMOLOGY IN ANTIQUITY
M. R. Wright

ANCIENT MATHEMATICS
S. Cuomo

ANCIENT METEOROLOGY
Liba Taub

ANCIENT MEDICINE

Second edition

Vivian Nutton

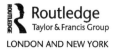

Routledge
Taylor & Francis Group

LONDON AND NEW YORK

First published 2004
This second edition published 2013
by Routledge
2 Park Square, Milton Park, Abingdon, Oxon OX14 4RN

Simultaneously published in the USA and Canada
by Routledge
711 Third Avenue, New York, NY 10017

Routledge is an imprint of the Taylor & Francis Group, an informa business

British Library Cataloguing in Publication Data
A catalogue record for this book is available from the British Library

Library of Congress Cataloging in Publication Data
A catalog record for this book has been requested

ISBN: 978-0-415-52094-2 (hbk)
ISBN: 978-0-415-52095-9 (pbk)
ISBN: 978-0-203-08129-7 (ebk)

Typeset in Garamond by
GreenGate Publishing Services, Tonbridge, Kent

Printed and bound by CPI Group (UK) Ltd, Croydon, CR0 4YY

CONTENTS

CONTENTS

ILLUSTRATIONS

FIGURES

MAPS AND PLANS

NOTE TO THE READER

All quotations from Greek and Latin have been translated into English by me, unless otherwise stated, and ancient titles have been given in English throughout. Ancient names have been generally given in their most familiar form, without any attempt at total consistency between a Greek and a Latinate spelling. I have often indicated also the modern name or general location of an ancient place. The exact dates of many ancient writers are rarely known, and only approximations are often possible. I have tried to be consistent in indicating all dates BC, but I have added AD only to dates where there might be confusion in the mind of the reader, especially in chapters that crossed the boundaries between the Hellenistic and Roman worlds.

Two features in the notes should be mentioned here. Square brackets around the name of an author, e.g. [Aristotle], indicate that the work cannot be attributed with any degree of certainty (and usually with none) to that author. Hence, for reasons made clear in the text, I refer to writings in the Hippocratic Corpus always as by [Hippocrates].

Second, the two main blocks of ancient medical material are cited in two different ways. All references to Hippocratic texts are with an English title, their book and chapter heading, and the volume and page number in the standard edition of Emile Littré (Paris: Baillière, 1839–61). By contrast, in order to save space, I have cited Galen mainly by the volume and page number in the standard edition of K. G. Kühn (Leipzig: K. H. Knobloch, 1821–33), adding, where possible, the page number of an accessible English version. Where necessary, I have occasionally referred also to an improved text in a more recent edition, usually in the *CMG* series. Texts not in Kühn have been cited by title, section and page in the relevant modern edition.

I have generally used standard editions of other ancient texts, indicating where necessary the name of the editor. I have not provided full bibliographical references to papyri, usually indicated by P., and to inscriptions, e.g. *I. Ephesos* or *Griechische Versinschriften*. Those with Greek or Latin who wish to check these documents in their originally published form should consult the list of abbreviations in Liddell, H. G., Scott, R. and Jones, H. S.

(1968) *A Greek–English Lexicon*, ed. 9, with Supplement, Oxford: Oxford University Press; and the revised *Supplement* (1996) ed. P. G. W. Glare, Oxford: Clarendon Press; or in the *Oxford Latin Dictionary* (1968–82) Oxford: Clarendon Press.

ACKNOWLEDGEMENTS

I have incurred many obligations in the writing of this book, which has taken far longer than I or the original editor of the series, the late Roger French, envisaged. Many parts of this have been presented at conferences or seminars around the world, and I am grateful for the comments and criticisms of the audiences on these occasions and, particularly, in London, Paris and Pisa. Several colleagues read and commented on the manuscript either in whole or in part: Elizabeth Craik, Jason Davies, Helen King, Cornelius O'Boyle, Thomas Rütten, Manuela Tecusan, Philip van der Eijk and Heinrich von Staden. Isabella Andorlini, Klaus-Dietrich Fischer, Ivan Garofalo, Mariaelena Gorrini, Ralph Jackson, Marie-Hélène Marganne, Innocenzo Mazzini and Gotthard Strohmaier kept me informed of very recent discoveries in their particular fields of interest, and allowed me to cite some of their work when it was still unpublished. Ralph Jackson and Nikolai Serikoff kindly provided photographs from their own collections. I also had the privilege of discussing many of the ideas in this book with two friends who, in their different ways, made a great contribution to the study of ancient medicine, Luis Garcia Ballester and Owsei Temkin. Neither, I am sure, would have entirely approved of some of my speculations, but both would have encouraged me in my aim of presenting to a wider public the recent findings of my own and others' scholarships.

This book represents the fruit of a long association with the Wellcome Trust and the Wellcome Institute for the History of Medicine, as it was called before its enforced dissolution in 2000. My academic colleagues, now within the Wellcome Trust Centre for the History of Medicine at UCL, have long tolerated my eccentric interests in our shared field, and a stream of research students and research fellows has ensured that my ideas have been constantly challenged. My secretaries, Frieda Houser and Sally Bragg, brought a certain degree of order to my life, usually to the strains of music. Jane Henderson undertook the major task of compiling the index. A generation of medical students has cheerfully listened to tales of Dr Galen and, although they may not credit it, has also taught me much about medicine and about presentational skills. Successive heads of the Department of Anatomy, notably Geoff

Burnstock and Nigel Holder, have encouraged my researches as part of the department's wider programme.

I have been fortunate to be able to rely on the resources of some of the finest libraries in the world, including those of the Institute of Classical Studies, the Warburg Institute and, the browser's ultimate paradise, the Cambridge University Library, and I acknowledge the kindness and helpfulness of their staffs. But this book would have taken even longer had it not been for the remarkable collections and the still more remarkable staff of the Wellcome Library. Whether in the Reprographics Department, where Chris Carter worked wonders with a camera and Catherine Draycott instructed me in the mysteries of the on-line catalogue; in the Poynter Room, where Richard Aspin allowed me to make use of innumerable manuscripts and where John Symons provided an unfailing source of recondite and precise information on the bibliography of the whole history of medicine; or in the main reading rooms of the library, I have always found kind, enthusiastic and cheerful colleagues, whose expertise I have shamelessly exploited over many years. The names of Nigel Allan, Eric Freeman, Robin Price, William Schupbach and Brenda Sutton can stand for the many friendships I have made there.

The writing of the book was begun in 2000 when I held a Fellowship at the Institute for Advanced Study at Princeton, a haven of academic tranquility at a time of great upheaval. I am grateful to the staff of the institute and to my fellow members for many valuable insights and discussions that forced me into much hard thinking, and rethinking. My visit to Princeton was made while I held a Research Leave Fellowship from the Wellcome Trust, whose support for my own work and for the history of medicine in general has been outstanding for many years. It is a pleasant duty to acknowledge the encouragement I have received from Peter Williams, Bridget Ogilvie, David Allen and their administrative staffs.

My greatest thanks go to my family and, above all, to my wife, who has read every word of this book in various drafts, and has improved its logic, accuracy and style throughout. As we both know, this is not the book I said I would write for her over thirty years ago, but it is still offered as a testament to her love and devotion over that period.

In making this revision I have incurred further debts to the friends and colleagues mentioned above, and also to Glenn Bowersock, Mark Geller, Peter Goode, Brooke Holmes, Caroline Petit, Laurence Totelin, and the reviewers of the first edition, particularly John Scarborough and Danielle Gourevitch. This revision is dedicated to former members of the Wellcome Trust Centre for the History of Medicine at UCL, whose enforced closure in 2011 was an enormous blow to all those interested in the subject.

ABBREVIATIONS

ANRW   H. Temporini and W. Haase (eds) (1974–) *Aufstieg und Niedergang der römischen Welt: Geschichte und Kultur Roms im Spiegel neueren Forschung*, Berlin: De Gruyter.

B.   J. Bertier (ed.) (1972) *Mnésithée et Dieuchès*, Leiden: Brill.

BGU   (various authors) (1919–) *Berliner griechische Urkunden*, Berlin: Weidmann.

CIE   *Corpus Inscriptionum Etruscarum* (1893–) Leipzig: I. A. Barth.

CIG   *Corpus Inscriptionum Graecarum* (1828–77) Berlin: Academia Borussica.

CIL   *Corpus Inscriptionum Latinarum* (1862–) Berlin: Reimer.

CMG   *Corpus Medicorum Graecorum* (1908–44) Berlin and Leipzig: Teubner; (1946–) Berlin: Akademie Verlag.

CML   *Corpus Medicorum Latinorum* (1908–44) Berlin and Leipzig: Teubner; (1952–) Berlin: Akademie Verlag.

Dbg   C. Daremberg and E. Ruelle (eds) (1879) *Oeuvres de Rufus d'Éphèse*, Paris: Baillière.

DK   H. Diels and W. Kranz (1952) *Die Fragmente der Vorsokratiker*, ed. 6, Berlin: Weidmann.

Dkw   *Galen: On Anatomical Procedures* (1962) tr. W. L. H. Duckworth, Cambridge: Cambridge University Press.

DNP   H. Cancik, M. Landfester and H. Schneider (1996–2003) *Der neue Pauly: Enzyklopädie der Antike*, 15 vols in 18, Stuttgart and Weimar: Metzler Verlag.

FgrH   F. Jacoby (1923–58) *Die Fragmente der griechischen Historiker*, Berlin: Weidmann.

G.   I. Garofalo (ed.) (1988) *Erasistrati Fragmenta*, Pisa: Giardini.

Gu.   A. Guardasole (ed.) (1997) *Eraclide di Taranto: Frammenti*, Naples: M. D'Auria.

IG   *Inscriptiones Graecae* (1877–) Berlin: Reimer.

IGLS   L. Jalabert and R. Mouterde (1929–) *Inscriptions grecques et latines de la Syrie*, Paris: P. Geuthner.

IGRR   R. Cagnat, *Inscriptiones Graecae ad res Romanas pertinentes* (1906–27) Paris: E. Leroux.

IGUR   *Inscriptiones Graecae Urbis Romae* (1968–) Rome: Istituto italiano per la storia antica.

ILS   *Inscriptiones Latinae Selectae* (1892–1916) Berlin: Weidmann.

L.   E. Littré (ed.) (1839–61) *Oeuvres complètes d'Hippocrate*, Paris: Baillière.

RE   A. Pauly and G. Wissowa (eds) (1893–1978) *Real-Encyclopädie der classischen Altertumswissenschaft*, Stuttgart: Metzler.

RIB   *The Roman Inscriptions of Britain* (1985–) Oxford: Clarendon Press.

SEG   *Supplementum Epigraphicum Graecum* (1923–) Leiden: Sijthoff.

St.   F. Steckerl (ed.) (1958) *The Fragments of Praxagoras of Cos and his School*, Leiden: Brill.

TAM   *Tituli Asiae Minoris* (1920–) Vienna: Akademie der Wissenschaften.

1

SOURCES AND SCOPE

History is an art of forgetting as well as of remembrance. Many of the voices of the past, especially of the losers in any conflict, can be heard faintly at best, and the further back in time we go the larger the gaps in our understanding. The two millennia or more separating us from the ancient Greeks and Romans mean that any comprehensive reconstruction of their ideas on health and healing is fraught with problems. The vicissitudes of the written word over the centuries have drastically narrowed the range of material to a mere fraction of what once existed. As a result, the fact of survival has given prominence to certain documents and has imposed a way of thinking about them that at times distorts the historical reality. By looking back in this chapter at this process of destruction, and by setting out in general some of the consequences for our understanding of the past, I hope to stress both the fragility of our historical information and the need to be open to alternative interpretations of what does survive.[1]

Yet to begin by talking of written records is to risk forgetting that much of Greek and Roman medicine never made it into writing at all, for in a society where literacy was restricted on the whole to the higher echelons of male society oral communication predominated. The 'little old woman' from whom Scribonius Largus bought a remedy for stomachache around AD 40 and the peasants in Tuscany and on Corcyra from whom, five hundred years later, Alexander of Tralles gained information about their drugs were almost certainly illiterate.[2] Many details of craft skills in particular – how to set a bone or remove a whitlow, how to recognise and cull healing herbs from the woods and fields, even how to diagnose a range of illnesses – were handed down by word of mouth and practical example alone, and were rarely committed to writing.[3] We can no longer know what precisely the botanist Theophrastus learned from talking to rootcutters around 330 BC, nor how, and more importantly why, trepanation, the removal of small circles of bone from the skull, was performed in prehistoric Greece.[4] We can only guess at many of the words uttered to repel illness by ancient exorcists, whose ministrations are derided by the author of *The Sacred Disease* in the fifth century BC and refused legal acknowledgment ('although some have gained benefit thereby') by a Roman

1

lawyer around AD 200.[5] We can do no more than speculate on the contents of the medical lectures delivered by Asclepiades of Perge in the gymnasia of his home town and at neighbouring Seleucia (S. Turkey) that contributed to the offical grant to him of a gold crown and citizenship from the one and a public memorial from the other.[6] Nor are we privileged to sit in on an ancient consultation or see an ancient operation taking place. They must be reconstructed imaginatively from case reports, educational treatises giving advice on what ought to happen, archaeological finds of instruments and drugs, and occasional artistic representations of an idealised moment.[7]

Moreover, writing of itself did not guarantee the survival of all that was copied down. It was not just the recipes scratched on to broken pieces of potsherd that were at risk of being destroyed. The fragments of once luxurious herbals and substantial medical tracts on papyrus recovered from the sands of Egypt bear equal witness to the deadly ravages of time and neglect.[8] Tantalising hints remain of an extensive literature now almost entirely lost. One would give much for the survival of a complete medical treatise by Diocles, Erasistratus or Asclepiades of Bithynia, for it would surely transform our views of these influential but controversial figures, whose opinions are preserved today only in the writings of others, often their opponents. Our understanding of even so famous a figure as Hippocrates would be enriched by direct access to the archives at Cos, allegedly used by Soranus of Cos for his *Life of Hippocrates*, or to the far less respectful conclusions of Andreas in his *The Descent of Medicine*, both works known only from passing references in a later biography.[9] Not just scholars but novelists and film directors could make much of the medical *Memoirs* of Dorotheus, with their gruesome story of a mummified child kept on display in Alexandria, or of the still more titillating reminiscences of Olympus, a doctor in attendance at the brilliant and short-lived court of Antony and Cleopatra in the 30s BC.[10] Often we owe our knowledge of the existence of a work solely to another author who denigrated it or used it for a non-medical purpose. The forty-eight books in which the doctor Julian expounded the *Aphorisms* of Hippocrates in the second century are mentioned only by his opponent, Galen; while a few words quoted by a later writer on grammar are all that have come down to us of a treatise on medical matters by his contemporary, the famous Latin orator and author of *The Golden Ass*, Lucius Apuleius.[11]

This disappearance of much of ancient medical literature is partly the result of the relative absence of suitable repositories where books might be kept safe for centuries. With the possible exception of temple collections, major libraries were few and far between, the creation of the super-rich and of monarchs such as the rulers of Alexandria in the third century BC or of Pergamum a century later.[12] The public library of Celsus at Ephesus flaunts the wealth, good taste and high imperial standing of its donor, Ti. Julius Aquila Polemeanus, consul in Rome in AD 110.[13] On the other hand, most private libraries were small and liable to dispersal. A carving on a doctor's

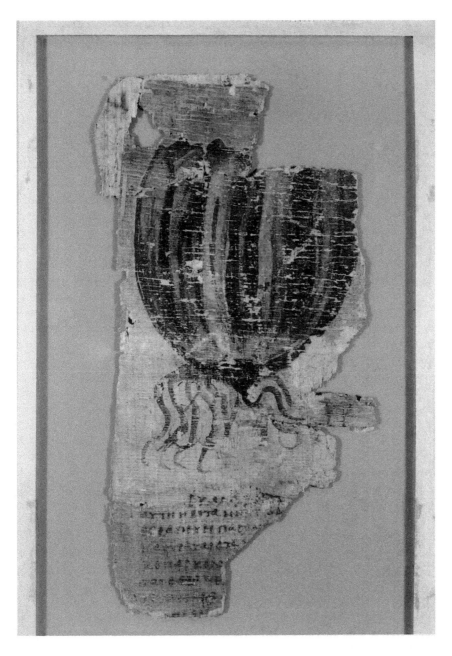

Figure 1.1 A page from an illuminated herbal, written on papyrus in Egypt *c.*AD 400, possibly showing *symphytum officinale*, comfrey. London, Wellcome Ms. 5753. Courtesy of Wellcome Library, London.

tomb from Ostia, the port of Rome, shows a mere handful of book-rolls, and Galen of Pergamum claims to have helped impoverished medical colleagues with the books and instruments that they could not acquire otherwise.[14] It is true that in Galen's day there was a flourishing market for medical books in Rome, where one might buy the 156 books written by an imperial doctor Tiberius Claudius Menecrates, who founded his own 'clear and logical' medical sect in the mid-first century, and Galen's wealthy friends could arrange to have copies made of his discourses to take back to Asia Minor or Palestine.[15] But most doctors may have owned at best a few brief handbooks or digests of earlier doctrines to supplement what they had learned by word of mouth or simply by watching others as they operated or expounded in theatres or public spaces.[16] The gulf between the book learning that Galen himself displayed and even what he expected of his accomplished physician was vast, to say nothing of those practitioners he dismissed as ignorant and incompetent. Indeed, he had almost to excuse to his audience his unusual passion for acquiring books on medicine, and for spending so much money on them.[17] Later legend credited him with having had copies produced on silk with embroidered lettering and with owning a rare treatise by the early philosopher Anaxagoras.[18] But Galen was the son of a rich architect, living in a rich city at a time of Rome's greatest prosperity and well able to find funds to buy or to have copied for him whatever interested him. Lower down the medical scale such bibliophilia was an expensive luxury.

In short, the survival of ancient medical literature depended on two related factors: the copying and recopying over the centuries of such writings, and the continued existence of individuals and institutions both interested in them and in an economic position to buy and preserve them.[19] Some treatises, such as Diocles' book *Anatomy*, may have been lost because they were thought to have been superseded by later developments; others, even when written by favoured authors such as Galen, because they were too specialised. The hazards of everyday life also played their part. Galen himself lost many of his books in the great fire of Rome in 192, and had to rely on copies owned by his friends in order to recover at least a part.[20] By 500 in the mainly Latin-speaking world, which stretched from Britain, Gaul and Spain round to modern Algeria and Tunisia, in a society impoverished as a result of war, conquest, high taxation and general economic collapse, books had become a rarity, and most of these were copies of the scriptures and theological works. A Latin medical culture that was still flourishing in N. Africa in 450, with writers such as Caelius Aurelianus and Cassius Felix, had come near to collapse as the civic institutions that had supported it weakened and crumbled away. The priorities of the churches and monasteries, to whose libraries we owe for the most part the preservation of classical Latin learning, were not necessarily those of doctors. In such circumstances choices had to be made of what to copy and preserve and what to leave aside. An erudite philosophical disquisition on medical theory on the model of Galen or a multi-volume survey of the whole of medicine was irrelevant when what was most needed was a short compendium that reduced medicine to a manageable compass and provided a restricted range of practical therapies within a single volume. This process is neatly illustrated by the fate of the *Natural History* of the Elder Pliny (d. AD 79), a massive compilation on the whole world of nature. Although manuscripts of this colossal encyclopaedia continued to be written, its medical sections enjoyed a much wider circulation in Late Antiquity and the Early Middle Ages in the form of separate abridgments, the so-called *Medicine of Pliny* and the *Physic of Pliny*.[21]

One consequence of this literary catastrophe has been the almost total disappearance of medical writings in Latin from the period before AD 350. The recipe book of Scribonius Largus and possibly the medical poem of Quintus Serenus, of uncertain date, are the sole survivors of works written by actual doctors, for both Cornelius Celsus, the author of *On Medicine*, and Pliny were wealthy amateurs.[22] This is not to say that the summaries and handbooks that remain from the Latin half of the Later Roman Empire should be dismissed, as Valentin Rose put it, as 'an entire literature for barbarians', for much of it was derived from more extensive learned writings, some of them even originally composed in Greek.[23] But the process of adaptation and, where necessary, translation produced a book that looked and read very differently from its sources. It allowed little room for alternative diagnoses or therapies, and even less for philosophical doubt: brevity, clarity and practicality were what was required.

A similar diminution in the amount of medical writing available occurs even in the far wealthier Greek-speaking, or Byzantine, half of the Later Roman Empire, although for different reasons and with a very different chronology. Intellectual activity outside theology appears almost to cease for a century from 650 onwards. Few books on medicine and science were copied then, and still fewer composed. But the process of attrition had begun much earlier than the seventh century, and was to continue for much longer. Whereas a Latin text that was still being read in 700 is likely to be available to us today, losses of Greek medical works continued steadily for several centuries more. This was in part the result of the triumph of Galenism. Although there were others who had earlier been interested in preserving and pursuing the teachings of Hippocrates, it was Galen's view of Hippocrates and of the Hippocratic Corpus that came to prevail from Late Antiquity onwards. He had defined what was genuinely written by Hippocrates and what was not, what was worth studying and what could be left aside, and his decisions were accepted to the point where Galenism and Hippocratism were viewed as identical. To the Greeks of mediaeval Byzantium, Hippocrates and Galen had become almost divine, worthy of being commemorated in fresco alongside patriarchs and prophets as heralds of Christian truth.[24] Their opinions carried a similar authority, and helped to marginalise and eventually to suppress competitors. Other traditions of learned medicine, most notably those of the Empiricists and the Erasistrateans, which had flourished from 250 BC for almost five hundred years, were now entirely lost, save for fragments preserved in the work of other writers. Methodist therapeutics were far better represented in late Latin texts such as Caelius Aurelianus than in Greek. Alternative views to those of the Galenists remained largely only in areas of medicine where Galen had said little – in gynaecology, with the Methodist Soranus, or in medical botany, with Dioscorides – or where, by chance, works written by others became attached to or were mistaken for genuinely Galenic treatises, e.g. *Medical Definitions* or *The Ensoulment of the Foetus*.[25] New material now being made available through the discovery of mediaeval translations of earlier Greek medicine into oriental languages (Syriac, Arabic, Hebrew and even Armenian) has not yet radically altered this picture, except by revealing Galen's largely unacknowledged debt to his Hippocratic predecessors, most notably Rufus of Ephesus.[26]

This process of destruction was also a consequence of the actual ways in which ancient books were produced, and of the need for successive recopying over the centuries if any particular treatise was to survive. Hippocrates, one often forgets, was more distant in time from Galen than Leonardo da Vinci or Martin Luther is from us; Paul of Aegina stands in the same chronological relation to Galen as Shakespeare does to the present – and we are assisted by the multiplying and stabilising effects of the printing press. The earliest Greek books took the form of a long, continuous book-roll, hard to write, and even harder to consult for a particular recipe or observation. From the second century onwards, the book-roll was gradually superseded by the codex, similar in form to our modern book. Those works that were not transferred to the new format, unless preserved accidentally in the ruins of Herculaneum or the sands of Egypt, were then lost. Greek handwriting also changed over the centuries, so that older manuscripts became less accessible to succeeding generations. The major change in Greek occurred from about 850 onwards, when the older, squarer and larger script was replaced by a smaller and more rounded hand with far more abbreviations. In the famous Vienna illuminated manuscript of Dioscorides' herbal, originally written in 512 or very shortly after, all the plant names and large portions of the text were eventually copied anew into a 'modern' Greek script around 1406, presumably because the original (and to modern observers more beautiful) handwriting was now difficult to read. The new script had the further advantage of requiring less parchment or paper, and in time drove out the old.[27]

It was in the course of this transition that the second great destruction of Greek medical texts occurred; those books that were now recopied were, on the whole, those thought to be of greater use or of greater authority. Many of the more theoretical writings of Galen that had been extant in the ninth century, when translations into Syriac and Arabic were made, seem to have disappeared soon afterwards. Big books, which were more expensive to produce, were in particular danger. Hunain ibn Ishaq in his search for Greek manuscripts of Galen around 850 already had great difficulty in finding copies of Galen's *On Demonstration* or of the three books of *On Erasistratus' Anatomical Knowledge*, and both are now lost entirely in Greek.[28] Rufus' large compendium of self-help medicine designed for the layman ('for those who have no access to a physician') and his treatise on melancholy also vanished at this time.[29]

Warfare and conquest played a part, as the Byzantine world shrank to embrace little more than W. Anatolia, Greece, Constantinople and S. Italy. How serious the loss of medical material was when Constantinople was sacked by the crusaders in 1204 is hard to determine, but it is clear that some ancient medical writings survived, only to disappear later, perhaps in 1453, when the Ottoman conquest of Constantinople led to the dispersal and loss of many other ancient Greek texts. The doctor–translator Niccolò of Reggio, who worked at the court of Naples in the first half of the fourteenth century, turned into Latin, on the basis of manuscripts obtained in Constantinople or in S. Italy, at least five works of Galen that are no longer extant today in Greek.[30] This gradual disappearance of ancient medical texts can be neatly illustrated by the fate of Galen's *On Problematical Movements*. Two translations were made into Syriac and one into Arabic in the ninth century, and a Latin translation was made from the Arabic by Mark of Toledo around 1200. It was still available in Greek in full around 1320, when it was translated directly from the Greek by Niccolò, and was quoted thirty or so years later by a Byzantine annotator. But so far no complete Greek manuscript has come to light, and the complicated printing history of Mark's Latin version easily persuaded scholars from 1540 onwards that this was at best a pastiche of Galen's original.[31]

The printing of Greek medical texts, which began effectively in Venice in 1499 with the Aldine Dioscorides and continued the next year with the first volume of a projected (but never completed) edition of Galen by Kallierges and Blastos, marks a turning point.[32] What remains available for consultation today is largely what was published between 1499 and 1540.[33] There are a few tantalising hints of manuscripts of rare works surviving briefly in isolated or inaccessible libraries into the sixteenth century, but these are more in the nature of travellers' tales and intellectual gossip than firm evidence.

The destruction of the written heritage of Greek medicine was effectively stemmed by the advent of printing; no treatise, once printed, has since been lost. The process of destruction has even to a certain extent been reversed over the last century. Leaving aside the remarkable discovery in 2005 of the Vlatadon MS of the works of Galen, papyrus finds in Egypt have revealed names and even works of writers otherwise unknown, and the opening up of libraries and collections in the Middle East has seen the recovery, albeit in translation, of some treatises lost for more than a millennium. One may continue to hope for more. But this partial resurrection, valuable though it is, should not disguise one essential fact. We possess today only a small

7

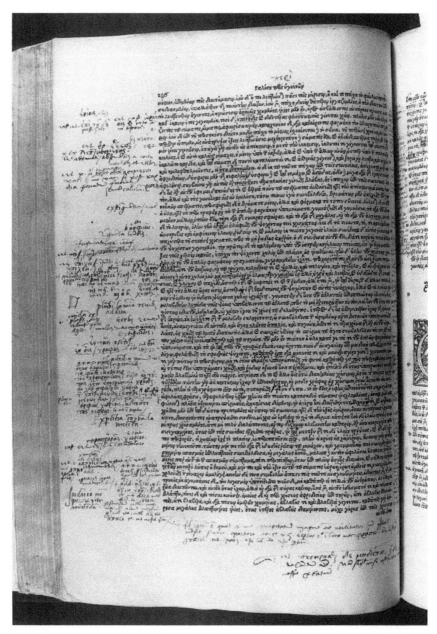

Figure 1.2 A Renaissance scholar's Galen. A page from the 1538 Basle edition of the complete works of Galen, owned by John Caius (1510–73). The margin contains notes and variant readings copied from books and Greek manuscripts Caius saw in England and Italy. Eton College, vol. IV, p. 286. Reproduced by permission of the Provost and Fellows of Eton College.

proportion of what existed in Greek in 850, itself a fraction of the literature accessible to Galen, and for much of Antiquity we have only fragments, titles or nothing at all. This shrinkage warns the historian of ancient medicine of the fragility of any generalisation based on surviving documentation, and imparts a note of caution to even the most definite of pronouncements. There are too many missing links within our surviving medical sources to invest total confidence in any hypothesis, and often the best that can be done is to lay out possibilities or define parameters. To talk of ancient medicine, Greek medicine, Roman medicine, or whatever title one might choose, gives to any pronouncement, particularly once set in print, a sense of comprehensiveness and finality that the evidence at our disposal scarcely warrants. The reader is advised to retain a certain scepticism, and to regard this exposition as an outline of possibilities rather than a detailed map.[34]

But if the fragmentary nature of our surviving sources renders a history of ancient medicine based largely on medical writers difficult, if not impossible, it also presents an opportunity and a challenge. For many aspects of health and healing one can consult documents produced by non-medical authors in non-medical contexts – lawyers, historians, poets, playwrights, to say nothing of Egyptian papyri and inscriptions in Greek and Latin from all over the ancient world. It is true that their information does not always correspond to the wishes or priorities of a medical writer. Galen in the second century was already lamenting that it was Thucydides the historian, not Hippocrates the doctor, who had left us an account of the great plague of Athens in 430–428 BC; the latter would not have left out any essential item of medical information, nor would he have used a terminology that was imprecise in crucial particulars.[35] But, one might reply, we would not then have had Thucydides' impressive analysis of the effects of the epidemic on Athenian society in time of war, or, much later and in obvious imitation of Thucydides, Procopius' searing account of the pandemic of 541–4.[36] Other authors allow us to see events at a more local level. An anonymous Syriac chronicler, describing a famine in the region of Edessa (now Urfa in modern S.E. Turkey) in 499–500, vividly depicts a community battling to keep going as the sick flocked in from the countryside to seek shelter and rest under the colonnades that had been turned into temporary hospitals. One's heart goes out to those unfortunates, 'wandering about the streets, picking up the stalks and leaves of vegetables, all filthy with mud, and eating them', and the children whose mothers had deserted them, ashamed because 'when they asked for something to eat they had nothing to give them'. Their fate is chillingly and briefly recorded: 'the dead lay exposed in every street'.[37]

As well as these memorable, and arguably unusual, events, many aspects of the daily round of the ancient doctor are revealed only incidentally in passing comments of other non-medical writers. A law-court speech of the fourth-century BC orator Isocrates graphically describes the loneliness and squalor of the sickroom, where a patient lies bedridden covered in pus, his angry moods driving away all his servants save for a single slave, and making it almost impossible for his solitary caring relative even to sleep. In such circumstances it is hardly surprising that less committed members of the family preferred to stay away from their dying, tubercular kinsman.[38] Several centuries later, perhaps around AD 370, an anonymous author composed in Syriac, the common form of the Aramaic language used in the Near East, an account of the lives of the two Christian doctor–saints Cosmas and Damian. He pictured them treating humans and animals alike in their surgery, and taking it in turns to go round the neighbourhood for weeks at a time or to stay at home minding the shop, details of routine medical activity not otherwise revealed by medical (or veterinary) writers.[39]

The orator and the hagiographer thus allow us to go beyond what is told to us by medical authors, who, in writing for fellow practitioners, had no need to provide information already familiar. Literary sources not only give us glimpses of the patient's view and of the social context of ancient medical practice, but also impart a richness and liveliness into the history of ancient medicine. They introduce personalities and human dilemmas into an otherwise austere and impersonal narrative, for ancient medical authors rarely describe themselves to their readers at length. The Hippocratic physician remains largely an anonymous (or, more strictly, pseudonymous) figure; the biographer of Theodore Priscian is condemned to making bricks out of straw.[40] Amid such aridity, one becomes grateful for the many self-referential asides of Galen, whose determination that the world should know who he was, what he wrote and what he believed achieved its purpose only too well.

Particularly for the Roman period, there is an abundance of information outside purely medical texts on which the historian can draw. Archaeological evidence can reveal not only the evidence of operations, both successful and unsuccessful, but also the instruments and even, very occasionally, the drugs that a practitioner had at his disposal.[41] The standing of ordinary doctors or healers in their communities, their training, their family backgrounds can be gleaned from the comments (and complaints) of their patients, from their tombstones and from the many other inscriptional records on display in an ancient city. At Ephesus in the second century AD an alert viewer might have observed carved in stone the results of an annual medical contest (with four classes of 'event'), as well as a decree from Rome confirming the various tax privileges accorded to doctors over more than a century and a half.[42] A large stone recorded the honours given to Attalus Priscus, son of Asclepiades, 'town councillor, temple official, guardian of the estate of Antonius, and a member of a dynasty of civic doctors', while yet another inscription proclaimed that the guardianship of the tomb of the civic doctor Julius was the responsibility of his fellow Jews.[43] Tombstones commemorate the successful and the less successful; from Aquilas, civic doctor at Synnada (now in central Turkey), who married his daughter into a family prominent for generations in the wealthy province of Asia and now linked to the Roman imperial administration in the 170s AD, to his near-contemporary Barbius Zmaragdus, a humble member of the College of Mars, at the N. Italian town of Aquileia.[44] The decree of the town of Halasarna on Cos honouring Dr Onasander around 180 BC describes at length the career that took him from a mere humble assistant in a country town to the capital city, and then to his own practice there, in which 'he did not hesitate to treat for nothing, if necessary', his old friends from the countryside.[45] By contrast, the numerous small funerary plaques in Rome of doctors, frequently ex-slaves, give little more than their name and profession.[46]

But inscriptions of the dead rarely give an insight into the habits of the living, and medical texts tend to stress the exceptional, the outstanding case, or lay down what should happen when faced with this or that ailment. They omit much because it was obvious to the intended reader; for example, how the Hippocratic physicians took down their case notes that were worked into the celebrated case histories that make up the seven books of the *Epidemics*.[47] We have to wait until Galen to find a doctor commenting on the possible confusion of information handed down only in badly handwritten copies (medical handwriting seems not to have improved over the centuries). One solution, favoured by Servilus Damocrates around AD 40, was to turn one's recipe into verse in the hope that the constraints of metre would impart a certain stability to its formulae.[48]

The best picture of what the average healer did may be gained from the papyri of Graeco-Roman Egypt, which extend mainly from the second century BC until the sixth century AD. They show us healers at work, summoned to carry out inspections of those injured in an affray or dying in suspicious circumstances, prescribing, running a family hospital, even writing their own books.[49] We have their tax assessments (and, for comparison, those of their fellow villagers or townsfolk) and even some of their private correspondence. A son writes to his mother to excuse his brother Marcus who cannot come home to attend a funeral because he is worried about leaving the not inconsiderable number of patients in his surgery.[50] We have traces of the books they read, or tried to find.[51] Some of the fragments once formed part of the works of learned surgeons and pharmacologists, sometimes beautifully illustrated on high-quality papyrus, a pleasure to handle as well as to view.[52] But alongside them we have also the so-called magical papyri, whose authors saw nothing unusual in claiming magical and divine assistance in treating disease.[53] Papyri written in Coptic, the language of the native Egyptians, also remind us that in their expansion the Greeks and, to a much larger extent, the Romans incorporated into their political structures regions and groups with different styles of healing, some, like the Egyptians, with medical pedigrees more ancient and with treatments arguably more effective than those of their conquerors.[54]

How far the evidence of the papyri can be applied to other regions of the classical world at other times is a vexed topic. Scholars are divided between regarding Egypt as a region with its own particular social and legal structures deriving from pharaonic times and seeing it as part of the wider world of Hellenistic Greece and Imperial Rome. Nonetheless, even if one must remain cautious about transferring Egyptian institutions to other parts of the ancient world, the papyri do provide the historian with an insight into the range and diversity of healing activities outside the great metropoleis. So, for example, the combination of native and non-native material found in a medical book from Crocodilopolis, compiled around AD 170, has a close parallel outside Egypt two centuries later in the Latin writer Marcellus, whose large handbook of practical remedies, *On Drugs*, expands the tradition of Scribonius Largus and Dioscorides to take in many of the herbs and healing practices of his native Gaul.[55]

Taken together, this material, medical and non-medical alike, gives the lie to the notion of a single medical system in Antiquity. It reveals such diversity that even the very concept of a history of 'ancient medicine' becomes fraught with interpretative difficulties from the very beginning. To think in terms of a Western tradition of medicine, as some historians have done, only complicates matters further, for what has been thought to constitute that tradition has altered from time to time, and, at the least, sets up a tension between a history of the past seen in its own terms or, teleologically, as steps leading up to the present.[56] But to recognise and openly acknowledge this problem is also to go at least some way towards its solution. Snapshots, which is what we have, can be used to evoke the past, and they are a better guide to it than a blank page. They require interpretation and careful discrimination, but they can be made to reveal information not always visible at first glance. Texts from across the centuries may also indicate long-term continuities as well as changes, as many of the examples already given in this chapter have shown. Besides, scholars have often shown how a variety of views might be accommodated together; how, for example, insights from the study of the language (or languages) of medicine can be linked with the evidence drawn from history, or even archaeology.[57] The work done since the 1970s, even if not always performed on traditional medical writings, has given a different texture to the historical weave from that of a generation ago.

These new developments, it is hoped, are reflected in the account that follows. Chronologically, it covers a period from the poems of Homer and Hesiod in the eighth century BC to Paul of Aegina around AD 620. Before the poets, we have only the evidence of archaeology and, several centuries earlier in the Greek world, the Mycenean tablets: after Paul, in both east and west, we reach a literary lacuna of over a century. The geographical focus is initially the Aegean world of the Greeks, with its subsequent extension into the Middle East and Egypt, and later the Roman Empire, based around the shores of the Mediterranean but including at its widest extent most of Britain and Europe as far north as the Elbe and the Danube. If these definitions are relatively uncontroversial, and dependent on the pattern of our written evidence, what is meant here by medicine is more arbitrary and problematic. This account looks at a range of healing practices and ideas, not all of which would be universally accepted, either then or now, as falling within medicine proper. From at least the Hippocratic Corpus onwards there has been a tension between those seeking to restrict the name and nature of medicine to one type of healing or one set of beliefs and those favouring, whether as patients or as practitioners, other methods and concepts. Some of them might be termed rational, and granted approval for that reason; others might be better labelled as alternative, complementary, religious or magical healing, with, depending on one's standpoint, pejorative or approving connotations; others might be thought of as a conflation of both sorts of healing. It is precisely this diversity that this book aims to capture, and it is not concerned with the precise label to be attached to any specific theory or therapy.

The choice of these chronological and spatial limits is also intended to dispel several traditional prejudices. The inclusion of information drawn from the languages of the Near East, Hebrew, Syriac and Coptic, serves as a reminder that the Roman Empire was more than a collection of speakers of Latin and Greek, and that medical practices do not necessarily abide within linguistic boundaries. I am also deliberately abolishing the border between the early Christian centuries and their non-Christian predecessors. Although, as we shall see, the coming of Christianity brought new perspectives and, in part, a new ideology of health and healing, the structures of the society in which it developed did not change overnight. There were many continuities. Centuries after the last slave doctor is recorded on an inscription, Christian lawyers in the sixth century were still determining the price to be paid for a slave who had studied medicine.[58] The medical legacy that Antiquity bequeathed to the Middle Ages and the Renaissance consists mainly of ideas from the fifth century BC as modified by scholars a thousand years later.

Above all, the extended chronology adopted in this book is meant to counter two long-standing prejudices that, linked together, have acted as a deterrent to the serious study of the medicine of Antiquity as a whole. The first is our admiration for the Greek miracle, the understandable wonderment at the intellectual excitement, new discoveries, new theories and new healing practices that characterise Greece and the Greeks in particular from 650 to 330 BC. Here, it is usually argued, are to be found the beginnings of Western science and medicine in its gradual emancipation from religious and folk healing: observation and argument replace prayer and panaceas.[59] It is to this period that the great majority of texts in the Hippocratic Corpus are to be dated, for their language, style and modes of thought fit closely with other intellectual developments in literature, history and philosophy. Indeed, it is in many ways the interaction between the practitioners of all these different genres that gives this period its special 'feel'. This sense of the excitement of the new is often extended to include the early Alexandrian anatomists, Herophilus and Erasistratus, who lived in the first half of the third century

BC and who were active in the similarly intellectually vibrant environment of Hellenistic Alexandria.[60] But this model of medical history, with its emphasis on new discoveries and new modes of thought, becomes difficult to apply to subsequent periods, when novelties are, allegedly, somewhat fewer and when doctors worked often with a sophisticated awareness of the importance of their intellectual traditions.[61]

Political and linguistic reasons might also be adduced for ending the story of Greek medicine in early Alexandria. Far from breathing the clear air of free democratic Greece, whose climate and geography, according to the author of *Airs, Waters and Places*, produced the best of all possible races, morally as well as physically, most of the surviving Greek medical writers lived under the domination of Rome.[62] Many of them were not properly Greek in that Hippocratic sense: whatever their nostalgia for the good old days of independent Greece, most had never glimpsed the Parthenon or set foot on Parnassus. Their Greek was the simpler 'common' language of the Hellenistic East, and, if they strove to reproduce the language of Demosthenes or Hippocrates, they then ran the risk of critical condemnation for artificiality. Nor were their morals above reproach, to judge by the Greek satirist Lucian's account of the life of a Greek intellectual in second-century Rome.[63] Historians have thus been able to dismiss their medicine as equally derivative, worthy, at best, of a brief nod in the direction of Galen, Soranus, Rufus, Dioscorides and the rest, before returning to the more interesting material from the Golden Age of Greece. They were thereby relieved of the obligation to brave the thousands of pages of Galen or the still more forbidding fastnesses of Oribasius or the Late Alexandrian commentators from the fifth and sixth centuries.[64]

If classicists who have chosen to write on Greek medicine have had relatively little to say about the Greek medical writers of the Roman imperial period, those who have written about Roman medicine have, until recently, been equally dismissive. This is in part the result of a second distorting preconception – namely, the false equation of Roman with Latin – which, although largely valid for the Roman Republic, is impossible to sustain for the following centuries. The Roman Empire was multilingual, and Greek culture in the first two centuries of our era was extraordinarily vigorous, reaching far beyond the confines of the Aegean. As examples, alongside that most Greek of Greeks Plutarch of Chaeronea (who nonetheless bore the Roman citizen name of L. Mestrius) one can point to the Alexandrian Jewish philosopher Philo; the geographer Strabo of Amaseia (from Pontus, N.E. Turkey); and the Egyptian astronomer Ptolemy; to say nothing of the Roman Emperor Marcus Aurelius, who wrote his *Meditations* in Greek. To confine the study of medicine in the Roman world (which is what I understand Roman medicine to mean), or even in Italy, largely to Latin texts is a major error of judgment, but one that has its roots in ancient Rome itself.

Writing in the 180s BC as part of his campaign against Rome's foreign enemies, the politician Cato the Elder warned his son in vigorous and colourful language against putting his faith in Greek immigrant physicians. His message was repeated at length, and with spectacular instances of avarice and corruption, 250 years later by the Elder Pliny, who argued strongly that medicine was intrinsically un-Roman, invented by the Greeks to the detriment of their Roman patients.[65] Like ornamental tables, medicine was an index of immorality, proof of society's descent from pristine virtue into the moral sink of Neronian Rome.[66]

Pliny's criticism did not lack evidence: his historical examples, and others found in more sober writings, were truly shocking. Furthermore, in subsequent ages, the near total absence of medical texts in Latin from the period before AD 400 appeared to confirm that this was not a subject with which students of Roman, i.e. Latin, culture need concern themselves.[67] At best it derived from Greek sources; at worst it was mere charlatanry and mumbo jumbo. Its most famous representative, Galen, himself a Greek-speaking immigrant to Rome, provided a doubly convincing proof of all that Pliny had said. His denunciations of earlier doctors in Rome, particularly Asclepiades and the Methodists, highlighted and confirmed their many failings and inconsistencies, while his own theoretical interests and repetitive *longueurs* exemplified all that Pliny and Cato had detested. In concentrating, as he so often did, on the theoretical principles that should determine therapy or on the hidden structures and workings of the body instead of offering clear and detailed guidance as to precisely what remedy would cure what condition, he could be accused of preferring empty words to effective physic. Even when he did provide this information, as in his drug books, his prolixity (already a cause for complaint in Antiquity) deterred those looking for a swift and simple answer. As for what came after him, this was easily consigned to oblivion as repetitive, reactionary, scholastic or worse. It contributed nothing new, being content merely to recycle the old in an appallingly bad style. Late Latin authors were frequently cursory and intellectually undemanding, Greek encyclopaedists and commentators over-long, over-theoretical and over-dull. In short, after the achievements of the Alexandrian anatomists Greek medicine was deemed to have passed swiftly into a terminal decline. Galen and his tribe of admirers could be assigned to the rubbish bin of history. What valuable insights into medicine they possessed they owed largely to their predecessors, especially Hippocrates, from whom Galen himself claimed to derive all the foundations of his medicine.

The later development of medicine only confirmed the wisdom of this neglect. Vesalius, Harvey and the chemical physicians of the sixteenth and seventeenth centuries were assumed to have destroyed Galenism, and notably its anatomy and physiology, as a valid medical system. By contrast, Hippocrates survived as a living symbol, if not entirely as a living voice, into the twentieth century. Hippocratic holism continued to be proclaimed and practised by wealthy clinicians, the Hippocratic *Oath* to be upheld as the touchstone of medical morality.[68] The long success of Hippocrates confirmed

15

the wisdom of neglecting Roman medicine in favour of concentrating on fifth- and fourth-century Greece. Not only was this the period that saw the creation of Western medicine, but many of the principles then formulated had remained eternally valid.

This description of a particular attitude towards Roman or late Greek medicine may seem somewhat exaggerated, a rhetorical riposte to the arch-rhetorician Pliny, although it is still not entirely absent from modern scholarship. But since the 1970s the general pattern of research into the history of ancient medicine has shifted considerably. A generation ago the central point of academic research into ancient medicine was very firmly the Hippocratic Corpus, and largely the small selection of texts thought to be linked closely with Hippocrates himself and signalled out for praise by the great nineteenth-century editor Emile Littré.[69] Indeed, until 1988 less than half of the Hippocratic Corpus was available in English, and some treatises, particularly those dealing with gynaecology, have yet to appear in the Loeb series or in an easily accessible English translation. Now, the fulcrum has moved to the Greek world of the Roman Empire. Not only has it been demonstrated beyond all doubt how much the historical picture of the achievements of early Greek medicine owes to the prejudices of Galen and, equally, of nineteenth-century scholars, but the role of Greek culture in general in the Roman world has been examined anew in its historical, archaeological and literary contexts. Ancient medicine, in particular, has been studied in greater detail and with greater care and attention than at any time since the middle years of the sixteenth century. The result has been an increased appreciation of the role and achievements of medicine in Classical Greece as well as in the Roman world, and the reappearance of much that had earlier been consigned to moulder on the furthest shelves of a classical library. This revival of interest has involved co-operation across a wide range of disciplines. Philosophers and palaeographers, epigraphists and epidemiologists, editors of texts and excavators of sites have all co-operated to recover and to explain anew this one aspect of the ancient world.

This survey, covering the long period from Hippocrates to Paul of Aegina, also incorporates one major conclusion from the world of social anthropology. There it has been argued convincingly that the pattern of modern Western medicine or healing cannot simply be transferred back to different centuries or different cultures to reinforce a neat distinction between rational and irrational, proper and improper, formal and informal, with the further implication that anything not in the first categories is not medicine or eligible to be studied as part of the history of medicine. Healing is better seen as a broad system of interaction between society and individuals over the meaning of health and the way it is to be maintained, regained and defined.[70] This definition allows historians an inclusive model for understanding the medical world of Antiquity that can embrace questions about the efficacy of herbal or surgical treatments as well as the role of religious healing. It can discuss the philosophical speculations of Galen alongside the practical farming of Cato, Hippocratic meteorology as well as Egyptian amulets. Such a comprehensive view of healing is not new. It could be found half a century ago in the preface to Henry Ernest Sigerist's *A History of Medicine*, a magnificent and melancholy fragment that began with prehistory and anthropology but had reached only the fourth century BC at its author's death in 1957.[71] A comprehensive history of medicine on the scale he envisaged would be a history of humanity of Galenic proportions, which is perhaps why it has never been attempted since. But that should not blind us to the breadth or value of that vision of medicine, or exclude a more modest attempt to survey the history of medicine not only as a system of ideas but also as a network of practices rooted within a particular society, overlapping, competing and changing with time. It is that historicity, as well as that diversity, that this study aims to convey.

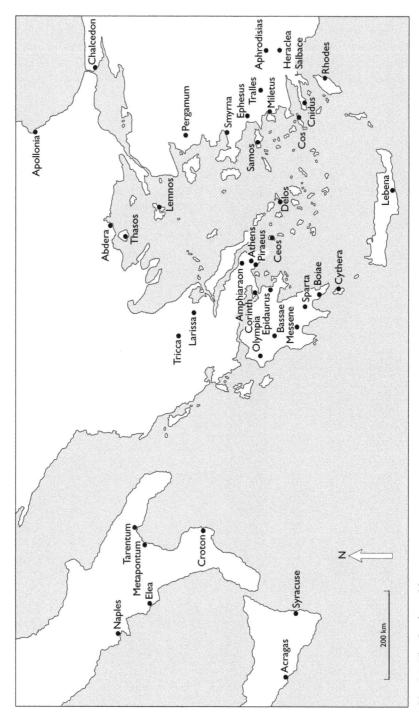

Map 2.1 The Greek world

2

PATTERNS OF DISEASE

The world of Classical Antiquity was in its geography and in the range of its diseases restricted compared with the world of today. Largely confined to the Mediterranean basin for most of our period, it was also relatively free from large incursions of outsiders bringing with them unfamiliar pathogens.[1] Traders might reach as far as China, Malaya and Zanzibar, and sail from N. Africa round the northern tip of the British Isles, but these were exceptions.[2] For the most part, home was around the inland sea, 'our sea' as the Romans called it. Even when the armies of the Roman Empire reached the Danube, the Elbe and the Tigris, and when soldiers from Spain, Syria and Dacia stood guard on Hadrian's Wall, mixing with vendors and camp-followers who had come from even further afield, from Commagene in modern Turkey or Palmyra in the Syrian desert, the pattern was not radically altered.[3] Travel was slow, whether on foot, on horseback or by sea, and fear of winter storms often closed the Mediterranean for weeks. Consequently, the world-view of the average man or woman was confined to the farm, the village or the nearest large town. Those who ventured from one part of the ancient world to another were relatively few. Only armies and, in the last two centuries BC, captives destined to be sold as slaves in the markets of Delos or Rome moved in large numbers over great distances.

Large-scale concentrations of population were also rare. Before 330 BC, only a few places, notably Athens, Corinth, Syracuse (Sicily) and Carthage (Tunisia), had more than 15,000 inhabitants. Many so-called 'Greek cities' would have had fewer than 2,000 persons living within their walls, with more beyond them in the surrounding countryside, but rarely exceeding 6,000 in all.[4] The number of large cities grew in the Hellenistic and Roman period, including Alexandria (Egypt), Antioch, Ephesus and Smyrna (all in modern Turkey), and Rome itself, whose population has been estimated at between 750,000 and 2 million by AD 10, but these were exceptional. Reasonably exact figures are hard to obtain even from the more detailed data supplied by Egyptian papyri, but those that have been proposed, based on a variety of types of evidence drawn from all over the ancient world, give a sense of the order of magnitude involved.[5] They confirm the earlier pattern: most of the population lived in what we would now term villages, rarely with more than 3,000 inhabitants, although site surveys in Italy and elsewhere have shown more evidence for an inhabited countryside than previously suspected. These populations fluctuated in response to a variety of circumstances. Archaeology seems to confirm a substantial decline in the population of mainland Greece in the last two centuries BC, mainly as a result of war.[6] Equally, the next two centuries show a marked increase in numbers everywhere, before the Antonine plague brought a sudden reduction, on the Egyptian evidence, of at least 10–15 per cent.[7] Population decline in Late Antiquity is a vexed subject; while many towns in Gaul and Italy appear to be contracting in the fourth century, Roman Britain seems to prosper longer, and in Roman N. Africa too a decline may not have occurred until the middle of the fifth century. By the mid-sixth century the inhabited area within the walls of Rome had shrunk considerably from what it had been five centuries before, with a population numbered in tens, rather than in hundreds, of thousands, perhaps only a quarter the size of that of contemporary Constantinople.[8]

We are thus dealing, on the whole, with small-town agrarian communities, 'where we all know one another – our family, education, wealth, and way of life'.[9] The opposed stereotypes of town and country, familiar in Classical Greek comedy and tragedy, or, in their later articulation by Cato, *c.*165 BC, and by the Elder Pliny in his *Natural History*, two centuries later, those of the shifty Greek city slicker and the virtuous Roman peasant farmer, should not be allowed to mislead.[10] Town and countryside were everywhere intimately connected. Galen's father, an architect, was also a landowner with a considerable personal interest in farming and the development of his crops and vintages.[11] Even when members of the urban elite moved on to a bigger city or, later, to Rome and the centre of power, as they often did, they would still retain their links with their home town or region and their estates there. Likewise many characteristic features of Greek medicine neatly show its rural antecedents. The careful noting of winds, seasonal changes, rain and temperature in the Hippocratic *Epidemics* finds its closest parallels in Hesiod's *Works and Days* or in Virgil's *Georgics*, poetic renderings of much practical farm-lore.[12]

The exact pattern of settlement differed from region to region: the villa farmland of Britain or N. France can be contrasted with the more clustered urban landscape of Italy, Sicily or the coast of Asia Minor (W. Turkey), the villages strung out along the Nile with the largely empty *tavoliere* of S. Italy or central Spain, the small farm settlements of upland Samnium (central Italy) with the ordered colonial market towns planted at intervals along the edges of the plain of the Po valley two hundred miles to the north, a coastal town in multi-cultural Campania, such as Pompeii, with a provincial village away from the sea or a major highway. But everywhere, cities, towns and villages were on a smaller scale than their equivalents today, their horizons more restricted, their population less mobile. While some areas, such as the English Fens, seem to have provided a more than adequate supply of foodstuffs for a wider market, most communities relied on self-sufficiency and adopted a variety of strategies to cope with seasonal and yearly changes in patterns of rainfall and fertility.[13] This was partly out of necessity, for the bulk movement of foodstuffs such as grain to ward off a potential famine was immensely expensive. When such transport was needed it was made possible only by the generosity of a wealthy benefactor or the exploitation of an imperial power, such as Athens or Rome, to keep the inhabitants of its capital regularly free from starvation and from any consequent political unrest.[14] The average farmer, living away from the coast, might well have echoed the words of a Christian bishop, Gregory of Nazianzus: any surplus was largely unprofitable, and any deficiency potentially catastrophic.[15] One bad harvest might be overcome, but a series of such harvests spelled death and disaster; the linkage (and at times confusion) of the two similar-sounding Greek words for dearth and widespread disease, *limos* and *loimos*, is more than word play. Going back at least to the poet Hesiod around 700 BC, it expresses an ever-present reality, the fine boundary trodden by the typical subsistence farmer of Antiquity between having enough to feed his family and a desperate search for anything to eat.[16] Galen reports the plight of the country folk of his own day, driven to eat roots, leaves and grasses after their own supplies had been taken away by force by the powerful men from the big city.[17] In the Gothic wars of the sixth century the population of central Italy, forced to subsist on acorn bread and little else, suffered severely from diseases of all kinds. Procopius' eyewitness account of their dried-up skin and their inability to gain nourishment from food, even when it had become available once more to them, is a masterpiece of shrewd observation and pathetic description.[18] At other times, peasant farmers might try to cheat in the amount of grain they delivered to the town in order to keep more back for themselves, or even refuse to come and sell their corn at all, avowedly for fear of catching the plague, but, in the eyes of the hungry townsfolk, in order to profit later from higher prices.[19]

Whether in town or countryside, malnutrition, the consequence of this precarious balance between the supply and demand, was a major factor in the general demographic outline of Classical Antiquity. Not only was there a relatively small margin for error in each year's harvest, but certain foodstuffs might become unavailable at various seasons of the year. Winter storms will have kept fishermen in harbour, and a shortage of fresh vegetables in the same season would have led to xerophthalmia and other deficiency diseases, particularly among the very young.[20] While the consequences of a long period of near-starvation may be reduced by a return to a consistently healthy diet, repeated famines will have had a more serious impact on general health. Although reliable statistics are hard to come by, there can be no doubt that the demographic profile of Antiquity was akin to that of a third-world country today, with an average life expectancy at birth between twenty and thirty.[21] But this general average masks several crucial variables. Each locality might have a very different disease and demographic profile, what Grmek has called its pathocoenosis, from its neighbour.[22] Some areas, particularly those close to malarial lowlands, were extremely unhealthy – and were known to be; in others, such as Tifernum in Umbria, one might see grandfathers and great-grandfathers in numbers. By contrast, big cities sucked in people from the immediate locality, and often from hundreds of miles around, to replenish a population that was unable to sustain itself naturally.[23]

Second, although there was a very high mortality among those less than one year old, those who survived that crucial period could expect to live into their thirties or forties, with around 5 per cent reaching 60.[24] How many of these would be women is unclear. Certainly, the specific problems associated with pregnancy and childbirth must have killed many women, although reliable estimates are impossible.[25] There are graphic descriptions of post-partum haemorrhage and infection, and the most substantial treatise on gynaecology, that of Soranus (around AD 100), offers detailed instructions as to ways of turning the child in the womb to avoid complications in the actual process of birth.[26] Nonetheless, the existence of instruments called the 'embryocrusher' or 'embryo-slaughterer' to help remove a dead child (or abort a live one) indicates that the precaution was not always successful.[27] Even after the birth, to judge from modern Africa, young mothers, themselves malnourished, would also be at high risk of disease and death, leading in turn to an imbalance between the sexes that would be increased by the practice of disposing of unwanted infants, especially girls and the handicapped.[28]

To integrate the varied evidence for disease in Antiquity into this general demographic background presents problems of its own. Ancient perceptions and descriptions of diseases and the ways in which they were then classified are frequently impossible to correlate with diseases reported in a modern medical textbook.[29] Sometimes this is because the category was far too broad: the ancient heading 'fevers', 'fiery diseases', could cover almost any condition in which the patient's body felt hot, while discussions of the way to treat 'tumours' included everything from cancer to carbuncles. In other instances, a disease itself may have mutated over the centuries to produce a whole series of related and possibly also short-lived strains, for example of viruses. The still-growing list of attempts to establish the identity of the Thucydidean plague exemplifies the difficulty, even when the information itself is relatively abundant and provided by an eyewitness who had himself caught the disease.[30] Far too often, even in a medical text, the information given is, to modern eyes, fragmentary, because the author either failed to observe certain symptoms that we today would regard as crucial or omitted details that were to him commonplace. The most extensive, although not the most elaborate, reports of individual cases to survive from Antiquity, those contained in the books of the Hippocratic *Epidemics*, are already selective in their presentation of signs and symptoms, focusing in particular on things that would, in future, enable the writer (and later his audience) to estimate the severity of a similar condition, forecast its outcome and, where possible, intervene successfully. Other data that might seem equally crucial to a modern diagnosis are excluded.[31] Especially in non-medical texts, an account often has been structured to emphasise things that are only peripherally diagnostic, such as the way in which a patient reacted to illness or the behaviour of the physician, which makes a modern diagnosis difficult, if not impossible. The tablets set up at various shrines of the god Asclepius, most notably at Epidaurus (S. Greece), often record at length the condition or conditions that brought a sufferer to seek help from the god, but their aim was not to act as a sort of medical case-book, but to extol the god's power to heal.[32] On other occasions the conclusions reached by the ancient witness may not fit easily with modern descriptions of the identified condition: biblical 'leprosy', for example, appears on walls and clothing as well as humans.[33] Palaeopathological surveys help to give precision, and bio-archaeology can be expected in future to add further information, but both disciplines have been relatively infrequently used on classical sites, and are, as yet, of only limited value in understanding the written evidence.[34]

Nonetheless, with these qualifications in mind, it is possible at least to sketch an outline of the disease profile of Classical Antiquity.[35] One may begin with a negative conclusion: given the age structure of the population, the degenerative diseases characteristic of the twentieth century will have been fewer in number. It is no coincidence that the longest discussion of such disorders occurs not in a medical but in a philosophical treatise, Plato's *Timaeus*, and is related at least as much to his concept of a world built up from, and capable of resolution into, mathematical shapes than to any medical information he may have gained from others.[36]

This is not to say that such diseases were unknown. Arthritis, in particular, has been detected in many skeletons, often of the relatively young, and many skeletons also show other conditions that would have caused chronic pain, perhaps for decades. It was also well understood that certain conditions were more likely to affect the old than any other group. Cancers, for example, except for so-called 'congenital' cancers, were said to be uncommon before adulthood, and many types of cancer before 'old age'.[37] Breast cancer was linked to the menopause, when blood that formerly flowed freely stagnated within the body and turned nasty. It was likely to be fatal, although Galen believed that, if quickly diagnosed, it could be cured by removing from the body the main causative agent, excessive black bile.[38] Cancer surgery was the province only of the able or audacious, and then only for superficial cancers. Indeed, unless one could remove the roots of the cancer entirely, it was thought that the patient's life might best be prolonged by avoiding the knife altogether.[39] Celsus was unenthusiastic about such drastic intervention, for, in his view, it was far more likely to damage than help the patient. He put his faith in a conservative management that did not provoke the cancer to develop further or move to an even more dangerous part of the body.[40]

But in general, rather than drawing attention to specific ailments of the elderly, ancient doctors saw the gradual physical and mental deterioration of old age as part of an inevitable process, a wasting away or the extinction of the flame of life.[41] Hence, it is not the infirm that we hear of, but the exceptions, the hale and hearty, such as the Elder Pliny's centenarian friend Antonius Castor, still pottering around his herb garden.[42] Galen's pair of active old men each had his own individual prescription for longevity. Dr Antiochus at 80 walked a daily mile or more to the Forum and back and to see his patients, while Telephus the schoolmaster lived to be almost 100 on his diet of boiled barley, honey, vegetables, fish, birds and bread, and a little wine, with a visit to the baths no more than once a week.[43]

Ancient writers are more informative about what we might term epidemic or widely communicable diseases, but their evidence presents a variety of different problems. On the demographic model already sketched out it might be expected that the population was on the whole too scattered to allow for frequent and widespread outbreaks of epidemic disease, which is loosely termed 'plague'.[44] Either the infective agent would not survive long enough to be transmitted to a non-immune host or there were enough potential hosts with immunity, either acquired through previous exposure or inherited, for the agent to be unable to reproduce itself.[45] This predicted pattern is confirmed by the historical record, for, although one can draw up a long catalogue of outbreaks of plague, these mostly appear to be only local in extent. For example, an epidemic in 278–276 BC covered apparently only Rome and Latium, and was ended by the exceptionally cold winter weather.[46] An epidemic in autumn AD 65, according to Tacitus, killed 30,000 within Rome, including members of the senate and nobility, but whether there was any link with the epidemics that a few years later raged north of the Alps is unclear.[47] This impression of largely local plagues may be simply the result of a failure in our sources, which concentrate heavily on Rome and Athens, to record developments on a wider scale. So, for instance, in his description of the great plague in 430 BC Thucydides concentrates on events in Athens and among the Athenian troops at Potidaea, but leaves vague its passage from Egypt and via Lemnos, and does not identify the 'other most populous places' that it struck, apart from the negative comment that the Peloponnese was only lightly touched.[48] Similarly, Livy records outbreaks of plague in Rome in 431 BC and 428 BC, but without any reference to the plague in Greece.[49]

On occasions, however, ancient writers do record diseases spreading over much wider areas. The Antonine plague of 166–72, which was in all likelihood smallpox, moved westwards from Persia all the way across the Roman Empire and even beyond the Rhine, carried, it was supposed, by the victorious Roman army returning from a campaign against Persia.[50] This is a plausible explanation for its transmission, although one need not go further and accept the ancient view that the army was in some way being punished by the god for sacking a temple of Apollo, or suppose that it had had the misfortune to march near the naphtha wells of N. Iraq, whose vapours turned the air poisonous.[51] An outbreak of a probably different disease is recorded by

Galen in 189, when its effects in Rome were intensified by several months of famine.[52] A further pandemic occurred in 250 and lasted for almost twenty years, moving from east to west, according to Cyprian, an eyewitness, sparing not a single city. Half the population of Alexandria is reported to have died, and at least one village was wiped out.[53] The plague of Justinian, which began in 541 in Egypt and spread as far as Spain, Trier and possibly Wales, is notable for two things. It is the first confirmed outbreak of bubonic plague (although it is, of course, not named as such) and it continued to flare up at regular intervals around the eastern Mediterranean, the most densely populated region, for a further two hundred years.[54]

Nonetheless, other factors support the notion that most outbreaks of infectious disease were local. In many of the sources an outbreak is linked to local famines, with a consequent lowering of resistance, and to periods of siege, as the historian Ammianus Marcellinus observed when besieged at Amida in AD 359.[55] Often, too, it is associated with armies, either in camp or moving en masse on campaign. Carthaginian armies in Sicily were ravaged by disease in 406 and again in 396 BC.[56] Both a Roman and a Carthaginian army were smitten by disease before Syracuse in 212 BC, and in 190 BC a Roman fleet was forced to weigh anchor and leave off operations in Lycia because so many of its galley slaves had fallen ill.[57] In 90 BC 17,000 men allegedly died among the forces of Octavius besieging Rome in the Roman civil wars between the supporters of Marius and Sulla.[58] The crowded conditions of an army camp are an ideal breeding ground for disease, and it is no surprise to find that even in the well-organised Roman army more soldiers were likely to be unfit for duty because of ill health (including contagious eye diseases) than because of wounds.[59]

An incident in AD 232 neatly illustrates the point, as well as showing ancient ideas about the causation and spread of such diseases. In that year the emperor Alexander Severus and his troops were encamped near the Euphrates frontier in N. Syria, where, so the contemporary Greek historian Herodian reports, all fell sick in the stifling air.[60] The troops brought from Illyrium suffered especially badly and many died, being accustomed to moist cool air and to more substantial rations than were being issued to them. The army was compelled to retreat to Antioch, where both emperor and men revived under the influence of the cool air and good water of the city.

A modern epidemiologist, called in to diagnose a mass outbreak of disease in a military encampment in the Mediterranean region, would immediately suspect some form of transmissible disease, such as shigellosis or another type of bacillary dysentery. The notorious 'camp fever', typhus, would probably be excluded from first consideration, as it requires a cooler climate for its vectors, lice, to flourish.[61] But an explanation would then be forthcoming in terms of insanitary living conditions, infected water or some form of pollution.[62] By contrast, Herodian, like ancient writers in general, ascribes this medical disaster in an army camp, almost a small town in itself, to poor diet and the

25

inability of the troops to adjust to a new climate and its hot, stifling air.[63] The water of Antioch restores them, not because of its purity and freedom from parasites, but because it brings about a change in the general make-up of their bodies: wind and water together counteract the heat and 'thickening' effect of the Syrian desert frontier.[64]

Herodian's brief comments reveal the gulf that separates modern medical explanations and priorities from those of the ancients.[65] He focuses on different aspects of disease, he has a different view of causation and his emphasis on habituation stresses climate rather than vectors, germs, bacilli, viruses and the like. In common with almost all medical writers of Antiquity, he explains illness on the model of an individual's interaction with the surrounding air; receptivity and resistance, strengthened or weakened by diet or lifestyle, are crucial in determining the response to bad air, however that may be defined or explained. On this schema the question why the air becomes bad is secondary; what is causing the pollution is of less importance than the knowledge that the air has become dangerous.[66] What matters, above all, is the ability of the potential sufferer to repel any harmful changes, an ability which, doctors advised, could be increased by a change of diet or, as one Hippocratic author recommended, by taking in less air through altering one's breathing pattern.[67]

This overwhelming belief in Antiquity among Greek medical writers that epidemic disease was the result of bad air stands in apparent contrast to the common use in Latin of words such as 'infection' and 'contact/contagion' to describe the process of the transmission.[68] Nasty things such as disease or heresy can pass from one person to another, rather as dye seeps across a piece of cloth or as a dirty finger leaves its mark on a sparkling white toga.[69] But this apparent contrast between Greek and Latin authorities does not mean that the Greeks lacked any notion of person-to-person transfer or that the Romans anticipated nineteenth-century bacteriologists in a belief in individual causative agents. Thucydides, in his Greek account of the Athenian plague, talks about the passage of disease from person to person without any hint that this opinion was unusual, and a range of Greek authors offers explanations for why one individual catches a disease from proximity to another sufferer and others do not. Both Latin and Greek authors take as their prime examples of diseases spread in this way phthisis (tuberculosis), psora (scabies) and 'ophthalmia', but they equally regularly exclude 'fevers' and they offer an identical explanation for the potentially illness-bringing phenomenon of the 'evil-eye'.[70] In their metaphorical descriptions of the process – and it is always difficult to decide how far any metaphor is a dead metaphor – Latin authors frequently talk of 'touching', Greeks equally frequently of 'sharing'.[71] Yet neither discuss the therapeutic consequence of these metaphors, the exclusion, temporary or permanent, of the infected carrier from social contact, for two good reasons. The remedies thought appropriate when dealing with infected animals could be applied only with the greatest of difficulty to humans. It is easier to kill an infected sheep in one's flock than an infected member of one's family, and, second, ancient society had neither the power nor the administrative structures to deal adequately with matters of public health.[72]

This last point may seem paradoxical to those familiar with the sewers and aqueducts of the Roman world, or even the simpler arrangements of earlier Greece, or with the system of publicly hired physicians we shall discuss later. Such provision undoubtedly helped lessen the impact of disease in an overcrowded town, even if, as Galen noted, the outpourings of the Roman sewers reduced the fish caught in the lower Tiber and its estuary to little more than scraps compared with the fat and healthy fish from its upper reaches.[73] But there is little hint that considerations of public health played a great part in their establishment compared with considerations of aesthetics, the donor's personal prestige and, particularly in Rome, the need to prevent disorder in the heart of the Empire. Regulations about the location of burial grounds outside the town walls or the touching or mutilating of corpses existed for religious far more than for sanitary reasons, although, as with Jewish dietary regulations, the former might bring consequent improvements to the latter.[74] Sabinus, Galen and others in the Hippocratic tradition of *Airs, Waters and Places* might offer excellent advice on the siting of towns, the breadth of streets and the importance of good ventilation in a house, and writers of architectural manuals such as Vitruvius (*c.*20 BC) endorse it, but there is no evidence that their views were ever followed.[75] Some of what they preached was common sense – the avoidance of swamps and marshes, fumaroles and stinking corpses – and it did not require a medical man to warn against such dangers, as any reader of Varro's advice to the farmer knew.[76] But the city as a political entity did not pursue a major role in matters to do with health, except for its own administrative purposes: doctors, for instance, would be needed to serve the army and to act as expert witnesses in cases of murder or serious injury. Except among the Jews and Christians, responsibility for health was a purely private matter for the individual and the individual's family. The Roman poor still crowded together in multi-storey tenements in the 'furnace-hot Subura', while, by contrast, the mansions of the rich Pergamenes (Galen among them) enjoyed a far healthier environment, being sited, as recent archaeological excavations have confirmed, half way up the great hill, above the stifling lower city, and open to gentle cooling breezes from the Aegean a few miles to the west.[77]

This environmental perspective also explains the scanty information given in our ancient sources on occupational diseases. That a connection might be made between occupation and health in Antiquity is clear from Galen, who talks about fishermen temporarily paralysed by striking an electric eel with their trident, and of professional scribes (such as could still be seen not long ago outside mosques in Turkey) blinded by continually writing in bright sunlight on reflective surfaces.[78] The pale face of the lead or silver miner, especially in Spain, is a commonplace among Latin poets, and Pliny the Elder reports how workers digging for minium devised small masks for protection (although his description of their use does not inspire confidence in their effectiveness).[79] One can only guess at the fate of the many slaves employed in the heavily polluted silver mines and smelters of Attica in the late sixth and fifth centuries BC (to judge from studies of the Greenland ice-cap, the period with one of the highest concentrations of lead yet found in the atmosphere) or that of those condemned by Roman judges to the mines of the Wadi Faynan (Jordan).[80] Some medical assistance might be provided (a Roman inscription records a doctor attached to a Spanish mining company), but it was probably not much.[81]

No less brutal and short will have been the lives of many slave labourers on the large estates of Republican Rome, often working in notoriously unhealthy regions, fed on stodgy but scarcely nutritious food, and, when ill, treated, if at all, with only the most general and basic of remedies.[82] In the early fourth century BC, when Plato sketched his ideal state in the *Laws*, he advised that free men and slaves were to be treated by different types of physicians. Slaves should be looked after by slave physicians, who would provide rough and ready treatment without explanation, like 'despots', not diligent doctors.[83] Whether domestic slaves in the households of the imperial family and wealthy senators in Late Republican and Early Imperial Rome fared any better at the hands of the slaves or ex-slaves serving as doctors, or even specialists, among the divisions of the household cannot be known.[84] An exceptionally regarded slave might be treated by the owner's personal physician, but it is more likely that, branded, beaten and worked almost to death, the only time that slaves saw a doctor was when they were to be sold.[85] Then a doctor might be called in to examine them, and to decide, for example, whether a suppurating ear would clear up or was a chronic or congenital defect that would reduce the price.[86] If they were handed over to unscrupulous gang-drivers, their life would be miserable and short.

Reconstructing the disease profile of Antiquity is hampered by the great difference between ancient and modern understanding of the concept of 'a disease'. Although diseases were occasionally viewed, particularly in a religious context, as if they had an existence of their own, most ancient doctors thought of them solely in terms of pathological processes taking place within the body over time.[87] They would have agreed with the Aristotelian author who wrote that disease implies motion whereas health is a state of rest.[88] In general, they viewed disease as something that affected an individual and had its origin in an individual's own physical make-up as affected by his or her lifestyle. Certain groupings of symptoms came very soon to be called 'diseases', and, particularly in the Roman period, there were sophisticated and, in terms of observation, impressive discussions of nosology. But even when the importance of these groupings became widely accepted, many doctors, particularly those in the Hippocratic tradition, regarded them more in the nature of guidelines, to be modified in the light of whatever was concluded about the individual patient. Equally, although it was accepted that certain symptoms or syndromes were 'pathognomic' or 'prognostic', characterising

28

particular types of illness, they were not considered to be the disease itself, merely indicators of deeper changes in the patient's constitution.[89]

Moreover, some ancient names for diseases were far from specific in modern eyes. The term 'phthisis', for instance, usually interpreted as tuberculosis, could cover a variety of other wasting diseases.[90] Sores, gangrenes and abscesses, some quite dramatically described, were all lumped together, and there was no guarantee that one author's terminology for pustules coincided with that of another. Galen's trenchant criticism of the 'younger doctors' who wished to introduce their own, at times more specific, terminology to describe disease points neatly to the difficulty of combining precision with wide intelligibility. The accuracy of their description, he believed, would be lost on those unfamiliar with their words, and there might be other and better ways of giving a clearer definition of a condition while still utilising the older and broader terminology.[91]

Nonetheless, despite the problems of identification, it is clear that many diseases familiar today were present in Antiquity.[92] Coughs, colds, pneumonia and pleurisy were common in winter; diarrhoeas in summer.[93] Jaundice and other liver infections are clearly described, as are a variety of parasitic infections of the digestive tract. Tapeworms, ascarides and in Egypt Guinea worms are all described as common.[94] In the absence of antibiotics, ulcers must have been a frequent sight, and, as Galen implies in his *Method of Healing*, formed a large part of the work of the average doctor and surgeon. But there were many other disfiguring skin conditions, including scabies, alphos and herpes, and the pharmacological writer Dioscorides gave more remedies for these conditions than for any other group.[95] Among them is 'lichen' or 'mentagra', a form of fungal sycosis said by Pliny to have been introduced into Italy only in the early first century AD.[96] The use of public baths, one of the essential signs of civilisation to the Romans, may have reduced some forms of dirt disease, but, one might suspect, also led to other cross-infections.

The most famous of all ancient skin diseases is leprosy (Hansen's disease), a chronic condition caused by *mycobacterium leprae* and affecting the skin and peripheral nervous system. Palaeopathological evidence for its existence in the Mediterranean lands is inconclusive before Hellenistic times.[97] Texts from Babylonia, Egypt and Israel from 800 BC onwards describing disfiguring skin diseases, which might include Hansen's disease, probably refer to psoriasis. More problematic is the biblical disease, za'arath, translated in the Authorised Version of the English Bible as leprosy, which is described as affecting not only the skin, but also house walls and clothing, and with an emphasis on its scaly (and fungoid?) nature.[98] The word 'lepra', which means in Greek 'a scaly disease', is mentioned in the Hippocratic Corpus, and a tract on 'elephantiasis', a Greek word that stresses the thickening of the skin and the bone changes in the disease, is ascribed to the fifth-century philosopher Democritus, although it was probably not composed until three or four centuries later.[99] When this disease entered the Mediterranean world was disputed, even in Antiquity. Pliny placed its arrival in the mid-first century BC, in the time of Pompey, whereas his slightly later contemporary Plutarch cited an earlier doctor, Athenodorus, who claimed that this disease only appeared in the late second century BC.[100] But there is good reason to believe that it was already being discussed around 250 BC by the doctor Strato, and an ointment against 'elephantiasis' was produced by the surgeon Archagathus, who lived at the end of the third century BC.[101] Contracts for the sale of slaves from Hellenistic Egypt often include clauses rendering the sale void if the slave is later found to be suffering from epilepsy or 'the touch', which has been interpreted as some form of leprous skin disease.[102] But for the most graphic and detailed descriptions of what is beyond doubt Hansen's disease we must wait until the Roman authors Aretaeus and Caelius Aurelianus.[103] The significance of this disease goes far beyond the merely medical, for the stories of leprosy in both the Old and New Testaments gave this disease a special prominence in Christian literature. The Gospels' account of Christ's meeting with lepers on the road implies that such sights were not infrequent, in contrast to what might be concluded from the ancient medical authors or the surviving palaeopathological evidence.[104] The discrepancy may be explained by the strong and lasting impact that the scaling skin and collapsed face would have on any casual observer, as well as by the range of modern conditions that might be included under the same ancient term.

Kidney and bladder problems also figure prominently in any ancient medical handbook, with a variety of explanations given for failure to urinate or for painful urination.[105] Several operations are mentioned for removing bladder stones, but all carried the danger of later infection if the incision failed to heal properly.[106] It is perhaps not surprising that some surgeons came to specialise in the treatment of fistulae, the consequences of continued ulceration, particularly in the perineum or the region of the anus.[107] Haemorrhoids, by contrast, were usually viewed as something good, a way for the body to evacuate excessive or harmful blood, and it is the ending of their bleeding that causes concern, for this might indicate that the bad blood was being kept within the body as a sort of hidden poison. Cystitis and abscesses of the urethra and prostate are also described, but cancers of the penis and the uterus do not appear until late in the surviving literature. Only the milder forms of sexually transmitted disease are recorded, such as those caused by *Chlamydia trachomatis*; whether the nasty and persistent discharge described as gonorrhoea corresponds to the modern condition is disputed, and, despite some vigorous advocates, venereal syphilis has not yet been conclusively identified in Antiquity. The various ulcers, chancres and swellings of the penis mentioned can be otherwise explained, and only a handful of skeletons have so far revealed signs of the characteristic lesions of the later stages of syphilis.[108] But it is still uncertain whether this was the result of a venereal or a non-venereal infection, although pathological changes in a foetus excavated in S. France do suggest the existence of the venereal form.[109]

For skeletal abnormalities our evidence, palaeopathological, textual and artistic, is far more extensive.[110] Fractures, vertebral arthroses and dislocations, both congenital and the result of trauma, are regularly found in excavations.[111] There is a classic description of humpback, almost certainly as a result of tuberculosis, in the Hippocratic treatises on *Joints*, and both it and *Fractures* describe a wide range of joint problems, although it is disconcerting to find what sounds like a Colles fracture of the wrist treated as if it were a dislocation (and then reported as hard to cure!).[112] Artistic representations, particularly sculptures, show a wide range of deformities, from dwarfism and acromegaly to club foot and (congenitally?) dislocated hips.[113] Gout was honoured with a satirical poem to itself within the corpus of works by or attributed to the Roman author Lucian. Its comic title, *Tragodopodagra, a Gouty Tragedy*, cannot obscure the torments faced by its sufferers.[114]

Eye diseases are also well represented in ancient art, and were sufficiently common to justify their own specialists. Glaucoma, trachoma and conjunctivitis were frequent, and Galen expected any competent surgeon to be able to cure a wide range of eye conditions, including growths on the cornea and eyelid.[115] The discovery of a set of oculist's instruments in a grave at Montbellet (France) has illuminated three ancient descriptions of an operation for cataracts, by Celsus, Antyllus and Paul of Aegina.[116] Whether the discovery of more than 300 stamps used to mark sticks of hard ointment for eye diseases (especially 'blear-eye', *lippitudo*) at many locations in Gaul, Britain and the northern provinces indicates that eye disease was more common there than around the Mediterranean is an open question.[117] Evidence from Egypt and the pattern of modern eye disease in the Levant suggest that it was not, while the discovery of a variety of surgical instruments alongside several of these oculists' stamps suggests that eye conditions were not the only ailments treated by these practitioners.

Other conditions leave no trace in the archaeological record, but are graphically described in both medical and non-medical texts – strokes and epilepsy (both ascribed to divine as well as more natural causes), migraines, headaches, and many nervous and mental disorders.[118] These might range from a feeling while lying in bed that somebody, or some demon, was attempting to throttle the life out of one (*ephialtes*), to paranoia or to a deadly hallucination that a servant was a large jar that should be tipped out of an upstairs window.[119] The boundary between madness and prophetic frenzy was always open to dispute, whether in paganism, Judaism or Christianity, and the melancholy of genius became a commonplace from Hellenistic times on.[120] Scenes of madness figure prominently in literature from early epic through Classical Greek tragedy to Latin poetry, and are related consistently to divine vengeance.[121] Particularly in texts from the Near East, including Jewish and later Christian literature, mental disorders are often ascribed to the intervention of demons, some of whom may even take up residence in the body.[122] Nonetheless, medical writers from Hippocratic times to Galen, a self-styled expert in the relationship between mind and body, resolutely proposed alternative physicalist explanations, even if they were in a minority.[123]

The largest group of conditions mentioned in our ancient medical texts is that of fevers, *puretoi* or *febres*, a broad term deriving from the feeling of fiery heat. (Since the thermometer had not been invented, temperature had to be judged purely from touch and the patient's own description of his or her condition.) In modern medical parlance, a fever is a symptom, and it is only one of the indications of a specific disease. In Antiquity, the fever itself was the disease, but, even so, it required further precision. Some fevers, such as the so-called 'shivering fever', were described in terms of their effects, but the most common taxonomy depended on their periodicity, whether the high temperature was constant or waned and then returned after one, two, three or more days. The pattern on which this is based is that of malaria, a disease generally of low-lying marshes or slow-moving rivers, spread by the mosquito. It is also characterised by an enlargement of the spleen and the liver, and by a recurrent pattern of attacks and remission.[124] The mathematical regularity with which this can be calculated and forecast, as well as its typical seasonal pattern of late-summer infestation, will have suggested to the Greeks that disease too was subject to the same ordered laws as the rest of the universe.

Of the three main Mediterranean forms of malaria, *Plasmodium vivax*, *P. malariae* and *P. falciparum*, the last is the most dangerous. Sometimes it brings about a rapid death, but often its debilitating effects – as, indeed, those of all forms of malaria – are long term, on both mind and body. Falciparum malaria has been present in Greece at least since the Neolithic period, but its incidence has not always been constant. Many areas that later became notoriously malarial, for example Boeotia and the Macedonian plain, were more densely populated in the fifth and fourth centuries BC than in the early twentieth century.[125] The southern coastal cities of Etruria had flourishing populations until the third century BC, while the Greek colony of Paestum in S. Italy, famous today for its magnificent temples, was located in an area that by the Early Middle Ages was a malaria-infested marsh. Hence, scholars long believed that earlier infestations of falciparum malaria in prehistory had been reduced as a result of climatic changes that controlled the mosquito vector, and that this strain of malaria became common again only in the mid- or late fifth century BC. Certainly, from then on there are enough reports of sound observations about the incidence of fevers and the behaviour of mosquitoes to suggest a considerable familiarity with malaria: upstairs rooms are healthier than those below (since mosquitoes are poor fliers); severe fevers are particularly common in a year with a wet spring and hot summer (which first creates large pools of standing water, an ideal breeding ground, and then dries them up, forcing the mosquitoes to seek other habitats); and sea marshes, as around Ravenna, are less dangerous than inland marshes (their salinity prevents the mosquito larvae from breeding).[126]

But while, in general, there is a correlation between poverty and the prevalence of malaria (and vice versa), particularly in low-lying areas near marshes or slow-moving rivers, the pattern of malaria is much more complex. Human intervention, creating farmland out of forest or driving roads on causeways across lowland, may paradoxically have increased the number of breeding sites for mosquitoes. At the same time, the fertility of many plain areas, particularly the Roman Campagna, will have encouraged farmers to remain, particularly if they had gained some immunity by early infection and reinfection, for the life of an upland farmer was scarcely better in terms of health and arguably worse in terms of prosperity. But once malaria had taken a firm hold it could defy all attempts to bring the land back into cultivation. The Pontine marshes, a heavily malarial area of woods and wetland in the Roman Campagna, had swallowed up several towns and villages long before the first recorded attempt to drain them, by Cornelius Cethegus in 160 BC, and continued to defy all improvers until Mussolini in the 1930s.[127] By AD 500, with the impoverishment of Rome itself, the whole Campagna was already slipping back to become one of the worst of all regions for malaria infestation as drainage channels became stagnant and fertile farmland became waterlogged.[128]

Malaria is certainly a more plausible explanation for the economic decline of certain areas of the Roman world than another commonly accepted culprit, lead poisoning.[129] Although skeletal analysis does show an increased presence of lead in Classical Antiquity over those from the second millennium BC, this is less than might have been predicted, given the substantial increase in lead production between 600 BC and AD 500 and the widespread use of lead for household objects and waterpipes.[130] Partly because the disease replicates the symptoms of many other diseases, clear descriptions of lead poisoning are rare. Nicander, in the second century BC, provides the earliest example, and only Paul of Aegina, seven centuries later, implies that the condition was widespread.[131] Vitruvius warned against drinking water from pools near lead mines, and also condemned the use of lead in water conduits, a ban supported by Augustus, although hardly enforced.[132] But free-flowing sources of water – taps were rare – would not have been greatly contaminated by lead, and the build-up of other deposits, especially chalk, on lead pipes would have reduced the danger still further. Far more dangerous would have been the boiling down of fruit juice in lead-lined containers to produce *sapa*, a procedure recommended by many culinary and agricultural writers to give a better flavour. Modern replications following Columella's advice have resulted in concentrations of 800 mg per litre, about 16,000 times greater than the recommended upper limit for drinking water.[133] But, although the wealthy upper class may indeed have been exposed to poisoning from *sapa*, claims for lead poisoning as an explanation of the behaviour of emperors or the population decline of the Roman Empire are greatly exaggerated.

Lead poisoning, however, was not the only hazard faced by the population from their food and drink. Much of the bread of Antiquity will have contained hard particles, and sometimes even pieces of grit, while other farinaceous mixtures were even worse.[134] Wheaten porridge Galen would have thought totally inedible, had he not had the misfortune, at the end of a day's hard journey, to come upon a group of peasants eating their meal. They generously offered Galen and his two young companions some boiled and moderately salted wheat porridge, prepared by the women on the spot. The result was flatulence, constipation, headache and eye disturbances. But, reports Galen, the peasants said that they regularly ate this wheaten porridge, even though it was, they admitted, rather heavy and indigestible – as anyone can see, says Galen scathingly, even without having eaten it.[135] He was also against the consumption of fruit of all kinds, both because he had himself been ill for a long while after eating even a little fresh fruit and because it was always liable to rot in a hot Mediterranean climate, especially apricots, peaches and nectarines. Apples allowed to ripen and then stored, if baked or steamed, might benefit the sick, he grudgingly conceded, but he shows no surprise at the practice of Asian peasants in feeding apples to their pigs. Unripe fruit was also a danger, witness Protas the rhetor, 'our fellow citizen', who fell ill after eating unripe apples and pears.[136] Finally, although the emperor Claudius may well have been deliberately murdered by means of poisonous mushrooms, as the historian Tacitus alleges, there will undoubtedly have been others who perished accidentally through mistaking a deadly variety for an edible one.[137]

To these hazards to health one might also add the ministrations of healers themselves. An Egyptian patient wrote to his doctor, wondering when his next visit would be, for he had been left alone unwashed and stinking of pus for several days.[138] There might be even worse consequences: the Elder Pliny condemned all Greek doctors for being allowed to kill their Roman patients with impunity.[139] This denunciation is a memorable exaggeration of a technical point in Roman law, but is given greater impact by inscriptions such as the lament of the husband of Aurelia Decia, 'rarest and most chaste of wives, whose death, at the age of 28 years, 10 months and 24 days, occurred in my absence through the fault of those who tried to cure her'.[140] Similar tragic tombstones record the premature deaths of Euelpistus, 'that most innocent soul, whom the doctors killed', and Ephesia Rubra, a devoted mother, hastened to her end by her doctors.[141] The husband of the 20-year-old Julia Prisca could only console himself for the mistakes of her physicians with the thought that death carried kings away likewise.[142] His grief would not have been diminished by the knowledge that at least some ancient doctors were willing to acknowledge a certain degree of medical responsibility for causing a patient's death or exacerbating their condition.[143] But their willingness to make this apology did not indicate a wholesale confession of their shortcomings but their consciousness of the difficulty of always reaching the right conclusion when dealing with so complex and individual a matter as the human body. Medicine, whether from the perspective of the patient or of the healer, was always a chancy business.[144]

So too were its consequences. It is easy to forget, amid the mournful tombstones to those who died before their time and the encouraging rhetoric of handbooks detailing the treatments that have proved effective, that many sufferers will have continued for years in pain and anxiety.[145] Hippocratic physicians say relatively little about chronic conditions, although the fact that they regularly talk of 'acute' cases implies that they were aware of the distinction, and it is not until the Hellenistic period that we find treatises devoted to long-term illness. Sometimes treatment was merely palliative, stabilising a broken limb in such a way as to permit some mobility, although not full use.[146] At other times, the physician might contemplate a course of treatment lasting months, if not years. Galen, for instance, claims to have treated successfully a sufferer from breast cancer by a year's course of purgation to remove the dangerous black bile from her body, and to have repeated the purgation once a year from then on.[147]

On the whole, ancient medicine depended on the recuperative powers of the body and the self-limiting nature of many acute illnesses. Long-term illness, which must have been the painful lot of many, is glimpsed only rarely, in the desperation of the woman with the issue of blood 'who had been ill for many years and had given her all to the physicians' striving merely to touch the hem of the garment of the famous healer passing through her village, or in the relief of an anonymous Syrian at being cured by divine intervention when thirty-six doctors had already failed.[148] Deep in the Peloponnese, Euandridas gratefully erected a fountain in honour of Hercules, the mighty healer, 'who favoured me, unlike my doctors'.[149] The cure tablets that adorned the walls of healing shrines around the ancient world present a sadly joyful litany of illness overcome; of blindness, paralysis, pains in the stomach and head, damaged limbs, strokes, mental disorders, all of which must have placed an intolerable burden on patients and their families until they were cured. One can only imagine the joy of Felix, a public slave in Rome, blind for ten months and abandoned by his doctors, when he was healed by the Bona Dea.[150] Accounts of miracles of Christian healing continue the traditional picture. One can appreciate the social as well as the personal inconvenience caused to the rich lawyer Innocentius by his anal fistula that had defied all the attempts of the best doctor and surgeon in his home town of Carthage.[151] The pool of Bethesda, like the Asclepieion of the Tiber Island in Rome and, one suspects, many other healing shrines, was filled with the cast-offs of society, the lame, the blind, the mentally infirm, asking for charity or waiting in hope for some means of a cure.[152] Their situation was far worse than that of the wealthy Roman philosopher Seneca or the Greek orator Aelius Aristides, whose substantial accounts of their own sufferings over many years are prominent in the literary record.[153]

With all this, our understanding of the reality of illness in the ancient world, whether at a personal level or as a background to the theory and practice of medicine, must remain partial at best. In this chapter much has had inevitably to be omitted and compressed. To bring together texts from different periods, different places and different traditions risks reconstructing an edifice that never existed, or that was not recognised by contemporaries. Demographical studies have relied heavily on tombstone inscriptions (overwhelmingly from

Italy and Rome) and on Egyptian papyri, which may carry with them their own distortions. Medical texts preserve as if in aspic information from past doctors and surgeons, yet the very process of accumulation may blur our understanding of what treatments were actually used or what diseases were generally encountered. One final example shows how the Greeks and Romans may have seen things differently, both from each other and from us. In the first century more than one author noticed that there appeared to be new diseases coming into the world, although they offered different explanations.[154] The Greek writer Plutarch imagined a dinner-table discussion precisely on this theme.[155] One speaker, a local doctor, produced as proof of the existence of new diseases Athenodorus' treatise on the *Epidemics* (both book and author are otherwise unknown), in which he claimed that rabies and 'elephantiasis' (probably leprosy) had been unknown before the time of Asclepiades in the late second century BC. This view was roundly attacked by another guest, Diogenianus, who was scathing about the Democritean (and Asclepiadean?) notion of atoms coming from outside our universe, bringing seeds of disease. In his view, all disease was the result of human diet: 'it is the disagreements of our food and drink with us or our mistakes in using them that upset our system'. There was only a small range of possible reactions: diseases were constant, and any so-called new diseases were the result of a failure of observation or of nomenclature. Plutarch himself followed a middle line. He rejected the notion of harmful things coming from outside, as well as Diogenianus' view of a perpetually static universe of disease. In Plutarch's view there were indeed new diseases, but with a simple cause. Primitive man had indeed suffered from dietary deficiency; but the luxurious lifestyle of modern Rome, with exotic foods arriving from all over the Empire and beyond, was far worse. It was not surprising that new and different diseases were engendered by a surfeit of luxury.

This little debate among cultivated Greeks offers an insight into ancient perceptions of health and disease. There was a general agreement that some things had changed, that there might be diseases previously unrecorded, but, at the same time, neither of the examples given would today count as an epidemic disease, while the modes of transmission of rabies and leprosy, cited as examples, are vastly different. For one speaker, the make-up of the universe, with its constantly shifting interaction between its atoms and pores, meant that the emergence of new diseases was always likely; for another, this was to mistake the reactions of an individual for a specific disease. For Plutarch, luxury and modern living were to blame. All of them saw disease in terms of the individual. Their ideas, their arguments, even their sources, can be traced back for several centuries. Together they stand for an approach to medicine that looks for causes and that involves debate and discussion, not just among doctors, but among all those with the time and the interest to participate. How this approach developed we shall now see in the rest of this book.

3

BEFORE HIPPOCRATES

In 1879 it was revealed to the learned world that the poet Homer had composed his *Iliad* while serving as deputy chief of the medical staff with Agamemnon's army before Troy. That he was a doctor was evident from the poem's remarkable emphasis on wounds and other matters medical; and his position as a staff officer was proved by his access to detailed information on the activities taking place on both sides of the front line. His vantage point, a little above the daily round of the actual fighting, showed that he was not serving on the battlefield itself, although he had seen corpses and casualties, and the position as chief of the medical staff would have denied him the leisure for writing available in a post only a little less senior. Although this conclusion reveals more about the organisation and prejudices of the Royal Saxon Army in which *Oberstabsarzt* Frölich served than it does about Homer, it points to one undeniable fact: the poet chose to include many medical details and to treat them in a sophisticated way.[1]

It is important to begin with Homer, not just because the Greeks themselves did, or because in his description of Machaon as 'a healer (*iatros*) worth many other men in cutting out arrows and spreading soothing drugs' he provided later doctors, neglectful of both the qualification in the second line and the military context, with a warrant for their sense of general superiority over the rest of mankind.[2] The Homeric poems afford us a glimpse of medical ideas and practices long before any of our strictly medical literature, and although their information cannot be taken back to the heroic days of Agamemnon and Odysseus, it can be used to illustrate what the poet's audience would have expected or taken for granted in the late eighth century. We may note the complex vocabulary for types of wound with which Homer expected his readers to be familiar, and the graphic descriptions of injuries, not all of which are the result of poetic imagination.[3] Frölich's belief that only a doctor could have written with such accuracy and technical precision underestimates both the necessity for a rapport between poet and audience, and, although he could not have known this in 1879, the methods of oral composition that lie behind the *Iliad* and *Odyssey* as we have them. Far from an acquaintance with medical terms and situations being the preserve of professionals alone, the poems demonstrate that many others had access to and understood this information. That there were already individuals recognised as healers with specific skills should not obscure the equally important fact that their knowledge was not kept entirely secret.

According to Homer, Machaon and his brother Podalirius come from a medical family and their knowledge of drugs descends, via their father Asclepius, from Chiron the Centaur. But in the *Iliad* both Machaon and Podalirius are portrayed in the first instance as warriors, chieftains leading their contingent from Tricca, Ithome and Oechalia, and playing their part in the fighting like other heroes.[4] Machaon's role in leading his men as 'shepherd of his people' does not depend on his medical abilities alone, and the adjectives that are applied to him are also given to other chieftains.[5] As a healer, he removes arrows, sucks out poisonous blood and applies 'soothing drugs' to the wounded Menelaus, with immediate success.[6] One might also imagine him bandaging the wounded, as other heroes do for their wounded comrades.[7] Podalirius, by contrast, is not seen in action, an omission rectified by a later epic poet, Arctinus, in his *Sack of Troy*.[8] While his brother attends to the wounds of Ajax, Podalirius, who can 'recognise the invisible and cure the incurable', observes the glint in the patient's eye that reveals the burdensome thoughts that will end in suicide.[9] We need not go as far as Alexandrian scholars who made the one into the prototypical surgeon and the other into the prototypical physician, for the poet's differentiation serves an artistic rather than a professional purpose. But Arctinus' divergence from Homer was noted, and easily explained: since wounds were what doctoring in warfare was largely about, it was hardly surprising that Homer should have concentrated on what was most relevant to his epic conflict.

More significant is the fact that both Machaon and Podalirius perform their actions without recourse to the gods: Machaon applies his dressings and Podalirius diagnoses Ajax's incipient madness without any mention of them. Indeed, when Apollo comes to treat the gods who have themselves been wounded in skirmishes he does so in the same manner and is described in the same words as Machaon.[10] Although this argument should not be pressed too far in dealing with a poem that relies heavily on formulaic language in its depiction of both gods and heroes, there is not a little humour in having the immortals treated by a god with the same means as Machaon used for his human patients. But the gods are not entirely absent from the human battlefield at the moment of healing. At *Iliad* 16,523, Glaucus, having just witnessed the death of Sarpedon, prays to Apollo to be healed of his own wound, and his prayer is answered.[11]

The role of Apollo in the plague that opens the first book of the *Iliad* is much more complex. He is the agent of both destruction and its cessation. He sends his arrows with the 'evil illness' to strike animals and men alike, because he is angry with the Greeks for roughly rejecting the request of his priest, Chryses, for the return of his daughter captured by Agamemnon. Apollo acts in response to Chryses' prayer for assistance, and, from then on, the ending of the plague is a matter for negotiation solely with the god. The reaction of the Greeks after nine days of death is to ask advice from a seer, priest or dream interpreter as to the precise cause of his anger.[12] There is no place for the *iatros* here, for the poet makes it clear that everyone believes in the divine origin of this affliction, and, as a consequence, that it is not an *iatros* but someone skilled in understanding the gods who is required.[13] Achilles, the spokesman for the Greeks, is in no doubt of the reasons for the god's anger: there has been some offence directly committed against Apollo. The Greeks have broken a vow, or have offered an unacceptable sacrifice.[14] At this stage, a more complicated chain of causation is not envisaged. Nevertheless, once the actual cause has been revealed to them by their own seer, there is both universal acceptance of this reasoning and agreement that only an appropriate apology to the god will persuade him to end what he has begun. Agamemnon's insistence on his right to compensation for giving up the girl obscures, but does not contradict, his willingness to concur with this explanation and this advice. The final expiation is twofold: the return of the girl to her father and sacrifice to the god. Only when both are completed does Apollo relent.

This belief that a disease affecting so many must have a cause that goes beyond the merely individual and must relate to the anger of some divinity or other can be found elsewhere in the Mediterranean, particularly in the Old Testament. When God is angry he looses his bolts against the sinful; when the Israelites, or their leaders, break their convenant with Jehovah they are punished with terrible diseases, which are only ended when satisfaction has been made.[15] Even in modern Western societies, familiar with the effects of pollution, malnutrition, infectious diseases, viruses, bacilli and the like, a religious or moral dimension is not entirely absent from discussions of epidemic disease, as the initial reactions to the spread of AIDS in the 1980s demonstrated.[16]

But the consensus of the Greeks before Troy that their epidemic was the result of divine anger does not prove that Homer and his audience attributed all illnesses to the gods. The assumption that Apollo, Artemis, Zeus or some other god might have sent a sickness on to a community or on individuals is one that was widely shared.[17] But there are traces of another view. The stinking and excruciatingly painful ulcer that led to the Greeks leaving Philoctetes behind on Lemnos is ascribed to an apparently natural cause, the bite of a water-snake.[18] At *Odyssey* 11, 171–3, the poet makes Odysseus juxtapose a religious and a non-religious reason when he asks his mother in the Underworld whether her death has been due to a long sickness or to being struck down by the arrows of Artemis. Hesiod in his *Works and Days* also offers alternative explanations. Misery, famine and plague may be sent from heaven by Zeus in order to punish those who act violently or cruelly, but the poet also conjures up a vivid picture of diseases roaming around the world, silently bringing mischief to mortals. Zeus might be in overall control, for he took away speech from these beings, but they move spontaneously, as and where they want.[19] There is no Greek Book of Job, pondering the causes of individual human suffering and prosperity before reaching the conclusion that the inscrutability of God's purpose in allowing these disparities is but one part of His majesty. Instead, we find a series of explanations that overlap with each other and that are chosen as appropriate to a given situation. Some involve the gods directly, others indirectly, others not at all.

The development of medicine in the ancient world has frequently been seen as the extension of the last category at the expense of the others, and there are good reasons, both ancient and modern, for adopting this interpretation. So, for example, when a comic dramatist c.420 BC displays a chorus of semi-divine heroes, 'the stewards of good and evil', threatening the unjust with a variety of diseases – coughs, bad spleen, dropsy, catarrh, scab, gout, madness, lichens, swellings and agues – we may suspect that part of the humour lay precisely in the conjunction of divine punishment for thieves and minor criminals with a sophisticated medical differentiation of types of disease.[20] But, as we shall see, this extension of the space occupied by non-theological explanation does not lead to a total exclusion of other possibilities, even among rationalist physicians, and many of the prejudices and reactions of the pre-Hippocratic Greeks continued to exert an influence on medical thinking and practice for many centuries.[21]

The Homeric poems also throw important light on the social situation of the doctor. Along with the seer, the armourer and the bard, the doctor is one of the craftsmen, 'servants of mankind at large', whose country 'knows no bounds', and who move from place to place as and when their services are required.[22] It is a way of life familiar from other documents from the contemporary Levant, particularly relating to royal households. Hittite, Babylonian and Egyptian texts show doctors moving from court to court, being summoned (or sent as part of a diplomatic exchange) to heal rulers and their relatives.[23] Against such a background, it is tempting to associate the grant of land to an *ijate* at Pylos in the Mycenean period with an attempt by a local lord to secure the residence of a healer among his dependants.[24] The career of Democedes of Croton in the sixth century can be in part interpreted in the same way, as he moved from S. Italy to Aegina, to Athens and then to the court of Polycrates of Samos in the 520s BC. He was taken as a captive to Persia on the overthrow of Polycrates, but he gained his freedom and great wealth by curing King Darius of a foot injury when his Egyptian healers had failed and, later, by treating Queen Atossa for a long and painful disease of the breast.[25] Two generations later, Apollonides of Cos became a court doctor to Artaxerxes I for thirty years, before being buried alive for having had intercourse with the queen's sister, a story told by yet another Greek doctor in Persian service, Ctesias of Cnidus.[26]

Egypt is seen as a major source of such healers.[27] Homer talks of it being the home of the 'race of Paion', where 'everyone is a healer' and 'the bountiful land produces many drugs'.[28] It is there that Helen goes to obtain from Polydamna, the wife of Thon, *nepenthes* and *acholon*, herbs to chase away the

sadness of Menelaus and Telemachus. Archaeology confirms the general existence of a traffic in medicinal substances between the Aegean and the Levant,
although beginning much earlier. Aromatic resins, opium, coriander, cyperus
and many other substances entered the Greek world from Egypt and the Near
East well before the time of the Homeric poems.[29] Many of the gynaecological
recipes in the Hippocratic Corpus contain Near Eastern ingredients, and it is
possible that we should seek a similar origin for the practice of fumigation,
applying sweet-smelling scents, in gynaecological disorders.[30] When and how
this transfer occurred is unclear in our present state of knowledge, for Greek
doctors themselves do not acknowledge any borrowing. And the traffic is
far from being one way, for there are references in Egyptian medical texts to
Cretan beans and other remedies that come from the Greek world.[31]

Whether an acquaintance with remedies also involved more than a casual
understanding of the theories behind them is a controversial question.[32]
Homer's exaggerated view of the ubiquity of Egyptian medical practitioners hardly suggests direct acquaintance, and a reminiscence of this Homeric
passage may lie in part behind Herodotus' comment that the Egyptians had
numerous doctors, each of them specialising in one sort of disease.[33] The
fourth-century writer Isocrates was doubtless not alone in tracing the origin
of medicine and pharmacology back to the Egyptians, although we may
wonder how much his rhetorical *tour de force* in praise of a long-dead Egyptian
monarch was acknowledged by his audience to have a basis in historical
fact.[34] Still more puzzling is Herodotus' claim that the Babylonians had no
doctors at all, but merely brought the sick out into the streets for them to
receive helpful advice from passers-by. If this is the testimony of an eyewitness, it would appear to involve a whole series of misunderstandings and
misapprehensions, as recent publications of cuneiform medical texts amply
demonstrate.[35] Babylonian medicine, it is clear, was still flourishing in the
fourth century in the Levant, if not for some time later.[36]

Herodotus' references to Egyptian and Babylonian medicine as somehow
distinct from the Greek form one piece of evidence in the complex debate
about their interrelationship and the ways in which a specifically 'Western'
medicine came to develop within sixth-, fifth- and fourth-century Greece. To
prove conclusively dependence or, still more, non-dependence is impossible
in the present state of our knowledge, and the arguments used on both sides
often derive their colouring from a conviction of the superiority of one civilisation over another.[37] To refuse to believe in a Nubian Hippocrates is seen as
denying all value to Egyptian medicine; to raise the possibility of Babylonian
influence on Greek medicine is considered tantamount to questioning the
existence of the Greek miracle. Merely to remark upon the difficulty of devising appropriate criteria for judging interdependence is to risk an accusation
of small-mindedness.[38]

It is, of course, likely that the Greeks took over some medical ideas and
practices from their neighbours, just as they took over some of their plants

and herbs.[39] Greek trading posts and so-called colonies were established around the Levant from the eighth century BC onwards, and scholars have pointed to influences, particularly from Babylonia, on Greek literature, art and religion in this early period.[40] There were Greeks who had visited these regions, even staying there for some time, and who were impressed enough by what they saw or heard to transmute it into a Greek form. One may not wish to place too much faith in the claim of Diodorus Siculus, writing his *Universal History* at the end of the first century BC, that the practice of incubation, a prime feature of many Greek healing cults, including that of Asclepius, originated in the cult of Isis in Egypt, but offerings made at the shrine of Hera on Samos (in the sixth century BC) do include figurines of a type associated with a Babylonian goddess of healing.[41] There are also parallels, to put it no stronger, between some Greek medical ideas and those found elsewhere in the Near East. The Egyptian belief that disease was caused by residues rotting within the body and that they required removal through purgation has its analogues in Greek medical texts, as has the emphasis in Babylonian medicine on the body's fluids (corresponding to 'humours') as a major determinant of illness.[42] Nor is it entirely fair to dismiss either type of medicine as lacking in rationality or devoted to supernatural explanations. Although both Egyptian and Babylonian doctors saw the workings of the gods in illness, the author of the Edwin Smith surgical papyrus offers his treatments without referring to the gods. Writers of cuneiform texts clearly differentiated between the two types of therapy by including on the same tablet instructions for the cure of a disease by an incantation priest or by pharmaceutical remedies and allowing for some choice between them. Even types of psychological distress could be treated in Babylonia with ordinary drugs and recipes, and eye diseases are frequently discussed in texts that contain both magical and medical remedies.[43]

But against this evidence for possible influence must be set the notorious unwillingness of the Greeks to learn other languages. Even Herodotus' account shows how even an intelligent man could be led astray by his own eyes and by his interpreters. Hence, there is no guarantee that a visit to the East would have resulted in anything but the most superficial acquaintance with non-Greek medical theory. The exchange of substances need not have involved any deep exchange of ideas beyond the most obvious instructions for use, and by the fifth century many foreign substances were so common that they had lost any links with their original Near Eastern medical context. Similarly, the two comparable doctrines are so broad that they could easily have been fashioned in more than one place, and, with one little-noticed exception, no Greek medical author either acknowledges dependence on or a possible derivation from a non-Greek source. Anonymus Londinensis cites Ninyas the Egyptian for the belief that there are two types of affection, congenital and acquired. The former are innate, the latter the result of residues and of the body's heat working on nutriment that has remained in the body without being properly absorbed.[44] This theory is certainly to be found in

Egyptian medical papyri, and one would like to know more about this mysterious Ninyas and when he lived. But it is equally significant that he is singled out as the holder of an opinion differing only in a minor detail from others held by doctors who were Greeks, and that his general approach is not recognised as being specifically Egyptian.[45] His presence in this list of medical opinions, however, does indicate a possible conduit of information, whether he wrote in Greek or was a native Egyptian whose views were transmitted through Greek intermediaries.[46]

Ninyas' theory is reported as merely one of a series of variants on the same theme. He is included among those who believe that diseases arise from the residues of nutriment (as opposed to some change in the body's elements). The list begins with Euryphon of Cnidus and Herodicus of Cnidus in the mid-fifth century BC, and includes names drawn from all over the Greek world, from S. Italy to the N. Aegean. Although it is possible, as has been suggested, that this idea of disease as the result of some form of residue came from Egypt, found a home among the doctors of Cnidus and was then transmitted around the Greek world, the geographical range of the doctors named and the variety of ideas they put forward suggest rather that this type of explanation need not have had a single point of origin.[47]

A more compelling argument for the independent development of Greek medicine is that the type of medical literature found in Greece differs considerably from that known elsewhere. While some treatises in the Hippocratic Corpus can be categorised as lists of drugs and therapies, many others are in the nature of exploratory arguments, debating with and criticising other authors. They raise theoretical as well as practical problems while seeking to establish some of the fundamentals of their art, and often range widely in their argumentation. They employ sophisticated reasoning, and, for the most part, within the sphere of medicine as they define it, there is no place for divine causation or divine cures.[48] While some of the material is clearly intended for private use, whether by an individual alone or in a small group of colleagues and pupils, other parts are equally clearly intended for a wider audience, if they are not in fact transcriptions of speeches delivered in public. This plurality of debate about first principles is not confined to the Hippocratic Corpus as we have it. The middle section of the Anonymus Londinensis papyrus takes the form of a list of the competing explanations for disease put forward in the fifth and fourth centuries BC.[49] Nor was a medical text something fixed and unalterable. One of the earliest written texts of which we have record, the so-called *Cnidian Sentences*, was already circulating in a revised form when the author of *Regimen in Acute Diseases* took issue with it in the late fifth century.[50]

It is, of course, possible that these confrontational features were also present in Babylonian or Egyptian medical texts, and that their non-appearance is simply the result of chance, for, indeed, one could produce many Greek lists of recipes and surgical techniques that resemble closely the arrangement and organisation of Near Eastern texts and that leave out any argumentative discussion of their underlying theory.[51] But the increasing number of tablets becoming available from Babylonia, and not least the very late commentary texts from Uruk, weakens this argument from silence, and nothing that we know of Egyptian medicine and Egyptian society leads us to expect the vigorous debates found in Greece. If there is influence, it is more likely to have been in specific remedies and practices than in theories, and the 'style' of Greek medicine, like that of Greek science in general, appears radically different from that known from elsewhere.[52] To say this, it should be emphasised, is not to denigrate non-Greek medicine in a priority dispute over the invention of medicine and medical thinking. In our present state of knowledge, proof of non-Greek influence is extremely difficult to find, and, if there was influence, its effects developed in a very different way from what is securely known about Babylonia or Egypt.

This competitiveness is related to a further feature of Greek medicine that marks it out from medicine in many other cultures – its openness. Although, as we shall see, there were guild-like groupings of doctors and constant attempts to define the constituents of the true art of medicine (and consequently to exclude those whose beliefs and practices did not fit this definition), the boundary between medicine and other investigations was, and remained, remarkably fluid. Medical ideas were discussed freely whether among a small group of acquaintances or in a public place, and once writing had become widespread, by 500 BC, medical books were available in towns such as Athens, Corinth or Miletus for any who wished to buy them. 'Physicians have written much', commented Xenophon somewhat snootily in the early fourth century.[53]

Important contributions to the theories and methods that should govern medical practice were not confined to those who bore the title '*iatros*', 'doctor'. Anyone who wished could join in the debate. Nor was the exchange of profitable ideas always in one direction, or to the liking of all parties. *The Art of Medicine* was written to defend medicine against those who disputed its effectiveness, while the author of *Ancient Medicine* strongly attacked those who introduced into medicine philosophical hypotheses.[54] One cannot imagine that he would have been greatly impressed by the attempt of his contemporary Metrodorus of Lampsacus, a pupil of Anaxagoras, to interpret Homer's *Iliad* as a giant physiological and cosmological allegory, in which gods and heroes represented parts of the universe or of the human body: Apollo, for instance, stood for bile; Demeter for the liver; Dionysus for the spleen.[55]

The early participants in these debates are often called the pre-Socratic philosophers, a somewhat misleading name, since many were the contemporaries of Socrates (469–399) and few were philosophers in the modern sense of the word. The earliest of them, in the sixth century, attempted to explain how the world came to be, pursuing 'an inquiry into nature'. For the historian of medicine their conclusions, which often stressed a single original substance, are less important than their method of approach and their geographical origin. Many of them were associated with the rich and, at that time independent, cities of Ionia (W. Turkey), and medical, historical and scientific texts from then on were often written in their local dialect of Greek, Ionic. Even though the inhabitants of Cos, the home of Hippocrates, used another dialect, Doric, and many of the writers in the Hippocratic Corpus appear to be associated with regions of Greece remote from Ionia, the works in the Corpus are all in Ionic.[56] In its turn, the language of the Hippocratic Corpus continued to be employed for medical writing for many centuries to come, and doctors often used the Ionic form of *iatros*, *ietros*, to describe their profession on their tombstones, even though the rest of their epitaphs were in the standard *koine*, 'common' Greek.[57]

The method of approach of these early thinkers was to look for natural explanations for phenomena; that is, explanations that did not involve the somewhat arbitrary intervention of divine powers. They were interested in causes, and in seeking to explain what they perceived around them. By using reason and argument they believed they could penetrate, like Arctinus' doctor, behind the visible to observe the invisible.[58] They assumed, also, that human beings, as part of the natural world, were made from the same material and behaved according to the same rules as everything else within it, although the parallels between the macrocosm of creation and the microcosm of mankind were not yet made fully explicit.[59]

Their desire to find a single explanatory cause for the universe was vigorously criticised by Parmenides (*c*.515–450 BC), one of a number of thinkers from the Greek-speaking areas of S. Italy and Sicily who contributed to debates across the Greek world.[60] Parmenides' vigorous logic in denying all motion and change, all coming into being and passing away in the physical world, compelled those who wished to defend empirical data either to produce a more subtle approach to monism or to argue for a plurality of eternal and immutable entities whose combinations and recombinations explained the mutability and diversity of all that could be seen around. Some of the favoured hypotheses predated Parmenides: the Pythagoreans, for example, believed that the basis of the universe was number, while the cryptic Heraclitus (fl. 500 BC), in whose system fire played the essential role, implied the permanent necessity of change. But the thinkers who followed Parmenides were more aware of the problems involved in any explanation involving change, and widened the scope of their investigations to look closely at the human body. So, for example, Melissus of Samos (fl. 450 BC) argued strongly, in part from the evidence of physiology, that everything was differentiated out of 'One-being', and that pluralistic explanations only involved additional (and unnecessary) bases of exactly the same kind as his own One-being. In so doing, he was almost certainly attacking the views of Empedocles (fl. 460 BC), who thought of the world as built up from four stable elements – earth, air, fire and water – whose potentially unstable combinations produced everything that could be perceived.[61] For Leucippus (fl. 435 BC) and Democritus (fl. 420 BC) the world was made up of atoms ('the uncuttable') and void. Anaxagoras, their slightly older contemporary, argued that the original mixture of the universe contained an immense diversity of ingredients, coming together in the form of seeds, each containing a part of everything else, and hence with the potentiality for growth and change. By the mid-fourth century the belief that disease was the result of some inadequate combination of 'elements' was extremely common, and no longer limited to philosophers. Although the list of such believers preserved in the Anonymus Londinensis papyrus begins with Plato and Philolaus of Croton, it also includes the doctors Polybus of Cos, Philistion of Locris and Petron(as) of Aegina, as well as Menecrates, a controversial and somewhat eccentric savant of the mid-fourth century, who wrote a treatise, *On Medicine*.[62]

These links between philosophy and medicine can be traced back at least to Parmenides, if not earlier to the Pythagoreans, whose ideas on appropriate living included a ban on eating beans.[63] The Pythagorean doctrine of numbers may have also contributed to the later medical doctrine of critical days, days of particular importance during the course of an illness, which were often expressed in terms of numbers from the starting point of the illness and which, at least in the higher numbers, would seem to have been based on very little clinical evidence. Parmenides himself was later honoured at his native Elea with a beautiful bust set on an inscribed base that declared him to be a 'student of nature' ('*physikos*'). It stood in a building with an unusual underground portico, and was erected to him by a medico-religious group, a *pholeon*, that traced its formation back to his lifetime. Some of its leaders bore the family name of Parmenides, Ouliades (which may be connected with the cult title of Apollo Oulios), and inscriptions on their (much later) statues also indicate that these men were also doctors. Another inscription may reveal the presence of a 'medical prophet' ('*iatroma{ntis}*'), a term otherwise first attested in the playwright Aeschylus.[64] Whether this apparent combination of philosophy, religion and medicine goes back to Parmenides himself is uncertain, but far from impossible, as our evidence for Empedocles shows.

Even if we discount as happy invention later stories of his cure of the plague at Selinus, enough remains to indicate that Empedocles was himself involved in medicine at a practical as well as theoretical level.[65] Not only did he promise in one poem to teach its addressee to 'learn all the drugs that are a defence against ills and old age', but he claimed that wherever he went he was followed by large crowds, 'some desiring oracles, while others, long pierced by grievous pain, demand to hear the word of healing for all sorts of illnesses'.[66] He was credited with a medical treatise in verse, and with another in prose, and the fragments of his surviving poetry show a deep interest in matters medical.[67] Empedocles is one of the philosophical authors attacked by the writer of *Ancient Medicine* for leading contemporary 'doctors and sophists' to believe that a sound grasp of medicine required speculative investigation into what mankind is.[68] According to one modern reconstruction of his career, he resembled a shamanistic wonder-worker far more than a frock-coated physician or a calmly contemplative philosopher, an interpretation that, even if exaggerated, challenges preconceptions as to how each of these activities might have been carried on in ancient Greece.[69] The new Strasbourg fragments also show how he managed to include within a single poem ideas that have often appeared to historians sufficiently disparate or disjointed as to warrant the editorial obelus as incomprehensible or at least a distribution between different works.[70]

Empedocles' theories covered the whole of human physiology and its changes from cradle to grave. He believed in four basic elements – earth, air, fire and water – whose different proportional relationships to each other explained the differences between substances. Blood was an almost perfect balance of the four elements, and from blood was formed flesh. Bone and sinews had different proportions, the latter being formed without any air whatsoever.[71] The eye contained all four elements, but vision depended largely on fire and water alone.[72] Digestion was, in part, a mechanical process: food was cut and ground by the teeth before passing to the stomach, where it then underwent a process of putrefaction, probably under the influence of the body's natural heat, before being sent to the liver, where it was turned into blood.[73] Heat, which Parmenides had equated with life, played a major role in Empedocles' view of the human body, being used to account for the differences between the sexes (males are hotter and better cooked than females) and to explain sleep (as a cooling process).[74] Blood was the agent of nutrition, and maternal milk was the result of the decomposition of superfluous blood. Although Aristotle later criticised him for his choice of metaphor, describing the process as one of cooking rather than putrefaction, Empedocles' basic idea that milk was formed from residual blood was widely accepted.[75] It is probable that he thought that semen was also formed in this way, although we have no clear picture of how he pictured the internal organisation of the body.[76]

In his considerable interest in and knowledge of medicine, Empedocles has a counterpart in another philosopher from among the western Greeks, Alcmaeon of Croton (S. Italy). Whether he flourished in the late sixth century BC or a generation or so later, in the second quarter of the fifth, is disputed. Tradition claimed him as a pupil of Pythagoras 'in his old age', but the textual and historical basis for this assertion is far from sound, and Alcmaeon's interests and the sophistication of some of his methods are better suited to the later date.[77] His medical interests can be best seen in his theory of health, which deserves quotation at length, even though its wording may not be entirely his own:

What preserves health is the equal distribution of its forces – moist, dry, cold, hot, bitter, sweet, etc. – and the domination of any one of them creates disease: for the dominance of any is destructive. Disease comes about on the one hand through an excess of heat or cold: on the other hand through surfeit or lack of nutriment; its location is the blood, marrow or brain. Disease may also sometimes come about from external causes, from the quality of the water, local environment, overwork, hardship or something similar. Health, by contrast, is a harmonious blending of the qualities.[78]

Here one finds the same type of explanation as given by Empedocles: health depends on a balanced mixture, but it is not a harmony based on specific proportion but on a complete blending together of all the body's forces. It is not elements but qualities or powers that need to be kept in balanced equality. Alcmaeon's scheme also allows for a greater flexibility: if once Empedocles' careful proportions are disturbed, then there is change for the worse, but Alcmaeon's 'equality' or 'fair shares' is not so strictly defined. In this programmatic statement Alcmaeon displays also a striking range of metaphors. 'Harmony' was an ideal of both Heraclitus and the mathematico-musical Pythagoreans, with whom Alcmaeon may have consorted in S. Italy, but 'equality', 'individual domination' or 'monarchy', and 'powers' or 'forces' also carry overtly political messages. 'Equality' was one of the slogans favoured by the incipient Athenian democracy, and 'monarchy' was its polar opposite. Likewise, a battle between forces within the body was a corporeal civil war, from which nothing but harm could follow.[79] The analogy between the human body and the body politic, as we shall see, was continued by many thinkers, and the notion of health as a harmonious, balanced mixture of opposites grew to dominate medicine well into the nineteenth century, if not down to the present day.

Alcmaeon's medical interests extended further into embryology and sex differentiation, and into a practical investigation of sensation. He concluded that the sense organs were linked directly to the brain by channels, and that loss of sensation could be the result of these channels becoming blocked, an insight that has drawn the approval of many historians, although they would not accept his further contention that the blockage was most often caused by the brain itself shifting its position.[80] He claimed empirical proof for his notion of channels, pointing to the void within (or behind) the ears, the nasal channels and the pores in the tongue, but saying nothing about touch. Although in this fragment he does not explain how the sensation of sight is transmitted to the brain, talking instead about the fiery, gleaming and transparent elements that are contained within the eye, his information on sight almost certainly derived from his knowledge of the optic nerve, for, according to the fourth-century AD commentator on Plato, Chalcidius, 'he was the first to dare to essay the excision of the eye'.[81] What is meant by this is not at all clear. It is unlikely that Alcmaeon dissected in any modern sense of the word, and it is doubtful on what grounds Chalcidius believed him to be the first to carry out a surgical excision of a damaged eyeball, if that is what he alluded to. It remains possible that he removed the eye of a slaughtered animal, although butchers will have preceded him in this, but Chalcidius may simply be reading back into Alcmaeon's mention of the conduit that we know of as the optic nerve his own understanding of a much later anatomical procedure.

Two other philosophers with medical interests flourished in the last third of the fifth century BC. Diogenes of Apollonia wrote on many similar topics to Alcmaeon, and seems to have been regarded by Galen as a doctor as well as a philosopher.[82] He believed that everything was in some way derived from air, including thought and sensation. Aristotle preserves a long report of his description of the blood vessels, along with that of the otherwise unknown Syennesis of Cyprus, the earliest such descriptions to survive in Greek.[83] Both are schematic, based almost entirely on what could be deduced from surface anatomy, and possibly from observing sacrificial victims, and are as much intended to support a thesis as to offer an accurately detailed description.[84] Diogenes' system consisted of two large parallel ducts, each serving one side of the body and linking with the testicles (or uterus). Surplus nutriment, i.e. blood, also passed from the spinal marrow to the spermatic vessels, where it became foamlike, probably through an admixture of air.[85] A believer in the idea of innate heat, Diogenes may also have seen semen as the vehicle of the soul. His long description of the vessels was superseded by that of Aristotle and the Alexandrian anatomists, but his hypothesis of a link between the spinal marrow and the testicles continued to be influential for centuries to come, for it suggested, if not guaranteed, a connection between the brain, the soul and the embryo. Leonardo da Vinci's famous drawing of coition still includes this hypothetical channel in the early sixteenth century.[86]

The second medical philosopher of the later fifth century, Democritus of Abdera, had an even more considerable and longer-lasting influence on medicine than Diogenes. An Alexandrian catalogue of his writings includes works on prognosis and on dietetics, and in one intriguingly called *Medical Opinions*, either the opinions were his own or those of others which he collected or criticised. He had medical followers well down into the period of the Roman Empire. Philo of Hyampolis, who is found in the first century AD discussing medical topics at Plutarch's table, is described as a Democritean.[87] Fifty years or so later, the sophist Timocrates of Pontus is said to have devoted himself to the study of medicine and to have become fluent in the theories of Hippocrates and Democritus.[88] A short summary of rules for foretelling impending death, the *Prognostics of Democritus*, circulated widely in Latin manuscripts of the Early Middle Ages, giving him authority as a seer as well as a doctor.[89] He gained an enduring reputation for anatomical studies from the famous (and apocryphal) story that when Hippocrates was summoned by the Abderitans to cure Democritus of his supposed madness, he found him surrounded by the bodies of animals he had just dissected in an attempt to discover the nature and seat of bile, the cause of madness.[90] Not only did Robert Burton publish his *Anatomy of Melancholy* in 1621 under the pseudonym of Democritus Junior, but one of the most important of early

49

modern studies of comparative anatomy, Marco Aurelio Severino's *Zootomia Democritea*, of 1645, expressly appeals to his example. The book's elaborate frontispiece depicts Democritus at work, writing up the results of his animal dissections.[91] The story is not without some basis in the surviving fragments of his writings. That Democritus had an interest in animal anatomy – although this need not have involved actual dissection – is evident from a report that he believed that animals could produce many young at once because they had multipartite wombs, a theory that was later applied to the formation of human twins by a Hippocratic author.[92] Elsewhere he argued vigorously for a sound lifestyle, with prevention rather than cure, as the basis for a healthy life, complaining that it was the soul that ruined the body by its desire for pleasures and wine.[93] Many of his other theories continued earlier debates. Like Alcmaeon, Democritus wrote about vision, dreams and sensation, and, although firmly believing in a world whose ultimate constituents were atoms and void, he attached great importance to *pneuma* (or air) as the vehicle of life, transmitted in semen. Seed was drawn from all parts of the bodies of both parents, not the male alone, to produce the embryo, whose sex was determined by whichever seed proved most powerful.

The significance of these debates among philosophers for the history of medicine is considerable. As we shall see in the next chapter, their ideas contributed to discussions among medical writers, whether about specifically medical themes, such as embryology, or more widely through the methods of argument they sought to employ. They were interested in change, and the causes of change; Leucippus, the teacher of Democritus, proclaimed that nothing was produced in an absurd manner, but everything came into being according to reason and necessity, with the implication that it was the philosopher's duty to investigate both these aspects.[94] Their use of argument and controversy was mirrored also in vocabulary and style. The language of Democritus has been discerned in more than one Hippocratic treatise, and the pregnant brevity of the *Aphorisms* and the less familiar *Dentition* and *Coan Prognoses* has a parallel in the oracular sayings of Heraclitus.[95] Other, less overtly philosophical influences were also at work. At least one Hippocratic treatise, *Breaths*, shows traces of the style of one of the so-called sophists, Gorgias (c.480–380), whose claims for the merits of his rhetorical education were derided by the philosopher Plato.[96] Nor should it be assumed that the flow was always in one direction, from the philosophers to the doctors, or that those who contemplated the problems of sickness and health in the body were never able to articulate them without philosophical assistance, and gave nothing in return. The author of *Ancient Medicine* vigorously rejects the dependence of doctors on natural philosophy, arguing that clear knowledge of the natural world can be gained only from medicine.[97] Many of the difficulties encountered in creating a cosmology or an anthropology on a large scale were shared by those attempting to understand the little world of the body. As we have seen, it is difficult to disentangle the medical from the non-medical concerns of more than one pre-Socratic philosopher, and even harder to decide which came first.

Medical ideas and medical vocabulary were not confined to doctors. The historian Herodotus' ways of thinking about historical processes and about the various nations with whom the Greeks came into contact have strong parallels within the Hippocratic Corpus.[98] Thucydides' description of the plague of 430 BC, even if not perhaps written in the form we have it until twenty or more years later, shows a considerable command of medical technicalities, and his wider approach to historical causation displays an acquaintance with the theories of contemporary medicine.[99] The follies and incapacities of healers became a common element of comedy; in the fourth century several plays were constructed entirely around this theme.[100] The tragedians put a variety of pathological cases on the stage, ranging from the blindness of Oedipus to the madness of Ajax and Agave, often using specifically technical medical language.[101] Euripides' Medea was called 'large-spleened', a word whose meaning had become obscure even by the time of Galen, who interpreted it to indicate the violence of her character.[102] The shared universe of medical ideas between tragedy and medicine was noted already in Antiquity. Clement of Alexandria, in the second century AD, drew attention to the similarity between the aims of *Airs, Waters and Places* and three lines of Euripides: whoever wishes to practise medicine properly, when they study disease, should look at the lifestyles of those who live in a city and also at its land.[103]

But the words and explanations of the dramatists did not always coincide with those in the Hippocratic Corpus. This is hardly surprising, since they were less interested in the phenomenon of sickness per se than in an analysis of its psychological, moral and philosophical role in human life. So, for example, Sophocles' tragedy *Philoctetes*, produced in 408 BC, sets out a harrowingly detailed description of illness. Philoctetes himself explains his festering leg as the result of a snakebite, as in Homer.[104] Only later is it revealed to him that his misfortune was part of some 'divine chance', the result of his inadvertent violation of a sanctuary and, we know as the audience, part of the gods' plan to keep him away from Troy.[105] He relies on a herb to keep the wound quiet until it is finally cured, as he hopes it will be.[106] But towards the end of the play it becomes clear that human intervention will not be enough. Even then, Philoctetes rejects Neoptolemus' assurance that he will be healed by the sons of Asclepius, Podalirius and Machaon, if and when he comes to Troy with the bow that will allow the Greeks finally to capture the city. He relents only when the god Hercules, himself both warrior and healer, reveals that he himself will send Asclepius from heaven to perform the cure.[107] It is tempting to associate this transition from a disease thought to have a purely natural cause to a divine healing at the hands of the god Asclepius with Sophocles' own personal beliefs, for tradition claims that he was involved in the cult of Asclepius at Athens, even at one point keeping the sacred snake in his own house.[108] But equally significant is the space initially devoted to a natural explanation: only when it is made clear that it cannot account for all that is taking place do we move away from human to divine healing.

That here and in his portrayal of the plague in his *Oedipus the King* Sophocles favoured religious over natural explanations, or that the historian Herodotus ascribed the impotence of the Scythians to a curse from the goddess Aphrodite, when the author of *Airs, Waters and Places* blamed it on the consequences of long riding in the saddle, is perhaps less important than their shared interest in understanding the phenomena.[109] Like the arguments among the philosophers, they reveal a variety of approaches, co-existing, competing and countering one another. Medicine is part of an ongoing debate involving doctors and non-doctors from all over the Greek world, from Sicily and S. Italy to the shores of the Levant. It is no surprise to find the views of Phasitas of Tenedus, an island in the N. Aegean, cited alongside those of Timotheus of Metapontum in S. Italy, Aegimius of Elis in S.W. Greece and Thrasymachus of Sardis (now in W. Turkey and possibly at the time of writing a part of the Persian Empire). The same author saw nothing odd in giving more space to Plato's opinions on the causes of disease than to those of any other author, medical or non-medical.[110] Even had we not the Hippocratic Corpus, it would have been easy to conclude that in fifth-century Greece medicine was a vigorous topic of public debate, controversial, challenging and multiform.

4

HIPPOCRATES, THE HIPPOCRATIC CORPUS AND THE DEFINING OF MEDICINE

Except for the Bible, no document and no author from Antiquity commands the authority in the twenty-first century of Hippocrates of Cos and the Hippocratic *Oath*.[1] They are regularly cited in both learned journals and the popular press as the standard of ethical conduct to which all practising physicians should adhere. In medical schools around the world students give assent to principles and words they believe go back to the Father of Medicine, and in the eyes of their prospective patients failure to live up to his prescriptions for competence and morality is the greatest of all medical sins. Revised, bowdlerised, set to music and made into a CD-Rom, updated or denounced, the *Oath* has made Hippocrates a familiar name even today, appealed to as the creator of the modern medical profession.[2] It may then come as a shock to learn that almost nothing is known of Hippocrates himself, that he is unlikely personally to have devised the *Oath*, and that several passages in the Hippocratic Corpus describe practices that would have involved a doctor breaking it, even assuming that he ever had sworn to it, which is itself unlikely.[3]

This discrepancy between what is generally believed about Hippocrates and what he may, in reality, have said or done is the result of three converging tendencies. The first is the understandable wish of Greeks and Romans to know more about the great figures from the past; the second, the gradual accretion, whether deliberate or accidental, of anonymous or suppositious treatises around more genuine writings; the third, the growth of a Hippocratic tradition of interpretation that emphasised the value of certain treatises above others and the consequent belief that these in particular came from the pen of the master. Together they allowed free rein to the imagination of those who wished to reconstruct the life of Hippocrates on the basis of information contained in texts in the Hippocratic Corpus.[4]

The Greek habit of composing imaginary speeches or letters by famous persons from the past as school exercises and public display pieces gradually blurred the distinction between the genuine and the false. A group of letters and speeches that on grounds of style, content and historical detail must have been composed at the earliest around 350 BC, and some perhaps over a century later, helped to fill out the otherwise brief data on Hippocrates' life.[5] They depict him as a wise sage, called in to cure Democritus of madness – and then refraining from intervention because he found him sane; a patriot who refused to take Persian gold to serve their king, the enemy of Greece; and a wonderfully versatile doctor, capable of treating both a monarch's lovesickness and the great plague of Athens (which Thucydides had deemed incurable). These stories in turn became part of the picture of the historical Hippocrates, so that, for instance, they played the dominant role in shaping Galen's understanding of the behaviour of the ideal physician and figured prominently in the only surviving substantial biography of Hippocrates from Antiquity, that written by Soranus around AD 100.[6] Other stories grew up around him, numerous busts were made of him, and Cos in the Roman imperial period even had coins struck bearing his image.[7]

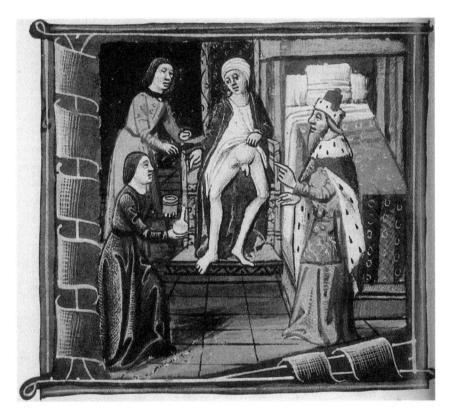

Figure 4.1 Hippocrates curing the plague of Athens. The mediaeval illustrator of the *Epidemics* imagines Hippocrates lancing an inguinal bubo as if he were dealing with bubonic plague. Dresden, Sächsische Landesbibliothek, Db 93, fol. 458r.

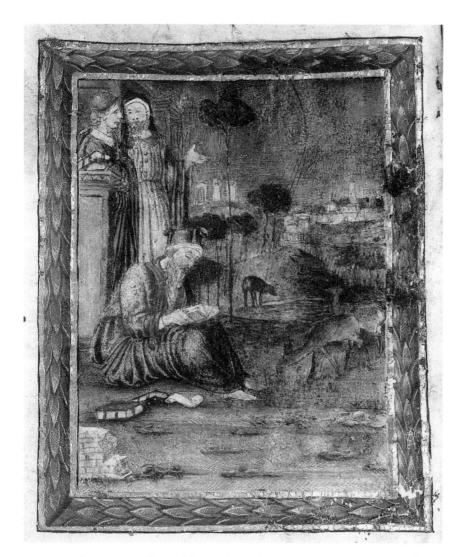

Figure 4.2 Hippocrates reading, while two bystanders argue. Opening illustration from a
   late fifteenth-century manuscript of the *Aphorisms* in Latin translation. London,
   Wellcome Ms. 353, fol. 3r. Courtesy of Wellcome Library, London.

In order to penetrate behind the legend, historians have usually adopted
the principle of giving greater weight to those testimonies that go back to
the lifetime of Hippocrates. So, for instance, the Athenian philosopher Plato,
writing his dialogue *Protagoras* in the early years of the fourth century but setting it fifty years earlier, around 430 BC, confirms that Hippocrates came from
Cos and that he already enjoyed a great reputation for medicine, comparable

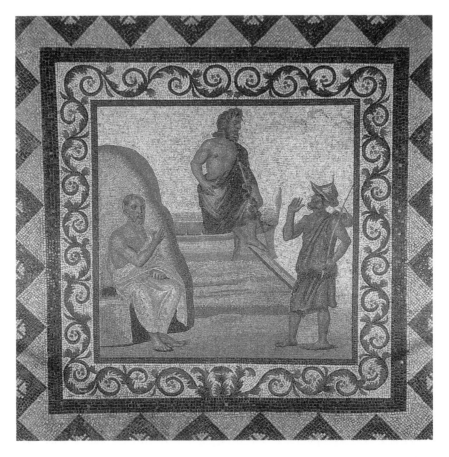

Figure 4.3 Hippocrates' dream. A mosaic from Cos showing Hippocrates seated, while a fisherman greets Asclepius as he disembarks. Second or third century AD.

to that of Polyclitus and Phidias in sculpture. His paradigmatic status is also shown by Aristotle's somewhat later use of his name in his *Politics* to show the need for precision in the definition of terms: Hippocrates is 'biggest' with regard to medicine but not to height. Plato, in the same passage in the *Protagoras*, also indicates that Hippocrates was an Asclepiad, a member of a family that claimed descent from Asclepius, and that he was teaching medicine for money. Far from restricting his medical knowledge to a family group, as suggested in the *Oath*, Hippocrates is portrayed as willing to accept anyone who wished to pay him to be taught medicine.[8]

What he taught them, however, is far more difficult to determine. In a passage in the *Phaedrus*, written at some point after the *Protagoras*, Plato again uses Hippocrates as an example to elucidate his concerns about a slightly different topic, rhetoric. Socrates, Plato's chief interlocutor, first announces that rhetoric and medicine share the same procedure; they both have to employ a logical method of division of the nature of their subject, medicine dealing with the body, rhetoric with the soul. When Phaedrus gives only lukewarm assent to this formulation, Socrates repeats his question in a different way: 'Then can you understand the nature of the soul intelligently without the nature of the whole?'[9] Phaedrus' response is a somewhat ironic assent: 'At any rate, if we're to believe Hippocrates, one can't even learn about the body without this method.' Agreement established, Socrates then demands more than the authority of Hippocrates; he demands 'true reason' as well. Only then does he go on to define the true (and ostensibly Hippocratic) method, which consists in determining whether the object is a single thing or multiplex, and, if the latter, dividing it up into its constituent parts and determining the relationship and interactions between them.

What Plato meant by this has been the subject of vigorous debate ever since the time of Galen, if not earlier.[10] He is not quoting Hippocrates directly, although Phaedrus' words certainly imply that Hippocrates spoke in general about the need to understand the nature of 'the whole', but he is using this famous figure of his own day to exemplify proper procedure in a discipline, medicine, parallel to that which he himself wishes to investigate.[11] The success of Hippocrates in medicine shows the validity of this method in practice: it is more than mere words. Nonetheless, Plato is here interpreting a Hippocratic statement for his own purpose, and, given Plato's formulations of the views of historical figures elsewhere in his dialogues, there is no guarantee that his interpretation agreed with what Hippocrates himself intended. For Plato, the crucial point is that Hippocrates employed a similar logical method in dealing with the body to that of the ideal rhetorician in dealing with the soul, and 'the whole' must be taken in the sense of the whole of the object under discussion.[12] Since Plato's focus of attention is on correct procedure, it is impossible to decide whether in considering 'the whole' and the interrelationship and interaction of its parts Hippocrates believed that illness in one part of the body could only be explained by looking at the body as a whole, its nutriment and its activities, or that the human body could be properly understood only in the wider context of 'the whole of nature'.[13] Both these (and other congruent) doctrines can be found in the Hippocratic Corpus, but to claim that one or other of them is mentioned here approvingly by Plato, or that this can then be used to identify a genuine treatise by Hippocrates, is to go beyond the evidence.[14] All that Plato is doing is to stress the accurate method employed by Hippocrates, and to insist that it requires supplementation from 'true reason' if it is to be more than highly effective empiricism.

This mention of Hippocrates in the *Phaedrus*, although disappointing in what it reveals about Hippocrates' ideas, is still valuable for the importance it assigns to him as the representative of medicine, even in his own lifetime.[15] More questionable is the report by Galen in his commentary on *Joints* that a younger contemporary, the doctor–historian Ctesias of Cnidus, took issue with Hippocrates for claiming that he could successfully reset a dislocated thigh, a statement that, if true, would imply that the text *Joints* and probably the closely related *Fractures* also were indeed written by him.[16] But Galen may be merely interpreting a comment by Ctesias, that a reset thighbone quickly dislocated again, in the light of his own belief in the Hippocratic authorship of *Joints*, and turning a general observation into a specific polemic against a particular text.[17]

The final pre-Alexandrian testimony to the beliefs of Hippocrates is both the longest and the most controversial, as it was already in Antiquity. The writer of the Anonymus Londinensis papyrus places the views of Hippocrates third in a list of those who believe that diseases arise from pathological residues of nutriment.

> Either because of the quantity of things taken or through their diversity, or because the things taken are strong and difficult of digestion, residues come to be produced. ... When the things that have been taken in are too many, the heat that produces digestion is overpowered by the multitude of foods and does not effect digestion; because digestion is hindered, residues are produced. When the things taken in are diverse, they quarrel with one another in the belly, and because of the quarrelling there is a change into residues. When they are very coarse and hard to digest, there is thus some impediment to digestion because they are hard to assimilate, and thus a change to residues occurs. From these residues arise breaths; when they move upwards, they bring on disease. This is what Hippocrates said, influenced by the following conviction.[18] Breath is the most necessary and the most important component in us, since health is the result of its free, and disease the result of its impeded, passage. We are like plants: just as they are rooted in the ground, so we are rooted in the air by our nostrils and by our whole body. We are like the (water-) plants called soldiers. Just as they, rooted in moisture, are carried now to this moisture and now to that, even so, we, being like plants, are rooted in air, and are in motion, changing position now here, now there. If this is so, it is clear that air is the most important component. On this theory, when residues are produced, they give rise to breaths, which rising as vapour cause diseases. The variations in the breaths cause the various diseases. If they are many (or violent), they produce diseases; if they are very few, they also produce diseases. Diseases are also produced by the changes in the breaths, in two ways, to excessive heat or excessive cold. Whichever way the change takes place produces (different) diseases.[19]

This is striking testimony from an apparently good, scholarly source that was both concerned to investigate the documentary evidence from the past and in a chronological position to be able to talk to those who had heard the great doctor themselves. Although the evidence is not as clear as one might want, there is general agreement that these sections go back to Aristotle and his pupil Meno, who compiled a list of the opinions of earlier physicians.[20] For this reason alone it carries considerable authority. But it presents a whole series of problems, and did so even as it was being copied out by Anonymus himself. A learned and intelligent doctor, Anonymus objected strongly to this characterisation of Hippocrates, interrupting the list of opinions with his own refutation of Aristotle's argument. He appended a series of quotations – the first, in a badly damaged portion of the papyrus, probably from *Diseases* 1, the second from *The Nature of Man* – to show that Aristotle should have placed Hippocrates in the opposite camp, among those who believed that disease was the result of imbalance.[21] Anonymus' response is in itself interesting, for while *The Nature of Man* held centre stage in the Hippocratic tradition represented by Galen, and was subsequently accepted as supremely authoritative, *Diseases* was certainly not among the treatises generally considered to have derived directly from Hippocrates and his closest followers. Indeed, it is never cited in any of the genuine writings of Galen.[22]

The fact that Aristotle's view so blatantly goes against later Galenic Hippocratism may be regarded as a strong argument in favour of it representing what the historical Hippocrates actually believed. A later observation by Galen confirms that Anonymus had not at this point misunderstood his source. Galen noted that although Meno, Aristotle's pupil, had listed several authors who believed that blood was the sole element in the body, he had included none who considered bile, phlegm and black bile as elements. The consequences of this omission for his own view of Hippocrates as the proponent of the theory of the four elemental humours Galen did not bother to pursue, brushing the anomaly aside with the truism that, of course, Meno could not put down theories that were either 'totally forgotten or inaccessible' to him.[23]

But those who wish to accept Aristotle's account face a major difficulty: nothing in what he says fits neatly in every particular with any surviving work in the Hippocratic Corpus. True, there are passages in *Regimen*, *Aphorisms* and particularly *Breaths* that come close to the ideas, and occasionally the wording, of this passage, but one must then also assume a substantial reworking by the doxographer in order to produce a succinct entry.[24] But even though he summarised the medical information in Plato's *Timaeus* in this way, it is very hard to believe that the vivid description of mankind as rooted in air, carried hither and thither like a water plant, is entirely his own or is derived from snippets of ideas found elsewhere in Plato or Aristotle.[25] It suggests that this entry is a composite, not corresponding to any single treatise, and including a section taken from a work that is now lost.[26]

But if, like the Platonic passage, this report proves largely unhelpful in deciding which, if any, of the treatises in the Hippocratic Corpus were the work of Hippocrates himself, it remains extremely valuable for two reasons: it confirms the importance of the man and his work within his own time, and, moreover, suggests that the so-called Hippocratic tradition, based on the theory of the four humours, was not one in which Hippocrates himself in fact believed. This theory Aristotle, quoting from *The Nature of Man*, ascribed to Polybus, who was believed to have been Hippocrates' pupil and son-in-law, and it is this relationship which may in turn have helped to associate the theory with the master himself.[27]

The Hippocratic Corpus as we have it is made up of sixty or so works written in the Ionic dialect of Greek.[28] The collection, in the form in which we have it today, goes back only to 1526, when the Aldine press in Venice printed the first edition of the complete works of Hippocrates in Greek, for no single ancient manuscript surviving today contains every tract from the collection, and many have only a small selection.[29] But it is also clear from the manuscripts themselves and from the work of ancient commentators and compilers of Hippocratic dictionaries that the great majority of the texts printed in 1526 were already circulating together under the name of Hippocrates by the first century AD, if not 300 years earlier.[30] Nonetheless, anomalies remain. One text, the so-called *Testament* of Hippocrates, is found in many Greek manuscripts and in a variety of translations, but was never included in the printed editions of the Corpus. By contrast, *Sevens*, which was regarded as Hippocratic in Antiquity, was effectively lost until 1837 and today appears within the Corpus mainly in the form of a Late-Antique Latin translation. A third treatise, *On Wounds*, was commented on by Galen and quoted later by Oribasius, but survives today only in the form of scattered fragments.[31]

The total number of treatises in the Corpus is also uncertain, for some were already wrongly combined or separated in Antiquity. Most scholars, for example, are agreed that *Generation* and *The Nature of the Child* once formed part of the same work, and, equally, that the seven books of the *Epidemics* were written at three different dates (books 1 and 3 around 410 BC; books 2, 4 and 6 around 400 BC; and books 5 and 7 between 358 and 348 BC) and, probably, by several different authors.[32] Some groups of books may have been written by the same author, such as *Airs, Waters and Places* and *The Sacred Disease*. Others were put together from the same material: a block of case reports in *Epidemics* 5 repeats almost verbatim cases in *Epidemics* 7, although neither version appears to preserve exactly the wording of the initial reports.[33] Elsewhere, separate chronological layers have been discerned within the same tract.[34]

Dating individual treatises is not easy.[35] There are a few sparse references to events whose dates are known from other sources, but usually a decision has to be made on grounds of the style of the language (just as a modern writer today uses words and sentences in a way that differs from that of the 1920s or 1970s); on (occasional) internal relationships, where passage X is copied from Y (thus for example *Aphorisms* is placed in the first half of the fourth century BC, since it contains traces of earlier writings); and on scholars' 'feel' for where a treatise might fit in relation to particular developments. This is far from infallible.[36] Nonetheless, it is very likely that the great majority of the treatises come from the period 420–350 BC, roughly corresponding to the active lifetime of Hippocrates. Others, such as *The Heart* and *Precepts*, are to be placed in the third or second centuries BC; *Decorum* has been given an even later date, the first or second century AD.

Where and when the bulk of the collection was assembled can only be conjectured. The tradition that Hippocrates gained his medical information from writings within the temple of Asclepius at Cos is demonstrably false; even more fanciful is the legend that, having done so, he burned the rest of the library to preserve his superiority.[37] One author in the time of Galen believed that at least part of the collection was written down by Hippocrates to preserve the oral doctrines of the family of Asclepiads that were in danger of disappearing because they were handed down only by word of mouth.[38] Cos figures scarcely at all in the Corpus, neighbouring Cnidus somewhat more, and various towns in north and central Greece still more prominently, which raises doubts about an origin on Cos itself.[39] Nonetheless, it remains likely that the collection was first assembled in broadly the form we have it at Alexandria in Egypt in the famous library of the Ptolemies, at a time when Cos was part of their empire. Certainly some texts were being studied there from around the 270s onwards by Herophilus, who may have had connections with Cos through Praxagoras. The discussions of writers of medical glossaries such as Bacchius and Zeuxis starting about 250 BC show that a Corpus had already been formed by then, although it may not have coincided entirely with what we know today.[40] The somewhat haphazard way in which materials were brought together and stored at the Alexandrian library would also explain, at least in part, the varied nature of the collection. Medical volumes crammed together on the library shelf could easily be attributed to a single author, particularly if more than one work was included on the same book-roll and if there was little or no indication of the original author's name.[41] The presence of even later Greek texts within the Corpus shows that the process of accretion lasted for centuries. A comparison between our Hippocratic Corpus and other works attributed to Hippocrates and surviving in Greek, Latin or Arabic shows that the name of Hippocrates continued to attract to itself a mass of spurious and pseudonymous material, often with next to nothing to do with what survives from the fifth and fourth centuries BC.[42] The ascription to Hippocrates, where it was made deliberately and not by an accidental confusion, was used in these works to give authority to their contents, and to suggest that their message went back to the very earliest days of medicine.[43]

Establishing which, if any, of the surviving Greek texts was actually the work of Hippocrates himself is, as has already been suggested, a difficult, if not an impossible, task, and scholars continue to disagree, as they have done since Antiquity. Aristotle's opinion differs from that of Anonymus Londinensis himself, and the selection of treatises used by the earliest writers of medical glossaries is slightly different again. What until the mid-nineteenth century were viewed as 'the genuine writings of Hippocrates' were defined as such by Galen in the second century AD on the basis of the tradition as he knew it and his own sophisticated investigations into language, style and content.[44] He based his argument principally on the authenticity of most of *The Nature of Man* and claimed to identify different grades of genuine material, from those penned by Hippocrates, through collaborative works and books by his pupils, to those that were merely in the Hippocratic spirit. But for all Galen's diligence and learning this was an ultimately circular procedure; Aristotle had already denied the reliability of its starting point.[45]

While one may lament the absence of agreement on the works composed by the great physician himself, this has paradoxically opened up the Hippocratic Corpus to scrutiny. Instead of concentrating on a small group of 'genuine' writings, scholars are now free to consider the Corpus in all its diversity of forms, doctrines and, indeed, purposes.[46] Some texts, notably *Aphorisms*, *Coan Prognoses* and *Dentition*, are little more than a series of easily memorable sentences, perhaps for use in teaching; others, such as *Breaths* or *The Art*, are public orations defending a particular medical point of view; still others, especially *Humours*, have attracted a charge of deliberate obscurity.[47] Some, such as *The Sacred Disease*, propound a definite thesis; some, such as *Diseases*, merely list a variety of ailments. *Affections* is written for the layman, *The Use of Liquids* for the practitioner with his own surgery. Some, particularly *Breaths*, are written in elegant prose; others, most notably the *Epidemics*, represent case notes at various stages of creation and selection.[48] No generalisation can cover all the texts, and no summary can do more than hint at the multiplicity of (often conflicting) theories they contain.[49] Together they show the gradual creation of a form of medicine that came to dominate Western medical thought and practice for centuries to come, as a source of theories, therapies and ideas on the way in which medicine should be taught, studied and put into practice.

That there were doctors who lived before Hippocrates is clear from the Homeric poems, and it is also beyond doubt that some of them were wealthy and enjoyed a certain prestige. One has only to glance at the beautiful statue of Sombrotidas, son of Mandrocles, from Megara Hyblaea in Sicily in the early sixth century BC or the equally fine relief of an unnamed doctor, now in Basle, some fifty years later to see that these were men of wealth and standing in their communities.[50] Equally, the evidence of archaic literature and art shows how doctors were expected to act and what methods they were expected to use.[51] They are shown touching the patient or bandaging, while the Basle relief (see p. 94) depicts cupping glasses for bleeding the patient.[52] Cutting and burning, procedures universally acknowledged to be painful, are the two techniques associated with doctors by authors as different as the philosopher Heraclitus and the playwright Aeschylus, and Plato adds to them incantations and drugs.[53] That on the whole doctors were appreciated for their services is also evident from the literary texts, even had we not the career of Democedes as a paradigm. Before he became the personal physician to Polycrates of Samos, he had been employed as a public physician – that is, a doctor in receipt of some public funds – by the island of Aegina and by the city of Athens, and, after his escape from Persia, he returned home to Croton, where, rich and respected, he married the daughter of the famous athlete, Milo. A later civil war saw him again in mainland Greece, in exile at Plataea with other defeated aristocrats.[54] But before the Hippocratic Corpus we have no surviving testimony from the doctors themselves as to how they saw their profession, and only then can we begin to place the *iatros* within the wider context of others offering health advice and healing.

From this abundant evidence it is obvious that in the late fifth century BC there was considerable debate and discussion about what constituted medicine and that the authority of the *iatros* was far from universally accepted. The author of *The Art* has to defend medicine against those who 'have made an art out of criticising the arts' and who denied the validity of medicine because some people recover without the aid of physicians while others die despite all their efforts. His argument is thus aimed at demonstrating that medicine is more effective than merely trusting to nature or to chance.[55] A similar approach can be found in *Ancient Medicine*, whose author, while accepting that if the art of medicine did not exist the treatment of the sick would be left to chance, demonstrates the absurdity of relying only on chance by pointing to the discoveries of medicine made through carefully conducted enquiry. In his view the art of medicine lies in an understanding of causes and in an ability to discriminate between what is significant and what is not.[56] What the *iatros* offers the patient is a deeper concern for causes, for the way things are linked together. Once these are understood, asserts the author of *Breaths*, one can administer whatever the body needs for recovery, a sentiment widely shared by other writers in the Corpus.[57] It is a claim that takes the notion of true healing beyond the mere application of remedies to the possession of an appropriate epistemology of health and disease. It takes for granted the possibility of a successful cure, and places the distinction between the good and bad practitioner in the understanding of the reasons behind the disease and its cure. An investigation into the causes of illness leads simultaneously to knowledge of the treatment. The more one knows what is causing illness, the more easily one can take steps to ensure recovery, prevent any further deterioration or, if the cause is such that there seems little hope of life, prepare the patient and the family for death.[58] Conversely, so it is claimed, knowing why a particular treatment works will assist the doctor in the future in his choice of an appropriate therapy, and, equally important, allows the patient to take responsibility for his or her own body, now viewed in a new way.

This argument, however, goes only part of the way to defining what medicine is about. While asserting its superiority over mere chance or to empiricism, it does not mark it off so clearly from the healing provided by those who might believe in causation but who employ non-Hippocratic methods of treatment, or whose understanding of causes is only partial or is antithetical to that of the Hippocratic doctor.[59] Some of the most famous tracts in the Corpus address themselves directly to this problem, while others discuss it implicitly or in a passing comment. *Ancient Medicine* takes the philosophers as its target, denouncing them in general, and Empedocles by name, for believing in ungrounded or foolish hypotheses.[60] Its author rejects all unitary theories of the body, for a unity could hardly feel pain or change from health to illness and vice versa, while he attacks theories of elements and opposites for their lack of an empirical basis. Far from deriving medical theories from wider notions about the nature of the cosmos, he believes that understanding the body through medicine provides the best way of understanding the world of nature.[61] Nature and the body are indeed linked, but his process of investigation is the reverse of that of the philosophers. He sees the body as a battleground for a multitude of hostile forces, sweet, sour, acrid and the like, which are most evident in foodstuffs and which he believes he can demonstrate to be at work within the body.[62] He accepts that in its early days medicine may have had a basis in simple experience (when one was ill one took whatever foods were thought to make one better), and that it was little different from cookery, but gradually, over a long period, doctors began to investigate just what it was that made one treatment superior to another, thus carrying out a form of research. The results of these investigations may not be entirely accurate and precise, but that is no reason to reject medicine as such.[63] One has only to compare its results, obtained by a sound method, with those produced in a different way to see that the doctor is aiming in the right direction. Acting on the principle that a certain eventuality is likely to happen 'for the most part' is better than inaction, and one can always make allowances for the lack of total certainty by leaving a wide safety margin in therapy.[64]

Similar claims are made elsewhere by authors who are seeking to distinguish their type of dietetics from those of earlier practitioners and of the gymnastic trainers. Physical exercise and proper diet had become fashionable in the middle years of the fifth century BC, when a science of gymnastics had been introduced by Herodicus of Selymbria. The author of *Ancient Medicine* sees this development as something positive, as a move towards a more widespread understanding of health and illness in proper medical terms, but he believes that Herodicus and his followers did not go far enough in their understanding of the effects of their training and diet.[65] Other writers in the Corpus were less charitable: the 'unnatural' lifestyle of athletes was remarked upon critically in *The Nature of Man* and *Nutriment*; at *Aphorisms* 1, 3, the word 'perilous' is used to describe it four times in only a few sentences.[66] Galen, much later, also enjoyed quoting the playwright Euripides, who denounced the follies of excessive training.[67] Aristotle shared some of this disdain, wondering whether the attainment of perfect health and fitness in the manner of Herodicus could really be called healthy living if it required so much abstention from all, or nearly all, the things that made human life enjoyable – a criticism that could equally be made of the precise regulations for health laid down by the medical author of *Regimen*.[68]

An even more vigorous attack is mounted by the author of *The Sacred Disease* against those who believed that epilepsy, mania and a range of other diseases were caused by the gods and thus needed to be treated by religious means.[69] He denounces those who use incantantions, prayers, chants and charms to communicate with the gods, 'magi, purifiers, wandering priests and charlatans' with their claims to piety and special knowledge. In many of their procedures they come close to what the doctor does: they prescribe special diets and bathing, and, of course, says the writer, if the patient recovers, that is due to the foods they have been given, not to any supernatural intervention.[70] Some of them resemble doctors in their mode of life, wandering the roads of Greece, seeking out patients, just like the doctor to whom *Airs, Waters and Places* is addressed, and they too attend to the patient's signs and symptoms, although they then interpret them differently. A madman foaming at the mouth has been made ill by Ares, god of war; nightmares are the result of the intervention of Hecate or Heroes; making shrill strident neighing noises shows the influence of Poseidon.[71]

This attack by the author of *The Sacred Disease* is threefold. He can accept the reality of some of his opponents' cures, while at the same time denying the causal connection that they have asserted: a patient has been cured by the drugs or diet they prescribed, not by the will of the gods. Incantations do not add to the effectiveness of the drugs already prescribed. Second, he can provide a better and simpler explanation for these diseases: an excess of bile or phlegm affecting the head.[72] Third, he accuses his opponents of impiety and irreligion, while at the same time proclaiming his own conviction of the divine nature of the universe.[73] Their claims that the body of a human being can be possessed and defiled by a god are blasphemous, for the role of gods is to purify, not to make impure. If it is true that they advertise their ability to bring the moon down to earth or cause storms and drought to cease (all activities that, as we have seen, were associated with Empedocles), then they can themselves be convicted of impiety for wishing to disturb the natural order of the heavens and for pretending to greater power than the gods themselves. Praying to the gods to come and assist them is a blasphemous attempt to manipulate the gods for personal reasons.[74] It detracts from the power and majesty of the divine that is revealed above all in the 'necessity' that binds everything together, and that allows the true doctor to understand the whole course of disease, from its beginning in the past to its development in the future.[75]

This author is not alone among the writers of the Corpus in opposing this new view of Nature and of the gods to the more traditional one that allowed the gods to intervene in the world, for good or ill, as they saw fit.[76] In his search for natural causes he sees himself as properly pious, and certainly far from an atheist. In this he can be compared with the author of *Regimen*, who in his last book explores the medical significance of dreams. Some are divinely sent, foretelling good or evil, and must be interpreted by 'those who possess the skill in dealing with such things'. These interpreters may also offer to explain the meaning of other dreams that are more closely related to changes in the body such as surfeit or deficiency. Sometimes they may even reach the right conclusion. But these dreams, claims the author, are really the province of the doctor, who can give instructions on the proper precautions to be taken. Prayers to the gods are good, but man should also lend a hand.[77] This is not a rejection of the gods, but a demarcation of spheres of effective action. These spheres may overlap. The patient should take note of the changes in the heaven and avoid chills and the hot sun, and, at the same time, offer up prayers to the gods to turn away the forthcoming evil.[78] Both here and in *The Sacred Disease* the author is broadening the space available for the doctor's intervention by stressing his particular competence in the medical market-place.[79]

Another way of claiming an advantage over other practitioners was to appeal to ethical considerations and to suggest that the knowledge that was on offer was based on more than mere technical expertise.[80] Indeed, one of the major requirements of the true practitioner is to know the limits of his ability, and to be prepared to hand over to others more skilled if necessary. The decision to treat or not is his responsibility, and, hence, he ought to know which cases are curable and which not, and, if the latter, how far any treatment might help to ameliorate them.[81] No blame was attached to a reasoned refusal to treat. At least one author in the Corpus believed that it was essential to reject any case judged to be incurable; another advised that a decision to treat should be accompanied by an announcement of the likely outcome.[82] Above all, the doctor must choose the treatment that is most effective, not that which is most dramatic and creates the best immediate impression. There is no point in finishing an operation with a wonderful display of bandaging if after three days the patient is still in pain.[83] Similarly, one must learn how to speak tactfully and effectively, both in public and at the bedside, and know which arguments are to be accepted and which critically rejected. Even the manner of one's disagreement with others offering treatment can help to create the right impression on those in search of a doctor.[84] Those who fail to live up to these high aims for medicine may still be considered doctors, albeit foolish ones; other patients may prefer to label them as charlatans or quacks and have nothing to do with them.[85]

Nowhere is this division between the true and the false doctor more clear than in the *Oath*.[86] This famous document falls neatly into two parts, one detailing the obligations of the swearer in receiving and transmitting medical knowledge, the other his obligations with regard to medical practice and his patients. Many of the so-called ethical aspirations in the *Oath* find general acceptance elsewhere in the Corpus; for example, the notion that the doctor should act to the best of his ability, 'to heal, or, at any rate, not to harm', and keep whatever information he has gained in the course of his practice secret.[87] The *Physician* mentions the special position of the doctor with regard to his patients, especially with women and girls, and there are references elsewhere to the need to keep the 'holy things' of medicine restricted to those who are part of the same medical community.[88] But other sections of the *Oath* go far beyond what is said in other treatises, and, at times, contradict them.

While a willingness to yield in treatment to others more qualified can be regarded as a valuable part of the make-up of the doctor, nowhere else in the Corpus is there the strict division between dietetics and pharmacology on the one hand and surgery on the other. The *Oath*'s ban on the use of the knife is absolute, even for a relatively minor procedure such as lithotomy.[89] The involvement of the doctor in prescribing poisonous drugs, and in 'taking the lead in giving such advice', would doubtless have been deprecated by most ancient doctors if it resulted in murder, but there is ample evidence of their willing participation in suicide and euthanasia.[90] Likewise, despite what is said in the *Oath*, *The Nature of the Child* contains a famous case of an abortion, while the prescription of pills, potions and pessaries to prevent conception or provoke abortion is found in medical writings throughout Antiquity.[91]

What makes the *Oath* different from all other documents on medical ethics and etiquette from Antiquity (and explains, in part, why most scholars are reluctant to attribute its authorship to Hippocrates, although they may disagree on when and in what circumstances it was in fact written) is its heavily religious tone.[92] Religion binds the disparate parts of the *Oath* together: the gods are called at the beginning to witness, and, at the end, it is implied, to punish the backslider. The middle sentence, 'In purity and holiness will I keep my entire life', employs words of deep religious significance. The doctor's whole life is to be guided by this religious ethic, within and without the sickroom.[93] He must refrain from all gossip, and from sexual relations, not just with the patient but with any members of the household, male or female, slave or free. He will protect his patient from 'harm and injustice', the latter going far beyond the former. Only by fulfilling the precepts of the oath will the doctor enjoy both his life and his art and gain an eternal reputation among men (words more familiar on a tombstone than in a working document).[94]

In this way, the *Oath* defines what medicine is, and what it is not. Even if it was not composed by Hippocrates, its circulation as part of the Corpus (and possibly its prominent position among the first treatises on the book-roll) ensured that it became widely seen as a summation of ethical practice – not always with approval.[95] Cato the Censor in the mid-second century BC saw it as proof of a sworn conspiracy by Greek doctors to harm their (Roman) patients.[96] But allusions to it on the tombstones of doctors from around the ancient world attest to its prestige and importance, and, by the fourth century AD, it had come to stand for the medical profession.[97] Only then do we begin

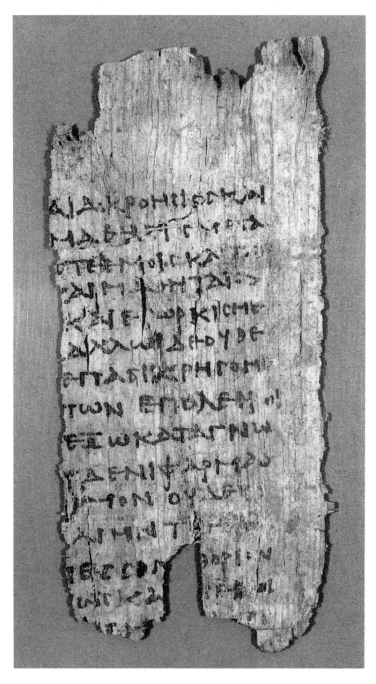

Figure 4.4 A papyrus of the Hippocratic *Oath*, written *c.*AD 275, P. Oxyrhynchus 2547 = Wellcome Ms. 5754. Courtesy of Wellcome Library, London.

to find secure evidence that the *Oath* was being sworn, but it does not appear to have been universally imposed anywhere for several centuries after this.[98]

Indeed, the tradition of writing on medical ethics in Antiquity takes, for the most part, a different line.[99] Whereas the *Oath* starts off from an ethical and religious base and then goes on to define what is expected of the doctor, most other authors, including notably Galen, adopt a more pragmatic approach. Good practice is effective practice: whatever contributes to that end is acceptable; whatever detracts from it is to be rejected. That the two approaches at times coincide is understandable, but this should not obscure the singularity of the *Oath*.[100]

The opening section of the *Oath*, dealing with the obligations of the taker towards his teachers and the art of medicine, is no less unusual. The aspiring practitioner, having taken the oath 'according to medical law'[101] and signed up, is to join the doctor's own family and to treat its members, and be treated by them, as a son or brother. He will be taught from books and orally and 'in every other way' – that is, with practical training and advice – and in turn he is to be willing to impart his knowledge to the members of his new family and to those who wish to enrol and take the oath. This document extends the obligations of the medical apprentice, in contrast to other apprenticeship contracts known for other crafts, far beyond the bounds of his education.[102] It imposes obligations on him that are lifelong and that extend sideways to take in the family members of his teacher. Even when, as must have been common, someone wishing to learn a craft – and one must never forget that doctors in Antiquity ranked as craftsmen – joined the household of his teacher, they did not thereby undertake to pass on that craft, free of charge, to their teacher's family or to support them in adversity.

It is tempting to set the *Oath* in a situation in which an earlier pattern of medical education is gradually breaking down. Medicine, which was once restricted to members of a medical clan, is now available to all who wish to learn it. They will be taught alongside the members of the clan (who will not be charged for their instruction). Whether they too must take this *Oath* is less clear: probably it is assumed that being brought up from an early age in a medical household will have been enough to impart the essential ethics of good practice, especially as the 'children of doctors' (a phrase used from Antiquity onwards for centuries to refer to younger practitioners) may well have been employed in doing simple tasks as assistants (bandaging, applying ointments, making up common remedies) from an early age, just as in other crafts.[103] Plato, indeed, claims that, whereas slaves who were to become doctors would have to be sent out to learn medicine, for the children of free-born doctors this is a natural process, since they are taught by their fathers from childhood.[104]

The strong family component within ancient medicine is not surprising; even today, a high percentage of medical students come from medical families. Hippocrates claimed descent from Asclepius, son of Apollo (according to a fabricated genealogy, his was the seventeenth, eighteenth or nineteenth generation from the god, depending on which variant story one follows), as well as from another healing deity, Hercules. Not surprisingly, legend also knew of many distinguished doctors in his family before him. The historian Theopompus, writing around 330 BC, confirms the tradition of a long-standing link between Cos and the family of Asclepius, adding that another branch of the family had never left Asia Minor but had stayed at Cnidus, a town on a mainland peninsula directly opposite Cos. This was the branch to which Ctesias allegedly belonged. A further tradition, reported by Galen, had it that there were once three 'choirs' of doctors, settled respectively on Cos, at Cnidus and on the neighbouring larger island of Rhodes, but that the third had become extinct, a story also alluded to by an earlier doctor, Andromachus, and by Galen's contemporary, the hypochondriac worshipper of Asclepius, Aelius Aristides.[105]

The existence of a strong family tradition linking Cos and Cnidus with descendants of Asclepius was confirmed in 1956 when an inscription from the great oracular shrine at Delphi was published. Inscribed in the fourth century BC, it instructed the members of the 'commonalty' of Coan and Cnidian Asclepiads how to identify themselves by an oath in order to claim the privileges accorded at Delphi to Asclepiads 'in the male line'.[106] One may legitimately doubt the validity of this divine descent, but this inscription proves that belief in it was of at least moderately long standing, and that it was accepted beyond the immediate region of Cos and Cnidus. But it should not escape notice that it is the male descendants of Asclepius, not doctors as such, who are the beneficiaries of the privileges. As we might surmise from the Hippocratic Corpus, and not least the *Oath*, not every doctor was a descendant of the god, and not every descendant a doctor. Whether at some dim and distant date in the past Greek medicine had been kept solely within a few families, as the *Oath* implies, is a matter solely for conjecture. If there ever was such a time, it antedated the Homeric poems, for, while concentrating on the healing activities of two Asclepiads, they also imply the existence of other healers outside the family.

By the time of the Hippocratic Corpus, then, medicine was no longer the preserve of a group of clans, if it ever had been, but a subject publicly debated and capable of being taught to anyone who wished to learn and could afford a master's fee. Its most celebrated practitioner was Hippocrates of Cos, whose reputation stretched at least to Athens and was soon to spawn a whole series of legends and documents to flesh out the details of his family and career. But while the achievements of the historical Hippocrates lent authority to the books that circulated under his name, he cannot have written more than a fraction of them at best, for, as we shall see, they contain a multiplicity of different doctrines.

What they do show is that within these varied writings medicine was being defined both for what it does and, even more importantly, for what it does not do.[107] It covers all aspects of the health of the individual, mind as well as body; it goes beyond mere chance; it believes in a logical causation that is independent of any divine intervention, for good or ill; it offers new ideas about the physical body; it avoids chants, charms and exorcisms; and it claims a basis in empirical fact and sound practice that rejects flimsy philosophical hypotheses.[108] That some of the authors in the Corpus themselves indulged in speculation or argued in ways that seem unconvincing; that many, if not most, doctors, and certainly very many of their patients, continued to leave a place for the gods within healing; that many of the writers themselves would have disagreed with one another on points both great and small does not detract from the overall message gained from a reading of the Corpus or simply from its very existence as a body of writings. One Late Antique writer on medicine was closer to the truth than he knew when he praised Hippocrates for collecting and weaving together the scattered ideas and observations of earlier doctors into a complete and coherent art of medicine.[109] Henceforth, certainly from the early third century BC onwards, the Hippocratic Corpus came to be seen as a standard against which other types of healing might be measured, and then approved or rejected.[110] In that sense, its eponymous hero Hippocrates can indeed be called the Father of Medicine.

5

HIPPOCRATIC THEORIES

When the Anonymus Londinensis papyrus was first published, in 1893, it created a considerable stir because it contradicted what had for centuries been the traditional understanding of Hippocratic medicine.[1] The immediate debate centred largely upon the so-called Hippocratic question, the identification of the source or sources of the ideas attributed in the papyrus to the historical Hippocrates, and upon the authorship, and by implication the reliability, of the doxographical sections that the anonymous author had taken over from Aristotle.[2] Less attention was given to the actual theories described in the papyrus, despite the fact that many of the authors named in it were previously unknown. That many of them flourished in the first half of the fourth century was a further reason to omit them from consideration in a study of Hippocratic medicine in the fifth. This excuse for neglect becomes less cogent, however, when one examines the Hippocratic Corpus as a whole (since many of the texts contained therein are likely also to come from the fourth century), and it is certainly out of place in any study of Greek medicine in general.

The Aristotelian section of the papyrus opens with the unequivocal statement, probably by the writer himself, that there has been a considerable disagreement (*stasis*) over just what causes disease. Some believe that diseases result from residues, whether produced pathologically or as natural bodily secretions; others from changes in the body's elements.[3] Although this emphasis on disagreement may simply be an heuristic device to assist in classification and can be found in many similar ancient lists of philosophical and medical doctrines, there can be no doubt that both here and in the Hippocratic Corpus is to be found a variety of competing solutions to the same question: what is disease or illness?[4] Yet it is also clear that there are many similarities between all the authors, whatever their theories and wherever and whenever they were active. All provide entirely natural explanations for disease and assume that whatever cause they have identified is a universal cause, applicable to all or most conditions. Some authors thought in terms of more than one cause: Ninyas distinguished congenital from non-congenital conditions, while stressing the effects of harmful residues produced from nutriment; Philistion held that there were three general causes, an imbalance between the body's elements, a failure of the body to function properly and external factors such as woundings, excessive heat or cold, and bad food.[5] But, whether single or multiple, these causes have a universal application, and can explain all types of disease.

Philosophers and doctors can be found on both sides of the Aristotelian division. Although those who attribute disease to residues, where they can be identified, tend to be doctors and those who believe in elements are mostly philosophers, this is not invariably so; nor can one make a sharp division between the two groups in terms of the level of abstraction of their theories. All pay close attention to natural phenomena, even if they interpret the relationship between the same phenomena differently. For Timotheus of Metapontum, as for the author of *The Sacred Disease*, some diseases arise in the head through the blockage of various passages, and the running nose and streaming eyes of the common cold are the body's natural way of unblocking them.[6] But for Aias it is the purging itself that is the cause of illness; the fewer the outflows, the healthier the patient.[7] In a similar reversal of the chain of cause and effect, Petron (or Petronas) of Aegina in the first half of the fourth century held that bile was produced only when the body was diseased, and thus was not, as most people believed, itself the cause of many diseases.[8] Other authors seem consciously to have modified the views of their predecessors. Euryphon of Cnidus, perhaps the earliest of those named, living around 450 BC, claimed that diseases were the result of residues left when the belly was unable to rid itself of all the food it had taken.[9] His contemporary, Herodicus of Cnidus, while accepting the theory of residues, denied that it had anything to do with the body's ability to evacuate, and claimed instead that the residues occurred because of a lack of exercise, with the result that food remained undigested until it turned into two forms of harmful liquid. Diseases differed according to the type of liquid involved and the site to which it flowed.[10]

A similar interest in diseases and their potential variety is ascribed to the even earlier authors of the *Cnidian Sentences* by the writer of *Regimen in Acute Diseases*, and by Galen in his commentary on the latter book. Galen suggested that they distinguished seven different sorts of imbalance of bile, twelve kinds of bladder disease, four of kidney disease, four of strangury, three of tetanus, four of jaundice and three of phthisis, a classification that both he and the Hippocratic author felt was too precise, especially when it led the authors to neglect symptoms that would be useful for prognosis.[11] Others disagreed, for there are several treatises in the Hippocratic Corpus, notably *Diseases* 2 and 3 and *Internal Affections*, that incorporate these or similar subdivisions. The author of *Internal Affections*, for instance, gives four types of jaundice, four of kidney disease, three of tetanus and three of phthisis.[12] Along with the gynaecological treatises, *The Nature of Woman*, *Diseases of Women* 1–2, and *Diseases of Young Girls*, these treatises form a group more interested in the general description of a disease than in its manifestation in the individual patient. They provide a straightforward listing of the disease, its symptoms, prognosis and therapy, without wider theoretical or professional considerations.

Because these treatises follow a similar pattern of arrangement to that criticised by Galen in the *Cnidian Sentences* and almost certainly drew on them or similar material, they have often been called Cnidian and associated with a medical 'school' at Cnidus, although they themselves provide no indication of any origin, author or sources. Whether this attribution can be justified, let alone used as the foundation for constructing a whole series of polarities between so-called Coan and Cnidian medicine (patient centred/disease centred; aetiology/classification; prognosis/diagnosis; organism/organs, etc.), is a matter of vigorous dispute.[13] The story of the development of the two groups, or 'choirs', of doctors on Cos and Cnidus (see p. 70) is a typical Greek invention to explain the presence of Asclepiads in both places (and their disappearance from Rhodes) and makes no mention of any theoretical differences between them. But the short stretch of water separating Cos from Cnidus was no Berlin Wall. The author of *Regimen in Acute Diseases*, who, as we have seen, knows and criticises Cnidian material, shows that its usage and influence were not confined to Cnidus itself, or, if he was himself a Cnidian, that there was disagreement among Cnidians themselves. Galen had no difficulty in assuming that Ctesias of Cnidus was familiar with Hippocrates' work on dislocations, and many texts in the Corpus display both so-called Coan and Cnidian emphases and types of organisation.[14] Most modern scholars, therefore, see this neat division between Cos and Cnidus as a creation of earlier historians, ancient as well as modern, projecting back their own conflicts into the past.[15] It has some value as a tool for classifying and analysing certain of the texts in the Corpus, but it is of only limited historical worth and may obscure as much as it clarifies the theoretical debates taking place in fifth- and fourth-century Greece.

The Hippocratic Corpus contains a multiplicity of theories that resemble in many ways those sketched by Anonymus Londinensis. *Breaths* endeavours to show that all diseases are the result of air, which has enormous effects within both the individual and the universe as a whole, even when it might not appear at first sight to be the obvious cause, as in haemorrhages and dropsy.[16] *Places in Man*, by contrast, comes close to the theory of Herodicus of Cnidus in its stress on the importance of seven types of flux originating in the head and causing illness at the point where they happen to settle.[17] In *The Nature of Man*, as we have already seen, can be found the theory of the four humours ascribed in the papyrus to Polybus, whose insistence on health as a form of balance is shared with many of the authors of other treatises.

Explicitly or implicitly, all the writers within the Corpus acknowledge that their topics can be explained on the same principles as the rest of natural creation, of which mankind is but one part.[18] When dealing with a dislocated forearm, one should endeavour to set it in a straight line, for this is its 'most just nature'; stretching out one's arm straight is something that one is 'compelled by the justice of nature' to do.[19] The author of *Ancient Medicine* insists that one can best learn about nature from the human body, while that of *Regimen* devotes its first book almost entirely to a discussion of the way in which mankind, like the rest of nature, is the product of the interaction of the two primordial substances, fire and water. Without this understanding of the body, it is claimed, any attempt at providing a suitable regimen is bound to fail.[20] *Fleshes*, similarly, begins with the need to relate the genesis of mankind to the genesis of the whole cosmos, but chooses a different pair of basic substances, the fatty and the glutinous.[21] That this correspondence between microcosm and macrocosm, to use later terminology, should not invariably be seen in narrowly physiological terms is also made clear at the end of this treatise, where the author explains the importance of the number 7 in the creation and development of the human body.[22] Similar cosmological and numerological speculations appear in *Sevens*, a tract with parallels in Ancient Near-Eastern literature, which has been variously dated between the late sixth/early fifth century BC and the first century of the Christian era.[23]

The specific phenomena of the natural world are regarded as strongly influencing the health and disease of the human body.[24] The author of *Regimen* declares it necessary for the doctor to become familiar not only with the constitution of his patient but also with the seasons of the year, the winds, the weather, the geographical region, the rising and setting of the sun and, indeed, the whole cosmos, 'from which arise diseases for men'.[25] *Airs, Waters and Places* is the most celebrated example of this geographical or meteorological medicine, although its author has a vastly different understanding of the make-up of the human body from that of *Regimen*.[26] In this treatise the travelling doctor is instructed on how to predict the sort of diseases he will find in any locality from its geographical and climatological situation. The inhabitants of a north-facing city, with cold winds and generally hard water, will be vigorous and lean, and any constriction affect the lower abdomen more than the chest. They will suffer, among other things, from pleurisy, eye inflammations and acute diseases: younger men will experience violent nosebleeds in summer; women may become barren because of the water and find both menstruation and childbirth difficult. After giving birth they will often suffer from phthisis, and their young boys from dropsy of the testicles.[27] This geographical determinism explains both physical conditions, for example the flabby white bodies of the inhabitants of S. Russia, and mental states. According to the author of *The Sacred Disease*, purely physical causes produce not only such pathological conditions as mania and epilepsy, the result of an excess of bile and phlegm, respectively, but also general psychological traits.[28] The pleasant situation of the inhabitants of Asia, living in an equable, well-tempered climate, neither too hot nor too cold, in a land where crops and animals flourish abundantly, means they lack courage and energy. Their life is just too easy, and this, in turn, accounts for their subjection to kings.

75

By contrast, the inhabitants of Europe, and especially mainland Greece, brought up in a slightly hardier and ever-changing climate, have developed the right combination of martial vigour and political independence. They are their own masters; their successes are their own, as are their failures. The key to all this is the diversity of the geography and climate of Europe, with its hills, plains, rivers and steppes, which explains the great diversity of its inhabitants, although all fall under the same general type that marks them off from Asiatics or Africans.[29] If some of this reads like political propaganda by a Greek recalling the successes of the Persian Wars or as ingenious speculation, the result of an idea pushed far beyond its limits, it is also in part based on acute and precise observation. The description of the barrenness of the Scythians derives from an eyewitness report, probably by the author himself, and may have a modern medical explanation in the high iron content of some of the local rivers.[30]

Even more precise are the climatological observations that make up the so-called *Constitutions* included in the series of books that form the *Epidemics*.[31] The most celebrated are those in the earliest block, Books 1 and 3, but similar observations can be found in all the remaining books, either as fragments or as presuppositions in the individual case histories. They are unusual in attempting to survey the range of diseases 'residing' in a particular town over the course of a single year and then to correlate them with changes in the climate. So, for instance, the very first *Constitution* in Book 1 begins with a description of the winds, rainfall and temperature changes on the island of Thasos in the N. Aegean.[32] There is an implication that it was, at least in part, as the result of a change in the prevailing winds in spring from southerly to northerly that people began to fall ill with slight fevers, haemorrhages, swellings around the ears and dry coughs. The author's comment that, in this generally healthy year, it was young men who attended the wrestling school and gymnasia who were most affected, and who also consequently suffered from painful swellings in the testicles, suggests that this disease was mumps. In *Epidemics* 6 a detailed account of the 'cough of Perinthus' (now Eregli, on the Sea of Marmara) opens with a date and the changes in the pattern of the winds: coughs began about the winter solstice, fifteen or twenty days after there had been frequent changes in the south wind, the north wind and the snow wind.[33]

Some of the individual case histories in *Epidemics* 1 and 3 provided data for the wider picture of disease put forward in the *Constitutions*; the author of the description of the Perinthine cough specifically refers to his own medical perceptions and activities when it was raging. The individual case histories as we have them say little or nothing about time, place or climatic changes, but that may simply relate to the way in which the cases are presented, and not to the collection of information that lies behind them.[34] Furthermore, even if we allow that not everyone was as interested in amassing this material or was as careful an observer and compiler as the author of *Epidemics* 1 and 3, there is ample evidence throughout the Corpus that he was not an isolated believer in the effects of wind and climate.[35] Anyone who, like the author of *The Nature of Man*, thought that widespread disease was the result of something nasty taking place in the surrounding air had to be aware of alterations in atmospheric conditions.[36] Writers as diverse as those of *Regimen* and *Humours* emphasised the need for the doctor to take note of everything going on around him that might in any way affect the patient.[37] The first part of the third section of *Aphorisms* summarises the diseases that arise as the year passes through the four seasons, paying particular attention to the winds and how they modify the basic seasonal pattern.[38] It may be significant that in this, the most famous of all Hippocratic treatises, three times as much is said about the diseases of season and climate than about the diseases to be encountered as the body itself changes through life.

In general, the Hippocratic physician explained illness as the result of something wrong with the body's system of fluids and conduits. Although the anatomy of a woman was different from that of a man, and brought with it an extra range of diseases and problems, the overall reasoning behind Hippocratic gynaecology made no distinction between the sexes. The advice of the author of *Diseases of Women 2* that one should take careful note of the nature, colours and age of his patient, as well as of her environment, could apply unchanged to the male, as could the emphasis on fluxes and on hot and cold.[39] Indeed, what was thought to take place within the female body was regarded as good evidence for less visible processes in the male. Observing the one provided support for theories that encompassed the other.[40]

Although there is no evidence for systematic dissection by any of the writers of the Corpus, there is no doubt that they had some basic understanding of the workings of the body and its internal organisation, even if this was limited and at times fanciful and, as yet, lacked any precise and agreed terminology.[41] So, for example, the word that later came to be used for 'vein' at this stage meant any blood vessel, and 'nerve' could be used to mean ligament and tendon as well as nerve.[42] But there is evidence that some doctors had seen some details of the inside of a human body: the descriptions of a humped back and of the spongy tubercles of a sufferer from tuberculosis clearly derive from observation, perhaps in an autopsy.[43] Likewise, among the proofs offered by the author of *The Sacred Disease* for his theory that epilepsy was caused by the build-up of phlegm in the brain cavity is one deriving from anatomy, the presence of stinking water inside the skull of an 'epileptic' goat.[44] That goats suffered from epilepsy was widely believed in Antiquity, perhaps because of the presence of 'staggers', whose symptoms resemble those of an epileptic fit.[45] Epilepsy might also be brought on by the weather, it was thought, for the warm south wind tended to make the brain moister, just as it allowed condensation or moisture to form on the inside of wine jars.[46] Elsewhere, writers also extrapolated from what they had seen inside an animal, and sometimes a diseased animal, to elucidate a similar human condition.[47] In

77

embryology, hen's eggs offered a model for understanding foetal development in humans, and ancient descriptions of the human womb closely resemble what could be far more easily seen in animals.[48]

The Hippocratic physiology of the body is based both on observation and on a wide range of analogies with the world around. The body's composition and processes are related to those visible elsewhere on a larger scale, for 'appearances give an insight into the invisible'.[49] So, for example, the author of *Regimen* begins with a long series of comparisons drawn from crafts as varied as gold-beating and forestry to confirm his theory that there is a constant toing and fro-ing within the body.[50] Similar analogies explain how individual organs work. The stomach is often viewed as a giant oven, with digestion as a form of cooking. The womb and the bladder are compared to a cupping glass, drawing fluids to themselves.[51] The making of cheese explains how fluids coagulate or separate out within the body.[52] The writers on gynaecology use a wide range of similes and metaphors to refer to the womb, particularly those of an oven, 'cooking' the embryo, and a jar.[53] It moves upwards and downwards as if in a tube, and, like a refractory pet animal, can be made to return to its proper home by inducements (sweet smells) or the reverse (driving it back by using foul-smelling substances).[54] How far these multiple analogies are to be pressed is more difficult to judge, since, taken together, they are not always consistent even within a single treatise. Their function, above all, is to provide an immediate support to the argument for whatever position is adopted. They are at one and the same time rhetorical and scientific devices, both explaining and convincing.[55] But they do not form part of what later would be seen as a properly logical argument, and, given the possibly oral delivery of much of this material before the public, they are perhaps best to be interpreted only in their immediate context. But their ubiquity also helps to explain why the ideal doctor is expected to understand how to distinguish a good argument from a bad, or when an analogy works and when it does not.[56]

What is present in the body's conduits (which should not be identified solely with nerves and the cardiovascular system) is regularly seen as the cause of illness.[57] Sometimes it is peccant matter, carried round until it settles on one spot; sometimes it is airs, fumes and gases; sometimes it is an evil fluid, a catarrh, for example, produced within the body; sometimes the problem is the result of a surfeit or deficiency of a fluid that, of itself, is generally beneficial.[58] These fluids or humours came to play the leading role in Hippocratic medicine. As explanations for disease they had enormous advantages. For the most part, they were visible either in illness, as pus or catarrh, or, like sputum, excreta and urine, in forms whose variations might easily be interpreted to show when illness was or was not present. Like a spring, they could be depicted as flowing down from the top of the body, the brain, through its other parts, bringing down with them as they did so material that would reveal an inner state otherwise invisible to the eye.[59] Where and in what manner they came to the surface (as a nosebleed or piles, vomit or a suppurating ulcer) was also considered significant as an indication of the site of a potential weakness within the body. Just as a stream would follow a course with least obstruction, so the flow of humours would seek out the easiest way of escaping from the body.

Above all, these bodily fluids were common and perceptible: 'we all experience them, and will continue to do so,' says the author of *Ancient Medicine*.[60] Their appearance, both regular and irregular, also suggested that the body had a natural tendency towards equilibrium in terms of both quality (the smell and colour of urine varied around a norm) and quantity – surplus food and drink taken in was then excreted as urine and faeces.[61] While at times this process might seem unnatural and dangerous, at others even so essential a fluid as blood was regularly expelled from the body without any apparent ill effects, as in small nosebleeds or, above all, in menstruation. Indeed, so 'natural' was the evacuation of menstrual blood that failure to menstruate came to be seen as a very dangerous symptom, and the beginning of the menopause marked for many doctors the almost certain onset of serious problems, as the blood that otherwise would have been removed remained stagnant and putrefying in the female body.[62] Although the days immediately before a period are associated with tiredness, headaches and sore throats, menstruation itself is seen as a good thing, not least when it apparently leads to the cure of other ailments.[63]

There was no fixed or agreed number of significant humours, but many of the authors in the Corpus ascribed particular importance to two fluids above all, phlegm and bile. As its Greek name implies, phlegm was originally a substance associated with burning or inflammatory disease: its cognates include 'flame', 'burn' and 'inflammation', which draws attention to the fiery redness of many lumps and swellings. By the fifth century it had come by a process as yet unknown to mean something cold, white and sticky.[64] 'All human diseases arise from bile and phlegm', claimed the author of *Affections*, a view shared by the writer of *Diseases* 1, who added the effects of externals, exertions, woundings, heat and cold. In the opinion of the latter author bile and phlegm were permanent constituents of the human body but they produced disease only under the influence of food and drink, heat and cold.[65] The author of *Airs, Waters and Places* and *The Sacred Disease* likewise regarded bile and phlegm as the two polarities of disease: the benefits of a cool dry summer for the phlegmatic are contrasted with its dangers for the bilious; phlegm causes epilepsy, bile mania.[66] The short text *Haemorrhoids* begins with a dogmatic statement that haemorrhoids occur when bile or phlegm settles in the blood vessels of the anus, causing them to heat and swell and to push out from the anus.[67] As Jouanna aptly remarks, a careful and accurate observation of the blood vessels is overlaid with an explanation that merely explains the visible by the invisible. Nor does it indicate in what way, if any, piles produced by one humour differ from those caused by the other.[68]

One of the reasons why the Hippocratic writers fixed on bile and phlegm more than on any other fluid is that they were both visible and easily associated with illness. Their external appearance is always nasty, and they are particularly obvious when the patient is ill or expels something that may be potentially harmful. The constant flood of mucus from a running nose, sputum coughed or spat out and white clouds visible in urine are all easily associated with disease, and their effects inside the body can be imagined equally well. Glutinous sputum can be easily imagined as blocking the passage of air around the body, or settling on a knee joint and causing arthritis. Bile, by contrast, appears in vomit and diarrhoea, and can be easily thought to destroy the internal surfaces and processes of the body in the same way as it interferes with proper digestion and stings the mucous membranes. Bile and phlegm are also seasonal in their occurrence; a winter cold can be contrasted with summer dysentery, both of which are more common, and also more often fatal, in two different age groups, the elderly and young children. The deaths of the elderly from winter respiratory diseases will have been as marked in Antiquity as it is now.[69] Such easily visible phenomena will have encouraged the belief in the potency of these two fluids.

Other fluids fitted into the same pattern of explanation. The author of *Ancient Medicine*, who rejected strongly the theory of elements, believed instead in a variety of forces within the body manifesting themselves to the senses largely in the body's fluids.[70] Thrasymachus of Sardis added pus to bile and phlegm, all three being harmful fluids produced from blood under the effects of an excess of heat or cold.[71] They were definitely pathological, to the extent that Thrasymachus viewed them as deformations of blood, but elsewhere the role of certain humours is far less clear. Philolaus of Croton held that all diseases originated through blood, bile and phlegm, but his phraseology leaves it open whether bile and phlegm are present in the body in a normal healthy state and are changed to dangerous substances only by developments inside or outside the body.[72] Within the Hippocratic Corpus, the author of *Airs, Waters and Places* described how the inhabitants of S. Russia were conditioned by birth and climate to be susceptible to phlegmatic diseases. But while they might have a natural excess of phlegm predisposing them to certain ailments and afflictions, being phlegmatic was not an illness of itself. Besides, the inhabitants of Asia and Europe also have phlegm as a normal humour within their bodies, just as they have a moderate amount of bile. It is not the fluid itself that is harmful, but its excess or deficiency.[73]

This sort of explanation we have already met in Alcmaeon and in other pre-Socratic philosophers, and it fits neatly with their concepts of health as harmony, balance and order. Indeed, so entwined are these notions in Greek thought that the Greek word 'kosmos' can, depending on its context, mean 'beauty', 'order', 'the world' or any combination of the three. It is no surprise therefore to find Plato in his *Symposium* putting into the mouth of the doctor Eryximachus the claim that the doctor understands 'balance' in human life more than anyone else.[74] Health can thus be thought of as 'eukrasia' (good mixture), 'harmony' or 'symmetry'; illness as its opposite.[75] It is not the individual components themselves that are to blame for illness – although some are more dangerous than others, for all are natural and thus part of the natural order of the universe – but the way in which they combine together.

But this raises a further problem for the definition of health and disease. Some Hippocratic texts see a clear break between being well and being ill. Even if there is some imbalance of the humours, only when the peccant material settles in one place, only when phlegm, for instance, blocks the passage of air around the body, is the patient ill.[76] Otherwise, health is the normal state. The third of the *Aphorisms* turns this argument on its head: it is not disease that is the rarity but perfect health. Even a trained athlete can only remain briefly at his peak, for any change, unless carefully governed, can only be for the worse: once the top has been reached, the only way is down. Even staying there is 'dangerous' (the word is repeated six times in a few paragraphs), and presents difficulties for those with a less than perfect constitution. Any alteration is potentially harmful, and it is the job of both doctor and patient to forestall as far as possible the consequences of any change.[77] *The Nature of Man* gives a similar explanation that places the onset of illness as soon as the mixture of the humours becomes unbalanced or when one humour becomes isolated and begins to flow on its own.[78] Human health is thus perpetually endangered.

But many other authors take a different approach to the idea of health as balance. In their opinion there is not one single point of balance, every deviation from which counts as illness, no sudden shift from being well to being ill, but a wide band in which a certain disequilibrium is allowed as well as the perfect equilibrium. Only when the imbalance becomes excessive, as when one fluid separates itself off from the mixture, does the individual become ill. The author of *Regimen*, for instance, sees the whole body as existing in a perpetual flux between its two elements, fire and water, and the physician must keep this flux within its appropriate limits. The long series of analogies that begins this work is intended to show how this constant flux is a feature of all natural activity.[79] The link here with the ideas of the philosopher Heraclitus is patent, and it has been suggested that this sort of theory was particularly associated with the Greeks of Asia Minor.[80] That of a more precise and potentially more stable balance was favoured by doctors coming from S. Italy and Sicily, influenced by Empedocles in particular. This is an intriguing suggestion, but one that, in the general absence of information on the place and date of composition of most treatises, risks being circular in its application.[81]

Nonetheless, there can be little doubt of the impact of Empedocles' theories on the medicine of his day.[82] The author of *Ancient Medicine* specifically criticised him, while *The Nature of Man* drew heavily on his ideas for what was later to be seen as *the* Hippocratic theory, that of the four humours.[83] Empedocles' belief in four cosmic elements, earth, air, fire and water, linked

with the four qualities, hot, cold, wet and dry, had great explanatory potential, and it is not surprising that theories of disease based on only three
humours fell out of favour.[84] But there was still debate over what should
constitute the four humours or bodily elements.[85] The author of *Diseases* 4
believed that they were water, bile, blood and phlegm, water being obviously
in excess in diseases such as dropsy or diabetes, but no other surviving author
seems to have followed him.[86] Both Petron(as) of Aegina and Philistion of
Locris in the early years of the fourth century emphasised the imbalance of the
four elements, hot, cold, wet and dry, but not of the humours as such. Petron,
in fact, regarded bile only as a product, not a cause, of disease.[87]

In a different formulation Menecrates, who lived in the middle years of
the fourth century, argued that the body was created from four elements, two
hot, blood and bile, and two cold, breath (*pneuma*) and phlegm. Their harmony produced health, their disagreement illness. Menecrates also believed
that if what he termed red bile was allowed to become stagnant and stale it
turned to black bile, which produced different diseases depending on where
it happened to settle during its course around the body – pneumonia in the
lungs, lumbago around the hips, pleurisy in the ribs and, if settled in the
bowels, *kausos*, an extremely burning fever throughout the body.[88]

Menecrates is among the earliest medical writers to consider melancholy or
'black bile' as a specific substance, and in his reduction of it to a degenerate
form of bile (or 'red bile') he may well be reacting to the theory of the four
humours put forward in *The Nature of Man*. As in many of the other treatises
so far discussed in this chapter, its author defined health and disease in terms
of balance and imbalance, this time of its humours:

> Health is when these constituents are in due proportion to one
> another with regard to blending, power and quantity, and when they
> are perfectly mixed.[89] Pain is experienced whenever one of these con-
> stituents is deficient or in excess or is isolated in the body and is not
> blended with all the others. For, whenever any one of these is isolated
> and stands by itself, of necessity not only does the place which is left
> become diseased, but also the place where it stands and floods causes
> pain and distress through being over-full.[90]

This is true, no matter what the age of the individual or the season of the
year.[91] It is something that can be proved to be both logically true and in
accordance with the workings of the natural universe around: 'necessity' com-
pels assent, and, in turn, guarantees at times 'the surest of prognostics'.[92] But
health is always a precarious state, affected by the air around us and by the
way of life that we lead, food, drink, sleep, exercise and so on. It is constantly
at the mercy of change, whether of the climate as the year moves from season
to season or of the ageing process.[93] It is also highly specific. Each individual
has his or her proper mixture that is unlikely to be widely shared, if shared at

all, and that mixture is constantly in danger of being altered for the worse by changes going on in the world around. But many of these changes are predictable, and, as such, can be prevented with suitable prophylaxis. If most fevers come from an excess of bile, and if bile predominates in summer and autumn, then one can take suitable precautions to reduce the amount of bile-making foodstuffs taken in; likewise the natural increase in blood in spring and early summer can be kept from damaging the body by taking steps to offset that increase.[94] It is true that one must take into account the individual's age and constitution, the season of the year, the type of remedy to be prescribed and a whole range of similar factors both in prevention and in restoring the body to its original balance, but this is not impossible, however complicated it might at first seem.[95] Indeed, this knowledge is available to everyone who wishes to take thought for his or her own health, 'the most precious of goods'. The individual's own judgment as to what is suitable for him or her, if made in accordance with the rules enunciated by the author of this tract, can go a long way to preserving and restoring health.[96]

In this treatise, more than in any other in the Corpus, is found a system of rules that fit together with almost mathematical precision and predictability, and that gain authority precisely because of the easy elegance with which they do so.[97] While on the one hand the author admits the difficulty of dealing with sickness and health in the individual – for it is the individual who falls ill, not an intellectual construct – he is also convinced that his scheme of understanding the body, if rightly followed, will lead to a substantial degree of certainty. He imposes two hard tasks on doctor and prospective patient. The latter is expected to take appropriate precautions at all times in order to avoid falling ill; the former is to understand the individuality of the patient in front of him in order to give advice and to heal. But neither task is impossible, and the writer's confidence was transmitted to later generations of doctors.

They were perhaps unaware of the problematic nature of the fourth humour, black bile or melancholy, because it slotted so neatly and so unobtrusively into place within a cosmology that was (or certainly soon became) widely accepted. The four elements, the four seasons, the four ages of mankind and the four types of fever could be extended almost indefinitely to include four tastes, four colours and, by the end of Antiquity, the four temperaments, the four cardinal points of the compass and the astrological signs in each quarter of the heavens. (The Middle Ages went on to add even further refinements, including the four tonalities and the four Evangelists.)[98] Given the prevalence of this scheme of fours, the question that should be raised is not why there should be four humours but why the fourth humour should be black bile rather than another fluid. One partial answer is that there was already a strong association of words relating to black bile with death and disease, and hence it could easily be made to stand in direct opposition to blood, which was generally associated with life and health. But this of itself does not explain the notion of black bile entirely, for until this treatise references to black bile itself as a specific substance are almost entirely absent, and when they are found they serve simply to distinguish this type of bile from bile of other types and colours. Earlier authors do not regard it as a separate humour.

What are found instead are terms such as 'melancholic', 'melancholia', 'being melancholic', all of them relating to some disease. These words are found both inside and outside the Hippocratic Corpus in medical contexts that often link them with a psychological state, whether anger or some form of madness. At *Aphorisms* 3, 20, 'melancholia' heads the list of typical spring diseases, and is immediately followed by madness and epilepsy; at 3, 22, the list is reversed, and 'melancholias' conclude the list of typical autumn diseases.[99] However, in *Airs, Waters and Places* 'melancholias' would appear to be largely physical conditions.[100] In both comedy and tragedy 'melancholic' words are used to describe destructive anger or madness.[101] Especially in pre-Hippocratic and folkloric contexts, 'black' may simply be used to emphasise the malignancy of the condition.[102] It need not imply the existence of a separate humour, but only a change in the form of the bile to become something peculiarly dangerous; the notion of Menecrates, already mentioned, that black bile is a deformation of red bile corresponds nicely to this earlier understanding. Similarly, his contemporary, Dexippus of Cos, who derived diseases from bile and phlegm, saw black bile as the result of changes occurring in a mixture of blood and phlegm.[103]

That the concept of black bile as a separate humour was relatively new at the end of the fifth century may also be gathered from the way in which the author of *The Nature of Man* refers to it as 'the so-called black bile', a formulation that implies that the term was, as yet, far from universally familiar.[104] This would then agree with the conclusion of most scholars that black bile came into existence to explain 'black bile diseases', and that its designation as a separate humour, as opposed to a type of bile, came later still.[105] Once hypostatised, its existence could be 'proved' by a variety of empirical observations (although, of course, none related to black bile in a totally pure form, but only to indications of its presence within the mixture of fluids within the body). One need only consider the dark colour of warts and naevi, the way in which blood changed colour and consistency to form a black scar on a surface wound and the occasional portions of dark blood vomited up to conclude that the body contained something dark and mysterious. Its effects could be explained on a neat scheme of antitheses. Compared with its polar opposite, the bright red blood that gives life, black bile could be regarded as largely destructive. But just as blood could be harmful at times, by becoming stagnant or excessive, so black bile could be associated occasionally with things that were good – by the third century BC the melancholy man of genius had become a commonplace which persisted for centuries to come.[106] Later Hippocratic authors, notably Rufus of Ephesus and Galen, wrote books expounding their own views of black bile and its significance for medicine, and, although its importance as a humour disappeared in the seventeenth century along with the theory of humours itself, melancholy continued to feature in medical discussions well into the twentieth century.[107]

Because of its own long and influential history, this theory of the four humours – blood, bile, black bile and phlegm – has dominated the history of Greek medicine. In consequence, *The Nature of Man* has come to stand not just for Hippocrates and the Hippocratic Corpus in general, but for all Greek medicine at whatever period. It has many features that merit such an exalted position. It is clear and consistent in its scheme; it is well and combatively argued, using both logic and the evidence of the natural world to refute its opponents; it unfolds a chain of causation that links the seasons to mankind and to each patient; it appreciates the importance of the individuality of each patient; it accepts the uncertainties of diagnosis and treatment while, at the same time, offering an overall method that, if followed correctly, offers as near certainty as is likely to be achieved; it takes anatomical considerations into account,[108] as well as the patient's whole environment; and it asserts the autonomy and superiority of the doctor over and against those, like philosophers, who offer attractive but unfounded speculations. In emphasising that health was a state of precarious equilibrium it both continues the early Greek interest in order and beauty as some sort of mean and ensures a role for the doctor in preventative as well as in curative medicine. Its Greek is also far more elegant and more accessible than that of most ancient medical treatises, let alone that of the Corpus as a whole. All these factors would justify the historian's high regard for the author of this treatise.

But, as this chapter has shown, that is far from being the whole story. Aristotle and his followers, who were in a far better position to know the truth than we are, believed that Hippocrates was not its author and gave credit for it to his student Polybus.[109] Even when it had later become firmly associated with Hippocrates, scholars such as Sabinus and even Galen himself believed that parts of it were written by another and far more fallible author.[110] The subsequent importance of this tract and its exposition of the theory of the four cardinal humours should not be allowed to disguise the fact that this was very much a minority view, even within the Corpus, and was, as we shall see, disputed by many later writers. If it shares many of its features with other treatises on medicine from the fifth and fourth centuries, it should not be forgotten that it also displays many others that are peculiarly its own, not least its anatomy and its theory of the four humours.

Deliberately relegating *The Nature of Man* to the status of one treatise among many emphasises the variety of ideas about health and illness put forward within the Hippocratic Corpus and by other doctors writing or talking at the time. They reveal an ongoing debate, a new understanding, if not a new discovery, of the body, with authors developing or contradicting the ideas of others, or putting forward totally new theories. Some writers are more philosophically inclined than others; others roundly condemn such idle speculation. Some favour what we might consider very odd notions indeed; others hold views that can easily be made to correspond with such modern ideas as homoeostasis and individual resistance to disease; others pay more attention to numbers than to the individual patient. But together they offer an insight into a vibrant intellectual world of Classical Greece in which authors from as far afield as Metapontum and Sardis, Cos and Croton debate the same questions, and formulate their own answers. The diversity of standpoints found in the medical writings of the late fifth and early fourth centuries is arguably greater than that in any other comparable block of Classical Greek literature. To concentrate on one theory or on those believed to be most closely associated with one man, Hippocrates, is to miss what are surely the most significant features of this medicine, its intellectual vitality and variety.

6

HIPPOCRATIC PRACTICES

Theoretical pronouncements notwithstanding, the Hippocratic physician was first and foremost a craftsman plying his trade.[1] He, and it was almost always he, might work from his own house, which thus served as his surgery or 'medical workshop', and remain largely within his own community, or he might, like Homer's craftsman–doctor, travel in search of patients.[2] He might practise alone, or in company with others, travelling around familiar territory or wandering further afield as a total stranger.[3] With one exception, his income depended on finding patients prepared to pay for his services, supplemented by whatever else he might gain from his property or estates, if he had any. That exception was some form of state service, whether as a doctor with the army or navy on campaign or as a so-called 'public doctor'. If Herodotus is to be believed, there was already a system of public doctors in Aegina and Athens by the late sixth century, for Democedes held such a post in both cities.[4] But there is then a gap in the historical record of a century or so, and the most detailed evidence does not appear until Hellenistic times. To judge from this later information, the presence of a public doctor was no welfare state *avant la lettre*. Certain physicians, in Athens chosen by the assembly, received what amounted to a retaining fee to reside in the community and be on hand to treat the citizens.[5] Whether their contract compelled them to offer treatment for nothing is a vexed question: their tombstones and the honorary decrees that record their distinguished service show that they did so at times, but it is more likely that free treatment was left to the doctors' own discretion than that it was legally imposed on them.[6] Social pressures in a small community might compel a doctor to treat the poorest citizens for nothing, but he is unlikely to have been willing to do the same always for the rich, or for non-citizens. Nor is there any need to assume that he had in the fifth century also the contractual duty of assisting at inquests or other official occasions on which a doctor might be called for (situations known from Graeco-Roman Egypt), or that the role of an expert witness in court was confined to public doctors.[7]

State service, however, was an option for only a small number of physicians; the others, along with midwives, bone-setters, herbalists and the like, had to rely on what they could gain by their own efforts. They faced competition, as we have seen, from various quarters, and it would be rash to assume that if self-help failed to work the patient always went out immediately to seek a doctor.[8] In such circumstances it was crucial for a doctor to make a good impression on his potential patient. He needed to be able to speak well, in terms of both content and style – the late text *Precepts* jokes that he should nevertheless avoid the flowers of poetry, since that might betoken time ill spent, away from medicine – to avoid being outclassed by those who were just good speakers.[9] First impressions counted for a great deal: a well-stocked and appointed surgery, a neat bandage on another patient, a sound pronouncement about the sort of disease likely to be met with in the locality, appropriate dress and behaviour, an avowed willingness to help, but, at the same time, a reluctance to go too far with rash procedures that might end up damaging or even killing the patient.[10] The comic poet Alexis joked that even one's dialect mattered: an Athenian doctor who prescribed beetroot using its Attic name would be despised, but a non-Athenian who used the Ionic or Doric form would be highly respected.[11] All these would help to create trust on the part of the patient, and trust, as the author of *Prognostic* stressed, was an essential element in the struggle against disease. In this struggle there were three protagonists: disease, patient and doctor.[12] It was up to the patient to choose whether to collaborate with the doctor or to fight his or her disease unaided. In turn, the doctor could not succeed without gaining the patient's co-operation, whether as informant or as the willing, competent and compliant recipient of his advice.[13]

How was this trust to be created and maintained? Ludwig Edelstein, in a famous chapter, pointed to the importance of prognosis in Greek medicine in the fifth and fourth centuries as the primary way in which the doctor could establish his credentials and, at the same time, protect himself against accusations of malpractice.[14] By being able to predict the likely outcome of a disease, and by announcing it beforehand to the patient's relatives and friends, he could gain obvious credit for a cure, particularly if things took the course he said, and, second, should the patient die, he had a strong defence if he had already announced that this was a likely outcome. Success in a doubtful case would add even more to his laurels; while failure would be better tolerated by a patient's family already prepared for the worst.[15]

But even within the Hippocratic Corpus one can find dissatisfaction with this 'tactical' use of prognosis as both advertising and insurance.[16] The author of *Prorrhetic* 2 opens his tract with an ironic account of splendid and marvellous cases of prognosis that he has witnessed or been told about. He describes doctors arriving at the bedside to give a second opinion and immediately predicting a recovery, but accompanied by paralysis or blindness, or, while passing through the marketplace, telling this or that trader that they will die or go mad.[17] A serious illness they might blame on a minor divagation from an athlete's training programme. This type of prediction and explanation the author rejects as mere 'mantic', 'divination', not true prognosis, and he strongly denies that this is what he himself is doing.[18] He is prepared to accept that some of these extravagant predictions do come true, but that is only because their maker has correctly identified and interpreted the important signs that any good doctor should know, or because the disease, which when the first doctor arrived had not yet established itself, has done so in the meantime, and is now easier to prognose. What matters, in his opinion, is accurate prediction, understanding the important indicators, and then drawing sober conclusions from them.[19] How one predicts has thus as important a role to play as what one predicts, and the patient is subtly warned against those whose claims might not be backed up by results.[20] This author, like that of *Prognostic*, allows the possibility of distinguishing between foreknowledge, prognosis in the strict sense of the term, and foretelling, but he regards such a distinction as irrelevant to medical practice. One cannot make a sound statement about the future without sound foreknowledge, and only a fool would choose to be swayed by the manner of the pronouncement rather than its potential accuracy.[21]

As this author implies, prognosis is more than a tactical device to impress patients: it is central to the practice of medicine as seen by many writers of the Corpus. It is essential to the understanding and treatment of the individual patient, ensuring that whatever is prescribed will be appropriate for that patient and his or her condition.[22] It is more than just predicting how a disease is likely to progress and whether the outcome is going to be favourable or unfavourable. It provides a way of controlling the disease, of modifying, if necessary, treatment in accordance with a predicted pattern, and of focusing on what each individual patient requires. It offers a claim to understanding that marks the doctor off from many other types of healers, and, if practised correctly, it enables the true doctor to intervene effectively and quickly even in the most dangerous of acute diseases.[23] In short, the doctor who professes the art of prognosis declares that his particular technique deals with the past, present and future of his patient, a bold claim incorporating what today would be termed obtaining the case history, diagnosis and prognosis.[24]

Advice on how to prognosticate appears in several different forms in the Corpus. Sometimes, as in *Aphorisms*, *Coan Prognoses*, *Dentition* and *Prorrhetic* 1, it is presented as short aphorisms, memorable sentences or apophthegms that can apply generally to all cases.[25] *Prognostic* and *Airs, Waters and Places* are avowedly longer guides to the practice of prognosis, the first treating it in general terms, the second specifically in a way that will prepare a travelling doctor for arrival in a new town. The *Epidemics* represent an intermediate stage, in which case notes are selected and organised according to their potential usefulness for prognosis. Individual case histories are rewritten in a form that allows them both to be incorporated within the *Constitutions* and to serve as a data bank for future comparison.[26] In addition, the author specifies what the doctor should consider the most significant features of any illness, the so-called signs, which the author of *Prorrhetic* 2 also judged to be an effective basis for a decision about the future course of a disease and the treatment of the patient.[27]

The author of *Epidemics* 1 gave a long list of such features: the common nature of all things and the particular nature of the individual; the disease and the patient; the regimen prescribed and the prescriber; the constitution of the heavens and the region, in general and in particular; the custom, way of life, practices and age; talk, manner, silence, thoughts, sleeping or not; dreams, plucking, scratching, tearing; exacerbations, stools, urines, sputa, vomit; the stages of a disease and its potential for crisis and death; and sweat, rigor, chill, cough, sneezes, hiccoughs, flatulence, haemorrhoids and haemorrhages.[28]

These symptoms lie at 'the threshold of the seen and unseen'.[29] Some of what should be looked for fits neatly with modern diagnostics and involves shrewd, careful and accurate observation, relying on all the senses: the pattern of the remission and relapse of fevers; any sudden change, especially in the altering of consciousness;[30] the sound; in both quantity and quality, of a patient's breathing; the possibility that a blow to one side of the head may show itself in an impaired function on the other;[31] the signs of suppuration and discoloration that portend serious wound infection; and changes in the way in which the fingers are held. The so-called *facies Hippocratica* (the 'Hippocratic face') that is described in graphic detail in *Prognostic* still remains an excellent indication of the imminence of death.[32] Other signs have fallen out of use, notably what has been termed 'carphology', the way in which a sick patient appears to pluck imaginary objects from the immediate surroundings, even though the phenomena can still be seen in hospitals and old people's homes.[33] Others seem to depend more on an underlying prejudice than on any clinical judgment. The often articulated belief, persisting into very recent times, that children born in the eighth month of pregnancy were almost certain to die whereas those born in the seventh generally lived is impossible to sustain on the basis of modern statistics of infant deaths, let alone in a society where the length and beginning of pregnancy were far from agreed or easy to determine.[34] Although numbers do play a role in establishing a prognosis, in this instance the numbers may be here to serve an exculpatory purpose: no one was at fault if this baby died, for it was born after the most unfavourable period of gestation.[35]

This emphasis on close observation of signs and symptoms, leading to an understanding of their cause and then to their recording as a guide to what might happen in the future, is not confined to strictly medical literature. The historian Thucydides follows such a pattern in his wide-ranging account of the plague of Athens, and demonstrates at the same time considerable acquaintance with the techniques and vocabulary of contemporary medicine.[36] Indeed, his whole history, with its emphasis on seeking an understanding of the causes of the conflict and its wish to make of it a record for future consultation in similar conflicts, shows that medical ideas might

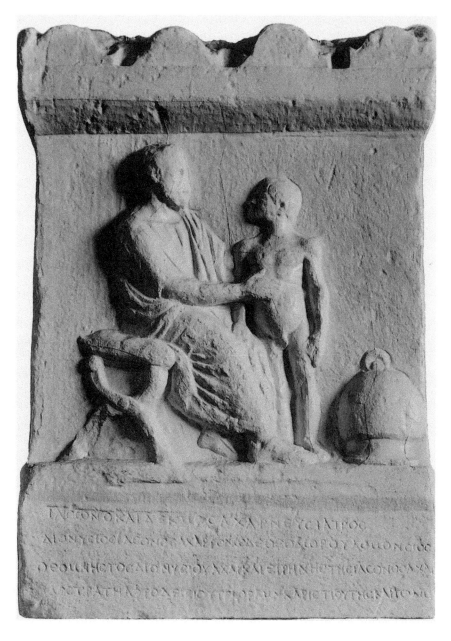

Figure 6.1 Marble tombstone of an Athenian physician called Jason, shown examining the swollen belly of a child. British Museum, Reg. No. 1865,0103.3. © The Trustees of the British Museum. *IG* 2² 4513.

have an impact among intellectuals that transcended a specifically medical theme.[37] Similarly, Plato attributes to the true statesman the same ability to understand the past and control the future as the doctor, and often uses analogies between medicine and politics.[38] It would, however, be unwise to attribute this influence solely to Hippocrates and to any single tract or group of tracts, for this prognostic tendency can be found throughout the Corpus and, as *Prorrhetic* 2 reminds us, was current among other doctors who have left no written memorial.

But the search for prognostic knowledge had its limitations, as may be seen in the case histories selected in the *Epidemics*. While a variety of symptoms are listed, even extending over several months, one of the aims of the author is to try to seek patterns of remission and relapse. He focuses on times of crisis, when the fate of the patient is being decided, at least temporarily, and attempts to measure the number of days between each crisis, presumably as a guide to linking various groups of fever symptoms together.[39] But there is no real case history: the past does not extend back beyond when the patient began to fall ill, and there is no general awareness that the patient's other illnesses at a different time might have had long-term consequences. Nor is the differential diagnosis performed along modern lines. Today's doctor seeks out distinctive symptoms in order to mark this cause of illness out from that, until a specific enough cause has been identified and it or its consequences can thereby be eliminated or forestalled.[40] The Hippocratic physician was less interested in distinguishing between diseases as such or in identifying a specific cause than in dividing important from unimportant symptom groups so as to discover the underlying inner changes within the individual body that constitute that person's disease. He was concerned with individual disposition, not individual cause. The differentiation occurs at the level of the patient, not the disease, for although all mankind reacts in the same general way to changes in weather or diet, the doctor must be able to separate the general from the individual and see just what is wrong with the individual patient.[41] In looking back, the doctor does not compare the past illnesses of the patient with the present, but, it is hoped, what the patient was like in health with what he or she is like in disease: the greater the divergence from this norm, the more gravely ill the patient.[42]

Once the doctor has established what is wrong with the patient, a decision has to be taken as to whether to treat or not. Although opponents of medicine might complain that doctors ought to be able to treat all sufferers, even those in severe distress, many, if not all, of the writers in the Hippocratic Corpus saw nothing wrong in refusing to intervene.[43] The author of *Prorrhetic* 2 forbade intervention when the patient had lost consciousness from a wound, or was delirious, or had suffered such a gash that recovery was unlikely.[44] For the writer of *The Art*, this was to acknowledge the powerlessness of the doctor in the face of some conditions, as well as avoiding unnecessary harm by futile intervention.[45] Plato, indeed, saw in this refusal an excellent example of true craftsmanship, a judicious acceptance of the limits of one's art.[46] Such a decision, however, still left the possibility open that someone else might judge the case curable, or at least capable of palliation. Some might think intervention a risk worth taking, for the patient might recover, and, if not, would have died anyway, and there were always social pressures to do something.[47] Even in a compound fracture, where success was extremely rare and where surgery might only exacerbate the situation, one might be forced to take action simply to avoid being thought incompetent.[48] But provided that treatment has not been recklessly or poorly carried out, the writers in the Corpus agree that the patient's death is no fault of the doctor. Nor is he to blame if the patient becomes bored with waiting for a fracture to heal properly and starts walking too early, with the result that the cure remains incomplete.[49]

Once a decision has been made to treat the patient the doctor has to decide on appropriate methods, including even surgery. Cutting and burning had long been seen as major weapons of the doctor, and the cupping glass figures prominently on the monument of the sixth-century doctor in the Basle Museum (Figure 6.2).[50] Despite the ban on cutting in the *Oath* and the willingness of the author of the *Physician* to defer to others experienced in dealing with war wounds, there can be little doubt that such procedures were expected of many practitioners.[51] Removing blood is a normal procedure for the author of *The Nature of Man*, and he gives a list of points where bleeding can be performed, advising that they should be opened as far away as possible from the site of the pain or swelling so as to avoid a major shock at the site and to prevent the blood from accumulating in the same spot.[52] Bloodletting, however, carried its own risks, and was practised only on those able to stand it. But, when necessary, and as a last resort, a patient might be bled so vigorously that he fainted.[53] Whether bleeding brought any therapeutic benefit was disputed even in Antiquity, and modern studies based on relatively rare conditions are unhelpful.[54] But swabbing the area to be cut with wine, as ancient doctors recommended, has been shown to reduce the chance of wound infection, and a small incision followed by cupping would probably have been reasonably safe.[55]

Cauterising with caustic drugs or hot irons, however, was very much a last resort, although the author of *Diseases 2* recommends it against a recurrent headache, and the author of *Internal Affections* claims that a series of twelve cauterisations at different points of the body will stop the flow of harmful bile and phlegm around the body. Some doctors used cauterisation for eye problems; others to help fix a dislocated shoulder in place.[56] But the risks were great. Too much use of the cautery might cause the scars to run into one another, or prevent the head of the humerus from fitting into the shoulder socket.[57] The outcome might even be fatal. Eupolemus from Oeniadae died covered in scars after various unsuccessful attempts to cauterise an abscess; the author sadly remarks that if other ways of stopping the flow of pus had been tried he might well have lived.[58]

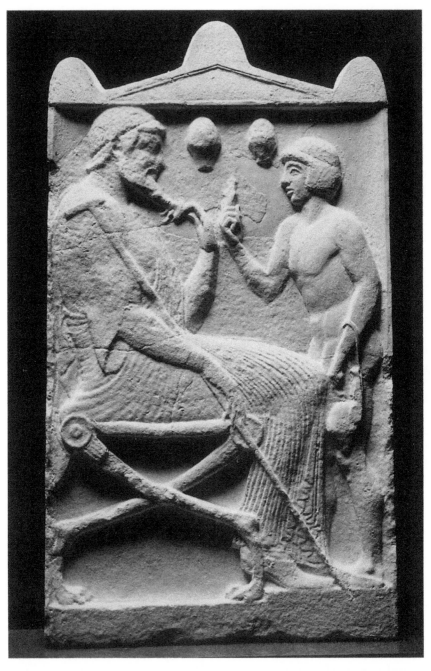

Figure 6.2 A Greek relief (*c.*480 BC) showing a doctor. The two objects are cupping glasses. Basle, Antikenmuseum Basel und Sammlung Lugwig, inv. BS 236. Photo: Andreas F. Voegelin.

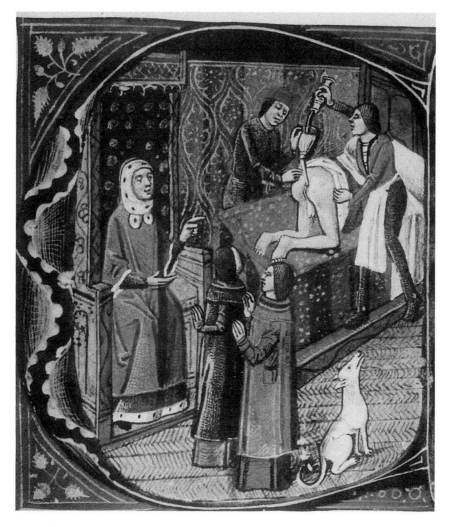

Figure 6.3 Galen orders the administration of a clyster. Dresden, Sächsische Landesbibliothek, Db 93, fol. 392v.

Where one might draw the line between sensible risk and reckless show-manship is neatly stated in *Joints*. In this book, as in *Fractures* and *Method of Reduction*, the author displays a broad understanding of the principles of orthopaedics.[59] He gives very sound advice about how to set simple fractures and how to reduce dislocation. He is annoyed with those who confuse a pain-ful but temporary hairline fracture of the epiphysis of a spinal vertebra with the far more troublesome dislocation of the vertebra, for his own knowledge of the spine is clearly based on long experience of touching, feeling and manipulating it. Treating slipped discs and dislocated elbows might be a matter of technique, but, at times, strength is required, from both the doctor and his assistant, supplemented even by instruments, a wooden beam or the Hippocratic bench.[60] This was a large bench, to which the patient could be strapped and braced while the dislocated limb was pulled upwards or outwards so that it could return to its original setting in the joint. Such a heavy piece of equipment could hardly be transported along the tracks of Greece, and shows how orthopaedic surgery was becoming urbanised.[61] The use of such machines or aids is recommended by the author of *Joints*, but he has his strong doubts about the wisdom of the procedure known as succussion. In order to reduce curvature of the spine, the patient is tied head down to a ladder, which is then dropped perpendicularly from roof height, either with the help of assistants or even using a block and pulley, but this is heavy and expensive. This procedure draws the crowds, eager to see the spectacle and not caring what the result will be. But, remarks the author sourly, he has never seen anyone benefit from this sort of treatment, which is little more than charlatanry.[62]

A similarly high level of practical expertise is also found in *Head Wounds*, where the author shows himself to be familiar with a wide range of skull fractures and with the practicalities of trephining (removing bone from the skull). He is aware of the injuries typical of a wide range of weapons and instruments, and of the relative dangers if the head has been hit at the front, side or back.[63] His use of a black solution smeared over the skull, left to soak in and then washed away to reveal clearly any fracture lines, is an ingenious and effective ploy when the extent of the injury is hard to determine, and one would like to know if this was the author's own idea.[64] But, although the author is himself experienced, he envisages some of his medical readers as less effective at operating in practice, and choosing instead to work alongside a specialist in trephining or wound surgery.[65]

His reader is expected to be able to diagnose, to apply bandages and poultices, but to be unwilling or unable to perform the actual surgery easily. His principal remedies are thus likely to have been the two standbys of diet and drugs. One of the distinctive features of Greek medicine is its insistence on dietetics as central to all therapeutics.[66] Indeed, the author of *Ancient Medicine* could even suggest that medicine originated in cookery and was developed over a long period by a careful observance of reactions to particular foods, even if the medical art now included more than this.[67] In its earliest form dietetics was concerned largely with the administration of foodstuffs in a hierarchy of liquids, gruels and solids to match the perceived degree of severity of the illness, and there are hints that, as in Babylonian and Egyptian medicine, the patient was initially kept without food or on the lightest of diets.[68] But Greek ideas on medical dietetics developed far beyond this in the middle or late fifth century BC.[69] Plato associated this development with Herodicus of Selymbria, whose expertise as a gymnastic trainer had led him to include both food and physical exercise in a regime designed for the improvement as well as the conservation of health.[70] If he is the Herodicus mentioned in the Anonymus Londinensis papyrus, which is far from certain on many grounds, he would have been acquainted with contemporary philosophical and medical ideas, and able to articulate them in a form acceptable to intellectuals.[71] Plato might disapprove of this 'new-fangled medicine which coddles disease', but many swiftly followed the fashion, including Democritus.[72] Indeed, Hippocrates was believed by later authors to have been a pupil of Herodicus and to have developed his ideas still further.[73] Certainly, texts preserved in the Hippocratic Corpus such as *Regimen*, *Nutriment* and *Regimen in Acute Diseases* place a high value on dietetics as the safest way of treating disease and recommend that the doctor should use diet from the very onset of the illness as part of the therapeutic process.[74] The author of *The Art* went so far as to consider the physician's skill in curing by diet the surest proof that medicine was an art, since regulating the balance between competing elements in this way was extremely difficult.[75] But, while one can accept that the scope of dietetics changed considerably in the lifetime of Hippocrates, the varied theoretical positions taken by the authors of these tracts suggest caution in attributing this to the influence of Hippocrates alone, and, still more, in using this evidence to prove that he had actually studied with Herodicus.

But the new dietetics also demanded an understanding of diet in a much wider context than before. It now encompassed far more than foodstuffs, and indeed embraced practically every aspect of one's lifestyle, including one's dreams.[76] It provided detailed and complex rules whereby one might regulate one's life in general throughout the year.[77] It now required for its proper performance a broad knowledge of cosmology as well as of medicine, and its demands for health to take precedence over all other considerations could have been put into practice only by a rich and leisured class, however much its advocates might claim to be writing for everyone.[78] The practitioner or his client now needed to know in greater detail how foodstuffs worked and how they fitted into a general picture. Hence, the author of *Regimen* listed at length what foodstuffs in his opinion cooled or heated the body, or were easily digestible or likely to lead to flatulence. In Book 3 he described the occasions when diet can be used to correct diseases brought on by over-exercise, and, reciprocally, how exercise can be used to modify the mistakes of diet.[79] Dietetics is not yet an entirely independent speciality, the third part of medicine along with surgery and pharmaceutics, but it is already on the way to achieving that status.

The therapeutic principles behind the use of diet are the same as those for bleeding and for drugs: indeed, whether to call a substance a food or a drug is at times almost entirely subjective. Given that the sick body is in some way out of balance, it must be brought back into balance either by removing whatever is in excess or by building up whatever is deficient. Cure is thus to be achieved allopathically, by the application of treatments that will have the opposite effect from the present condition.[80] Hence the importance of the lists of the qualities of foodstuffs given by the author of *Regimen*, and of the innumerable 'powers' assigned to foods in *Ancient Medicine*.[81] The actions of drugs are seen as contributing to the cure of a disease only in so far as they help to restore the balance in concert with other types of therapy and can be related to the requirements of the individual. Formulae such as 'If you wish to use' or 'You may use' and the regular reiteration of the need to refer any therapy to the patient's ability to withstand any of its side-effects give the doctor a substantial freedom in deciding which, if any, drugs to administer. This relativity thus can be distinguished from the treatment offered by 'rootcutters' and 'druggists', who provided specific remedies for a condition, allegedly effective no matter what the age or sex of the patient. Given this lack of differentiation, it is no wonder that the same word for drug, *pharmakon*, could be used to indicate a substance that could both kill and cure.[82]

Hippocratic pharmacology, however, presents a variety of problems of interpretation.[83] It is not that the more than 380 plant names in the Corpus and the much smaller number of animal and mineral substances cannot be identified, for most of them can, at least generically.[84] Nor is the difficulty that we are ignorant of the ways in which many or all of these substances work: scammony, for instance, is a familiar purgative, pomegranate rind an astringent, dill a carminative that would indeed 'relax the stomach'.[85] The juice of the squirting cucumber contains elaterin, a powerful cathartic, which is likely to have had some effect when prescribed as an aid to bringing on a birth quickly or as an abortifacient.[86] But sometimes the fit between ancient practice and modern herbalism is less exact. Some substances are not always prescribed for the purposes for which a modern herbalist would use them: linseed oil, a familiar laxative, is not recommended as such in the Hippocratic Corpus, but is used as a drink for 'uterine suffocation', as a clyster for 'uterine disorders' and in an ointment to soften the uterine orifice in order to correct sterility.[87] In none of these uses would it have produced the desired effect: it would lubricate and perhaps soften, but it would not cure sterility or diseases of the womb. Many of the animal substances recommended would also be unlikely to bring any direct benefit, or only over a very long term: the eating of goat's liver as a cure for menorrhagia would restore levels of iron and reduce anaemia but not immediately.[88]

This is of particular relevance when dealing with women's diseases, for the gynaecological treatises contain a long series of remedies for amenorrhoea, menorrhagia and other uterine complaints.[89] In this they differ from many other medical treatises, where a listing of diseases and their treatments is limited at best. The pharmacological treatment of women's diseases is also often strikingly different from that for men, containing far more exotic ingredients and what is known in German as *Dreckapothek* – foul, often excremental, substances. While the value of many drugs recorded in the non-gynaecological treatises can often be demonstrated with the aid of modern pharmacognosy, this is less true for the therapies for women's diseases. Here it is often their symbolic function that takes precedence: the same types of plant used in ritual purification, such as squill and agnus castus, fumigate and clean the womb. Dirt, which pollutes, is also magically powerful, and may be required to overcome the polluting menses.[90] Even the squirting cucumber, whose purgative properties are well established, may have been used as an emmenagogue or an oxytocic as much for symbolic as for practically evaluated reasons: its capacity to eject its seeds forcefully made it an appropriate plant to use when wishing to expel an unwanted conception, an afterbirth or a suppressed menstrual period.[91]

Drugs, then, may have been used in therapy for reasons other than those approved of by a modern pharmacognosist, but, given the placebo effect, even substances that are, in modern terms, clinically inert may be of value when given (and accepted) within the right environment.[92] The anthropologist's notion of a healing act being more than diagnosis and therapy, but focusing on the rituals and expectations of all the parties, can be easily applied to the ancient world, and especially to the conjunction of drugs and incantations.[93] Modern ideas of chemical efficacy, although not to be despised, may tell us very little about the effectiveness of cures, and still less about the relative merits of a variety of suggestions for curing the same condition. Placing a hot-water bottle over one's forehead is still a common home remedy for a headache, but we would draw the line at venesection and cautery, however much one might imagine it to help.[94] Other drug treatments combine the obviously efficient with a symbolic reasoning. Pains in the loins (thought to be the result of excess) can be cured, according to one of the *Coan Prognoses*, by giving the patient doses of hellebore, a violent emetic: he will then vomit up frequent and copious amounts of 'foamy stuff', entirely appropriate for a region close to the genitals.[95]

But even if a plant or mineral was recognised as having medical value there were many variables that might reduce its effect in any given case. As the author of *Epidemics* 2 put it cryptically:

We know the characteristics of drugs, from which ones come which kind of things. For they are not all equally good, but different characteristics are good in different circumstances. In different places medicinal drugs are gathered earlier or later; also the preparations differ, such as drying, crushing, boiling and so on †(I pass over most things)†; and how much for each person and in what diseases and when in the disease, in relation to age, appearance, regimen, what kind of season, what season and how it is developing and the like.[96]

This represents both a claim on the part of the doctor to specific knowledge, that of how to adjust the drug accurately for the individual patient, and an acceptance that there might be many obstacles in the way of achieving this aim.

This consciousness of the limitations of drug therapy may explain several features of Hippocratic medicine. On the whole it operates with broad categories – purgatives, caustics, emollients and so on – which thus allow for a wide range of specific alternatives in treatment.[97] Dosage is rarely precise: 'as and when necessary' is a common and far from foolish stipulation, and the amounts to be taken cannot always be expressed in a modern notation of grams and grains.[98] The size of a 'bean' was as much a variable as the amount of oil-and-wine mixture into which soda, castoreum or sagapenum and asphalt were stirred before being given to expel a troublesome afterbirth.[99] But two points should be borne in mind here. There is evidence from the early drug recipes in the Corpus to suggest that a substantial margin of error was allowed for, and that treatments that seemed to reduce that margin were stigmatised as very dangerous, even when they continued to remain in the literature – Petron's fever treatment (see p. 73), for example, is commented on very unfavourably by later authorities, although they continue to record it.[100] Second, most of the herbal substances employed, with a few exceptions such as hellebore, were not likely to be immediately toxic and their side-effects might appear only very gradually after a prolonged course of treatment.[101] In acute diseases, which are for the most part what concern Hippocratic doctors, consideration of such side-effects would be unnecessary or irrelevant, for the patient would have either died or recovered long before they showed themselves. Nonetheless, the doctors themselves are aware of the possibility of failure and of iatrogenic disaster, whatever its cause, and are at times willing to hold up their own mistakes for censure.[102]

But how far did their ministrations extend across the whole community of the Greek city, free, slave and non-citizen alike? Although Plato in his *Laws* made a theoretical division of doctors into slaves and non-slaves, each treating their own group, he also accepted that the free-born doctor would also treat the non-free, a situation confirmed by texts across the Corpus.[103] The cases in the *Epidemics* include one of a newly bought slave and another where the patient had been branded as a runaway.[104] Socrates, according to Xenophon, expected the average slave-owner to call in a doctor whenever one of the slaves fell ill.[105] The *Epidemics* also shows members of all classes of society being treated by the doctor, from a potter, a carpenter, a vinedresser and a sailor right up to a ship's captain and a local magistrate.[106] In the (later) texts in the Corpus that deal with the problems of payment for services, it is expected that some of these humbler patients will not be able to pay much, or indeed anything at all, and that in such circumstances free treatment is both called for and, ultimately, profitable as establishing the doctor's kindness, generosity and love of his art.[107]

Women are also treated in the *Epidemics* by male physicians, and the gynaecological treatises of the Corpus were almost certainly written by and for men. The author of *Diseases* 4, which concerns digestion, also reveals himself to have been the author of *Generation* and *The Nature of the Child*, and is in all probability the source of much information preserved in *Diseases of Women* 1.[108] At the same time, there is also an understandable reluctance on the part of women to talk about their intimate problems directly with a male physician.[109] Phaedra's nurse in Euripides' play *Hippolytus* draws a distinction between some injury that Phaedra ought to discuss with the male doctor and a more specifically female ailment for which she and the women in the chorus can offer help.[110] But whether there were women doctors and what that might mean in the context of fifth- and fourth-century Greece are matters of considerable controversy. The story of the first *obstetrix*, Hagnodike, recorded by the Roman author Hyginus about AD 150, is an obvious aetiological myth.[111] According to Hyginus, there were no such practitioners in Athens because women and slaves were forbidden to learn the art of medicine until Hagnodike, 'a pupil of Herophilus', who disguised herself as a man. When later tried for this crime and in danger of being condemned to death, she was saved by the protests of the Athenian mothers she had attended. Their husbands in the Areopagus relented, and the law was changed.[112] The chronological, legal and social difficulties in Hyginus' account defy any amount of special pleading to turn it into historical fact. It is also largely irrelevant in a society when, as often elsewhere, assisting at birth was not always a full-time occupation and where such craft-type skills were gained by attendance, observation and experience far more than by going off to study with a famous teacher.

More credence has been given to Plato's comment that elderly women, mothers themselves and beyond childbearing age, were the only ones to act as midwives, *maiai*, in late fifth-century Athens, and that they possessed their own special knowledge of herbs, chants and charms to assist in the birth process or to procure an abortion.[113] The second part of this comment is undoubtedly true, but the first does not fit entirely easily with what is recorded in the Hippocratic Corpus. There is plenty of evidence for male doctors attending births (and not only in difficult cases, for they report their experiences with 'normal' pregnancies as a guide to distinguishing anything abnormal) and even carrying out vaginal investigations themselves.[114] But they also seem to have made regular use of the knowledge and experience of such women as Phanostrate, '*maia* and doctor', whose funeral monument, from the late fourth century, is a masterpiece of elegance, a sure sign of wealth.[115] There is no doubt that Phanostrate's expertise as a 'doctor' (*iatros*, exactly the same word as for a male doctor) was seen by those who set up her monument as extending beyond that of a *maia* (although in what way remains unclear), and it is plausible to think that other women who are said to be 'doctoring' patients did more than just attend to births, perhaps dealing with a wide range of complaints of women and children. As with male practitioners, one can imagine a spectrum of activities that ranged from part-time work as a birthing attendant, through giving advice in earlier stages of pregnancy, to dealing with a whole range of conditions, not just those confined to women or children. The wife in Xenophon's *Household Manager* had the task of watching over the health and treatment of her husband's slaves, and presumably made no distinction between them on grounds of their gender.[116] Where one drew the line between a *maia* and a 'mediciner' was a personal one, since there were no laws that defined either profession.

A more difficult question is whether Phanostrate's medical attentions were given solely to women, children and members of her household, or whether males might seek her out. One should not exclude this possibility, for there is later Roman and Hellenistic evidence that suggests that some women also treated men, although social pressures and expectations would have restricted any such services to only a few men.[117] Xenophon's housewife, and one suspects many others like her, had the overall responsibility for the health of all the household, and would have been the first person called on to treat minor injuries and 'normal' ailments. There are also later references to women making and selling their own remedies in public, and not just for 'women's diseases'.

Had Xenophon's housewife been able to read, she too would have been able to draw on the therapeutic procedures outlined and discussed in the various treatises of the Hippocratic Corpus.[118] She would have been at home with many of its analogies, of the body's fluids bubbling, congealing and mixing together as in a kitchen;[119] of the doctor, like the good cook, knowing just at what crucial point, or crisis, to intervene; of the procedures for treatment, part written, but often empirically observed and handed down within the family; and of all the myriad of things that might go wrong when dealing with refractory material. She too, like many of the writers of the Corpus, would proceed optimistically, expecting events to happen in a regular pattern, and she too would exercise all her senses in running a proper household.

What is striking about the therapeutic practices within the Corpus is their great variety, akin to the variety of theoretical explanations contained in it and the relative freedom given to the practitioner to choose between them. While one can talk of a hierarchy of preferred treatments, they have not as yet developed the rigid stratifications of later periods. Dietetics has not yet taken the central place in therapeutics that it was to occupy a century or so later, and the decision whether to operate surgically or not is left to the individual's conscience and his understanding of his own ability with the knife. Philanthropy, and a generous safety zone, may have encouraged the doctor to intervene even if he could not offer any lasting benefit. But, above all, there is an awareness of the individuality of the patient. It is not just that, for many authors, the difficult part of medicine is being able to judge precisely what is happening in each patient, to distinguish the individual from the general, and from that starting point to choose the most appropriate therapy for each patient. It is also that human beings do not always respond to doctors in the ways in which books say they ought, and that even the best treatment may fail because of mistakes or negligence on the part of the patient. The Hippocratic writers were always aware that patient care, one might say, depends for its success both on the quality of the care and on the quality of the patient.

RELIGION AND MEDICINE IN FIFTH- AND FOURTH-CENTURY GREECE

On a remote hilltop in southern Greece stands one of the most beautiful of all ancient temples. The temple of Apollo at Bassae was built by the architect Ictinus at the expense of the small town of Phigaleia around 425 BC.[1] The cost of building this temple, transporting the marble a considerable distance up the mountain and arranging for carving and decorations of superb quality would have been enormous, certainly, one might imagine, far more than the resources easily available to an unimportant town in the middle of a war. Pausanias, our ancient informant, links the dedication to Apollo Epikourios (the Bringer of Help) with dedications made in Athens at the same time to Apollo Alexikakos (the Warder-off of Evil) in an endeavour to put an end to the great plague.[2] Pausanias' instincts, if not his arguments, were sound.[3] Plague, as the historian Thucydides had already noted, has an impact upon religion as much as upon medicine. Just as a sick individual might have recourse to a god for assistance, so the leaders of a community suffering from a widespread disease might appeal for divine aid or advice. In 426, when there was a recurrence of plague at Athens, the authorities took advice from an oracle and purified the island of Delos, sacred to Apollo, by removing from it all dead bodies, forbidding all future burials on the island and reinstating a long-decayed festival of Apollo and Artemis.[4] At about the same time, the shrine of the daughters of Leos, who had delivered Athens centuries before from plague, seems to have been refurbished after years of neglect. Outside the city, in the deme of Melite a shrine was set up to Hercules Alexikakos (the Warder-off of Evil), whose cult statue was carved by Ageladas, one of the leading sculptors of the day.[5] And, within a decade at most, a completely new healing god had been introduced into Athens, Asclepius.[6]

The burgeoning of the cult of Asclepius in the late fifth century BC is arguably as significant a development in the history of medicine as the contemporary ferment of medical theories that were later included in the Hippocratic Corpus. Asclepius came to be seen as the healing god *par excellence*, and the methods of healing favoured in his cult, principally incubation (seeking visions while sleeping in a temple), have often been regarded by historians as typifying all religious healing in ancient Greece and Rome. But, this chapter will argue, it would be wrong to view this development as a conservative reassertion of traditional values in a world where religious explanations for illness were being replaced by others that stressed connections within the natural world. The relationship between religious and secular healing, and between their practitioners, is far too complex to fit a neat opposition between religion and medicine, not least because, as we have already seen, Asclepius and his family were described in literature as secular healers, and, if Ludwig Edelstein was right in his speculations, they gained divine status precisely because of their healing skills.[7]

The earliest stories about Asclepius are confusing and conflicting. Homer mentions the hero Asclepius and his two sons Podalirius and Machaon in the *Iliad*, where they are said to rule over the inhabitants of Tricca, Ithome and Oechalia.[8] Hesiod, writing about the same time, and the slightly later author of the sixteenth *Homeric Hymn* also associate him firmly with Thessaly, where Tricca is situated.[9] But in historic times Ithome and Oechalia were well-known places in Messenia, in the southern Peloponnese, and there was a tradition, of uncertain antiquity, that claimed that a Messenian was the mother of Machaon, if not of Asclepius himself.[10] There was a major healing sanctuary around the tomb of Machaon at Gerenia, and a sanctuary dedicated to his sons at another Messenian town, Pharae.[11] Ancient and modern scholars have tried to resolve the discrepancy, some by discovering an ancient Tricca in Messenia, others by transferring the other two names to Thessaly, or by multiplying the number of divinities called Asclepius. None of these solutions is satisfactory, and it may be wisest to assume that the legend developed in the archaic period with two independent foci.[12] There was yet a third tradition that linked Asclepius with Arcadia in the northern Peloponnese, where he was said to have been brought up as a foundling.[13] The question was not even settled by divine intervention, for, although a poem circulated in Late Antiquity in which Asclepius himself declared that he had been born in Tricca, the oracle of Apollo had pronounced centuries earlier that, although his mother Coronis was a Thessalian, his birthplace was, in fact, Epidaurus. This decision, made in response to a query from an Arcadian, was probably given soon after 369 BC, when Messene was refounded as a city-state after decades of Spartan domination.[14] Although Apollo's decision appears to have satisfied most Greeks, who were by now very familiar with Epidaurus as the most important centre of Asclepius cult, the older traditions lingered on, particularly in Messenia, where the shrine of Asclepius at Messene itself was unusually located right in the middle of the city, as befitted a citizen, not an incomer.[15]

By favouring Epidaurus, the Delphic Oracle was responding to a new situation that had developed over the previous half-century or more. Epidaurus is not mentioned in the earliest versions of the stories about Asclepius, and the account of the Epidaurian legend given by the Roman traveller Pausanias bears all the hallmarks of a late fabrication to explain why Coronis, the daughter of a Thessalian king, should give birth to a son several hundred miles away from her home.[16] For the Roman geographer Strabo, Tricca was the earliest and most famous temple of Asclepius, and Epidaurus merely a celebrated healing shrine.[17] But although there is evidence for an early expansion of the cult, perhaps through association with other local healing cults – Strabo mentions a shrine of Triccan Asclepius at Gerenia in Messenia, and Herondas the mime-writer, around 275 BC, claims that Asclepius had come to Cos direct from Tricca – the shrine at Tricca remained largely local in focus and clientele.[18] On this evidence, the early cult of Asclepius in Thessaly, although concerned with healing, remained largely local in focus and clientele.

By contrast, from the mid-fifth century onwards the cult in its Epidaurian form spread widely, with obvious benefits for Epidaurus itself. The major shrine of the god grew ever richer in consequence. Thrasymedes of Paros was commissioned around 375 BC to carve the cult image, made of ivory and gold and half the size of that of Olympian Zeus at Athens. The round marble Tholos housed two paintings by the famous painter Pausias. Around 350 BC Epidaurus was so wealthy that it could contract with the architect Polyclitus, the builder of the Tholos, to design what to Pausanias was the most elegant theatre he had seen, as well as one of the largest in the ancient world.[19] Games in honour of the god, involving musical and dramatic events, as well as athletic contests, attracted competitors from all over the Greek world.[20]

Our most detailed evidence for the way in which the new cult spread comes from Athens and Attica. The shrine at Zea, in the port of Piraeus, was probably set up around 420 BC, since the implication of Bdelycleon's plan in Aristophanes' *Wasps* to send Philocleon to the island of Aegina to be cured by Asclepius is that in 422 BC, when the play was first performed, this was the nearest temple to his home.[21] When the shrine on Aegina was itself founded is unknown, but it too may not have been of any great antiquity, or, if it was, it was not so important that the cult spread quickly across the bay to Athens itself.

Asclepius arrived in Athens only in 420/419 BC, and was soon joined in his sanctuary on the south side of the Acropolis by Hygieia, although the building of the sanctuary itself, and the planting of a small surrounding grove, was not completed for at least half a dozen years.[22] Distinguished private citizens were among the earliest supporters of the new cult, including the playwright Sophocles, who composed a famous Paean in honour of the god. Popular tradition soon credited him with the introduction of the cult itself into Athens and with being the actual host of the god.[23] In 399 BC the reminder of the dying Socrates to his friends that he still owed a cock to Asclepius excited no surprise as to the object of this obligation, although how it had been incurred and what precisely Socrates meant by it remain obscure.[24] Although the initial impetus towards the introduction of Asclepius into Athens came ostensibly from a private individual, Telemachus, civic involvement is also clear almost from the start.[25] The decision on the siting of the new shrine required official endorsement in the face of a protest by the city's Heralds, and although the first clear-cut evidence for the city's official control of the shrine does not appear until the 340s, this may have begun much earlier.[26]

Athens was not the only city to welcome this new god and the various members of his family, including Hygieia, Panacea and Epione. By the middle of the fourth century his cult was established in many parts of the Greek-speaking world, from Cyrene on the coast of Africa to the island of Thasos in the N. Aegean and from Asia Minor in the East to Sicily in the West.[27] Associations of worshippers of Asclepius are known from across the Greek world from the fourth or third century BC until the third century AD.[28] No other divinity in Classical Greece made so swift or so effective a transition from a mainly local to a pan-Hellenic deity.

Particularly striking is the way in which the cult of Asclepius both co-existed with other cults and superseded them. At Athens, it established links with the Eleusinian Mysteries even before reaching the city. The god stopped at Eleusis on his way to Athens to be initiated into the Eleusinian Mysteries, and, perhaps by 400 BC, a festival called the Epidauria was included in the festival of the Mysteries themselves.[29] Worshippers of Asclepius associated with those of two other local Athenian healing divinities, Dexion and Amynos; the already existing shrine of Amynos may have encouraged the building of that of Asclepius immediately adjacent to it.[30] But elsewhere co-habitation or co-operation was a prelude to annexation. Recorded dedications to Athena Hygieia on the Athenian Acropolis, for instance, cease around 420 BC.[31] On Crete, the shrine of Asclepius at Lebena seems to have been earlier dedicated to Achelous and the Nymphs, and it is possible that before the building of the great temple at Cos in the fourth century the site had formed part of the temple or precinct of Cyparissian Apollo.[32] At Gortys in Arcadia, whose shrine and history has been taken to exemplify the development of Asclepius cult, construction of the shrine of Asclepius was begun in the fourth century in an area already identified with healing. Archaeologists have identified, a short distance above the temple, an older building, probably dating from the fifth century, which may once have been dedicated to the deities of the spring.[33] Even at Epidaurus the original deity of the remote spot where the Asclepieion was built was Apollo Maleatas, whose shrine stands a little way off on a nearby hill. But by 500 BC Asclepius was already becoming the dominant partner.[34] The same pattern of the son of Apollo taking over the healing functions of his father can also be seen at Corinth, Erythrae (on the coast of Asia Minor) and the island of Paros.[35] Why, when and how this takeover took place can be only dimly discerned; although the cult of Asclepius at Corinth may be among the earliest known, dating from the early fifth century, that at Erythrae may not have come into operation until a century later, and that at Paros later still.

But one should not exaggerate the dominance of Asclepius. For one thing, Asclepius was a latecomer, as the siting of his temples demonstrates. They are rarely found within the main religious area in a town centre. Sometimes, as in the Piraeus or at Delos, they are located at the edge of the sea; elsewhere they stand on a river bank outside the walls, and sometimes they are separated by several miles from the town itself. The great temples at Cos and Pergamum are a stiff walk away from the main settlement, beautifully situated amid their groves and with a panoramic view. The temple of Epidaurus is even further away from its town, and few of the thousands of tourists who nowadays visit the remains of the shrine even know of the town's existence, let alone take the opportunity to drive the six or seven miles to see it. The isolation of the temples of Asclepius prompted Plutarch to ask why they should be found in such remote spots, and to suggest that there might be healthful reasons for isolating the sick from those inside the town.[36] Only at Messene is a major Asklepieion located in the centre of the town's main sacral areas, surrounded by all the institutions of public life. But here, as we have already seen (see p. 105), the god was a fellow townsman, allegedly born there and honoured by his fellow citizens in the very centre of their rebuilt town. The god's role here is far more that of a local tutelary god, protecting his own, than that of a universal healer, which may account for the absence of any building specifically devoted to the curing of the sick.[37]

Asclepius co-existed as a healer with many other similar cults. Apollo in particular never lost his functions as a healing god. The inhabitants of Phigaleia dedicated their new temple to Apollo the Bringer of Help, even though there was already a tradition of Asclepius worship in that part of Arcadia.[38] The cult of Apollo Iatros (the Healer) was particularly prominent in the Black Sea region at colonies founded from Miletus in Asia Minor.[39] Indeed, almost simultaneously with the expansion of Asclepius worship within mainland Greece, the cult of Apollo the Healer (Apollo Medicus) was being introduced to Rome in 433 BC.[40] Further south in Italy the cult of Apollo Oulios (a word of doubtful origin, but certainly connected with matters medical) flourished, most notably at Elea/Velia, where the philosopher Parmenides is described as being a descendant of the god, and where a series of doctors bore the name of Oulis.[41] In Attica a wide range of healing deities continued to attract suppliants. An oracle of Apollo from Delphi in 348 ordered the Athenians to sacrifice for the sake of their health to Zeus the Most High, Hercules and Apollo the Protector.[42] Girls and young women made their healing vows to Artemis, Apollo's sister, at Brauron, while a shadowy figure called the Hero Healer was worshipped at a variety of sites both in the city of Athens itself and around Attica, at Marathon, Rhamnous and Eleusis.[43] Who he was was, even at the time, a matter for local conjecture, for he was variously known as Amphilochus, Aristomachus, Oresinius and even Amphiaraus. Amphiaraus, however, had his own sanctuary, with its own incubation rooms, far to the north-east of Attica near Oropus, and it may be the proximity and accessibility of this shrine that prevented the cult of Asclepius from gaining any major foothold in Boeotia.[44] But even if

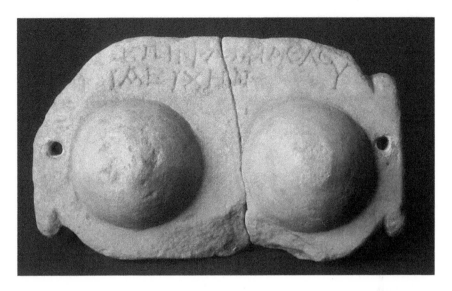

Figure 7.1 A votive offering made to Eilythuia, the Greek goddess of childbirth, Paros, *IG* 12,5,193. London, Science Museum, A163983. Photo © Science Museum/Science & Society Picture Library.

local gods were often aligned with Asclepius and his family, it is important to remember that any divinity had the power to protect and to heal, and that sufferers from illness had a very wide choice of divinities to whom they could appeal for assistance. The author of *Regimen* mentioned Zeus, Athena, Apollo, Hermes, Earth, Sun and the Heroes as healers who might be invoked to avert disease.[45]

Nonetheless, the marked expansion of the cult of Asclepius and his family at the end of the fifth century BC is striking, as is the enormous wealth that was quickly amassed by some of the sanctuaries.[46] It was a development encouraged by one of the highest religious authorities of Greece, the Delphic Oracle, and it cut across many of the more local healing cults. While the devastation wrought by the plague of Athens may plausibly be invoked as a catalyst, this cannot be the whole story, for there had been plagues before, and there would continue to be so again.[47] One might also ascribe some weight to the effectiveness of Epidaurian propaganda, as well as to a spirit of competition among cities to emulate one another in the provision of a shrine, but all this may not be enough to account for what, on the face of it, is a sudden expansion of Asclepius cult.[48]

Above all, we should not underestimate the effect that any cures allegedly performed by the god would have had, not just on the patients themselves, but on all who saw them recovered and restored to health, or who read their testimonies inscribed on tablets around the sanctuary walls. Those from Epidaurus, which form the most extensive group of cure inscriptions to survive, must represent only a selection of the accounts given to the priests or guardians of the shrine and then carved onto the temple wall in a long consecutive series of case histories.[49] Their purpose is to encourage, convince and warn. Health is attainable through the god, even in circumstances so incredible that believers themselves might laugh at the thought.[50] The god, like other gods, could punish those who offended against him or his sanctuary, but he was also prepared to heal even those whom he had punished.[51]

Most of the cure inscriptions are reports of chronic sickness cured by divine intervention: paralysis, facial blemishes, blindness, 'lice', swellings and a failure to conceive are all mentioned, but one story tells of a broken goblet put back together again by the god, and another of the rediscovery of a lost child.[52] Asclepius also appears to have a monopoly on curing three- and five-year pregnancies.[53] Later cure inscriptions, from the shrines in Rome, Pergamum and Lebena, tell similar stories.[54] The walls of the shrines were also hung with tablets and representations of parts of the body that were healed, some in terracotta or stone, others in bronze, silver or gold – hands, feet, legs, arms, ears, breasts, genitalia, as well as images of the whole invalid.[55] Many of these too suggest chronic diseases, but it would be wrong to conclude that only those suffering from such illnesses were ever treated or that there were not some whose first resort in any illness would have been to the god. Anthropology offers many suggestive parallels from other cultures for why an individual might choose to be healed by a god rather than another type of healer, and one should not in these circumstances make a strict division between religious and non-religious cures.[56]

At the shrine suppliants would purify themselves at a sacred spring, before offering an appropriate sacrifice, and then, wearing white robes, undergo a second purification before entering the *abaton* or an *adyton*, 'the inaccessible', words that stress that it is a building barred to the normal visitor.[57] Only those prepared to meet the god or to serve him as a priest were allowed to enter or to find out what actually took place within. A man called Aeschines, who climbed a tree to see if he could see what was happening when the suppliants were asleep, was punished by falling on to a fence and nearly losing his sight.[58] The *abaton* itself was a long porticoed edifice with distinctive individual rooms: when no such building existed, as in the early years at Athens, it was enough to sleep within the temple itself or perhaps even its precinct.[59] If the suppliants were fortunate, while asleep they would receive a vision from Asclepius. In it sometimes the god himself appeared and healed them by acting as a physician or surgeon; sometimes it was one of the sacred snakes or dogs who appeared to lick or enter the person; sometimes the dream itself was a mere riddle and required further assistance to be understood. On waking, the sufferer might be completely recovered, all paralysis or swellings gone, but sometimes the god had given instructions that needed to be interpreted by a priest or temple guardian and then followed up before a cure was secured. Many of the treatments find parallels within contemporary medicine, but others were perhaps selected for public display precisely because of their striking divergences from it.[60] But to think of the healing encounter solely in terms of medical techniques is to miss the context in which it takes place – the physical setting, the sacred spring, the sacred grove (even if, as at the Asclepieion at Athens, it could have hardly amounted to more than three or four trees),[61] the sacrifices and the reassurance offered by the memorials, whether inscriptions or cultic recitations, that this was a place where healing was available.[62]

The Epidaurian inscriptions imply that the patients spent only one night at the shrine, but that may be to press the evidence too far, for it emphasises the moment of cure, not the time spent at the shrine. Indeed, two sufferers had left Epidaurus on their first visit without being cured, one of them, a woman, being carried back almost to her home in Pherae (N. Greece) before the god appeared to her and cured her. On another occasion, about 300 BC, a celebrated poetess was sent by the god to bring a writing tablet from Epidaurus to a blind man living many miles away at Naupauctus across the Corinthian gulf. On receiving the tablet he found that he could see, and set up a shrine to Asclepius in his home town.[63] But, in general, the tablets emphasise the activity of the god within his own temple. The many pilgrims who made the journey to Epidaurus in person often travelled hundreds of miles, from Thasos, Lampsacus (now in N.W. Turkey), Mytilene, Cnidus and Epirus, as well as from less distant places.[64] By 300 BC, then, to judge from the Epidaurus tablets, the shrine already had a pan-Hellenic reputation: within little more than a century the cult centre there had changed from one of merely local significance to the greatest healing shrine of Classical Greece.

Inscriptions, dedications and archaeological remains thus testify to the ubiquity of healing shrines in Classical Greece, as well as to the burgeoning of the cult of Asclepius after 421 BC. The pattern of healing offered by the god, by incubation and dreams, is not unique to Asclepius cult: the traveller Pausanias commented on the parallels between it and the procedures he saw at the oracle shrine of Trophonius at Lebadea in N. Greece, while the cult buildings of the oracular and healing shrine of Amphiaraus near Oropus are almost identical with those of Epidaurus.[65] But one should not forget that any deity could choose to heal, and that the making of vows, prayers and sacrifices for healing at some local temple must have been far more common than a lengthy pilgrimage to a distant shrine of Asclepius. But what was arguably new about Asclepius was his concentration on healing; here was a deity that was a healing specialist and nothing else.[66]

A hurried reading of *The Sacred Disease* might suggest that this new arrival offered strong competition to the practitioners of secular healing and that human doctors viewed the arrival of Asclepius with as much concern as they did that of travelling exorcists. The near total absence of any reference to doctors among the inscriptions from Epidaurus is well known – the only one recorded there is possibly of Roman date, and may have served as a priest.[67] But this lack of epigraphic testimony at Epidaurus is largely irrelevant: the cure inscriptions declare who was treated, not who had treated them, and few of the funerary inscriptions from the environs of the shrine mention the deceased's occupation.[68] It is not entirely fanciful to suggest that for the biggest festivals Epidaurus, like certain other cities, arranged for doctors to be present to attend to the ailments of those who had travelled a long way, but perhaps this too was left to the power of the god.[69]

But if the inscriptions from Epidaurus are silent about the relationship between doctors and the shrine, the Athenian evidence suggests a considerable degree of co-operation. In the third century BC it was already an 'ancestral custom' for the physicians who were in the service of the state to make a sacrifice twice a year to Asclepius and Hygieia on behalf of themselves and the patients whom they had healed.[70] Whether a beautiful relief from the city Asclepieion, datable to the middle of the fourth century, should be associated with this twice-yearly sacrifice has been much disputed.[71] Six men are depicted in an attitude of prayer before Asclepius, Demeter and Kore (the last two also the deities most associated with the Eleusinian Mysteries): inscribed in crowns beneath the relief are the names of five men and their patronymics, and the same names were originally carved also above the relief.[72] One of them can be identified with a celebrated Athenian physician, Mnesitheus, and two more are the sons of another, Dieuches.[73] The relief is of a type associated with dedications, but there is nothing to link it with public physicians, and it might be best to regard it as merely another private dedicatory plaque and offering to the god. The shrine's inventories, which list dedications of surgical instruments, cupping flasks and medical writing tablets, show that doctors were among those who made offerings to the god (who in time became a sort of patron saint to their profession).[74] Two dedicators are explicitly called physicians, one giving a gold and cornelian ring, an object of considerable value.[75] Both have been identified, on grounds less than secure, with priests of the shrine, but, although doctors are known to have been priests of the god elsewhere and at later periods, this does not otherwise appear to have been the case at Athens, and there are other non-medical candidates for the office. But there are better grounds still for associating doctors with the cult of Asclepius. At Athens, when official honours were given to a Rhodian, Pheidias, for his work as a public physician in 304–303, the state secretary was instructed to arrange for the marble plaque to be erected in the Asclepieion.[76] If this was not an isolated instance – and there is nothing to suggest that it was – the walls of the shrine and its precinct would have formed a veritable 'Doctors' Corner', where one might read of distinguished practitioners from the past. The excavations at the Temple of Asclepius on Cos have also revealed a remarkable collection of decrees in honour of physicians, some erected by the town of Cos or other smaller places on the island, others by other cities further afield in gratitude for Coan doctors who had served them well.[77]

All this suggests that notions of hostility between human and divine healers have been much exaggerated. The author of *The Sacred Disease*, far

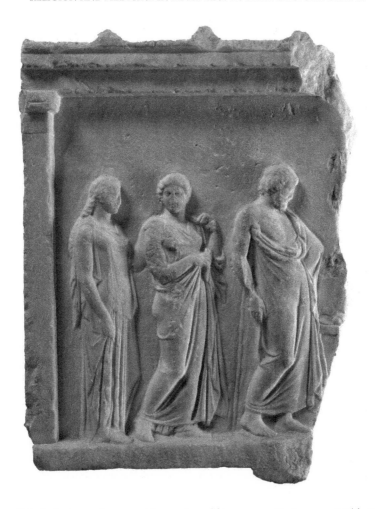

Figure 7.2 Asclepius and two goddesses. Late fifth century BC. Inv. no. 1346, National Archaeological Museum, Athens (photographer Kostas Xenikakis). © Hellenic Ministry of Culture and Tourism/Archaeological Receipts Fund.

from denying the gods any role in healing, professes his own high notion of piety towards them. He approves of the types of purification offered by most shrines, whereby the divinity washes away the stains, faults and impieties of everyday life. He even appears to concede the propriety of making a dedication to a god if one's condition were the result of some divine punishment (perhaps for violating a sanctuary unwittingly) – although, of course, his investigation into epilepsy and mania has convinced him that these conditions have a purely natural cause. He is prepared to allow sacrifice, prayer and supplication to the gods, while at the same time rejecting purification by blood or similar unholy procedures, or burying a purificatory object in the ground, on some lonely mountain or in the sea.[78] His attack is not directed against temples and shrines as such – for in them the decision to heal or not to heal is left to the divinity – but against those who claim to be able to drive out demons and compel the gods to do their will by means of chants and charms.[79] He attacks providers of holy healing who wander from place to place claiming a personal, non-institutional relationship with the gods. Their assertion that they can in some way order the gods to do what they want is truly impious, for it detracts from the majesty and power of the gods.[80]

The ostensible context of *The Sacred Disease* is that of an older conception of the relationship between the gods and healing at variance with newer opinions that stressed the organisation, order and beauty of the natural world and the possibilities that were now open for the reasoned understanding of its processes.[81] As we have seen, it is not an atheistic attack on the possibility of divine healing. Its author could well have accepted the division, enunciated by the playwright Euripides, of diseases into those caused by the gods and those that arose spontaneously, while at the same time seeking to broaden the scope and increase the doctor's understanding of the second category.[82] He would perhaps have agreed with the author of *Regimen*, who divided dreams into those that were divine and required religious interpretation and those that were firmly within the sphere of the doctor.[83] This author's assertion that 'prayer is good, but, while invoking the gods, one should also lend a hand' is no cynical denigration of prayer, but fully in line with his later recommendation to invoke appropriate divine healers and to employ dietary means together to ward off disease.[84]

In time, this development may have assisted the creation of a new orthodoxy within medicine. In the sixth and early fifth centuries healers could act like Empedocles as roving shamans, and the boundaries between magic and medicine were almost non-existent.[85] By 350 BC, however, barriers had arisen. Not that doctors rejected totally some therapies that others might consider magical, for chants, charms and so-called sympathetic or white magic all continued to be used, to a greater or lesser extent, within medicine.[86] Parallels with religious purification may indeed have assisted patients to respond to medical purification and purging, whatever their doctors might have said.[87] Rather, those practitioners who relied primarily on such procedures for their cures were now marginalised, or at least excluded from the new idea of medicine and the appellation of *iatros*.[88] Where the line was to be drawn still differed from individual to individual, and from case to case, but the rhetoric of orthodoxy insisted that a line could, and should, be drawn between the activities of the magician and those of the physician. How far this distinction was followed in practice is unclear, and is less significant than the fact that the magician was used as one of the defining boundaries of what was appropriate behaviour for the physician. 'I am not a mantic diviner', asserted the author of *Prorrhetic* 2, thereby distinguishing his method of medical forecasting from theirs.[89]

From this perspective both the Hippocratic Corpus and the rise of Asclepius cult are part of the same phenomenon, the defining of orthodoxy over against a magical alternative. In religion magic was credited with the potential to disturb the proper relationship between gods and men. It operated outside the formal religious channels for communicating with the divine; and it thereby posed a threat to civic order.[90] The rise of Asclepius cult was one way in which the divine power to heal could be channelled for the benefit of both city and individual patient. Those who offered religious healing outside these channels, such as the travelling priest and the exorcist, became marginalised, and their religious credentials were called into question. Even when it was accepted that they had the power to interfere with the natural workings of a divinely created world, this was condemned for its individualistic rather than its communal deployment. Skills so powerful, and so privileged an access to the gods, must be constrained within the framework of civic life. Thus, Telemachus' mainly private foundation of the shrine of Asclepius at Athens was gradually assimilated into the official religious environment of the city, and may have been subject to some civic control from its inception.

In this process Asclepius came to symbolise not just the power of the gods to heal and save but also the art of medicine itself as contrasted with other healing alternatives. Asclepius possessed the skills, talents and attributes of the good human doctor.[91] For a doctor to reject Asclepius and his healings might also be for him to reject the very things for which medicine was thought to stand. In this way religious and secular healing reinforced rather than opposed each other.[92]

8

FROM PLATO TO PRAXAGORAS

The Roman author Celsus praised Hippocrates as the first to separate medicine from the 'studium sapientiae', the study of wisdom, or, as we would say, 'philosophy'.[1] If he intended by this to suggest that after Hippocrates medicine and philosophy went their separate ways, and that neither learned or borrowed from the other, he was considerably mistaken.[2] Even as some of the texts in the Hippocratic Corpus were being composed, the philosopher Plato was making use of medical data for his own philosophical purposes, as well as putting forward an explanation for illness that was to have a long-lasting impact on the intellectual world.

We have already seen that Plato referred on several occasions in his dialogues to Hippocrates as the leading representative of medicine of his day, and in his *Second Letter* he mentioned his own acquaintance with the doctor Philistion of Locri.[3] His letter expressed the hope that Philistion would be allowed by his master, the tyrant Dionysius II of Syracuse, to come to Athens, although whether he ever did so is far from clear.[4] Plato is known to have made three visits to S. Italy and Sicily, in about 387, 367 and 362 BC, and may well have met with Philistion on any of these occasions. However, the authenticity of this letter has been frequently called into question, and a link between the two men could easily have been a later rationalisation of the ways in which some of Plato's theories come very close to those of Philistion as reported in the Anonymus Londinensis papyrus.

Philistion believed in three general causes of disease, which he then subdivided. The first (internal) cause was an excess or a deficiency in one of the four 'forms', hot, cold, wet and dry. The second (external) was the presence of wounds or sores, or the result of an excess or deficiency of external heat and cold, of inopportune changes from one to the other, or simply of wrong nutriment. The third and last cause was some impediment to the flow of air into or out of the body.[5] In his *Timaeus*, Plato produced two explanations that are very similar to the first and last of Philistion's: imbalances and irregularities within the four elements, and the failure of air to move properly into and out of the body. Where there is no breath, the body begins to rot; where there is too much, the air forces its way through where it should not, and causes painful swellings, sweatings and distortions.[6]

But Plato is not simply repeating Philistion; alongside breath or air he sets the far more traditional pair of bile and phlegm. His second cause goes even further in its apparent independence from what others had said before him. The Platonic body is built up from the four elements, earth, air, fire and water, which form the building blocks from which everything else is created. Flesh and sinews are formed from blood – itself the direct product of 'digested' food – and its constituents, and the 'viscous oily substance that comes from the sinews and flesh' nourishes the outer part of the bones, while a pure substance nourishes the marrow.[7] When this process is working correctly the patient is healthy. But it can go into reverse. The flesh can decompose, the blood become bitter, and bile, serum, phlegm and the like can then destroy the whole body. Instead of nourishing the body and benefiting from one another, they are carried round the body in the veins, spreading destruction and decay in mutual conflict and strife.[8] When the fluid that binds flesh and bone together dries out, the corrupted substance crumbles away and flesh and bone become separated. When the very marrow becomes affected, through some excess or deficiency, even more serious diseases occur. The deeper and more advanced the degeneration, the less the chance of recovery.[9]

Whether this concept of what might be termed diseases of decomposition is Plato's own or draws on an earlier philosopher or doctor is not clear.[10] It creates a powerful image of the body going into reverse, almost spontaneously. Earlier in his argument, Plato had explained growth and decay as the result of the vigour of the triangles that, in his mathematical universe, lay at the very foundation of all matter. When young and fresh, their edges are sharp, capable of prevailing over those that occur in food and drink, and so cutting up that material into its basic constituents, which can then be distributed efficiently around the body in blood as nutriment. The new triangles can attach themselves to the appropriate parts of the body and cause it to grow. Conversely, as we grow old, the triangles become blunter and lose their cutting edge; they themselves become more easily divided, and the body descends into old age. When the bonds of the triangles that make up the marrow can no longer hold together, they come apart, releasing the bonds of the soul, which flies off. This is the normal process of ageing and death. To what extent, if at all, the same process is followed in diseases of degeneration is far from obvious, and Plato does not explain what triggers such diseases.[11]

The descriptions of these diseases are all the more striking because they reverse the whole construction of the body so carefully and purposefully organised by Plato's Craftsman (the Demiurge or Creator). From marrow, the most important of all tissues, is formed the brain, and other parts are enclosed in bone to form the spine; after bone is formed flesh, which is carefully distributed around the body according to the design of the Creator. Because solid bone and thick flesh inhibit sensitivity, he reduced the thickness of the bones of the skull surrounding the brain, the seat of the intellect. The consequent loss of protection and the possibility of increased pain is more than outweighed by the gain in sensitivity.[12] The neck, through which only very tiny channels go upward to the head, further protects the brain from the deleterious polluting effects of the mortal elements of the soul which are located further down in the body.[13]

Plato's description of the human body in the *Timaeus*, which exercised a powerful influence over later thinkers, owes less to his acquaintance with the internal anatomy of the body (or with earlier writers on this theme) than to his own preconceptions about the soul. In the *Republic* he had exploited a complex series of mutually reinforcing analogies between the city and the soul to argue that there were three parts to the soul, concerned, respectively, with reason, spirit or energy, and desire. In the later *Laws* he drew parallels with the doctor's knowledge and practices to support the authority of the philosopher to legislate for the unhealthy city.[14] Just as in the healthy or just city all its citizens had to work together, each doing his or her appropriate task and, in Plato's view, guided by the wisdom of the philosopher rulers, so in the healthy person all parts of the soul must co-operate together under the guidance of reason. Just as the much more numerous third portion of the state always endangered its good working, so in the body uncontrolled desire had a damaging effect on reason and, in the end, its own well-being.

In the *Timaeus*, a mythic account of reality, this tripartition is extended further by locating each part of the soul in a specific part of the body.[15] The highest part of the soul is placed in the brain, the energetic part in the heart, and the lower, appetitive part in the belly, where can be found the liver, stomach and spleen. Plato does not make clear the detailed physiology of these lower organs, although he makes the liver the chief controller among them, just as his picture of the heart and its vessels is highly schematic. It was left to later scholars, Galen in particular, to correlate the tripartite soul with three largely independent bodily systems, the brain and nerves, the heart and arteries, and the liver and veins. Plato does not go this far, not least because a clear-cut distinction between the venous and arterial systems had not yet been drawn.

Plato's linkage of soul and body in the *Timaeus* also introduces a physicalist strain into his explanation of diseases of the soul. Simply by being located in the body, the immortal soul is hampered in its activity, and affected by both nature and nurture. Some psychic disorders are the result of bad upbringing, but others have a physical origin. Morbid humours, in particular bile and phlegm, send out vapours, which have a different effect depending on which part of the soul they reach. Madness (*mania*) and stupidity may both have their origin in changes in the body: alterations in the marrow, for instance, affect one's perceptions of pleasure and pain. If this is so, the correction of these mental or psychic aberrations must involve treatment of the underlying physical condition. So from one's earliest years one should receive a suitable physical and mental training, with appropriate regimen and gymnastic exercises, in order to keep the physical body as healthy as the mind. Drugs are not recommended by Plato, except as a very last resort.[16]

The medical sections of the *Timaeus*, then, are far from lacking in interest. They show a non-medical man, Plato, utilising ideas that, as we know from both the Hippocratic Corpus and Anonymus Londinensis, were at the forefront of medical debate at the time in order to write his own account of the creation of the human body and to explain some of its mental or psychic defects. His subsequent influence brought these ideas to a wide audience, and they, in turn, were developed by commentators who might themselves introduce further medical arguments and evidence.[17] Galen, as we shall see, was convinced that Plato had studied medicine with Hippocrates, and that Plato's notions of the body could reveal much about the teaching of Hippocrates that was otherwise unclear from the Hippocratic Corpus.[18] But, even if Galen's belief in Plato the medical student is largely his own invention, other more sober commentators brought their own medical information to bear on philosophical problems.[19] The celebrated (and disputed) passage about Alcmaeon's introduction of anatomy, for example, is preserved today only because a late Latin commentator on the *Timaeus*, Chalcidius, used it to explain further what Plato was doing in his account of sight (at 67d–e).[20] Unlike modern medical historians, Chalcidius was not concerned with what Alcmaeon had actually done (even if he could have found out), but only with the relevance of his theories to those of Plato.

Plato's pupil, Aristotle, the son of a court physician to the King of Macedon and an Asclepiad on both his mother's and his father's side, continued this interest in matters medical, although in a very different way from his master.[21] He posited a continuum between doctors and natural philosophers: most natural philosophers in their account of the world had also to consider medicine, while the more thoughtful physicians grounded their medical theories upon the principles of natural philosophy. He himself attacked problems that might be called medical, particularly in relation to psychology, while, at the same time, drawing on medical data to exemplify and to support his position in debates with philosophers.[22] He himself brought into harmony both the medical theories about opposites and the philosopher's ideas about elements, and, in particular, the four basic elements, the hot, cold, wet and dry. In the Aristotelian universe medical theory, and most notably the four-element theory of *The Nature of Man*, could find a secure home. The human body was built up out of the four elements, and its natural processes could be explained by Aristotle's physical principles. The inner heat of an animal was, so to speak, an 'internal fire', and the main function of air or pneuma was to cool this heat and prevent it from getting out of control and damaging the organism. The brain, Aristotle believed, acted as a refrigerator to cool down the fiery heart, the seat of the single and unified organic soul.[23]

Aristotle, like Plato, established his own school, the Lyceum, in Athens, where he and his pupils embarked on a wide-ranging and ambitious

programme of empirical investigation. They collected and studied information on the whole world of nature and of human endeavour, from records of
the constitutions of the various city-states and the opinions of doctors, to
botany and mineralogy.[24] This enterprise was backed by influential patrons.
Aristotle had worked first at the small court of Assos (now W. Turkey),
before becoming the tutor of the future Alexander the Great. The support
of Alexander allowed Aristotle to exploit immediately the conquests made
by his army as it traversed the Persian Empire as far as the mountains of
Afghanistan and the plains of the Punjab between 334 and Alexander's
death in 323. The conquering troops were accompanied on their marches by
scholars who kept records, measured distances and sent back to Aristotle in
Athens specimens of the new minerals and plants that they found.[25]

Aristotle himself was passionately interested from his earliest years in
what we would now term biology and zoology. He collected information
on a wide range of animals, birds and fishes, even going so far as to perform
systematic dissections on at least fifty different kinds of animal. He was as
well informed about the development of the chick in the egg as about the
habits of bees or the feet of the ostrich.[26] His credo, as set out in his treatise
The Parts of Animals, is a stirring call to investigate the natural world, 'for
every realm of nature has something marvellous about it'.[27] He was prepared
to acknowledge that looking at the constituent parts of bodies, blood, flesh,
bone, vessels and so on, might easily appear disgusting and shameful, but
that was only if one concentrated on the individual building blocks and not
on the whole house, or form. If one did that, then one would see the beauty
of the craftsmanship of nature, and one would derive great pleasure from
being able to discover and recognise the true causes of things. In particular,
one would quickly become aware that 'in the works of nature, purpose, not
chance, predominates'.

Aristotle is here committed to the study of biology in accordance with his
general philosophical principles, and the primary object of this study is not the
individual detail of any part but their composition as a whole. In particular, the
abundance of his information served to confirm one of Plato's central tenets in
the *Timaeus*, teleology – or, in Longrigg's words, the doctrine of internal finality within nature – although Aristotle did not commit himself to his master's
belief in a comprehensive and conscious design on the part of nature.[28] One
studied the natural world, not only for what it was itself, but in order to gain
insights from more accessible, albeit also transitory, material than was possible
from the contemplation solely of the precious and divine heavenly bodies. That
knowledge was more pleasing, but inevitably only partial; it needed to be supplemented by the empirical study of the things on earth.

These included animals, living beings, of which humans were only one.
Aristotle's project aimed at encompassing all of them, 'noble and ignoble
alike'. There is thus no specific anthropology in his writings, no treatise
devoted to an examination of the human body by itself. This would have

been an extremely difficult task, as he himself admits, for 'the inner parts of the body are unknown, especially those of man', but also an unnecessary one, if the requisite information that contributed to the overall understanding of nature could be obtained by other means. Analogy with other animals provided that means, 'looking at those animals which have parts similar to those of humans'.[29] Since at this time there were strong taboos in Greece against interfering with a human body, let alone dissecting it, human anatomy was out of the question. That of animals, birds and fishes was not, and Aristotle refers often to his own investigations (and to those of others, including, almost certainly, Diocles) into their organisation, structure and, above all, functions.[30] His results are far more detailed and wide-ranging than those of his predecessors, although at times his account is not easy to follow. His description of the vascular system, for example, both includes new observations and omits (or misunderstands) much that we might consider obvious. His description of the heart as having three chambers continues to divide modern interpreters into those who believe that Aristotle erred in what he saw when he carried out his dissection and those who argue that it is Aristotle's starting point for the description that differs from ours, not his observation.[31] His notions that the hearts of large animals, such as horses, had a bone within and that the number of chambers in the heart was related to size are a nice blend of fact and misunderstanding.[32] But there are times when Aristotle got things wrong beyond any dispute. Because he failed to find any blood vessel extending to the brain, he concluded that the brain in all animals was bloodless.[33] His belief that females have fewer teeth than males, and fewer cranial sutures, may be based on incomplete observations, but was also influenced by his underlying conception of woman as an inferior and somehow incomplete version of man.[34] But his mistakes are relatively few in comparison with his accurate descriptions of phenomena in the living world, and do not detract from the example he set to others (and to their patrons) of the value of such empirical research. He raised big questions about the whole process of life, from movement and sensation to ageing and sleep, although almost all that he himself wrote specifically on medicine has disappeared.[35]

His influence, which was substantial, took many different forms. Through his teaching of logic at the Lyceum, Aristotle created what might be described as the scaffolding for future intellectual debate, emphasising correct logical argument and the importance of a proper definition of terms in any exposition of medical or scientific material. In turn, by setting medicine and the human body within the wider system of the cosmos he allowed a dialogue about the causes of the natural processes within the body to be conducted at a deeper level of explanation. We can trace a whole series of debates with Aristotle over the interpretation of medical phenomena from his immediate pupils through to Galen, whose own influential systematising depends on a basically Aristotelian epistemology and on a combination of data drawn from the Hippocratic Corpus and Plato and inserted into a world of Aristotelian physics.[36] Aristotle's successor as head of the Lyceum, Theophrastus (c.371–287), not only included many medicinal plants in his *Enquiry into Plants*, but also wrote short tracts on such obviously medical topics as sweating, fatigue and giddiness. Other Peripatetics such as Strato of Lampsacus investigated questions that were to have repercussions for later physicians, while, conversely, medical notions about the brain came to play a major role in philosophical discussions on the soul.[37]

Aristotle refers several times in his zoological treatises to a book that he had written, entitled *Dissections*, which contained figures and drawings of dissected animals.[38] The relationship of this treatise to one written by his contemporary, Diocles of Carystus, is a moot point. In the opinion of Galen, Diocles was the first to write a specific treatise on (animal) anatomy, and he used the evidence of his dissection of mules to make inferences about the human womb.[39] But it is not easy to determine when Diocles, 'second in time and fame to Hippocrates' and 'a younger Hippocrates', lived and worked, since all we have of his writings are fragments and reports preserved by much later authors.[40] Most recent scholarship would put him as a contemporary of Aristotle, but their precise relationship is unclear.[41] Neither refers to the other for certain. It is true that Diocles' idea that in the womb there were 'breastlike outgrowths ... made with forethought by nature to give the embryo practice at sucking the nipples of the breast' partly resembles a theory expressly criticised by Aristotle, but he does not mention Diocles as its author.[42] Conversely, the statement in Anonymus Bruxellensis 44 that the heart has four chambers has been interpreted as a direct contradiction by Diocles of Aristotle's view that it had only three, although, once again, Diocles is not mentioned and the hypothesis that he is the critic is far from proven.[43] Even the clearest citation of Aristotle, in an attack on his theory of seed, turns out on inspection to be problematical, for the relevant passage could be the work of the compiler, not of Diocles.[44] Nevertheless, it remains likely that Diocles' work as an anatomist and embryologist overlapped with that of Aristotle, some of his writings being available to Aristotle, other parts written in reaction to him.[45]

But anatomy was only one part of his activity, and perhaps not that most familiar to his contemporaries. The titles of his books, for example *Gynaecology, Bandaging, Treatments, The Surgery* and *Affection, Cause and Treatment*, give only a hint of the variety and the extent of their contents. What survives today from them indicates that he ranged widely over all aspects of medicine, and that it was this comprehensiveness that gained him comparison with Hippocrates. In surgery he was credited with the introduction of a special spoon-shaped instrument for the removal of arrowheads from a wound.[46] He wrote on poisons and on vegetables, as well as a *Rhizotomikon*, a treatise on plants with medicinal properties; one of his remedies has recently been found in a prescription from Egypt written in the sixth century AD.[47] His discussion of fevers emphasised the importance of critical days, the days

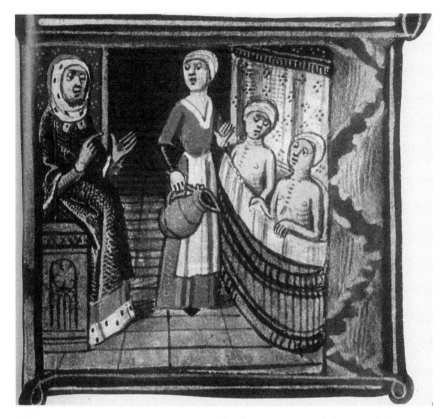

Figure 8.1 Ancient bathing as a treatment for fever, as imagined by a mediaeval artist. Dresden, Sächsische Landesbibliothek, Db 93, fol. 581v.

on which a fever might be expected to change crucially for better or worse, for remission or relapse, and he paid special attention to those that were multiples of seven.[48] There are obvious parallels here with the Hippocratic *Epidemics*, and Diocles' own *Prognostic* falls clearly within the same tradition as the Hippocratic treatise of that name, but proof of direct acquaintance with any specific tract from the Corpus is elusive.[49]

Diocles' overall theory of health and disease, typical of that of learned medicine in the fourth century, is marked by an increased methodological sophistication. He believed strongly in causation, and ascribed the internal causes of disease to some excess or deficiency within the body's four elements and the four primary qualities.[50] He accepted four humours, blood, phlegm, bile and black bile, which arise from nutriment and are differentiated within the blood vessels through a process of alteration by innate heat.[51] He paid particular attention to *pneuma* ('breath' or 'refined air'), which spread through the body's vessels to effect voluntary motion. The blockage of *pneuma* was

123

especially serious, and the cause of a variety of diseases. If its passage round the body was blocked by congealed phlegm within the aorta, it resulted in epilepsy and apoplexy.[52] More frequent was the interruption of the flow of *pneuma* taken into the body via the pores of the skin as a result of an excess of bile or phlegm. Phlegm cooled and compacted the blood, whereas bile caused it to boil and curdle. This obstruction not only caused fevers and headaches, but also brought on melancholy when it affected the heart, the source of the 'psychic *pneuma*' of the body.[53] Diocles' interest in *pneuma*, although many details remain obscure, confirms the growing importance of this substance among philosophical and scientific writers of the fourth century, as he links it both to mental states and to physical disorders. But there is not yet a systematic doctrine of *pneuma*, such as we find in the next century.[54]

Like many writers in the Hippocratic Corpus, Diocles emphasised the individuality of the patient, as the body changed over time, with the seasons of the year, the weather and the process of ageing. Health was the restoration of the individual's natural balance by appropriate treatments.[55] This was not always easy: for example, since male semen was drawn from the brain and spinal cord, frequent intercourse was potentially dangerous as the body might not be able to replace such vital fluid easily and quickly.[56] Women were even more at risk, for they had, of course, their own diseases, as well as those they shared with men.[57]

Although Diocles wrote on pharmacology and bandaging, his major interest in therapeutics was in diet and exercise – Galen was particularly enthusiastic about his advice on gymnastics, on which he considered him a real expert.[58] It was a skill Diocles may have inherited from his father, for he expounded his ideas on the use of oil in anointing and rubbing the body in a book entitled *Archidamus*, which was also his father's name.[59] His largest treatise on the subject was his *Hygiene*, in which he considered in a sophisticated manner the problems of prescribing diets.[60] The effects of foodstuffs cannot always be predicted from a knowledge of their properties, and, vice versa, it is not always possible to explain why a particular food has produced the effect that it has. On the whole, experience is here a better guide than theory, and one will make fewest mistakes if one assumes that what normally happens when a particular food or drug is given is caused by the whole nature of its substance, i.e. by the specific interaction of all its constituents together. To assume that foods with apparently similar individual properties, for example of hotness or pungency, will always work in a similar way is often refuted by experience.[61] Diocles is not here rejecting the possibility of an enquiry into causation, as the later Sceptics or Empiricists were to do, but acknowledging the practical difficulties of constantly carrying out such a procedure in dietetics. Indeed, while on some occasions such an enquiry might add to our understanding and to the plausibility of dietary prescriptions, in the great majority it would be unnecessary for the proper treatment of the patient.

Diocles, along with his contemporaries the Athenians Mnesitheus and Dieuches, the Coans Praxagoras and Phylotimus, and Pleistonicus, constituted a group of physicians and writers whose beliefs Galen thought essential knowledge for any competent practitioner.[62] None of their writings has survived intact today, and it may be doubted how much even Galen had of their books within his own library. Certainly the average physician in Rome would have had little chance of buying copies of the complete works of Mnesitheus, and it is probable that Galen was expecting him to use a manual that presented the opinions of earlier doctors in the form of a doxographical summary of their views on particular diseases. An impression of what such a manual might have contained can be gained from the anonymous treatise on acute and chronic diseases generally referred to as Anonymus Parisinus, so called because it was first edited from a manuscript in the Bibliothèque Nationale in Paris.[63] Written probably in the first or early second century AD, it lists the views of 'the ancients', and specifically Hippocrates, Diocles, Praxagoras and Erasistratus, on the cause or causes of a range of diseases, including epilepsy, ileus and tetanus. Discussing pleurisy, for instance, the author reports that Erasistratus believed that it was the result of an inflammation of the membrane on the inner side of the ribcage, whereas Diocles thought that it was due to some obstruction in the veins around the pleura. Praxagoras, however, considered it was an inflammation of the extremities of the lung itself. This anatomical precision is then contrasted with the view in the Hippocratic *Places in Man* that ascribed pleurisy to a flux moving from the head to the chest.[64] After causes comes a description of the symptoms, followed by recommendations for treatment. The general organisation is clear and simple, and the treatise is short and relatively easy to use.[65] One can see how such a document could fulfil Galen's demand that the competent practitioner (and, indeed, his learned patient) should familiarise himself with the main outlines of the ideas of the major authors among the 'ancients'.

What links Galen's classic writers together, and the reason why later commentators often labelled them as 'Dogmatics' or 'Logical Physicians', was their belief in the use of reason to establish a chain of causation.[66] Mnesitheus, for example, 'second to none in his methodical practice', was alleged to have followed closely Hippocrates' method of division in determining the causes of disease.[67] They all believed in the importance of humours and elemental qualities, although what they meant by these terms is not always clear, however much Galen, our major source, might insist that they shared his opinions. Even when, like Diocles, they accepted four cardinal humours, they did not always agree with Galen on what these were or how they came into being.[68] Others understood the same Greek word in very different ways. Mnesitheus used the word 'humours' or 'chymes' to refer to savours, and called bodily fluids 'chyles', without apparent differentiation.[69] Praxagoras identified eleven different humours, including a 'vitreous humour' responsible, among other things, for the shivering fever; Phylotimus may have spoken of even more.[70] Galen, wishing to claim both of them as forerunners, explained that they were merely giving precision to what Hippocrates had said. By contrast, Rufus of Ephesus, another Hippocratic, clearly saw their ideas as divergent.[71] Galen looked back to these 'ancients' also to support his views on the need to treat the whole patient rather than just the affected part. He may well be right in this, although his further claims that they appreciated the importance of venesection and of prognosis are far from assured.[72] Even Galen had to admit that they relied on prognosis solely to decide who was likely to recover and who was not. Mnesitheus, for example, announced that a craving for onions at the onset of 'pneumonia' indicated a future recovery, a craving for figs death.[73] Even if one accepts his (and Galen's) argument that these cravings reveal the underlying constitution of the patient, this is still a long way from Galenic prognosis as the essential guide to diagnosis and treatment, and one may doubt the basis on which Mnesitheus made this sweeping assertion.

These 'ancients' are also praised for their therapeutics. Dieuches is credited with discovering a means of applying dangerous drugs in a relatively safe way, no bad thing in view of what Praxagoras and his pupils at times advocated – hellebore, a very powerful emetic, whether taken orally or in a pessary.[74] Despite the risks involved in its use, hellebore in both its black and white varieties was continuously prescribed down to the twentieth century, not least because its effects were very obvious and because it might work when all else failed.[75] But hellebore was at least less deadly than Praxagoras' treatment for ileus, which, in some extreme cases, might involve even more violent emetics to remove impacted residues, a 'contrived death' as the later Methodist writer Caelius Aurelianus scathingly described it.[76]

Although a later author claimed that Praxagoras had brought dietetics to perfection, his contribution is represented only briefly in the surviving fragments of his writings, by contrast with Mnesitheus and Dieuches.[77] Like Diocles, they put diet at the very forefront of medical therapy in a way that was far more sophisticated and more thoroughly argued than the brief hints in the Hippocratic Corpus, and showed an acquaintance with the wider world beyond the Aegean. Their writings and their practical example are an important contribution to a development that led to dietetics being placed on the same level as surgery and pharmacology in the battle against disease; indeed, some placed it above them, on the grounds that dietetic medicine plays a role in preventing as well as in curing disease.[78] Mnesitheus was famous for his careful description of diets for children, while Dieuches was quoted by Oribasius verbatim and at length on the preparation and use of foods.[79] Some of his advice reads extremely practically today. It is useless to offer those taking to the sea for the first time a remedy against vomiting. Indeed, if one's stomach is disturbed, vomiting may actually help, but then one needs to take light and gentle food. Until one has gained one's sea legs it is unwise to gaze upon the tossing waves. But the best way of all to prevent seasickness is to take on board a bunch of thyme or another sweet-smelling substance to counter the stench that is always to be found on board ship.[80]

Their interests were continued by their slightly younger contemporary Diphilus of Siphnos, whose book *Diets for the Sick and the Healthy* covered a wide variety of foods, including cherries, damsons, nuts and mushrooms, both in their natural state and in their cooked forms. His comments on mussels, oysters and salt fish, to which he devoted a whole section, or possibly even a separate book, were much less enthusiastic, for he thought they had little or no nutritional value.[81] His treatise, however, is not cited by any medical author, unlike that of Phylotimus, which extended to at least thirteen books, and recommended likewise a range of diets for use in both sickness and health.[82] Phylotimus preferred pears to apples, and raw leeks to cooked ones, which he thought fibrous and difficult to chew. He had even less time for olives. Black olives were very oily, hard to digest and likely to produce a feeling of nausea for some time, whereas white olives kept in brine, although more digestible, were liable to engender a sharp, acid humour, like the yolk of an egg.[83]

Along with an interest in diet came an interest in anatomy, although what precisely Dieuches did in his dissections to gain the approval of Galen is unknown.[84] For Praxagoras and his pupils, however, the evidence is clearer. They not only meditated on the processes within the body (Pleistonicus thought digestion a sort of putrefaction), but they also examined its structures, for example the womb, the heart and the blood vessels. In doing this, presumably in animals, they provided an important bridge between Aristotle and the human anatomy of the Alexandrians.[85] Praxagoras, for instance, was both the teacher of Herophilus and influenced by many of Aristotle's ideas, although there is no evidence that he ever studied in Athens at the Lyceum.[86] Nor should we expect this. Like Phylotimus, who later became chief magistrate of Cos, he came from a distinguished Coan medical family that claimed descent from Asclepius and that was to remain prominent in the public life of the island for several generations to come.[87] Cos was and remained the centre of his medical world.[88]

The influence of Aristotle can be seen not just in Praxagoras' decision to dissect and to write at least one book on his discoveries, but also in his belief that the heart was the seat of the soul and the brain a mere outgrowth of the spinal cord, a doctrine he shared with his pupils and for which he claimed anatomical proof.[89] He posited that the arteries became progressively divided as they passed through the body until they collapsed inwards and became tiny 'nerves'.[90] He attempted to distinguish between the veins and the arteries (which had formerly both been called '*phlebs*', the word that later applied only to the veins), the arteries beginning in the heart, the veins in the liver. He then made the further assumption that the veins carried blood, the arteries only *pneuma*.[91] These findings and theories may not be entirely Praxagoras' own. Galen, our major source for his beliefs, reports that his father Nicarchus

127

also thought that the arteries carried only *pneuma*, and Diocles, as we have seen, was certainly interested in the role of *pneuma*.[92] But even if the ideas were only partly his own, it would appear to have been Praxagoras who worked out and justified their implications. The distinction between veins and arteries, and the link he claimed to have observed between the arteries and the nerves, allowed him and his pupils to raise further questions about the movement of the arteries, which he called the pulse, and about the source of the *pneuma* within it.[93] Was it all produced in the heart? Or was some of it also drawn in from all over the body? How was the actual pulse produced?[94] What was the relationship of the actual pulse to the beating of the heart itself? For Praxagoras pulse and heartbeat were independent of each other, and pulsation differed from similar movements of the arteries, such as tremor or palpitation, by being natural, not the result of some disorder.[95] Most significantly for the future development of medicine, Praxagoras was the first to see in the pulse a valuable diagnostic aid and to take the movements of the arteries as an index of changes going on elsewhere in the body. How he himself used the pulse to identify diseases is not made clear by the sources, and what survives of ancient pulse lore or sphygmology suggests that a sophistication of both diagnosis and terminology had to wait until his pupil Herophilus.[96]

Nonetheless, Praxagoras' discovery had profound consequences, and it was perhaps for this reason that he was regarded in Antiquity as one of the great figures of medicine. At least one statue was erected in his honour, which around 30 BC became the subject of an epigram by a distinguished man of letters, Crinagoras of Mytilene. Its eight lines convey in high-flown couplets the image of the great physician:

> Phoebus' son himself, anointing his hand with All-heal, rubbed the pain-killing science of your art into your breast, O Praxagoras. Therefore however many pains arise from long fevers, however many when the flesh is cut, you have been taught by gentle Epione to apply remedies enough. If mortals had had such physicians, the ferryboat would never have crossed over with its load of corpses.[97]

With Diocles, Mnesitheus and the other medical writers discussed in this chapter, we begin to glimpse for the first time individual named physicians instead of the anonymity or pseudonymity of the Hippocratic Corpus. They are often also consciously reacting to their own medical heritage, and can be seen to be building on and developing earlier ideas. Although we still remain ignorant about much of their doctrines and their relations with one another, and although it is clear that even that which we have may not correspond exactly to what they said or wrote themselves, the history of medicine from now on can more easily be written in terms of individual achievement and personalities.[98] They remind us that medicine in Classical Greece did not end with the Hippocratic Corpus, and that the interrelationship between medicine and philosophy was far more fruitful than the strictures of the author of *Ancient Medicine* might suggest.[99]

9

ALEXANDRIA, ANATOMY AND EXPERIMENTATION

Few episodes in the history of ancient medicine have been so well studied as the rise and development of human anatomy in the first half of the third century BC.[1] Herophilus and Erasistratus are rightly famous for their pioneering investigations that, for the first time in the Western tradition of medicine, revealed many of the hidden structures of the human body.[2] But this concentration solely or even largely upon the achievements of these two men in anatomy and physiology is not without its dangers. There is a tendency to forget that their dissections were performed within the wider pattern of their activity as physicians, and, even more, that what might be termed investigative or experimental anatomy based on human beings was carried out only for a limited period and in a limited area.[3] Although anatomical demonstration by means of a skeleton or surface musculature continued longer in medical teaching, especially at Alexandria, anatomical experimentation, whether using humans or animals, seems to have died out well before the end of the third century BC and not to have been revived until the late first or early second century AD.[4] When discussions of anatomical and, especially, physiological phenomena appear in later Hellenistic texts, they are largely, if not entirely, based either on chance observation or on the data provided by these early anatomists. The achievements of Herophilus, Erasistratus and the less familiar Eudemus thus mark not only the beginning of Greek human anatomy but also, paradoxically, its ending, leaving historians to account for its restricted temporal and geographical development.

As we have seen, the second half of the fourth century BC saw a vigorous interest in describing and interpreting a wide range of diverse natural phenomena. Aristotle and his followers, to say nothing of Diocles, had dissected animals, birds and fishes to gain a wider understanding of the world of nature, while Praxagoras' investigations into and speculations about the pulse led to further consideration of the physiological processes within the body.[5] Euenor, an Acarnanian doctor resident in Athens in the 320s, is said to have called the horns of the uterus the 'coils', although whether this was as a result of animal dissection or his experience with difficult births is far from clear.[6] The theories of these medical thinkers were elaborated with the aid of reason, but within a new epistemological space, that of the visible.[7] The influence of these developments on the anatomists of early Alexandria can be easily surmised. Herophilus is said to have been a pupil of Praxagoras, presumably on Cos, and tradition linked Erasistratus with the school of Aristotle through his alleged master, Theophrastus of Eresus.[8] At one level, then, the decision to cut into a human body is an understandable extension of a technique of investigation that had become relatively commonplace in Greek intellectual circles; from seeing the internal structures of a bird or a sheep to seeing those of a human being had thus become a small step.[9]

But it was a step fraught with problems, not least because it breached a long-standing Greek taboo on touching, let alone mutilating, a human corpse. Religious laws imposed a ban on interfering with a dead body, and continued to do so in Greece long after the arrival of human anatomy.[10] Although by now it was widely believed, especially among intellectuals, that the soul was something transient and immaterial, residing merely temporarily within the body and leaving it, at death, an empty physical shell, this view was not accepted by most Greeks, for whom the corpse continued to represent an individual human being.[11] Studies of the introduction of human dissection into Renaissance Europe and elsewhere have revealed the strength of the reluctance to interfere with a human corpse, and there can be little doubt that such a repugnance was also widespread among the Greeks.[12]

But there was one area of the ancient world where this taboo apparently did not exist. The Greeks had been familiar since the days of Herodotus, if not long before then, with the common practice among the Egyptians of removing the major organs of the dead and storing them in large jars before proceeding to mummify the body. Herodotus expresses a mixture of fascination and disgust at this strange procedure, and other travellers sent back similar reports.[13] Alexander the Great's conquest of Egypt in 332–331 BC brought the Egyptians under Greek rule, and his foundation of the city of Alexandria 'by Egypt', just west of one of the mouths of the Nile, was a symbol of Greek domination. This was a Greek city, created to be a military as well as a political strong point in the newly acquired land. Although it later became a cosmopolitan giant, in its earliest years the relationship between the Greeks and the native Egyptians was far from equal. The Greeks were firmly in control; the administration, economy and culture of the city were entirely in their hands; and for a long while native Egyptians were barred from obtaining Alexandrian citizenship.[14] Added to the common Greek urban prejudice against those who lived and worked in the countryside, this would have helped to create an apartheid mentality, which regarded the natives, and particularly Egyptian peasants, as almost sub-human. If they showed no abhorrence at what was, to Greek eyes, the mutilation and desecration of their own dead, there was little reason why the Greeks should be concerned about what happened to Egyptian corpses.[15]

Whether Herophilus or Erasistratus owed anything more to Egyptian mummifiers than the freedom from the Greek taboo is controversial. Those who seek a non-Greek origin for human anatomy and for an understanding of the internal organs of the body can rightly point to the sophisticated Egyptian anatomical vocabulary and to the technique of the Egyptian mummifiers in opening up the body.[16] But there is no clear evidence that Egyptian mummifiers carried out any systematic investigations into the human organs they removed or that their cutting open of the corpse served any purpose other than the ritual preparation for burial.[17] Egyptian medical authors and practitioners, if one may judge from what little survives of their medical texts, did not make use of the information provided by the removal of bodily organs to create new theories or provide further justification for old ones. While there was nothing to stop Greek anatomists from observing Egyptian mummifiers in action, without an interpreter to explain what was being done (for the Greeks were notoriously reluctant to learn the language of others) many of the details of their procedures would have remained obscure.[18] Contacts between leading Greek intellectuals and Egyptians in early Alexandria were slight at best, and, even as these developed over time, no evidence for any linkage between medicine and mummification emerges. Mummifiers and medics remained separate professional groups.[19] At most, then, the Egyptian practice of mummification would have provided an encouragement to break a Greek taboo in pursuit of an intellectual challenge that had been foreshadowed in medical and scientific discussions for at least a generation.

Alexandria under the early Ptolemies offered a remarkably supportive environment for intellectual innovation.[20] The example of Aristotle in his close relationship with Philip of Macedon and Alexander undoubtedly encouraged their successor monarchs to invest in culture and science. The new courts, especially in Alexandria, Antioch and, later, Pergamum, attracted intellectuals of all kinds, poets, sculptors, mathematicians and doctors. Their presence should not be taken simply as a sign of a disinterested love of culture on the part of the ruler: it served also more practical purposes – propaganda, warfare and the supervision of his general health.[21] When the savage persecutions of the Alexandrians by Ptolemy VIII in 145–144 BC drove many intellectuals to become refugees, they were eagerly welcomed elsewhere in the Greek world, with the result that, as one contemporary put it, Alexandria became the teacher of Greeks and barbarians alike.[22]

It was Ptolemy I who, perhaps around 300 BC, established the two intellectual institutions that gave Alexandria its great reputation as a cultural centre, the Museum and the Library (or rather libraries, since there was more than one in the city). If Galen is to be believed, Ptolemy endeavoured to obtain by fair means or foul copies of everything written that he could find. Once in Alexandria they were placed in one of the royal libraries, where they were catalogued by a distinguished series of scholar-librarians. It was probably in Alexandria, as part of this process, that the writings that form our Hippocratic Corpus were first brought together.[23]

Of still greater significance was the creation by Ptolemy I of the Museum, the 'Hall of the Muses', near the royal palace. This was a community of scholars and intellectuals who, in return for fulfilling their duty to the Muses (and their monarch), were provided with lodgings and free meals for life.[24] They included poets and critics, mathematicians and geographers, and, although in later centuries the range of the membership was extended to include government officials, it still retained its prestige as a cultural centre.[25] There was an interchange of ideas between the members of the Museum: the poet Callimachus shows an awareness of contemporary medical discoveries, while, as we shall see, the theories of Herophilus and Erasistratus depend in part on the new scientific and technological developments of others.[26]

While there is no evidence that the members of the Museum were obliged to teach or lecture, their very presence attracted students wishing to converse and study with the great men of the time in a vibrant intellectual atmosphere.[27] The pupils of Herophilus constituted his 'household', which implies that they lived communally, but not necessarily within the Museum.[28] Where he carried out his anatomical investigations is also unclear. If we accept Longrigg's attractive suggestion that he dissected within the protecting walls of the Museum, the corpses would thus have become a sort of sacrifice to the Muses (the religious character of the Museum is shown by the fact that its head was a priest, nominated by the ruler), and any violent opposition to their performance would perhaps have been reduced.[29]

Royal involvement (probably through both Ptolemy I and Ptolemy II who ruled 282–246) extended beyond mere protection, for official permission would have been required for these anatomies to be carried out even on the bodies of condemned criminals. If, as Celsus reports, the criminals were still alive when they were handed over to the anatomist from the royal jails, high-level approval would have been still more imperative.[30] Proof of Celsus' claim is, however, not easy to find, especially as many of the reported results could have been obtained from a combination of human dissection and animal vivisection. Galen, who might have been expected to mention Alexandrian vivisection, not least because he wrote one tract specifically on the practicalities of (animal) vivisection, says next to nothing about this human precedent.[31] Most later Galenists, whether in Byzantium or in Islam, never refer to human vivisection, and the exceptions, John of Alexandria and Agnellus of Ravenna, may be indirectly dependent on Celsus or his source.[32] The most strident condemnation of Alexandrian vivisection, by the Christian theologian Tertullian in the early third century, could be easily dismissed as a vivid exaggeration by a committed opponent of all dissection.[33] But, in general, Celsus shows himself to be well informed about Hellenistic anatomy and surgery, and his claims are made within the context of a Hellenistic academic debate about the value of anatomy. Given also that the later pharmacological experiments of Attalus III of Pergamum and Mithridates VI of Pontus were certainly made on living subjects, there is no

reason a priori to reject the possibility that some of these anatomical investigations were carried out on living humans, especially if, as criminals, they
might be thought to have forfeited their humanity and their rights and to be
making, by their suffering and death, a form of expiation and compensatory
contribution to the general good.[34]

Even if the reports of vivisection are rejected as polemical exaggeration,
there is no doubt that systematic research into the internal anatomy of the
human body was first carried out in Alexandria by Herophilus of Chalcedon.[35]
Of Herophilus' early life nothing is recorded, save for a period of study with
Praxagoras, which may have introduced him to the writings of Hippocrates.[36]
But although his familiarity with them even led some later doctors to believe
that he was the author of the Hippocratic treatise *Nutriment*, he was no slavish
Hippocratic. He took a critical view of Hippocratic prognosis, and, although
he based his physiology and pathology on the theory of humours, his interpretation did not necessarily agree with that of *The Nature of Man*.[37] His
interest in the meaning of Hippocratic words and technical terms fits nicely
with his penchant for giving striking names to some of the anatomical structures that he discovered. The calamus scriptorius (a pen-shaped groove in the
brain), the torcular ('wine-press', for the junction of the veins of the head),
the choroid plexus of the brain (so-called because it resembles membranes
wrapped around a foetus), the styloid 'pen-shaped' process of the skull, the
duodenum ('twelve fingers long') and perhaps the pineal gland ('pine-cone')
are all terms coined by Herophilus.[38]

His anatomical studies covered the whole of the body, from a careful
enumeration of the coats of the eye and the first detailed description of the
human liver and possibly the pancreas, to the male and female reproductive
systems.[39] He continued an interest of Praxagoras' by studying the nervous
and the vascular systems, distinguishing between veins and arteries anatomically, as well as functionally, by noting the greater thickness of the arterial
coats.[40] He may have been the first to recognise the significance of the hepatic
portal system, and he was acquainted, at least partially, with the valves in
the heart.[41] He seems to have rejected Praxagoras' opinion that the arteries
carried only *pneuma*, spirit, the vehicle of sensation, in favour of a belief in
a mixture of blood and *pneuma*.[42] Centuries later, Galen was impressed with
his work on the nervous system, by which he revealed the various coverings
of the brain and distinguished between its ventricles, as well as displaying a
detailed knowledge of several of the cranial nerves.[43] Although much of this
anatomy was carried out on animals – his description of the womb is that of
an animal, while that of the *rete mirabile* is based on an ungulate – several of
his comments, and his deliberate use of comparisons when talking about the
liver, prove that he indeed dissected humans too.[44]

The emphasis in later authors on his anatomical discoveries has tended
to obscure the fact that they formed only one part of his activity as a medical practitioner and writer. They provided information that could then be

turned to more practical purposes – his dissection of the womb, for instance, contributed data for his book on midwifery, in which he discussed, *inter alia*, multiple births and uterine prolapse.[45] His division of the nerves into motor and sensory nerves and his investigation of their co-operation with muscles in voluntary motion have a clear medical value when dealing with cases of paralysis.[46] Above all, his studies provided an anatomical justification and explanation for pulsation, which he considered of crucial importance for diagnosis.[47] To this end he constructed a portable water-clock by which to time the pulses, and delineated a whole series of different pulse types, classifying them by size, speed, vehemence and rhythm, using a vocabulary that has many parallels with music theory of the period.[48]

In contrast to his anatomical researches, what is known of his therapeutics can be characterised as traditional rather than radical, certainly by comparison with Erasistratus. In the eyes of Galen, his anatomical discoveries served largely to confirm the therapeutic truths that he derived from Hippocrates. Herophilus supported blood-letting and treatment by opposites, although expressing a judicious caution about the possibility of always identifying the proper cause with certainty.[49] But his refusal to discuss therapies in terms of the four primary qualities, hot, cold, wet and dry, seemed to Galen a drastic, and unnecessary, reduction in the number of options available to the physician.[50] He believed firmly in a liberal use of medicaments – 'the hands of the gods', he called them – for almost any disease, and contributed to the establishment of the Alexandrian tradition of complex pharmacology.[51] His most notorious, and most dangerous, remedy was the very potent hellebore, which he compared to a very brave general in its ability to stir up all the inward parts of the body before marching out in the vanguard.[52] But he also praised other ways of keeping fit, for 'without health one's skill remains invisible, one's strength unused, one's wealth worthless, and one's speech powerless', and a statue in his memory was adorned with gymnastic equipment.[53] In short, the range of therapies he used and the variety of topics on which he wrote should dispel any impression that he devoted all, or even most of, his time to dissection. That was only one part of medicine, which he defined as 'the science of things relating to health, of those relating to disease, and of those that relate to neither one nor the other'.[54] Medicine thus covered the whole spectrum of physical conditions, and provided the means both to preserve and to restore well-being.

By contrast with the generally favourable verdict of posterity on Herophilus, his contemporary Erasistratus of Ceos was, and remains, a much more controversial figure. Neither when nor where he lived can be established beyond all doubt. There is no need to believe that he was affected by a local law of his island that allegedly ordered all those over 60 to be put to death, and Galen's claim that he performed 'more accurate' anatomical dissection only at the end of his life, when he could devote all his time to anatomy, although plausible, lacks any objective support.[55] Although both his father, Cleombrotus, and his teacher, Chrysippus of Cnidus, were linked with the Seleucid court, there is no clear proof that Erasistratus himself was active there rather than at Alexandria.[56] Although he was later renowned as the doctor who treated the lovesick Seleucid queen Stratonice, his name appears only at a late stage in the evolution of the story.[57] The tradition that he was, in some way, a student of Theophrastus in Athens, or of another Peripatetic, Metrodorus, cannot be substantiated either, and may simply be an attempt to explain his use of ideas and practices deriving from philosophers and scientists.[58]

None of his writings survives in more than fragments, few of them copied word for word. Even when they are cited directly, they have mostly been manipulated by one side or another in later debates to prove or disprove their case. Galen, our single most extensive source, was ambivalent about him, to say the least. On the one hand, he had little but praise for his work as a dissector of the brain and heart, quoting with approval Erasistratus' comparison of the neophyte investigator to an untrained athlete:

> As soon as his mind begins to work, he becomes confused and bewildered, ready to withdraw from his investigation in a state of mental fatigue and exhaustion, like untrained runners in a race. But with constant practice, pursuing research, not just in an hour or so, but unceasingly throughout his whole life, he comes to penetrate whatever topic he chooses, reaching his goal by persistent enquiry into everything that might be relevant.[59]

Erasistratus appears to have been the first to discover all the valves in the heart and to have examined their workings in considerable detail before concluding that they were there to prevent any reflux as the heart expanded and contracted 'like a smith's bellows'.[60] He traced the pathways of both veins and arteries, concluding that each system split into smaller and smaller veinlets and arterioles that finally joined together, but with so tiny an aperture that blood could not, under normal circumstances, pass from one system to the other.[61] His investigations of the human brain led him to change his opinion on the point of origin of the nerves, at first locating it in the *dura mater* but later within the brain itself.[62]

Galen was equally impressed with his experiments, even going so far as to repeat some of them in order to confirm or reject his conclusions. There is no doubt that Erasistratus sometimes used experimentation as a way of resolving problems.[63] He inserted a cannula into an artery to discover whether pulsation was a property of the arterial tunics or the result of *pneuma* being driven into the arteries by the beating heart.[64] On another occasion he showed that there were invisible effluvia from animals by keeping a bird in a vessel without food for some time and then weighing it together with the visible excreta and comparing this with its original weight.[65]

But, on the other hand, Galen rejected with scorn many of the conclusions that Erasistratus drew from his dissections and experiments, using disagreements between later Erasistrateans to point up the failings and inconsistencies of their master. His polemic was at times devastatingly unfair. Erasistratus' reluctance to believe in the theory of humours as expressed, in Galen's view, by Hippocrates in *The Nature of Man* was interpreted as a wholesale rejection of humours; his refusal to accept the universal application of a Platonic 'directed' teleology as a failure to acknowledge any purposeful organisation within the body.[66] That there were others, such as Anonymus Parisinus, who included him among their list of physicians worthy of mention for their views on a variety of diseases was not enough to counteract Galen's biting criticism and secure the survival of his writings much beyond the second century AD.[67]

In part, this was because, unlike Herophilus, Erasistratus did not fit easily into a line of development running directly from Hippocrates to Galen's own teachers. He wrote no commentary on Hippocrates, and, where influences can be discerned, he owed far more to Aristotle and his school than to Plato.[68] His intellectual exuberance led him to wide-ranging investigations and to challenging conclusions, not all of which were easy to reconcile with earlier ideas about the body. What is most striking about him is his willingness to take over into his medicine a variety of concepts and techniques that were being proposed and put into practice by a range of contemporary scientists and engineers. Far from relying on and repeating the written texts of his medical predecessors, he created his own vision of the body in part from the ideas of non-medical men. By contrast with Herophilus, whose descriptions of the body give the impression of something static, Erasistratus emphasised the body as a living and functioning organism, explicable in terms of mechanics and physics.[69]

Mechanical analogies can be found throughout Erasistratus' writings.[70] The kidneys, liver and bladder act as filters.[71] The stomach grinds and crushes ingested food like a corn-mill, producing sensations of hunger if it continues to grind on after the food has been finely milled.[72] Growth and nutrition are mechanical processes, in which the essential nutriment and *pneuma* are distributed around the body by means of an invisible threefold rope of vessels, nerves, veins and arteries, which gains strength and flexibility from their interweaving.[73] Bone, flesh and even the brain substance are then produced as *parenchyma* from this nutriment, which is distributed in part by a vacuum process. To fill the void left by the nutriment that has been taken up, more nutriment is drawn in, since a continuous void is impossible.[74] Humoral fluids are present in the body, but they cause harm through blockages or overflow rather than through inducing qualitative changes.[75]

Many diseases were thus the result of some mechanical failure, which is why Erasistratus' treatises on fevers, paralysis and perhaps those dealing with dropsy and the spitting of blood all included an exposition of the relevant anatomical data.[76] Dropsy, for example, was the result of the scirrhosis of the liver, which felt as hard as a stone and which allowed only the thin watery part of the blood to pass into the veins.[77] Erasistratus' experience of treating those suffering from paralysis and mental disorders both encouraged him to investigate the anatomy of the brain and was enhanced by his discoveries.[78]

More controversial was his belief that fever and inflammation were the result of blood seeping from veins into arteries, which, in the healthy body, contained only *pneuma*.[79] To the obvious objection that, when cut, arteries bled, Erasistratus replied with an ingenious interpretation based on contemporary physics. Like the passage of blood or *pneuma* from aorta to ventricle within the heart, so too the appearance of blood in the arteries could be explained on the principle of the vacuum.[80] Just as blood or *pneuma* moved from one chamber to the other and then outward as the heart valves opened to allow it to flow into the space left vacant by the expelled material, similarly, when an artery was cut, the *pneuma* within it escaped and blood was drawn into it from the veins to fill the vacuum.[81] Whether Erasistratus derived his theory from Strato of Lampsacus or from observing some of the machines created by Ctesibius is less important than the fact that he saw this as a mechanical process within a system that connected veins and arteries by tiny capillaries.[82] Normally, in health, blood could not pass from one system to the other. But when the artery was cut, *pneuma* within it escaped, a vacuum was created and blood flooded in to fill the empty space. In other circumstances it was not an absence of material, but an excess, that was responsible for blood passing from veins to arteries. Within the veins there might be such a build-up of pressure of blood, 'stirred into motion like the sea moved by a gale', that it forced its way through the capillaries into the arteries.[83] Erasistratus concluded that this seepage of blood would then produce fever or, indeed, according to another report of his opinions, all manner of diseases.[84]

For Galen, this doctrine of infiltration was ludicrous and unnecessary, a perversion of sound anatomical observation for misguided clinical ends. It was open to refutation both by logic (and Galen mercilessly exposed the many weak points in its theoretical basis) and by experiment. Galen's repetition of the experimental insertion of a cannula into a ligated artery showed, he claimed, the falsity of any belief in pulsation as a mechanical process within the arteries as opposed to something transmitted within the coats of the arteries.[85] He also criticised Erasistratus for his failure to adapt his therapeutics to his theories by avoiding all mention of venesection as a swift and effective means of removing excess blood.[86] In its place, Erasistratus favoured diet, drugs and the use of bandages to move the blood away from the swelling and to prevent more blood accumulating.[87] But, at the same time, when pressed, Galen was prepared to acknowledge Erasistratus' concern for his patients, his careful attention to diet and drugs (including a dislike of strong purgatives) and his unwillingness to resort to drastic action that might have more serious consequences.[88] Nonetheless, Erasistratus was prepared to take risks. If bold treatment was called for in dealing with a dropsical patient he was prepared to promote a massive evacuation from the body, a procedure he admitted occasionally ended in death.[89] On another occasion he is said to have 'daringly' removed the covering flesh and membranes to apply drugs directly to the liver.[90] But, in general, he stressed that one was more likely to have success by gradual means, to which the patient might become accustomed, than by drastic intervention.[91]

Erasistratus aroused controversy already in his lifetime. Yet he was also an authoritative figure whose writings and influence survived for centuries.[92] Galen had access to several of his books, apparently at first hand, which he then used to convict contemporary Erasistrateans in Rome of a lack of fidelity to their master's teachings.[93]

But if there is good evidence for the survival of his therapeutics, even if only in a misinterpreted form, it remains uncertain how far his interest in experiment and dissection was carried on by others both during and after the lifetime of Herophilus and Erasistratus. Within the Hippocratic Corpus there is a short text, *The Heart*, which contains a description of the heart, whose hidden membranes, 'a piece of craftsmanship most worthy of description', would appear to include at least the semi-lunar valves.[94] When and where this tract was written cannot be determined with certainty. Its language suggests a Hellenistic date, but the fact that its author seems to mention one set of valves, not the 'inlet' valves discovered by Erasistratus, and thinks of them in terms of 'stays', 'cobwebs' and 'fibres', not little doors, suggests that he was writing either before or in ignorance of those discoveries.[95] Nor is there evidence of a link with Herophilus or any other Alexandrian, and indications of influence from Stoic philosophy are suggestive at best.[96] While it is tempting to envisage this author carrying out an Aristotelian programme of animal dissection (for his description of the heart is likely to be that of an animal and he unambiguously recommends an experiment on a pig to show how tight the epiglottis fits), not even this is certain.[97] There are no obvious school affiliations, and no references to the work of others. All that can be said is that the author claims to be a very skilful anatomist who thinks about the wider consequences of his theme, and that, whatever his date, he is apparently working away from any obvious centre. For such a man to remain ignorant of the discoveries of Herophilus and Erasistratus might seem implausible, and hence a date in the 270s is most likely. But – and this cannot be overemphasised – our knowledge of medicine and medical groupings at this period is so fragmentary, and our understanding of the process whereby new ideas and discoveries were transmitted so fallible, that this is at best a very fragile conclusion.[98]

Another anatomist, Eudemus, was also a contemporary of Herophilus and Erasistratus, although where he lived and wrote his treatise on anatomy is uncertain. Galen praises him as a practical dissector, although one far from reliable in his conclusions, despite his technical ability.[99] Eudemus prepared a description of the bones and investigated the pancreas and the nerves, as well as the transit of the vessels in the umbilical cord from the foetus to the womb.[100] He may have seen and described the horns of the uterus, but it is more likely that, in this instance, Galen was referring to another doctor, Euenor.[101] Even less reliance can be put on Wellmann's attribution to him of a fragmentary papyrus from the first century BC. Its division of nerves into motor and sensory postdates Herophilus, while its mention of the nerves in the brain and those issuing from the spinal cord continues a debate begun by Erasistratus.[102] But it is impossible to tell from the badly damaged pieces whether this was an independent record of new dissections or, more likely, a short summary of results achieved much earlier.

This evidence for a keen interest in investigative dissection in the first half of the third century BC, whether performed on animals or, in Alexandria, on humans, stands in sharp contrast to what follows. Galen's list of anatomists has a large gap between Eudemus and Marinus, who flourished at the end of the first century AD.[103] Rufus of Ephesus, who had visited Alexandria, lamented that, in his own day, the late first century AD, one had to learn the parts of the human body from observing the surface anatomy of a slave and dissecting an animal, whereas 'in the old days this was more correctly taught on man'.[104] However, the absence of interest in systematic dissection should not be mistaken for a disdain for anatomical knowledge. Celsus' discussion of dissection in his preface depends on an earlier writer (or writers) for whom the question of whether or not to dissect still addressed a practical possibility.[105] Likewise, at the beginning of the first century BC Apollonius of Citium chided Hegetor and contemporary Herophileans for their inconsistency in proclaiming the value of anatomy while failing to apply it in their practice.[106] He himself rejected dissection in favour of experience, both his own and that of others, rebutting Hegetor's anatomical explanation of a dislocated hip solely by a close interpretation of passages from Hippocrates.[107]

But even as Celsus and Apollonius participate in a debate about the value of anatomy, they reveal a shift in the focus of dissection away from the investigative and experimental. They report no new discoveries, no new experiments. Even for those who regard it as essential, anatomical knowledge is subordinated to a wider medical purpose, providing a basis for such ongoing concerns as pulse diagnosis and surgery.[108] The argument of its defenders is expressed pragmatically: if one knows human anatomy well, one will be better able to treat disease and apply remedies. The general ethical objection to human dissection as unnecessarily cruel is countered only by the argument that benefits to the future innocent outweigh the harm done to a few criminals.[109] The epistemological difficulties raised by the Empiricists (see pp. 149–52) and acknowledged by Cicero are not answered in Celsus' prologue: the case for anatomy remains simply at the level of practical advantage.[110]

The perception of dissection as cruel, irrelevant and unnecessary, a perception 'accepted by most people' according to Celsus, helps to explain the decline of Erasistratean anatomy, especially if it was accompanied by social and political changes that gradually put an end to the 'frontier spirit' of early Alexandria. There was never any formal institutionalisation of the sciences, including medicine, in Antiquity comparable to the universities and medical colleges that in the Middle Ages and Renaissance provided the stability that ensured the continuation of ideas and practices from one generation of researchers to another. It is rare that an interest in one particular aspect of research, in mineralogy or statics for example, is continued with any intensity for more than a generation or two. The shift away from anatomy from 250 BC is an instance of this, although this is not the whole story.[111] That royal protection was ever formally withdrawn is unlikely, but the arguments that might justify supporting those who wished to experiment on criminals became ever weaker.[112] Once the relevant data had been established by Herophilus and Erasistratus there was less need to repeat inhumane investigations in order merely to confirm what was already known. Some argued that new anatomical information might be found as easily by chance as by systematic anatomy, for a trained observer would not let the slightest thing escape his notice.[113] Alternatively, one might acquire all necessary anatomical knowledge from reading about it, becoming, as Galen scathingly put it, like a steersman who navigates solely from a book – and just as dangerous, in his view.[114] Others, and they were the majority, disagreed with this condemnation of book learning, and their objections still form part of a continuing debate today about the role and methodology of human anatomical dissection in the training of a modern medical student. Those who champion the need for dissection of human corpses in order to understand the human body and to become a better doctor are now opposed by those who argue that modern technology has rendered obsolete many of the doctor's former skills and that the simulated reality of an interactive video of a living body can teach the student far more than any dissection of a dead corpse. The Hellenistic dilemma is still with us today.

10

HELLENISTIC MEDICINE

To devote a chapter to the history of medicine in the Hellenistic Greek world, apart from anatomy and the coming of Greek medicine to Rome, might be thought unduly quixotic. Few original treatises survive, a situation characteristic of Greek literature of this period in general. The very success of Hellenistic scholars in commending as models the writings of earlier Greek historians, poets and orators militated against their own survival. What followed the Golden Age came to be seen as degenerate, lacking in originality or serious purpose, produced by ivory-towered pedants, akin to twittering birds in a cage and about as useful.[1] In philosophy, the later triumphs of Aristotelianism and (neo-)Platonism left little space for their opponents, the Epicureans and Stoics.[2] In medicine, Galenism emphasised the link with Hippocrates at the expense of other theoretical developments in the Hellenistic world, and, since what later writers thought the most significant results of the work of Hellenistic pharmacologists and surgeons could be easily incorporated into more up-to-date treatises, there was little reason to preserve the original books themselves. The literary remains of Hellenistic medicine have thus to be reconstructed almost entirely from the fragments preserved by others, with the constant dangers of deformation and misunderstanding. The traditional skills of the philologist, the precise decipherment and interpretation of an ancient text, must be exercised on material that rarely allows certainty.

Yet from a different perspective this historical enterprise takes on a less gloomy aspect. Although many details are inevitably gone beyond recovery, new trends, new developments and new opportunities can be discerned, without which the history of later Graeco-Roman medicine cannot properly be understood. New types of evidence begin to appear in abundance, notably the Egyptian papyri and the inscriptions set up in cities around the Greek world, especially in Asia Minor. If for the fifth and fourth centuries we are largely dependent for our information on medical treatises, speeches, histories and plays, the balance shifts in the Hellenistic period towards the non-literary evidence. No one city dominates; even Alexandrian medicine takes on a different appearance when viewed from a town several hundreds of miles up the Nile valley. Nor is there a block of contemporary material, such as the Hippocratic Corpus, on which attention can be easily focused. The resulting pattern is both more varied and more impressionistic.[3]

If the fourth century BC was the time when dietetics developed as an almost independent part of medicine, the Hellenistic period saw the rise of pharmacology to a similar status. Alexander's conquests and the growth of Alexandria to be the major entrepôt for the import and export of rare substances from Africa and India saw a massive increase in the range of herbs and spices becoming available.[4] Aristotle's pupil and successor Theophrastus (c.371–287), as well as displaying a wide interest in many aspects of biology, also wrote extensively on plants, including medicinal ones, combining information he obtained from rootcutters with his own observations and experiments.[5] His listings of plants are more extensive than those in the Hippocratic Corpus, and the number of new substances recorded in medical and botanical texts continued to increase for several centuries more.

This interest in new drugs was accompanied by a more sophisticated understanding of their workings. Diocles has been credited with introducing the important notion that drugs worked through their properties, or potentialities in the sense of the word used by Aristotle.[6] In a poison, for instance, the transmitted venom, although relatively small, had the potentiality to bring about enormous changes within the body of the host. Erasistratus developed this notion further when discussing antidotes either in a separate tract called *On Causes* or, more likely, in a large work dealing with the properties of poisons.[7] The exact effect of the bite of a poisonous snake, the cenchrines, he discovered by performing an autopsy.[8] But it was the followers of Herophilus, more than the Erasistrateans, who most developed medical botany.[9] Although none of their works survives in full, both Andreas of Carystus (d. 217 BC, who was one of the personal doctors to Ptolemy IV of Egypt) and Mantias (fl. 120–100) were regarded as significant authorities, and their portraits were included among those of the great pharmacologists in the opening pages of the Vienna manuscript of Dioscorides, of c.AD 512. Andreas was praised by Dioscorides in his preface as one of the two most accurate writers on medicinal roots and plants – the second being Crateuas – although others were less convinced of his personal experience.[10] Mantias' expertise lay in the production of compound remedies, although he was not the first to make such preparations.[11] Another pharmacologist, Apollodorus (fl. 280 BC), was regarded by later writers as the author of the first specific study of poisons. He is likely to have been among the sources on which the poet Nicander of Colophon, about 100 years later, drew for his own two works on pharmacology, his *Theriac* and his *Antidotes*.[12] Written in a highly ornate and mannered style, these two poems describe both animal venoms and poisonous plants. *Antidotes* shows a remarkably detailed knowledge of the specific action of plant toxins, but those from animals are less clearly differentiated or understood.[13]

143

The transfer of medical material into a didactic poem – and Nicander was neither the first nor the last to do this[14] – shows something of the cultural context in which learned medicine was developing. Nicander required an audience that could appreciate his linguistic *tour de force* as well as the interesting technical information that his poems contained.[15] In his virtuosity he followed the example of the leading poet of third-century Alexandria, Callimachus, who incorporated into his own poetry some of the latest ideas set forth by medical authors and practitioners. His contemporary, the epigrammatist Posidippus, devoted one section of his poems to some at times graphic descriptions of medical cures, the *Iamatika*.[16] Pharmacology also found royal patrons and practitioners. Attalus III of Pergamum (ruled 138–133 BC) allegedly carried out pharmacological experiments with poisons on his own slaves.[17] A more celebrated royal experimenter was Mithridates VI of Pontus (132–63 BC), who allegedly protected himself against poisoning by taking small doses of poison until he was habituated to it. He gave his name to a famous compound drug, Mithridation, which was claimed to be a universal cure because it included all known antidotes.[18] His remedies were taken over by Pompeius Lenaeus, the freedman of his conqueror, the Roman general Pompey, and thereby entered the Roman orbit.[19] Mithridates was in contact with another famous medical botanist, Crateuas (fl. 90 BC), whose large book was among the very first to be illustrated with drawings of the plants themselves.[20]

The abundance of new drugs and new botanical techniques also led to problems for the user. Heraclides of Tarentum, around 70 BC, wrote a tract devoted specifically to the proper preparation and testing of drugs, which he dedicated to Antiochis, in all likelihood the same person as the woman doctor honoured with a public statue in the main square of her home town of Tlos in S.W. Turkey for her remarkable medical knowledge.[21] Heraclides was the author of another recipe collection, entitled *The Soldier*, which may have dealt with military medicine.[22] Others composed works on cosmetics and beauty aids, of which the most celebrated was one allegedly written by Cleopatra, Queen of Egypt (ruled 51–30 BC), although her authorship is as unlikely as the later tradition that she taught Galen pharmacology.[23]

Another area of medicine where major developments can be discerned only dimly was surgery. The anatomical discoveries of Herophilus and Erasistratus led to new techniques and new instruments, and Alexandrian surgeons in particular gained a great reputation for their work in dealing with fractures and dislocations.[24] Palliative surgery, particularly for congenital malformations such as club-foot, aimed less at curing the condition completely than at allowing the patient to live a relatively normal and pain-free life.[25] Whether it also lessened the stigma of deformity is a more difficult question.[26] The Roman author Celsus provides us with many details of splints and other mechanical aids devised in this period to help recovery from surgery or injury, and it is tempting to place also at this time the beginnings of a trade in specialised medical instruments, although most continued to be made by

144

the local blacksmith.[27] Some idea of the complexity of Alexandrian surgery can be gained from the so-called commentary of Apollonius of Citium on the Hippocratic *Joints*.[28] Apollonius, who was active at the court of one of the Ptolemies, either in Cyprus or in Egypt around 90 BC, goes far beyond his Hippocratic text in his discussion of hip dislocations, which he illustrated with drawings and diagrams.[29] The surviving manuscripts of his work, especially the so-called Nicetas codex of around AD 900, contain later reworkings of his drawings, but their close relationship to Apollonius' originals and to his text is clear.[30] Apollonius' book is more a meditation on the Hippocratic treatise than a commentary in the strict sense of the word. Some of the Hippocratic passages are passed over in silence; others merely provide the spur for a discourse of Apollonius' own.

But by taking *Joints* as his starting point, Apollonius shows himself to be writing within a trend that set special store by the writings of Hippocrates. This can be traced back at least to Herophilus, who discussed sections of the Hippocratic *Prognostic*, although probably not in the form of a running commentary.[31] Some of his pupils composed glossaries, dictionaries of words found in the Hippocratic Corpus that were hard to understand, in an endeavour to interpret what were clearly seen as authoritative writings. Others struggled to make sense of the signs and abbreviations found in some manuscripts of the *Epidemics*. It is, however, doubtful whether these medical scholars also composed detailed commentaries explaining the text line by line and word by word as part of their teaching of their students, and there is nothing to suggest that they were concerned with what modern scholars have called the Hippocratic question, the identification of those works written by the master himself.[32] What is certain, however, is that this growing interest in Hippocrates was not confined to a small group of Herophileans.[33] A papyrus fragment from Tebtunis in Egypt, written at the end of the third century BC, appears to quote *Regimen*, and may well come from an early discussion of this tract.[34] Heraclides, and others in the so-called Empiricist school before him, also used some of the mysterious sayings of Hippocrates to claim that they alone were the true followers of his teaching and that he valued empirical evidence above all else.[35]

The idealisation of Hippocrates as a medical authority in this period also gave rise to, and was in turn influenced by, biographical invention. The letters and speeches within our Hippocratic Corpus, all of them spurious, describing or purporting to derive from incidents in his life, date from this period. They emphasise Hippocrates' wisdom (witness his non-treatment of Democritus), his shrewdness (in his cure of King Perdiccas of Macedonia) and, above all, his patriotism.[36] Hippocrates speaks on behalf of his native island of Cos against the Athenians wishing to enslave and punish it; he intervenes in Athens to cure the great plague (an incident unknown to Thucydides); and he refuses the substantial reward offered to him to go and treat the King of Persia, for this would be to help the enemy of the Greeks.[37] This creation of a biography

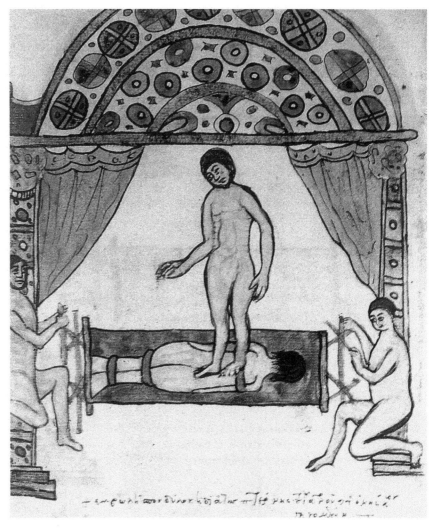

Figure 10.1 Reducing a dislocated spine by traction. From Apollonius of Citium, Bologna University, Ms. 3632, fol. 428v., a fifteenth-century copy of the Nicetas codex.

for a figure from the past is typical of the scholarship and belles lettres of the Hellenistic period, and it is only in recent years that the fragility of this seductive 'evidence' has been fully appreciated.[38]

How Hippocratic texts might be used in a more general way and how a new consensus about the doctrines of the historical Hippocrates was in the process of formation can be seen in a work in a very different genre, the *Problems* ascribed to Aristotle, which quotes directly from *Airs, Waters and Places* and includes other Hippocratic allusions in the discussions of

146

medicine that occupy a large part of the work.[39] When this collection of scientific questions and answers was first put together is a matter of some controversy. Part of it may go back to Aristotle's day, if not to Aristotle himself.[40] But if it had been entirely composed in the third quarter of the fourth century BC its sophisticated use of Hippocratic material, striking enough as it is, would stand out still further, and would demand a complete rethinking of the growth and development of Hippocratism.[41] In fact, considerations of language and philosophical influences suggest that a date around 250 BC for most of the *Problems* is far more likely. This would still demonstrate the importance of Hippocratic theories, while allowing time for a Hippocratic Corpus to be formed and used within the Hellenistic environment of Alexandria and perhaps also Athens.[42]

Whatever their precise date, the *Problems* provide a rare insight into views on medicine in the period after the Hippocratic Corpus. Only the first section, according to the subtitle, is devoted to medicine, but this is misleading, for medical themes occupy the first fourteen sections, and recur frequently after that, sometimes repeated in a different context or examined from a different perspective. Some problems are put forward very brusquely, and are answered in the form of a second question: why is it that great excesses cause disease? Is it because they engender excess or defect, and because it is in these, after all, that disease consists?[43] Others constitute almost little treatises in themselves. One can thus learn why cabbage is used to clear a hangover; and why diseases such as phthisis, ophthalmia and scabies, unlike dropsy, can be easily transmitted to susceptible contacts.[44] To the question of why those pre-eminent in the arts, music, philosophy and the like are clearly of a melancholic or atrabilious temperament, the author responds with a long disquisition on the effects of black bile and the meaning of temperament that was taken up by a whole string of authors from Antiquity onwards.[45]

The collection as a whole displays a consistent approach to both the theory and practice of medicine.[46] The human body is situated within the Aristotelian universe of the four primary qualities and the four elements. Illness is largely the result of excess or deficiency, which explains also why doctors cease treatment once the patient has been restored to health by the rectification of any imbalance.[47] Constant attention to diet and exercise, though, is valuable because they enable the body to reduce any potentially dangerous excesses, and hence lessen the chances of illness.[48] The body is always liable to imbalance as a result of its natural mixture or temperament, and each temperament is prone to particular types of diseases and conditions, in both mind and body. In particular, the body is affected by the seasons, location, winds and all the sorts of changes familiar to any reader of the *Epidemics* and *Airs, Waters and Places*. So the Ethiopians and Egyptians have bandy legs and frizzy hair because they are burned up by the sun, and northerners are on the whole more warlike and courageous than southerners. It is potentially more dangerous to live in a low lying or marshy district than on a mountain – witness the pallor of the faces of the marsh dwellers – and a city whose streets are swept by brisk healthy breezes is more healthy than one in which the air is confined and stagnant.[49] The one possible exception to this basically humoral explanation of disease is plague, which affects all who in some way associate with those already suffering from it and which cannot easily be fitted in to a schema based on individual temperament. The author does raise the possibility that this is the one disease to which everyone is liable, no matter what their individual make-up, but he appears to prefer a slightly different solution. Plague affects anyone in a poor state of health: it takes advantage of an already-existing situation.[50]

In these *Problems* the understanding of disease and therapy is firmly allopathic: one reduces excess and restores deficiency to bring the body back into equilibrium. Herbs and other therapies are thus chosen because they produce particular effects. The compilers then go on to ask a series of questions about how certain drugs or procedures work as a class, for example styptics or cautery, and about how and why the doctor prescribes others in ways that at first sight seem to go against the general rule or that appear to contradict one another.[51] It might seem strange that in a quartan fever, an obviously hot disease, one should stuff the patient with food. In fact, explains the author, the whole aim of the treatment is to douse the flame of the fever, for, just as a large fire in a forest will swallow up smaller camp fires, so by making the body even hotter by feeding it, its own heat will consume away the fire of the fever. Once that is done, the temperature will drop as the amount of food is reduced.[52] Another question relates to two different therapies for the same condition. A bruise can be cured by applying either thapsia, a hot drug, immediately, or a cold bronze ladle some time later. The explanation given is that both bring about the same result but by different means. Both aim to stop the blood from congealing into a bruised swelling: thapsia by heating the body immediately so that the blood does not have time to congeal; a cold ladle by chilling the surface of the skin to such an extent that it freezes, thereby preventing the heat of the swelling from escaping outwards. Returning inwards, it heats the congealed blood, which becomes liquid again and flows away from the affected spot. Later on, another suggestion is tentatively made: the bronze ladle may have on its surface imperceptible traces of rust, which has a medicinal effect.[53]

The range of questions and answers is extremely wide. Sometimes they deal with details of daily practice. How can one diagnose an abscess? Answer: perhaps by pouring boiling water over it, which will reveal whether it is an abscess or some other type of swelling (a somewhat desperate and painful solution, one might think).[54] Or why does one need to remove poultices at regular intervals? Is it to prevent them losing their effect?[55] Sometimes they concern the physiology of normal bodily activities – sexual activity, seeing, speaking, touching or the consequences of lying down in particularly uncomfortable positions.[56] They deal with climate as well as drugs, the changes in the smell of urine after having eaten or drunk certain foodstuffs as well as mental aberrations.[57] Some of the questions fall into the category of things that everyone ought to know; others raise intelligent questions about phenomena that the author has observed and thinks require an explanation if they are to be brought into line with the overall schema of explanation. In general, they are formed within a society familiar with the general humoral and allopathic doctrines that can be found within the Hippocratic Corpus and among the authors listed by Anonymus Londinensis.[58] They show how widespread these general notions were, and how apparent anomalies might provoke enquiry and explanation.

The Aristotelian *Problems* also acts as a salutary reminder that thinking about medicine did not stop with the Hippocratic Corpus, nor was confined to doctors. The followers of Aristotle and Theophrastus continued to discuss medical phenomena such as breathing, while both the Epicurean and Stoic philosophers utilised, and possibly developed, new medical theories in explaining the interrelationship of body and soul. Epicurean physics could be invoked to explain the phenomenon of contagion.[59] The Latin Epicurean poet Lucretius devoted much of the final book of his poem *On the Nature of Things* to a discussion of disease, and of plague in particular. He places the origin of plague in putrefied air, either acting directly on an individual or poisoning the waters, crops and animals on which mankind relies, but his explanation for why the air becomes putrefied involves Epicurean notions of 'seeds', some giving life, others causing destruction and disease.[60] Whether Lucretius was relying on earlier Epicureans such as Demetrius of Laconia (fl. 120 BC), who is said to have discussed medical themes, or on more recent physicians in Rome is disputed, but is far less significant than his sophisticated use of medical examples to explain and justify his own philosophy.[61]

The growth of philosophical groupings or sects in the Hellenistic period has a parallel in medicine, for later physicians in Antiquity often described the development of medicine in this period in terms of schools and sects. What is implied by these terms is far from clear.[62] Some of the Herophileans were thought of as constituting a 'household', tied to an individual, whereas some 'schools' enshrined a tradition based in a certain location, such as the philosophical schools of Athens.[63] Some of these groupings were short-lived, others more enduring: doctors claiming to be Democriteans or Erasistrateans survived well into the Roman period.[64] Almost always, however, the word 'sect' is best interpreted as a shared ideology rather than any official institution and hierarchy. But, as in philosophy, there was no easy means of securing adherence to the doctrine of the sect in every particular, and there were ample opportunities for individual interpretations of the words of one's distinguished predecessors.[65]

The most extensive and durable of these Hellenistic medical sects was that of the Empiricists.[66] Its founder was a dissident pupil of Herophilus, Philinus of Cos, around 260 BC, although it claimed an even earlier authority in Acron of Acragas in Sicily, a contemporary of Empedocles in the mid-fifth century.[67] Its leading adherents in the Hellenistic period came from all over the Greek-speaking world, from Alexandria itself, the home of Serapion (fl. 225 BC), whom some believed was the real creator of the sect, to Antioch, Cyrene, Tarentum and Naples, a reminder that even after the Roman conquest of Italy the Greeks of S. Italy remained fully a part of the intellectual life of the E. Mediterranean.[68] Later in the Roman world some Empiricists became closely associated with Sceptical philosophy, but although the arguments of the Sceptics will have provided useful ammunition for the Empiricists in their debates with other doctors, the fragments of the earlier Empiricists show that they drew on a much wider range of writers.[69]

The Empiricists gained their name from their theories, not from their adherence to a specific teacher, such as Hippocrates, Erasistratus or Praxagoras.[70] In particular, they rejected any investigation into the causes of disease as both unhelpful and irrelevant, mere dogmas.[71] It was unhelpful, because those who sought to cure disease by eliminating its cause frequently disagreed over what it was they should be seeking, and irrelevant because, even if the patient could be indeed cured by deciding, for example, to restore a bodily balance, the same result, the recovery of the patient, could be achieved more swiftly and effectively by other means.[72] They were prepared to concede that some diseases had a physical or natural cause for which an appropriate treatment could be devised, but other successful cures seemed to be purely the result of chance or of an individual decision or inspired action – a sudden desire for a drink of water or, when stranded on a mountain, the application of a leaf of a plant growing nearby to an animal or insect bite.[73] In such circumstances to trace a chain of causation would be complex, time consuming and possibly fruitless. What counted was effective treatment. Sometimes what was needed was immediately obvious, sometimes one had a flash of inspiration, but in many cases one knew what would be likely to work simply from having had prior experience. Successful repetition of the cure would lead to a conviction of the value of a particular treatment 'for the most part', and close examination of all the circumstances of the cure might offer even greater precision in the future. The more experience the doctor had, the better he was likely to be; just as for the carpenter or the cobbler, practice made perfect.[74]

This experience need not be entirely that of the individual doctor himself. Case histories, the codified record of previous success, played an important role, providing a wider data bank for future use.[75] The Empiricists were particularly keen on recording information on drugs and their effectiveness, drawing on, and at times criticising, the work of the Herophileans.[76] The weakness of experience, so their opponents alleged, was that it dealt only with the past: when faced with an apparently new condition or new circumstances (such as having to treat an illness while on a journey away from home or without one's regular supply of remedies) the Empiricist doctor had to start effectively from scratch and resort to a method of trial and error. Such criticism was countered by the principle that, having observed carefully the conditions of a new case, the doctor should choose whatever therapy had worked in 'similar' circumstances. It was accepted that this was not the same as the certainty that could be gained from dealing with an identical case, but it provided a good starting point. Swift action, taken cautiously, might be of far greater benefit than lengthy ratiocination.[77] How effective this treatment might be depended on three things, the so-called 'tripod': accurate observation, a well-stocked library or, more often, a collective memory of what had worked in the past and an understanding of the virtues and limitations of similarity.[78] If the similarity was not sufficiently great, then the chances of a successful transition were greatly reduced.[79]

It is precisely this understanding of the epistemological difficulties of similarities that lies behind the Empiricists' rejection of anatomical investigation in the fashion of Herophilus and Erasistratus. They did not deny the findings of anatomy; they merely questioned its relevance and the need for its repetition. They saw no justification for cruelty or for mutilating a corpse if the knowledge that was thereby gained could be obtained by other means, by chance observation of a dead body or during treatment.[80] Indeed, careful observation of patients avoided the greatest problem with anatomy, that what was revealed in a dead body might be irrelevant to the cure of the living. The living body functioned differently from a dead one, and one courted disaster by applying information taken from a corpse to the treatment of a living patient. There was thus no longer any need to carry out such a barbaric procedure, since all the most useful information had been obtained by the earliest dissectors.[81]

Despite their name, the Empiricists were more than empirics. Indeed, their philosophy, their insistence on accurate observation, 'autopsy' (seeing for oneself), and recording of symptoms, signs and syndromes, their openness to new ideas and techniques, not to speak of their reverence for Hippocrates, the empirical observer, all indicate that their leading members were among the most learned doctors of their time.[82] Galen acknowledged the great merits of Heraclides of Tarentum, high praise in itself and entirely justified, even though he then proceeded to use Heraclides' disagreements with other Empiricists over the meaning of the pulse or the value of observations to cast doubt on their whole enterprise.[83] Heraclides wrote substantial books on dietetics, internal and external treatments and at least two major collections of drug recipes, appropriate works for a man said to have been trained by the distinguished Herophilean pharmacologist Mantias.[84] He was a more than competent surgeon. According to Celsus, he invented a technique for gently separating with the knife an eyelid that was adhering to the eyeball, although Celsus himself had never seen anyone successfully cured by this means.[85] His prescriptions for curing a large variety of ailments continued to be cited into Late Antiquity, although Caelius Aurelianus, our major authority, generally mentions them only to warn others of their dangerous consequences, and is likely to be citing them at second hand from the much earlier Soranus of Ephesus.[86] And Heraclides' explanations of Hippocratic sayings combined medical awareness with a fine sense of Greek style, which is not always true of other commentators.[87]

That Heraclides himself was sensitive to the difficulties and dangers of therapy is clear from his comments on his predecessor, Andreas of Carystus, whom he contrasted with Hippocrates. Hippocrates, as his writings showed, was extremely experienced and passionate for the truth; Andreas, on the other hand, was bombastic and unpractised, a charlatan who unthinkingly copied down details of plants he had never even seen. In a telling simile, Heraclides likened Andreas and others of his kind to public criers who give out a detailed description of a runaway slave without ever having set eyes on him. They take down details from those who know the slave, but would be unable to recognise him themselves, even if he were standing next to them. Their words function like a mere charm.[88]

Galen, who preserves this caustic comment of Heraclides, associates Andreas with one of his own bêtes noires, the grammarian Pamphilus of Alexandria (fl. AD 60), whose lists of plants and animals contained a mixture of learned and folk remedies.[89] Galen himself scornfully dismissed this as largely nonsense and mumbo-jumbo, refusing to have anything to do with lists of remedies drawn from basilisks, elephants and crocodiles. In his dislike for these strange concoctions he had a predecessor in Erasistratus, who had warned against the rash use of strange animal products such as the bile of the elephant or the crocodile.[90] But others no less eminent, such as Andreas and his near-contemporary, the Empiricist Serapion of Alexandria, drew the line differently between what was acceptable and what was not. Given his theoretical commitment to recording what worked or what had often been said in the past to have worked, it is easy to see why Serapion could have noted down a therapy for epilepsy that included camel's brains and bile, hare's heart, sea-turtle's blood and crocodile dung.[91] Similar remedies can be found in the learned tradition as well as in the so-called magical papyri. Much of this lore was taken over by such pharmaceutical writers as Sextius Niger (fl. 20 BC), and reappears in particular in the medical sections in the *Natural History* of the Elder Pliny.[92]

That a good deal of this material goes back at least to Greek circles in Alexandria in the first half of the third century BC is highly likely, and it can be associated with such supposititious works as that of Democritus' *On Antipathy and Sympathy*.[93] It includes Egyptian and Persian lore, with an appeal to a long tradition of the magi, and it would be wrong to exclude a Greek component in this amalgam.[94] That knowledge of it spread widely can be gathered from the magical papyri (although most are from much later periods), and from the circulation of writings attributed to exotic figures such as Bolus of Mende and Ostanes the Persian magus.[95] It serves as a reminder that the Hellenistic world now included, within an overall Greek administrative and political framework, other cultures that had maintained their own traditions of healing. The strong Babylonian belief in the power of demons to cause illness is recorded on cuneiform texts well into the Hellenistic period, and undoubtedly contributed to the wider notions of demonic possession that are found in both Jewish and early Christian writings.[96] Jewish prophets, 'holy men', were believed also to have the power to heal, and these wandering healers were a common sight in Hellenistic Palestine.[97] Alongside a more ascetic linkage between healing and proper religious belief and practice there were Jewish stories that ascribed a knowledge of herbs, chants and charms to some of the great figures from their past, most notably King Solomon.[98] In Egypt embalmers continued to remove the major organs of the dead, and their speciality of clystering had its own adherents and professionals. In an apprenticeship contract from the late first century, drawn up in Greek, an apprentice clysterer is promised an income for life, should he succeed in learning this technique.[99]

Although one can point to these varied traditions, and to an interchange, at least at the level of drugs, between Greek and non-Greek, the precise nature of this interaction remains very uncertain. Although there is some evidence for influence from the Greek upon some of the Egyptian medical texts kept in their major temples, the learned Greek medical texts and medical papyri show very little influence from Egyptian medicine.[100] Galen's inclusion of two remedies said to have come from an Egyptian temple at the major religious site of Memphis is a rare instance of such borrowing.[101] But far from implying any systematic search for effective native remedies, this citation merely shows the great variety of sources upon which Galen and others like him could draw for allegedly effective remedies. Galen makes no distinction between this remedy from an Egyptian temple and those he credited to Euschemus the eunuch, Orion the groom, Pharnaces the Persian rootcutter, Aristocrates the schoolmaster, Epaphroditus of Carthage, Protas of Egyptian Pelusium and Simmias the crowd-puller.[102]

Whether any of the medical institutions of the non-Greek world were taken over by the successors of Alexander is an even more puzzling question. Evidence survives in quantity only from Egypt, and would seem to indicate that there the centralised organisation of Pharaonic doctors survived at least in part. We read of a Tatas, 'a royal doctor', who, like the 'royal scribe', would appear to be a district official, probably attending to the Greeks or royal officials in his locality.[103] The Greek settlers to whom land was assigned after Alexander's conquest paid a special medical tax, perhaps to pay for doctors such as Tatas, but evidence for the continued payment of this tax after the Roman conquest is very dubious.[104] The historian Diodorus, writing at the end of the first century BC but basing himself on much earlier writers, says that 'the doctors' received subsistence allowances from the community in return for providing free treatment for soldiers and those on, presumably official, visits.[105] A similar tax is known for some Greek cities (although it was far from universal), but since papyri record doctors' fees and other sources of income the stipend of a 'royal doctor' was likely to have been relatively basic and would have been supplemented from other sources. Besides, a close reading of Diodorus makes it clear that his free treatment was not universal but restricted to a group of officials away from their headquarters.

Around 140 BC a courtier, Chrysermus, is recorded as ἐπὶ τῶν ἰατρῶν at Alexandria. Some scholars have thought that he was 'in charge of the doctors', but, more recently, Fridolf Kudlien, stressing that there is no other evidence that Chrysermus was a doctor, has interpreted the title to mean that he was in charge of the 'medical taxes'. Both meanings are possible in the Greek.[106] If Chrysermus was indeed in charge of the doctors, he could be considered the Ptolemaic equivalent of the 'chief doctor' or 'chief of the doctors of Upper and Lower Egypt', who seems to have been the head of the medical hierarchy in the Pharaonic period. That such a post continued under the Greeks may be implied from the tone in which Athenagoras, the *archiatros*, or 'chief doctor', wrote to the mummy-dressers and priests of the Fayum at some point in the first century BC demanding that they release the body of an assistant whom he did not want to be mummified.[107] But Athenagoras, as a leading physician, almost certainly at court, may have adopted this tone of superior authority with everyone, and did not rely on any official line of control to have his way.

Elsewhere in the Hellenistic world, the title of *archiatros* was applied to the personal physicians of the ruler. The earliest instance of its use so far known is in a religious dedication made on behalf of Apollophanes, chief doctor to Antiochus III, the Seleucid ruler. Apollophanes served at least three monarchs, and had acted as friend and tutor to the young Antiochus. He was a member of the royal council and played a leading role in unmasking the conspiracy of Hermias at the beginning of Antiochus' reign. A fragment of a letter to the people of Cos from Antiochus, probably in 197–192 BC, praises Apollophanes' services to him, and extols his merits as a physician.[108] He may have been the inventor of a complex vegetable theriac used by Antiochus against the threat of poisoning and reported by both Pliny and Galen. According to Pliny, this recipe was transcribed in verse on the walls of the Asclepieion of Cos, a pretty story if true.[109] Apollophanes' career can be paralleled from other courts. We have already encountered Andreas, killed in the tent of Ptolemy IV on the eve of the battle of Raphia in 217 BC; and Papias of Amisus was chief doctor, councillor and secretary to Mithridates VI of Pontus in 102–101 BC.[110] Slightly older than Papias was Craterus, 'first friend, chief doctor and keeper of the queen's bedchamber' under Antiochus VII of Syria.[111] Stories of their involvement with politics abound, whether the poisoning of a monarch or, a celebrated and much reworked tale, the medical discovery of the love of Antiochus I for his stepmother Stratonice and his subsequent acceptance as co-regent with his father around 294–292 BC.[112]

These royal physicians stood at the apex of a very disparate collection of practitioners. At the other extreme were the travelling doctors, wandering the roads of Greece or Judaea, touting their wares and their skills. Between the two came perhaps the majority of doctors, resident in one place for a long while, either using it as a base for touring or, increasingly, setting up small medical dynasties.[113] Egyptian papyri show doctors paying their taxes as farmers in their villages and an inscription in both Greek and Latin from S. Italy from the first century AD mentions a doctor's estate and orchard.[114] Both papyri and inscriptions place the doctor on the same level as village crafts-men. Around 200 BC two small towns in central Greece, Myania and Hypnia, came to an agreement that they would jointly pay for the services of 'one doctor and the other craftsmen', who had previously been supported solely by the Hypnians.[115] Given the small size of these communities, it is hardly surprising that the doctor is rarely among the top layer of the wealthy in a wider area, unless in royal service. But neither is he ranked among the low-est. In Cyrene *c*.300 BC the public physician is placed on the same level as the public teacher and the public trainer in archery, riding and hoplite-weapons, wealthy enough to be among the 10,000 with full citizen rights, but well below the political elite.[116] Even on Cos, where names of medical families can be traced for several decades, only one physician is to be found among the highest contributors to the *epidosis* tax. The others are of the 'middling sort', respectable but hardly outstanding.[117] Besides, in a society where the wealthy lived entirely on the income derived from others, as landlords or as slave-owners, having to work oneself for pay or reward was an indication that one did not properly belong to the elite. The Roman Cicero's praise of medicine as a liberal art, superior to shoe-making, is strongly qualified by his comment that it was suitable for those of an appropriate rank in society.[118] Seen from the perspective of a subsistence farmer, the life of a doctor might well appear eminently desirable; from that of a leading citizen of Athens or Alexandria, it was little better than that of a tradesman.[119]

One reason for this may be simply that there was a superfluity of doctors and not enough wealthy patients. Leaving aside the competition from other forms of healing, doctors are found at times in remarkably large numbers. It is not only in Antioch or Alexandria that one might expect to find many doctors, perhaps even organised into a medical guild, but even in much smaller towns.[120] Around 250 BC at Metapontum in S. Italy at least seventeen 'active' doctors, all members of the 'first workshop', were cursed together by an unknown person, either a disgruntled patient or ex-colleague or, for 'first' implies more than one, a member of a rival practice. An archaeologi-cal survey of the town and its dependent region suggests that at its peak, around 350 BC, there were around 40,000 inhabitants, perhaps two-thirds of whom lived outside the city.[121] A century later the town was in decline, with perhaps only half that number of inhabitants. Even at the larger figure, the ratio of doctors to potential patients is high, and it becomes still higher if the smaller one is adopted, one for every 1,200 inhabitants. That such ratios are far from implausible can be shown from the statistics for doctors and surgeons in seventeenth-century Tuscany or in Elizabethan England.[122] But they set a limit to the sort of income that could be obtained from medicine. Only those with access to the wealthiest of patients, at court or in a major metropolis, could hope to amass a fortune simply from treating the sick.

As the example of Myania and Hypnia just mentioned shows, it was also possible for some doctors to be paid by the community as well as by individuals. This system of 'public doctors' goes back to the fifth, if not the early sixth, century, as we have seen, but the fragmentary early references can now be supplemented by the copious evidence of inscriptions drawn from around the Greek (and later Roman) world from the Crimea to Egypt, and from S. Italy to Sicily. The earliest datable inscription comes from Athens around 322/321 BC; the latest so far discovered was carved in the wilds of upland Turkey as much as seven hundred years later.[123] Although many details remain obscure, the outlines of the system are clear. A doctor might be appointed a civic doctor after a period of residence or after having given evidence of successful practice elsewhere.[124] Dr Antipater was for some time a public doctor at the smaller town of Halasarna on the island of Cos before being summoned to take up a similar post at the town of Cos.[125] The island seems to have been at the centre of a medical network, for many of the doctors who were employed in this way in the Hellenistic period had Coan connections.[126] Hermias, for example, was chosen by the Coans and sent to the Cretan town of Gortyn, which had asked them to provide a doctor.[127] Other public doctors were sent for personally by an embassy from a city or by a letter of invitation.[128] When in 219 BC the surgeon Archagathus of Laconia was invited to Rome and given citizen rights and a surgery at public expense, this Italian city was acting in a similar manner to contemporary Greek cities.[129] The length of a doctor's service in a community varied: some towns may have offered only an annual contract, but there was always the possibility of renewal. The record is held by Menocritus of Samos, who, after some time in Rhodes, moved to become a public doctor on the island of Carpathos for more than twenty years.[130]

Others saw an appointment as a public physician as merely one step in a career that would lead to more profitable employment either in a bigger city or with wealthier patients. On his departure from his post the doctor would usually be given an official testimonial in the form of an honorary decree of the council or the inhabitants. In language that is often identical with that in medical texts instructing the doctor how to behave, it praised his learning, diligence and good conduct.[131] It set out the various privileges that the doctor had been given, such as the right to own land (a rarity for a foreigner), freedom from local taxes, a front seat at the theatre, a gold crown or even a statue.[132] In a society that was keenly interested in honour and status, such privileges would not be regarded as trivial, and they would express the community's approbation as effectively as any salary.[133] Honorary decrees, almost by definition, stress the unusual events in the doctor's career, such as serving on a campaign, rescuing a city from a disastrous epidemic or giving public lectures in the town gymnasium.[134] Public lecturing, however, was not always viewed with total approval. Some authors, usually patients, were chary of what they thought was mere advertising, warning their readers to beware the flashy instruments, the rhetorical flourishes and the showmanship of the speakers. Even the medical author of *Precepts*, while encouraging doctors to perform well and lecture in public, warned that too many flowery quotations from poetry should be avoided as a sign of misdirected learning.[135]

It was not only public physicians who received such honours. Other doctors who had given long or meritorious service in a community, or to a particular group, might be equally rewarded by a decree or, more rarely, a public statue. Dr Antipater's pupil and later assistant Onasander came with him to the town of Cos, where he treated former patients from Halasarna who sought him out, and he continued to do this even after he had opened his own private practice in Cos. Although he was not a native of Halasarna, he was honoured by the members of the district for all that he had done for its citizens. This included at times treating some of them for nothing (although he took money and retainers from others), which was regarded as particularly virtuous, since many of them were very ill and required considerable attention, out of which he might have expected to make a fair amount of money. Such kindness, allied to what was considered effective treatment, deserved the reward of an honorary decree erected in the temple of Apollo next to that of his master.[136]

The striking thing about this decree is not only its length and detail, but the way in which its sentiments and vocabulary link with three late treatises in the Hippocratic Corpus, *The Physician*, *Precepts* and *Decorum*. These are to be placed, on grounds of content and style, no earlier than 250 BC, and arguably considerably later. Whatever their date, they mark a distinct difference from the deontological texts of the fifth and fourth century.[137] They are concerned with what might be termed problems of medical etiquette, not least the question of fees and joint consultations. The physician must behave in a dignified manner, neither aggressive nor obtuse, for sour looks, roughness, arrogance and vulgarity are disagreeable. He must be philanthropic, kind and gentle, mindful of the benefits he may himself have received.[138] In appropriate circumstances he must remit fees to those who cannot pay, an act of charity that can only be to his advantage, in two ways. He will increase his own reputation and create in his patients the right frame of mind to aid their recovery. Similarly, discussing fees at the very beginning of a case is often a bad move, for this adds to a patient's worries, particularly in an acute case.[139] As the author put it in a pregnant aphorism, where there is love of man there is also love of the art.[140] A willingness to call in a second opinion and a refusal to disagree in front of the patient also help to distinguish the good doctor from the bad.[141]

Decorum (a more literal translation would be 'Good Form') is perhaps the very latest of the texts in the Corpus. It sets up the true doctor as a man of virtue and wisdom: indeed, 'between medicine and wisdom there is no gulf'. As a result, the true doctor is 'the equal of a god', keeping his whole practice directed to 'decorum and good repute'.[142] The purpose of the text is to instruct the doctor in the behaviour that will set him apart from the flashy charlatan wandering the markets from city to city with garish clothes and appurtenances.[143] Much can be gained simply from the way the doctor comports himself; he should be serious but urbane, slow to rush into confrontation, moderate in everything, gracious in conduct and capable of holding his tongue when need be. He does not chatter with those who are not fellow doctors, but says only what the situation demands, clearly and firmly. He is respectful towards the gods, for he is conscious of the frail powers of medicine – unlike the quack, who is only too easily inclined to mistake a spontaneous cure for the result of his own intervention.[144] The author then proffers advice on activities that will lead to a good reputation. The doctor should always be well prepared, with a range of recipes well memorised so that they can be instantly prescribed. Visits to the patient should be fairly frequent, so that one can observe quickly any changes taking place and act upon them. One should try to remain cheerful with the patient, even hiding many of the details of the case, if necessary, but should be prepared to chide or console. It is worth announcing one's forecasts to all those who have an interest in them, so that no blame can be attached to any failure. Indeed, because patients are often inclined not to follow their doctor's recommendations, it is advisable to leave a well-trained student or assistant with them to take charge of their therapy. In that way, the doctor can be confident of finding out about any significant changes as soon as they occur, and of ensuring that the patient follows his prescriptions. By acting methodically in this way, any blame for failure will be less and the chances of success will be much improved, with a consequent gain for the doctor's reputation.[145]

When and how these short tracts on medical behaviour came to be included in the Corpus when others such as the *Testament* of Hippocrates were not is difficult to establish.[146] But it is clear that the presuppositions of their authors reflect the institutions of medicine that were being created during the Hellenistic age: official posts, sects, medical associations and the formation of agreed bodies of knowledge considered essential for a physician that included many new ideas and techniques. The figure of Hippocrates emerges as the representative of the medical profession *par excellence*, although, as we have seen, agreement as to what Hippocrates stood for was far from universal. There were others who offered alternative ways of healing, and, arguably, they too increased in both number and variety during this period; but this does not alter the fact that Hellenistic doctors and surgeons constituted a more defined and self-conscious group than in the fifth and fourth centuries, with generally acknowledged obligations to one another as well as to their patients. We can discern this development, which may have begun earlier, thanks to a shift in the bias of the evidence away from medical tracts and literary anecdotes and towards epigraphic or papyrological documents that reveal the wider development of bourgeois civic life in the Hellenistic world.

But, more important still, it was in this period, from 330 to 30 BC, that Greek medicine moved out of the largely Greek world of the Aegean, S. Italy and Sicily to become the dominant medical system of the whole of the Mediterranean.

11

ROME AND THE TRANSPLANTATION
OF GREEK MEDICINE

The assimilation of Greek medicine into the Latin-speaking world of central Italy, and thence over time into Western Europe, is one of the most momentous developments in the history of medicine. A system (or a collection of systems) of medicine in one society was transplanted into another with a different language, culture and political structure, and was enabled thereby to become the basis of the Western medical tradition. Without this development Greek medicine might have remained on the same level of importance to us as that of the Babylonians or Egyptians, an interesting, if somewhat tangential, object of historical study. In Latin dress, Greek medical theories continued to be studied, applied, challenged and defended in Western Europe well into the nineteenth century. Mediaeval Western Europe knew of Hippocrates and Galen only in Latin, and even when bilingual editions of Greek texts were produced from the sixteenth century onwards it was largely the Latin version that was read and commented upon, not the Greek. Indeed, some Greek medical authors, although familiar to learned doctors in Western Europe from the sixteenth century on, were never printed fully in their original language until the twentieth century, and were studied almost entirely in Latin translation.[1]

Some aspects of this original process of assimilation cannot be placed in any secure historical context, but they cannot be overlooked simply for that reason. The development of a Latin technical vocabulary, so crucial for the spread of ideas, has been well described by many recent historians, who have pointed to the variety of ways in which Greek terms were taken over into Latin – by transcription, by translation to an existing equivalent or by a new creation on the model of an existing Latin term of similar form or meaning. They have studied how Latin authors depicted and classified diseases and their treatments or expressed the complex nuances of a Greek medical style in a somewhat less flexible grammar and syntax. They have examined the different registers of the usage of terms, in both medical and non-medical treatises, in prose and in verse, in order to gauge the extent to which this technical language was used in Latin society at various dates from the third century BC until the sixth century AD.[2]

For the historian of medicine, certain of their conclusions are of great significance. They show a steady development of a technical terminology over the centuries alongside a continuing use of Greek writings as models or, very often, as the basis for Latin renditions. The process of adaptation often involved the intelligent interpretation and rearrangement of his Greek original by the translator to produce something more than just a Latin paraphrase.[3] There are indications, too, that some authors wrote both Latin and Greek.[4] Second, although some specialised words remain almost entirely within a technical context, the great majority of medical terms and ideas appear widely across a range of literary and historical texts, which indicates a similar openness and accessibility of medical learning in the Latin-speaking world, as in the earlier Greek. Although the degree to which medical technicalities are used varies considerably from writer to writer – Cicero, for instance, while expressing similar admiration and friendship for his doctors, is far less at ease with medical theories and terminologies than is Seneca a century later – this cannot hide the general familiarity with such terms among writers of all sorts and conditions.[5]

Most significant for the historian is the linguists' conclusion that there already existed a substantial, sophisticated and wide-ranging technical vocabulary of medicine in Latin in the late third century BC, when the playwright Plautus was including medical jokes in his plays.[6] By the time the Elder Cato wrote *On Agriculture*, the earliest surviving manual to contain specifically medical information in Latin, around 160 BC, he could use Greek-based words unselfconsciously, despite his publicly expressed hostility to all things Greek. Whether this body of material entered into Latin only in the generation preceding Plautus or derived from much earlier contacts with the Greek-speaking world cannot be determined for certain on our present evidence, but it at least imposes caution before accepting the Romans' own stories about the transfer of Greek medicine to Rome.[7]

As we shall see, these stories leave out the rest of Italy and concentrate on a direct interchange between Rome and the Greek East. They say nothing about the medicine practised within the Greek-speaking cities of S. Italy, from the Bay of Naples southwards, although from the time of Pythagoras and Parmenides to Heraclides of Tarentum and beyond, doctors and thinkers from this area had an enormous influence on the development of Greek medicine.[8] By the first century BC wealthy Romans were visiting this region for recreation, and at Velia/Elea, for health.[9] Over many other aspects of medicine in the Italian peninsula darkness inevitably remains. What sort of medicine was practised by the two Ac(h)onii at Perugia in the first century BC can hardly be deduced from their bilingual tombstone in Latin and Etruscan.[10] Neither can much be concluded from the famous liver of Piacenza, which suggests that a certain degree of anatomical skill accompanied the art of the Etruscan *haruspices*, without, however, proving that this was more than high-class butchery.[11] In these areas the typical healer was either, like Lucius Clodius of Ancona, a *circulator*, travelling from town to town selling his wares, or someone who combined doctoring with farming and other pursuits.[12] By the second century AD, however, these regions, now more prosperous and urbanised, present a picture typical of the rest of Italy: some healers have a public salary for their services; others appear as holders of civic offices, such as that of *sevir*, a minor religious official; few, if any, are from the urban elite.[13]

One area, however, displays significant peculiarities, the highlands of central Italy, the home of the Marsi, whose reputation as snake-charmers and healers lasted for many centuries. They were reputed to possess magical powers; they could sing a snake to sleep and extract its venom, or allow it to rest within their tunics without coming to harm. They came down from the hills to Rome, where they could be seen cutting off the heads of snakes and preparing their exotic remedies. They were the experts, as even Galen was prepared to acknowledge, and they were consulted with respect, and even fear.[14] They represent a different type of healing from that of Cato's peasant farmer, but one that need not have been no less effective. They had their equivalents elsewhere in the Roman world, in the Thibians, the Psylli and the Nasamones, wild men from the backwoods of Paphlagonia and the fringes of the African desert whose prowess with snakes and antidotes was truly wonderful.[15] This is rural medicine, almost oblivious to the offerings of an urban culture, and still surviving today in similar conditions in the Italian mountains.[16]

The earliest references to any Roman involvement with the Greek world of health and healing are not concerned with secular healing, but with the importation of new gods to defend the Roman state during an epidemic. We have already encountered the introduction of the cult of Apollo the Healer in 433 BC, but it was the arrival of Asclepius that attracted most attention from later writers.[17] In 293 BC, after three consecutive years of plague in Rome, it was revealed, after a priestly consultation of the Sibylline Books, that the epidemic could be halted only by summoning Asclepius from the shrine of Epidaurus. The next year a formal embassy, led by Quintus Ogulnius, was dispatched there by the Roman senate; the god himself consented; and, in the form of a snake, he was conveyed to Italy. When the boat carrying the ambassadors put in at Antium, south of Rome, the snake swam ashore and took refuge in a temple of Asclepius, with its sacred grove. Our most detailed historical source, Valerius Maximus, imagines that the ambassadors were afraid that the snake would remain at Antium, but after three days the snake returned on board. On reaching Rome the snake once again slipped away, and took refuge on the Tiber island, where a temple was erected for him. The plague, needless to say, stopped 'with miraculous speed'.[18]

Several features of this account deserve notice. First, the introduction of Asclepius and his cult to Rome is a formal act by the Roman state, not an ostensibly private initiative, such as those of Telemachus at Athens or Archias at Pergamum.[19] The advice to seek the help of this god is provided

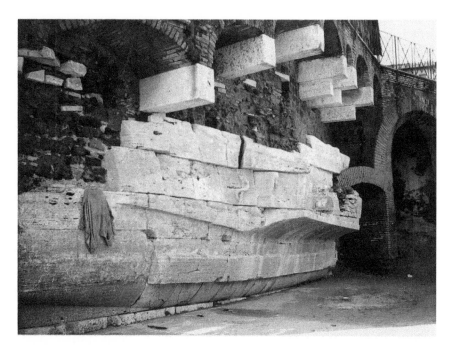

Figure 11.1 The tip of the Tiber island in Rome, the site of the temple of Asclepius, carved into the shape of a ship's prow, from which the god descends in the form of a snake.

in the most awesome manner, from the Sibylline Books, as interpreted by official priests. Second, the Roman story leaves out of consideration any possible developments taking place within Italy; it emphasises the direct link between Rome and Greece. The epidemic in Rome is a matter only for the Romans, and their decisions relate only to their own city. Only when the god goes ashore at Antium is there a hint that the cult of Asclepius was already known in neighbouring regions of Italy.[20] Without the evidence of archaeology we would not know that visitors were already flocking in large numbers to a healing shrine at Fregellae (central Italy), although we cannot be sure whether, at this early date, it was already a centre of Asclepius cult rather than dedicated to a more local god.[21]

Third, the position of the sanctuary on the Tiber island corresponds neatly to the liminal position of many Greek shrines of Asclepius. It is neither in the city, being surrounded by water on all sides, nor outside it; indeed, the dubious status of the island itself made it an appropriate resting place for a foreign deity worshipped with foreign rites.[22] It is also a shared site: according to Ovid, the senate dedicated on the same day two temples on the island, one to Asclepius, the other to Jupiter.[23] Votive offerings and the scanty building remains show that this was a very popular sanctuary in the Late Republican period, although less is known of it in subsequent centuries. By AD 50 sick slaves were in effect being dumped on the island by masters unwilling to go to the trouble and expense of looking after them, and the emperor Claudius had to issue a decree against this inhumane practice.[24]

What our literary sources do not tell us, but has been revealed by archaeology, is that similar healing sanctuaries were common in central Italy, often near springs. At many of them, sufferers dedicated votive offerings in the form of terracotta models of the affected part of the body – feet, hands, eyes and sexual organs in particular. Incubation may even have been practised at a shrine at Lavinium, not far from Rome. Although the form the cult of Asclepius took in Rome is assuredly Greek, the arrival of Asclepius can also be interpreted as an index of the assimilation of Roman Italy as a whole into the Greek world.[25]

The Romans' own history of the introduction of human medicine parallels that of Apollo Medicus and Asclepius in several ways. It stressed two inter-related things: medicine was Greek and it had been imported into Rome only with the approval and authority of the Roman Senate. This momentous development took place almost in a historical vacuum, for a lack of background knowledge hampers our understanding of the arrival of 'the first doctor', the Peloponnesian Archagathus, son of Lysanias, in 219 BC. Citing Cassius Hemina, a historian whose *Annals* were composed around 150 BC, Pliny, writing 200 years later, reports that Archagathus was given rights of citizenship as well as his own workshop, bought at public expense at the Crossroads of the Acilii. He was successful at first, being called 'the wound-man', but, because of his violence in cutting and burning, he was soon nicknamed 'the executioner', and the medical arts came to be loathed, and all physicians likewise. Archagathus returned to Laconia, leaving medicine, according to Pliny, with an evil reputation in Rome that was well deserved – and that persisted even into his own times.[26]

Once again the Romans are acting collectively, and in a manner that corresponds to that of a Greek city when employing a public doctor, although Pliny does not give Archagathus this title.[27] Whether Hemina was right to call him 'the first of the doctors' is impossible to determine, not least because he, like Pliny, wished to set up an opposition between Roman healing practices and those of the Greeks.[28] There may well have been healers already in Rome whom a modern historian would wish to classify as 'doctors', but Hemina reserves the epithet for the practitioners of Greek medicine.[29] He is not seeking to make a distinction between the theoretician and the craftsman, for Archagathus is expressly said to have been a 'wound-man', and a wound-plaster devised by an Archagathus is mentioned by later Latin authors and in a Greek letter to a doctor Dionysius in Egypt.[30] Rather, Hemina is emphasising a distinction between Romans and Greeks: whatever healing skills the Romans themselves might have possessed, they did not count as medicine, since that was a purely Greek import.

Hemina will have certainly been familiar with the public utterances of the Elder Cato (*c*.234–149 BC), who made a political career out of a strident hostility to all things foreign, and especially Greek.[31] In a work he wrote for his son, perhaps between 180 and 173 BC, he warned him against the corrupting influence of the Greeks, and especially their doctors, who had sworn an oath to kill foreigners by their medicine; what is worse, they even were prepared to exact a fee from patients before killing them.[32] 'Keep away from doctors', Cato's advice to his son, is not a condemnation of all forms of medicine or of all those with healing skills, but only of the Greeks or those who follow them. He approves of the Roman way of healing, by which the head of a household took responsibility for the health of all its members, animals included. He himself is said to have kept a notebook in which he wrote down prescriptions and diets for his household. This medicine is confined to the household: it is not bruited abroad, or traded for cash; and, so Cato claimed, it is effective, for it kept him and his family hale and hearty for many years.[33]

What sort of medicine Cato would have used is made clearer in his treatise *On Agriculture*, a manual that covers all aspects of farm management from ploughing to the health of slaves and animals.[34] It consists largely of herbal remedies, sometimes accompanied by chants and charms, and even ritualistic performances: a cure for intestinal and stomach worms, based on pomegranate blossoms, fennel, frankincense, honey, wild marjoram, and wine, ends with the injunction that the patient must climb up a square pillar and jump down from it ten times, before going for a walk.[35] In strong contrast to Hippocratic medicine, with its references to the sacredness of the art and the need for the patient to consult a proper physician, these remedies are accessible to all. The power to heal resides in the drug and its accompanying procedures, not in any specific expertise by the doctor; the rules for the incantation or medicine can be given to and used by anyone, from the head of the household to his slave herdsman.

In its content, this medicine is typical of folk medicine in many societies, and it would be unwise to claim that where the same sort of remedy is prescribed by Cato and by a Hippocratic author this indicates that Cato adopted it from the Greeks. But there are many details, not least Cato's choice of words for measures and for plants, and occasional passages where he does seem to be relying, at least in part, on Greek medical sources. Despite his powerful rhetoric, Cato allowed Greek concepts, Greek words and Greek practices into a domain, the care of the body and the treatment of illness, that, when writing to his son, he had most desired to preserve from the Greeks. Yet the very extent of these borrowings also helps to acquit Cato of hypocrisy, for, rather than assume that he was entirely responsible for taking these Greek ideas over into Latin, it is easier to believe that this process of assimilation, to judge from the linguistic evidence, had already been going on for some time.[36] Besides, by promoting effective remedies taken from Greek writers he was also making them available to his fellow countrymen so that they need no longer seek the assistance of charlatans and potential murderers.

This arrival of Greek medicine in Rome forms part of two wider developments, the Hellenisation of Italian culture generally and urbanisation, in particular the growth of Rome, from a small town around 300 BC to a great metropolis by 100 BC.[37] The stereotype of the Roman peasant farmer–soldier, presented most vigorously by Cato, was becoming in this period remote from the reality of life in the teeming, plebeian city of Rome itself. The wealthy had their private gardens, and the poor, in their barrack blocks of houses, might grow their herbs in windowboxes or go hunting for them in the green spaces outside (and even inside) the walls, a sight that has not entirely disappeared today.[38] But this is a very different way of life from that on the farm or in a village in the hills of Latium. Cato and, after him, Pliny bewail the decline of old Roman virtues, the collapse of morality and the potential ending of the very things that made Rome great. Their lament for the world they have lost gains its force precisely because of the increasing remoteness of the Golden Age, for this enables an even stronger contrast to be drawn between an ideal past and the ugliness of present reality.[39] At the same time, it also minimises the extent to which in certain areas of Italy (and beyond) herbal remedies, domestic medicine and only occasional contact with an expert (in the sense of specialist) healer continued to be the norm.[40]

Although Rome's political and military involvement with the Greek world dated only from the late fourth or early third century BC, when the Romans and their allies were drawn into conflicts in S. Italy and Sicily, cultural and trading contacts existed well before this. It was the further extension of Roman political interest across the Adriatic into Epirus and Macedonia, and, in the second century BC, further afield still, to the rest of Greece, Asia Minor, Syria and Egypt, that finally opened up Roman culture and politics to the full impact of Hellenisation. As the armies of Rome conquered or came to control the Greek world, Rome's culture became more and more Greek, whether this took the form of literary transmutations of Greek themes and even Greek plays, the import of Greek statues and furnishings, or the employment of Greek doctors. It was a process that was viewed as a paradox: 'captured Greece took the wild victor captive, and introduced the arts to peasant Latium', wrote Horace, and others echoed him.[41] Rome, it was felt, although winning the war militarily, had in fact lost the peace. Hence the vigour with which Cato and his supporters denounced those whom they saw as responsible for this failure and for the new tensions introduced into Roman political society as a result of the enormous wealth amassed by those who had commanded or simply served in the East.[42] Pliny even goes so far as to claim that when the Romans expelled the Greeks from Italy, long after Cato's death, they did not spare Greek physicians.[43]

Cato's opposition to Greek medicine is part of his broader attack on the phil-hellenes, and, sure enough, many of the Romans who show an interest in Greek medicine or who employ Greek doctors can be firmly located on the other side of the political divide from Cato. Archagathus' workshop was situated at the Crossroads of the Acilii, a family prominent in their support for things Greek (and later opponents of Cato), and the two consuls for the year 219 BC, L. Aemilius Paullus and M. Livius Salinator, shared similar interests.[44] Governors, generals and wealthy Romans acquired personal physicians in visits to the East, who in their turn acted as mediators between conquered and conqueror. Athenagoras of Larisa, himself a member of the local elite of his city, was honoured by Cos as the doctor to Cn. Octavius, who had been sent in 168 BC to regulate the affairs of Greece after the war with Perseus.[45] A similar decree was erected at Athens in honour of a doctor Ammonius, who is likely to have been a member of the suite of Sp. Postumius Albinus, who undertook a similar mission in Greece a generation later in 146–145 BC.[46]

By the middle of the first century BC it had become almost *de rigueur* to employ a Greek physician. Artemidorus, a doctor from Perge, having acquired Roman citizenship around 80 BC through the intercession of C. Cornelius Dolabella, governor of Cilicia, the province in which Perge was situated, almost immediately joined the staff of Verres, the governor of Sicily in 80–79 BC.[47] Dr Asclapo of Patras, 'a man of kindness, learning and fidelity', was recommended by Cicero to his friend Sulpicius Rufus as a valuable companion in Achaea in 46 BC.[48] Other doctors also seem to have come to Italy as a result of campaigns in the East. L. Manneius Menecrates, 'the wine giver', a doctor recorded on a tombstone from Atinum in S. Italy in the first century BC, hailed originally from Tralles in Asia Minor, but was then adopted by a Roman citizen at Atinum, Q. Manneius.[49] Where and when the two men met can only be guessed at, but their relationship shows that the introduction of Greek medicine was no longer confined to the metropolis. Precedents from Hellenistic Greek cities almost certainly lie behind the action of Julius Caesar, perhaps around 49 BC, in conferring Roman citizenship on any doctor practising in the city of Rome, and, scarcely a decade later, behind the granting to all doctors and teachers throughout the Empire of immunity from conscription and from having troops billeted upon them.[50] In 23 BC or shortly after, following his dramatic cure by an ex-slave doctor, Antonius Musa, the emperor Augustus is said to have granted tax immunity for ever to all practitioners of medicine.[51] The number of immigrant doctors who took advantage of this generosity to become full citizens and the procedures whereby one proved one's qualifications as a doctor or a teacher are both unknown. Nonetheless, the frequent repetition of the grants of immunity by a variety of subsequent emperors suggests that such generosity was not always appreciated by those who had to pick up the tax burden avoided by the doctors.[52]

These developments had one important consequence for the practice of medicine within Rome, and arguably within the Latin world as a whole. They fixed an enduring image of medicine as something Greek, or, if not purely Greek, something un-Roman, the province of immigrants, foreigners, slaves and ex-slaves.[53] For all Cicero's approval of medicine and his commendations of his Greek physicians, for all the wealth that could be acquired by treating a rich senator or, later, the imperial family, medicine was not a career for a proper Roman.[54] By contrast with the Greek East, where there were medical dynasties and, even occasionally, doctors drawn from wealthy families, the practitioners of medicine in Rome were at best parvenus, and, far more often, drawn from what in law were the very lowest sections of society, slaves and ex-slaves. Although the figures are a little distorted by the abundance of information provided by inscriptions coming from the emperor's Roman household of slaves and ex-slaves, scarcely 10 per cent of doctors recorded epigraphically from Italy and the western Latin provinces of the Empire before AD 100 are Roman citizens; over 75 per cent are either slaves or ex-slaves; and fewer than 5 per cent bear a non-Greek name. Although the percentage of citizens and of non-Greek names rises over the next two centuries, the general pattern remains the same.[55]

Literary evidence confirms that of the inscriptions. Doctors from the eastern provinces are common in Rome and further west, and continue to move there throughout Antiquity. A doctor from Phrygia, who had spent many years in Gaul, was martyred at Lyons in AD 177; Galen, an immigrant himself, inveighed against his compatriots who came to Rome to escape the detection of their medical crimes; and a Greek physician turned up in Spain at the end of the fourth century.[56] Even after the disappearance of the great households of slaves and freedmen that characterise Imperial Rome in the early first century, slaves and ex-slaves continue to be found in large numbers. One emperor, possibly Domitian in AD 93–4, fulminated against those who, in order to make money, sent their slaves half-trained on to the street to practise.[57] For centuries, Roman law codes continued to fix prices for slaves trained as doctors, even if by the sixth century their numbers must have been very few.[58] The likelihood that doctors were slaves or ex-slaves also provided the occasion for a rare Roman legal joke. Around 170 the Roman jurist Julianus ruled that the formal ties of obligation between master and ex-slave should not encourage the master to be perpetually ill in order to monopolise the freedman's medical services for free.[59]

This low legal personal status of medical practitioners in Italy and the western provinces, and the general perception that medicine was something foreign, cannot have helped the prestige of the art of medicine there, even if few potential patients had ever read the Elder Pliny's magnificently malicious account of the crimes and follies of the medical profession, Hippocrates included. Pliny does not deny that some Romans had an interest in medicine, the Rubrii and Calpetani, for instance, but he is convinced that their brand of medicine was something different from and superior to that purveyed by the Greeks.[60] His hero is the centenarian Antonius Castor, still pottering around his herb garden, living proof of the value of Roman herbal medicine.[61] But, like Cato before him, Pliny distinguished between remedies and those who proffered them. The long sections relating to the body and to remedies in his *Natural History* are avowedly based far more on Greek sources than on Latin, and aim to convey that learning to his fellow Romans.[62] This is not a sign of compilatory schizophrenia on the part of an author whose individual pronouncements are at variance with the data he purveys. Rather, by taking this information out of the exclusive hands of Greek practitioners he is removing its dangers by allowing it to be used by Romans whose moral viewpoint will ensure its proper and effective use. Roman possession of Greek knowledge thus produces a better type of medicine.

This tension can be felt even in the eight books *On Medicine*, written in Latin by the wealthy Roman Aulus Cornelius Celsus as part of his much larger encyclopaedia of *Arts*.[63] Celsus acknowledges the merits of the medicine developed by the Greeks over several centuries and now planted in Italy. This 'health-giving profession' has been followed by 'no ordinary men', from Hippocrates onwards, in a continuous chain down to his own time.[64] Surgery, which became an independent part of medicine only after Hippocrates, was developed by the Alexandrians before coming to Rome, where Tryphon, Euelpistus and Meges, the most learned of them all, made great contributions.[65]

Even when he opposes some Greek medical doctrines, most notably those of Asclepiades and Themison, Celsus does not indulge in verbal assaults deploring their Greekness. He himself has a remarkably wide acquaintance with Greek, and especially Hellenistic, medicine and surgery, quoting many unfamiliar authors and using in his vocabulary a large number of technical terms derived directly from Greek.[66] His anatomy, pathology and therapeutics are avowedly Greek, although he does not hesitate to put forward his own opinions in the course of describing a 'rational' approach to medicine. Yet, at the same time, despite his considerable book learning and his own experience of treating illness he never once calls himself a doctor or identifies himself with that profession. He tells us neither how he obtained his learning nor in whose company he saw some of the cases he reports.[67] There are both social and intellectual reasons for this reluctance. The true practice of medicine is incompatible with the indecent pursuit of '*quaestus*', monetary gain: for all his knowledge, Celsus and many of his intended audience were and remained gentlemen, interested at least as much in warfare and agriculture as in medicine.[68] Like Cato, Celsus implies that one should confine one's medical attentions to one's family and friends, and certainly not attempt to treat large numbers of patients all over town, for one would not be able then to give them the individual attention so necessary for a cure.[69] He acknowledges that an expertise with useful plants and herbs can be attained by many who are illiterate; indeed, he regards this type of healing as the norm, the product of popular knowledge consolidated into tradition, which may contradict and surpass the evidence of the written word. But such knowledge is not enough by itself: rationality is needed above all.[70] It is the Greeks who have created the art of medicine as Celsus knows it, and who, by separating it off from the study of philosophy, have enabled it to develop as an independent discipline.

169

He acknowledges the benefits that this change has brought, but at the same time he keeps a certain distance from it.[71] He is not afraid to criticise or to treat his Greek authorities with independence and a certain scepticism, especially since individual variables may render useless even the most cogent of their generalisations. But as well as posing theoretical objections he raises a more fundamental ethical question. Medicine in the Greek fashion is itself a product of immorality, the consequence of a decline into luxury and idleness, necessary only because the world itself has become corrupt. In turn, his vocabulary stresses Roman virtues, 'a sense of decency' and moderation.[72] His book, although based on a considerable acquaintance with Greek materials, is produced very much within a Roman environment: it presents the results of Greek learning but in a way that still reveals some of the prejudices of Cato and Pliny. For all his considerable knowledge and understanding of his Greek heritage, Celsus expresses a distinctively Roman point of view.

Yet this hesitancy towards medicine, even on the part of one so knowledgable as Celsus, should not be allowed to mislead. Medicine as practised and discussed by the Greeks was established firmly in Rome by the late second century BC. Despite public expressions of reluctance, Roman patients proved willing and eager to use Greek doctors to treat their ailments, and practitioners of medicine from the eastern Mediterranean flocked in increasing numbers to Rome.[73]

By far the most influential immigrant medical practitioner of Late Republican Rome was Asclepiades of Bithynia. Born at Cius (Prusias ad Mare) in Bithynia (modern N.W. Turkey), he is alleged by Pliny to have been an unsuccessful teacher of rhetoric before turning his hand to medicine.[74] He then came to Rome, where he enjoyed an enormous reputation, based on shrewd advertisement and apparently amazing cures.[75] When he made this move is far from clear. Cicero, in his dialogue *On the Orator*, which has a dramatic date of 91 BC, makes the orator L. Crassus speak of having enjoyed his services as friend and doctor in the past, when Asclepiades used to defeat his medical competitors by his eloquence, and above all by his expertise.[76] If this means that Asclepiades was already dead by 91 BC Cicero's silence about him in his letters from the 60s and 50s is easily explained, and, given that Asclepiades is said to have died at a great age, he will probably have come to Rome in the 120s, if not earlier.[77] But this then puts the dates of Themison, his pupil, very early, and leaves an uncomfortable gap between him and other Asclepiadeans such as Antonius Musa in the 30s BC, and still more between him and Thessalus, who modified Themison's doctrines around AD 50.[78] On the alternative and older interpretation of the passage in Cicero, Crassus was referring solely to his own treatment, and his comment on what Asclepiades used to say (*dicebat*) does not imply that Asclepiades was no longer active in Rome but refers merely to the period when he was close to Crassus. On this lower chronology, Asclepiades may certainly have lived into the 70s, 60s or even 50s BC, 'the age of Pompey', which is where Pliny locates him.[79]

170

But whether the bulk of his activity in Rome took place in the late second century BC or thirty or forty years later, there can be no doubt of his impact on Rome or the importance of his theories. Pliny ascribes his outstanding success to the gullibility of his Roman patients and the power of his rhetoric, which could awaken the dead, or nearly dead, but others, notably Celsus and Caelius Aurelianus, adopt a more sympathetic tone.[80] Certainly he attracted pupils to Rome from around the Mediterranean, from Sicily, Epirus and Syria.[81] In Greek sources he is regularly cited as the last representative of the so-called Dogmatic physicians before Galen, and doctors who bear the title of Asclepiadeans can be found in Gaul, and even in remote Asia Minor in the third or fourth century.[82] Yet what he said and taught comes to us only at second or third hand, and often through hostile witnesses.[83]

Asclepiades believed that the body was built up of invisible particles, and that health was a function of their free and balanced motion through theoretical pores in the body. Disease resulted from an imbalance, a blockage or a flood. Once the cause was established, treatment followed logically, and there was no need for an excessively complicated nosology or symptomatology. That did not mean a neglect of careful observation and description, for Asclepiades seems to have delighted in pointing out the mistakes in others' characterisations of particular conditions. Whereas some doctors believed that inflammation of the nerves was far more dangerous and painful because nerves were more sensitive than flesh, he denied that they had any sensation at all, a typical exaggeration according to Galen.[84] The Empiricists' belief in the merits of observation without theory he considered nonsensical, and the explanations of other theoreticians variously defective. Although he was familiar with many of the writings in the Hippocratic Corpus, writing studies, and perhaps even commentaries, on the *Aphorisms* and on *The Surgery* and criticising earlier authors for misunderstanding some of Hippocrates' language, he used the Corpus more as a storehouse of practical information than for its theories.[85] He commended the description of a spontaneous dislocation in *Joints*, which corresponded to what he himself had seen, but he rejected explanations for disease in terms of an imbalance or a bad mixture of humours. He was also opposed to those who argued in favour of functions determined by teleological purpose; nature, he argued, often acted dangerously. Whereas Galen later spoke of the attraction and expulsion of nutriment to and from the body in terms of natural faculties purposefully organised by nature within the body, Asclepiades invoked mechanistic explanations in terms of an evolution of the corpuscles towards a finer, warmer or more rarefied state. His mechanistic and materialistic explanation of kidney and bladder function owed much to earlier Hellenistic thinkers, notably Erasistratus and Heraclides of Pontus, and Galen was almost certainly right to include him among the Epicureans because of the similarity between his ideas and their conception of an atomic universe.[86]

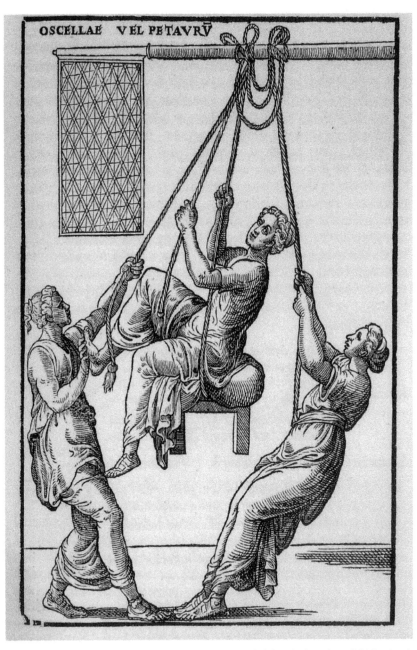

Figure 11.2 Gentle exercise on a swing, as recommended by Asclepiades of Bithynia. An illustration from H. Mercurialis, *De Arte gymnastica*, Amsterdam, A. Frisius, 1672, p. 217, a Renaissance treatise that reintroduced into medicine ancient ideas on exercise and physiotherapy. Courtesy of Wellcome Library, London.

What gained Asclepiades his reputation in Rome, however, was less his theories than his therapies. His slogan 'swiftly, safely, pleasantly', an adaptation of ideas in the Hippocratic Corpus, and his liberal use of wine and gentle exercise were as notorious among later opponents as they will have been congenial to his patients. He was famous for championing five types of basic therapy: regulating the intake of food and of wine; massage; ambulatory exercise; rocking appliances, to provide passive exercise for those unable to indulge in more strenuous activity; and bathing, to which he paid particular attention, devising a sort of 'hanging bath' for passive hydrotherapy.[87] None of these therapies was entirely new – Celsus criticises him for behaving as if he were the sole inventor of the use of massage in therapy – but their combination and his almost total reliance on them constituted a challenge to earlier practice, which he stigmatised as a study in death.[88] Some of his advice appears eminently sensible: he warned against an overindulgence in very cold baths, recommended music in the treatment of mental illness, and insisted that the doctor should pay as much attention to the whole process of convalescence as to the immediate treatment. Other therapies, most notably his liberal use of wine, appeared to his opponents as little more than craven attempts to cosset and indulge his wealthy patients.[89]

This charge is almost certainly exaggerated, for Asclepiades was prepared to use a wide range of remedies. While he was wary of using certain powerful drugs such as hellebore, and restricted the use of a common remedy, oxymel, a mixture of vinegar and honey, to curing snakebite, he was not opposed to drug treatment as such, although some believed that he was.[90] He still used clysters to purge the bowel, though not so frequently or violently as his predecessors. But his treatments could be painful if need be. Celsus describes the initial stages of his treatment for fever as akin to torture.[91] Even Caelius Aurelianus, a Methodist with no reason to discredit his predecessor, shows him using emetics and clysters, venesection, tapping for dropsy and even pharyngotomy.[92] This is eminently reasonable, for an author who wrote on wounds and wound treatments, as Asclepiades did, is unlikely to have shunned the knife completely.[93]

In Asclepiades Greek medicine in Rome found its earliest celebrated exponent. He wrote in Greek, although his message was largely to a Roman audience and his abilities were recognised across the linguistic divide. He was a success, all are agreed, in part because of the sheer force and independence of his personality. His example undoubtedly encouraged others to come to Rome and Italy to seek their fortune. The activity of Asclepiades in Rome marks the moment at which Greek medicine can be said to have been effectively transferred there. Henceforth, despite their differences of theoretical emphasis, despite their very different legal and social structures, medicine in the Greek and Roman worlds must be considered together as part of the same intellectual universe.[94]

12

THE CONSEQUENCES OF EMPIRE

Pharmacology, surgery and the Roman army

The transformation of the Roman world under Augustus (ruled 31 BC to AD 14), the heir of Julius Caesar, was not just a political transition from Republic to Empire, from the effective rule of the Senate and people of Rome to an autocracy hiding behind traditional terminology. It was also a social and geographical revolution as Roman imperial power was extended to the Rhine, the Danube and the Euphrates. Whether in N. Italy, Gaul or Asia Minor, local elites were assimilated, in a variety of ways, into the wider system of Roman government and Roman culture. The city of Rome itself was changed almost beyond recognition as marble public buildings replaced brick and apartment blocks took over from cottages. The population of the city grew enormously, and the city's boundaries had to be extended with all due religious pomp and ceremony. Amid this flood of immigrants (a veritable river Orontes, sneered one satirist) came Greek doctors, from Thebes (whether the town in Boeotia or Egypt is not clear), from Nicaea, Laodicea, Smyrna and other less prestigious towns all over the eastern Mediterranean.[1] They sought fame and fortune in the metropolis, in Italy, in the more Romanised provinces of the West and, in a few cases, even on the very fringes of the Western Empire.[2] The passage of Greek medicine into the Roman world was now so complete, with the same theories and often the same medicaments circulating in Latin as well as in Greek, that one can now truly begin to talk of Roman medicine as something that could be found across the Empire without any distinction of language.

At the very apex of the ambitions of medical practitioners was now the imperial household, the emperor, his family, their friends, advisers and, particularly in the first century AD, the ex-slaves (or freedmen) who acted as imperial secretaries. Becoming the personal physician to one of these grandees was, as will be shown later, a sure path to wealth and influence, for one's family as well as oneself. But even the suggestion of imperial approval could be used to promote a theory or vindicate a novel drug. Paccius Antiochus, on his deathbed c.AD 30, described his wonderful painkilling remedy in a letter to the Emperor Tiberius, who then arranged for it to be available in public libraries for all to read.[3] A generation later, Thessalus of Tralles addressed a somewhat boastful

174

letter to the Emperor Nero, denouncing the harmful precepts of Hippocrates and proclaiming the virtues of his newly created medical sect.[4]

How these imperial connections might work in practice and how the expansion of the Roman Empire had an impact on medicine are neatly illustrated by the career and writings of a Latin writer on pharmacology, Scribonius Largus. Largus dedicated his *Drug Recipes* to one of the most powerful of the imperial freedmen, C. Julius Callistus, in late 47 or early 48.[5] Although he was probably not one of the emperor's own physicians, Largus had good court connections – he gives details of the favourite dentifrices of Augustus' sister Octavia and the Empress Messalina, as well as drugs used by Augustus himself, Tiberius and the mother and grandmother of the Emperor Claudius – and in 43 he participated in Claudius' British expedition.[6] He describes a herb he had found near Luni in Etruria while waiting to embark with the emperor's household troops. Whether he was there as an army doctor on a short service contract or was brought along as the private physician of a general or leading courtier is unclear.[7]

His links seem strongest with Sicily. Largus refers in passing to an exotic remedy against snakebite carried by Sicilian huntsmen, and to the rare pointed trefoil growing there. He records a recipe against rabies presented to the town of Centuripae by his own teacher, a celebrated local physician. He himself was less than convinced of its value in rabies, but reports that he had used it effectively against other bites and stings.[8] As an educated Sicilian, he would have been bilingual in Latin and Greek. As well as his Latin drug book, and the, now lost, Latin medical books once presented on his behalf to the emperor by Callistus, some of his prescriptions survive in Greek, preserved among Galen's quotations from other Greek pharmacologists of the late first century. Whether these once formed part of a work written in Greek by Largus or had been translated from the Latin is disputed, but, whatever their origin, these recipes show the ease with which Latin and Greek information could now be interchanged.[9]

Largus' unpretentious book is full of interest. Its 271 *Recipes* are divided into three main sections. The first and largest group (1–162) is organised according to diseases, going from head to toe, from headache and epilepsy to gout; then follow thirty-seven antidotes against poisons, bites and stings; and the book concludes with plasters, dressings and soothing salves – the typical drugs used by surgeons.[10] Largus mentions 249 vegetable, forty-five mineral and thirty-six animal substances, drawn from the Mediterranean region or imported from further east or from Africa via Alexandria.[11] They range from the humble carrot to the exotic aloe, from fenugreek to ginger, from butter to the electric ray or torpedo fish, recommended for constant headache (perhaps migraine), since the continuous application of electric shocks would dull and ultimately remove the pain. A similar treatment, allowing the fish to attack the patient's feet and shins as he paddled in the sea until the painful area became numb, is claimed to have cured an official at the court of the Emperor Tiberius of pains in the legs.[12]

Most of the substances Largus employs can be found in modern herbals and have phytotherapeutic properties. His compound remedies often show a judicious combination of ingredients that would bring some benefit to the sufferer. His recipe for quinsy, for example, prescribed for the mother of the Emperor Claudius, would make a good analgesic; while his dentifrices contain abrasives, whitening agents and spikenard to improve the breath.[13] Recent chemical studies of recipes in other authors or of drugs found in excavated material confirm that such compounds were not merely chance agglomerations. A pot of face-cream from Roman London, still showing the finger-marks of its owner, would have been an effective cosmetic, and its composition can be paralleled from the traces of ointment preserved in Roman drug-jars in Mainz.[14] A recipe in Galen for a dark ointment against cuts, bruises and black eyes 'as used by an Olympic victor' stands comparison with some of the home remedies of boxing corner-men, since it contains substances that would deaden pain, reduce swelling and provide a quick and relatively flexible scar that would stem bleeding.[15] The contents of pills and ointments found in a shipwreck off the coast of Tuscany also show a nice combination of domestic herbs with others more exotic.[16]

Many of Largus' recipes come from authoritative sources, such as his teacher Vettius Valens or Meges the surgeon, and are found in other medical manuals; others have a more exotic or dubious pedigree.[17] Largus paid a substantial amount to 'a little old lady from Africa', who had cured many inhabitants of Rome of stomachache with a concoction of hart's horn, myrrh, pepper and wine. On another occasion he had heard of a wondrous remedy against epilepsy that was being touted on the island of Crete by a shipwrecked foreigner. He sent along a friend, a Cretan doctor from Gortyn, who handed over a large sum of money only to find that this marvellous remedy was simply a piece of hyena skin wrapped in cloth. Largus engagingly reports that he has not yet been able to try out this remedy, and hopes he never will, although he has, with some difficulty, already procured a hyena and had it skinned, for it is best to be prepared for all eventualities.[18]

All this might suggest that Largus was a credulous fool, unable to distinguish between quackery and proper pharmacology, but this would be unfair. His aim is to discover what works, and he can be scathing about what he calls 'superstition' and 'unprofessional conduct'. Ambrosius, a doctor from Pozzuoli, near Naples, was the author of a recipe to break up a bladder stone into sandy fragments that could be easily passed in the urine. Ambrosius recommended that the drug should be compounded by a person who was not wearing an iron ring and who used only a stone pestle.[19] This symbolism of stone and iron Largus dismisses as 'mere superstition'. Similarly, when a man recommending a remedy against epilepsy that involved the brain of a young deer added that the deer should be killed with a dagger which had just killed a gladiator, Largus was evidently disgusted – although he still includes the advice.[20] But remedies against epilepsy that involve drinking one's own blood or drinking blood out of the skull of a dead gladiator, or, even worse, consuming a portion of the gladiator's liver, he condemns as falling 'outside the *professio* of medicine, even though some seemed to have gained benefit therefrom'.[21]

This striking phrase, the *'professio* of medicine', is his final claim on our attention, for throughout his recipe collection, and especially in his long *Preface*, Largus expounds a view of pharmacy as part of medicine that has, rightly, been called a distinctive contribution to medical ethics.[22] In his opinion medicine is a unity; and just as there can be no proper surgery without dietetics, and vice versa, so neither of these can be practised except to the detriment of one's *'professio'* if pharmacology is excluded. There are pragmatic as well as theoretical reasons why a doctor should learn about drugs. While doctors stand around learnedly arguing over a diagnosis, lesser men, 'of no reputation and far removed from the discipline of medicine, and nowhere near the *professio* of medicine', step in and gain a reputation for effectiveness. Besides, the promise of a treatment that does not involve cautery or the knife brings in paying customers. Doctors who dispute the value of drugs in treatment do so for a variety of reasons; they may misunderstand or misrepresent the views of an earlier authority; they may know nothing about the composition of drugs; or, what is worst of all, they may want to keep their own knowledge secret from their competitors.[23]

But what is this *'professio'* that so inspires Largus? Although it is tempting to translate the word as 'profession' in our modern sense, its primary meaning is that of a public declaration.[24] It is a shared declaration, which goes back to Hippocrates, 'the founder of our profession', and to the Hippocratic *Oath*. Just as a soldier on swearing the oath of allegiance takes on obligations, so too the doctor by his declaration, his *'professio'*, imposes on himself duties within the discipline of medicine. Bound by the 'lawful oath' of medicine, the doctor will not give a poisonous drug to his enemy in war; but he is not prevented from killing him in battle as a good citizen. Above all, the doctor's duty is to heal, not to harm. If Hippocrates forbade damaging the unborn child, 'the father's uncertain hope', how much more care should the doctor take with human beings once born? Although some have said that the doctor should avoid all contact with poisons and the like, this is going too far. The true doctor must know their names and what they look like, simply in order to avoid or combat them; but knowledge of how to prepare them is against all right and justice in one's profession.[25]

Those who know about such things are the drug sellers, *pharmacopolae*, who are most akin to doctors, yet at the same time most distant from their ideals of virtue.[26] This is understandable since in all the arts and sciences one can always find an adversary in the profession that is most like one's own. Largus adopts a somewhat patronising tone to these rivals. They are dismissed as 'humble folk', useful when their remedies work, 'most execrable' when they do not or lead to death.[27] Hence, behind Largus' optimistic description of the doctor as a sort of saint one can detect the outlines of a more familiar and a less virtuous affair, an intra-professional quarrel.

Largus' preface is a plea for a Hippocratic ethic within medicine. It transmutes the Hippocratic *Oath* into Latin and sets it in a specifically Latin context.[28] Whether his plea was ever heard we cannot tell. Apart from the citations of his recipes in Greek, only Marcellus of Bordeaux, writing at the end of the fourth century, shows any clear acquaintance with his book, and manuscripts of it seem always to have been very rare.[29] Very different is the fate of another contemporary writer on pharmacology, Pedanius Dioscorides of Anazarbus (Anazarba, S.E. Turkey), whose five books in Greek *On Materia medica* attained canonical status in Late Antiquity.[30]

Dioscorides had studied pharmacology at Tarsus, the major city of his region, where there appears to have existed a strong tradition of pharmacological teaching that continued for at least a further fifty years.[31] His references to specific habitats of plants or to major entrepôts are overwhelmingly concentrated on the Greek-speaking world of the Aegean and the Levant. The few mentions of places further afield, such as the Balearic Islands, India or Britain (for its mead), are more likely to derive from the reports of others than from his own travels. This distribution of named sites presents a problem for those who wish to interpret his reference, in his *Preface*, to having travelled a great deal in 'a soldierly life', to indicate a period of military service. If, as he claimed, he had used his travels to observe native plants, he shows very little acquaintance with those from regions where the Roman army was mainly stationed, along the Rhine and Danube, in Spain or N. Africa. However, he may have served in Syria or, less likely, Egypt, or perhaps enlisted for a short while in the Armenian wars of 55–63.[32]

His aim was to provide as complete a listing of medicinal substances as possible, derived not only from a reading of earlier authors such as Crateuas or Sextius Niger, but verified, where possible, from his own experience or from that of others whom he had interviewed personally.[33] His own expertise emerges clearly in his comments on gathering, preparing and storing herbs in order to achieve maximum efficacy.[34] His interest was first and foremost in the intrinsic medical value of the substances, and he was not setting out to provide, like Scribonius Largus, merely a handbook of remedies for specific conditions. His list is thus far more extensive: it includes just over a thousand substances, of which around 700 are plants. He gives a succinct description of each plant, its appearance, its properties and its uses, whether in human medicine, on animals or around the house.[35]

Crithmon (also called critamon), for example, probably to be identified with samphire, is

a shrubby little herb about a foot high, with thick leaves, which grows in rocky and maritime areas. It is full of fat whitish leaves, like those of purslane, yet broader, longer and with a salty taste. It bears white flowers and a soft fruit akin to *rosemary*: sweet-smelling, round. When dried, it splits to reveal a fruit like wheat. It has three or four roots, as thick as a finger, fragrant and with a pleasant taste. The seed, roots and leaves, boiled in wine and drunk, are effective in easing painful urination and curing jaundice; they also induce menstruation. It is used as a vegetable, eaten either boiled or raw, and is also preserved in brine.[36]

Dioscorides' book is organised first by categories, animals, minerals and plants (further divided into roots, pot herbs, fruits, trees and shrubs), and then arranged according to their effect on the body, since, he explained, those seeking a remedy for a particular condition would be more likely to find it in a section dealing with similarly active drugs than by hunting alphabetically through a long list of plants.[37] His unusual emphasis on drug affinities, however, was not always welcomed. While later authors, such as Galen, acknowledged the comprehensiveness and wealth of practical detail to be found in Dioscorides, many found its organisation difficult to follow. Some copyists reverted to familiar practice and rewrote the whole book with the substances in alphabetical order within the larger divisions. Others assembled lists of synonyms or added the names for the plants in a variety of languages, such as Dacian. All this helped Dioscorides and his herbal to become the bible of medical botany and to exercise an enormous influence on pharmacology and botany well into the seventeenth century.[38]

Dioscorides' sophisticated understanding of medicine and pharmacology stands in sharp contrast to that of Pliny the Elder, who included even more extensive information on drugs in his *Natural History*. This is avowedly a compilation, drawn from a multitude of Greek and Latin sources, prepared for the benefit of the wider public and offering both interesting information and practical self-help medicine. Later generations of physicians, beginning with Niccolò Leoniceno (1428–1524), declared their exasperation with Pliny's errors of copying and misinterpretation, contrasting them with the precision of Dioscorides and Galen.[39] But Leoniceno and his successors had Greek and Greek texts at their disposal, a situation that was not necessarily true for Pliny's intended audience or for his readers in the later Latin and mediaeval worlds.[40] For them it was Pliny's accessibility and apparent comprehensiveness that mattered.[41] He took his remedies from all types of authority, whether botanists such as Theophrastus, medical writers such as Heraclides or Sextius Niger or the less reputable heirs of the Persian magi, whose methods he deplored as much as the theorising of Greek physicians.[42] His range of substances is even greater than that of Dioscorides, incorporating herbs from as far afield as Britain and Ethiopia.[43] This growth of knowledge Pliny acknowledges with a mixture of pride and caution. In his view medicine, as we have seen, was introduced to Rome only in the third century BC, knowledge of mineral drugs perhaps even later and the art of making compound remedies not until

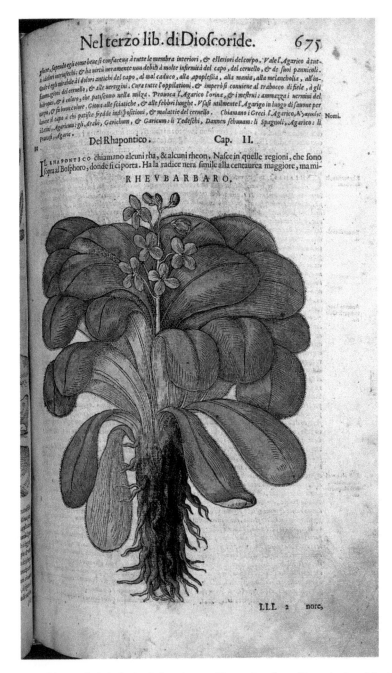

pliore, sapendo egli come bene si confacena à tutte le membra interiori, & esteriori del corpo. Vale l'Agarico à tutti i dolori intrinsechi: & ha virtù veramente non debili à molte infirmità del capo, del ceruello, & de suoi pannicoli. Onde è egli mirabile à i dolori antichi del capo, al mal caduco, alla apoplessia, alla mania, alla melancholia, all'infiammagioni del cernello, & alle uertigini. Cura tutte l'oppilationi, & imperò si conuiene al trabocco di fiele, à gli hidropici, & à coloro, che patiscono nella milza. Prouoca l'Agarico l'orina, & i mestrui: ammazza i uermini del corpo, & fa buon colore. Gioua alle sciatiche, & alle febbri lunghe. Vsasi utilmente l'Agarico in luogo di sauone per lauare il capo à chi patisce fredde indispositioni, & malattie del cernello. Chiamano i Greci l'Agarico, Ἀγαρικόν: i Latini, Agaricum: gli Arabi, Garichum, & Garicum: li Tedeschi, Dannen schwuam: li Spagnoli, Agarico: li Francesi, Agaric. Nomi.

Del Rhapontico.　　　Cap. II.

IL RHAPONTICO chiamano alcuni rha, & alcuni rheon. Nasce in quelle regioni, che sono sopra al Bosphoro, donde si ci porta. Ha la radice nera simile alla centaurea maggiore, ma mi-

RHEVBARBARO.

LLL 2　　　nore,

Figure 12.1 Dioscorides' rhubarb. A Renaissance illustration from Pietro Andrea Mattioli's Italian translation of Dioscorides, ed. 3, Venice, V. Valgrisi, 1568, p. 675. Courtesy of Wellcome Library, London.

the first century BC, following Pompey's defeat of Mithridates and the translation into Latin of some of the learned king's recipes by Pompeius Lenaeus.[44]
Roman power had made this accumulation of knowledge possible, yet at the
same time it had introduced dangerous luxuries that would lead to the neglect
of the simpler, more effective and morally purer bounties of Nature.

Pliny's comments on the development of compound medicines in this
period are borne out by the fragments of contemporary writers on pharmacology, such as Andromachus the Elder, a Cretan who became personal doctor
to Nero.[45] He was famous for his universal antidote, *Galene*, which replaced
the Mithridatium of Mithridates in popular esteem. It now contained more
ingredients, sixty-four as opposed to forty-one, with a higher proportion of
opiates and minerals, and with the original lizard flesh replaced by that of a
viper. Andromachus wrote his recipe in the form of a poem in eighty-seven
couplets, possibly, as another pharmacological poet Servilius Damocrates
argued, because verse was a better medium for preserving exact details than
prose, but also because it gave clear proof of the composer's cultural aspirations and abilities.[46] Andromachus' verses were later turned into prose by his
son, another Andromachus, probably an imperial physician later in the first
century. Galen judged the younger Andromachus harshly as a mere compiler
who lacked the ingenuity of his father and the precision and clarity of his
teacher, Asclepiades Pharmacion, whose ten books of external and internal
remedies Galen considered the best drug book available.[47] That did not, of
course, prevent Galen from taking over, often verbatim, large sections of the
three books of the younger Andromachus on external, internal and ophthal-
mological drugs.[48] Another pharmacologist and royal physician, Statilius
Crito, was also a major source for many recipes recommended by Galen, not
least for cosmetic purposes, where Crito had drawn upon a treatise on cosmetics allegedly written by the greatest beauty of her age, Queen Cleopatra of
Egypt.[49] The Galenic Corpus also contains an unusual survivor of a type of
pharmacological writing that must once have been common. Its anonymous
author, a Greek from Asia Minor who had migrated to the capital, describes
to his brother the almost wondrous virtues of a single plant, the centaury,
that he had found suitable for almost every kind of illness, from headache
and stomach pains to wounds and rabies. It could be used both internally and
externally, and was a true panacea. Indeed, until he had seen its results, he
had himself doubted whether it could be as effective as it was said to be. But
unlike Dioscorides, he makes no distinction between the two main types of
centaury, and gives only a brief botanical description.[50] Living in Rome, with
access to good networks of information and to drugs imported from around
the Empire, some specially gathered by imperial rootcutters, these men
formed a pharmacological elite. The development of treatises on *Substitute
Drugs*, listing what alternatives might be used if those originally prescribed
were unavailable, shows that their high aims and complex combinations may
have been difficult to achieve in the provinces.[51]

Crito, Dioscorides and Scribonius Largus had more in common than phar-macology: they had all seen service in the Roman army.[52] The wars of conquest in the last century BC, especially under Augustus, had firmly planted Roman forces along the edges of an empire that ran roughly from the Rhine and Danube in the north to the Euphrates in the east and the Nile valley and the Sahara in the south. Further campaigns in the first and early second century resulted in the takeover of much of Britain and Dacia (modern Romania), and pushed the Roman frontier further east to the Tigris. Although there had been conquests on such a scale before, by the Persians and by Alexander the Great, to name but two, and cities such as Carthage or Athens had put into the field substantial armies, the military situation in the late first century BC was different from anything that had gone before. Citizen troops raised only for the campaigning season and fighting close to home were superseded by long-serving professional forces composed of citizen legionaries and non-citizen auxiliaries. Campaigns were taking place many hundreds of miles from Rome and Italy, often in regions where the natives were not only decid-edly unfriendly but living in settlements that a Mediterranean dweller would scarcely call a town at all. It was no longer possible to follow the standard procedure of returning one's wounded, after treatment on the battlefield, to their own homes or leaving them behind in a friendly town.[53] New measures were called for.

By AD 14, the new Roman army, concerned as it was with the pacification of conquered territory as much as with further conquests, was largely resident in legionary fortresses or in much smaller and more exposed auxiliary forts.[54] Transitory tents and temporary billets were replaced by permanent bases con-structed of wood and stone. A standard plan for the fortresses was adopted that included a *valetudinarium* or hospital in a relatively quiet sector of the camp. This was usually a large rectangular building (that at Neuss, W. Germany, measures 89 m by 50 m) around a central court with small rooms opening off on both sides of a corridor running right round the building. There were also two or three much larger rooms, one of which probably served as an operat-ing theatre, as well as store rooms and kitchens.[55] To judge from the layout of surviving remains, careful attention was paid to lighting, latrines and water supply: at Inchtuthil, in Scotland, the beds were placed in cubicles in such a way as to avoid draughts as far as possible.[56] These hospitals were for the Roman legions, citizen troops. The forts of the non-citizen auxiliaries were much smaller, as befitted their smaller units (1,000 or fewer, compared with 5,600 men in a legion), and do not always appear to have been provided with hospital facilities. Where they were, they either reproduced the form of the legionary hospital on a smaller scale, as at Housesteads on Hadrian's Wall (N. England), or, more often, they formed a smaller rectangle with an operating room and cubicles along one side of a corridor, as at Fendoch (Scotland).[57]

Some healing plants could be grown in the hospital garden or collected nearby, but other drugs and materials were supplied from further afield.[58]

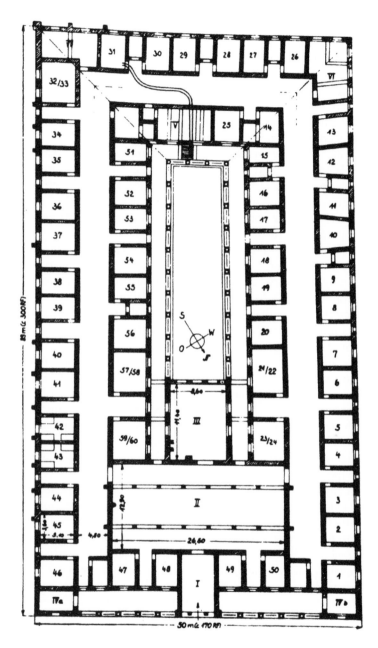

Map 12.1 The legionary hospital at Novaesium (Neuss, Germany). Built in stone *c.*AD 50, it served the 5,600 citizen soldiers of the sixteenth legion. The sick were brought into one of the large halls, which may also have been an operating room and dispensary, and slept in small cubicles off the corridor, which reduced draughts and noise.

Stamps on barrels for (medicated?) wine found at Aquincum, near Budapest, declare that they had been imported 'duty free for the account of the hospital of the 2nd Adiutrix Legion'. Wine flavoured with horehound was imported to the fortress of Carpow in Scotland for campaigns in the early third century, as Italian wine had been to Caerleon in S. Wales a century or so earlier.[59] An Egyptian papyrus records a contract in AD 138 for the making of blankets, 'plain white, six cubits by four ... with finished hems', for the hospital of a legion stationed in Cappadocia on the eastern frontier.[60]

Information on those treated in these hospitals is scanty. The plans of Neuss and Fendoch suggest that the number of cubicles coincided with the number of centuries in a legion or cohort; depending on the number of beds in each cubicle, this would give a possible occupancy rate of 2.5–5 per cent in normal conditions, and perhaps double that in an emergency. At Hod Hill, in Dorset, England, constructed during the initial phase of the Roman conquest in AD 43, when more fighting was expected, the excavator suggested that between 12 per cent and 20 per cent of the troops might be accommodated in the building he posited as a hospital.[61] But not all the inmates would be suffering from wounds inflicted by the enemy. The notion that the army operated a triage system on the battlefield, treating the lightly wounded on the spot, others in tents in the rear of the field and the more seriously wounded in the hospital of the legionary fortress, is a pleasant fiction.[62] Fighting rarely took place conveniently close to a military hospital. The permanent fortresses in Africa, at Lambaesis (S. Algeria), and in Britain, at Caerleon, Chester, York and, more briefly, Gloucester and Inchtuthil, were many days hard marching from where hostilities might be foreseen. Even where, as on the Rhine and Danube, the fortresses were much closer to the frontier, the legions and auxiliaries frequently campaigned well beyond it. The seriously wounded were far more likely to have died on the way home, long before they reached the comfort of the hospital for an operation or convalescence.[63]

And, in any case, invalidity is not exclusively the result of set fighting. At Vindolanda, an auxiliary fort near Hadrian's Wall, the duty roster for 18 May, AD 90 (?) shows that thirty-one out of 752 men were unfit for duty: fifteen were ill, six were injured (uolnerati) and another ten were suffering from eye problems.[64] Nor need even the injuries have been inflicted by the enemy: injuries due to accidents while drilling, or simply while patrolling the Wall, would also come into this category. There were other hazards, too. Claudius Terentianus, serving in the Egyptian fleet, was ill on board his ship, the Neptune, with food poisoning for five days.[65] At the fort of Künzing in Germany, deposits from the latrine have revealed the presence of an internal parasite, whipworm, often associated with contaminated pork.[66] One might surmise that medical assistance was also offered to some of the inhabitants of the canabae, the shanty towns around many forts where traders and the ordinary soldiers' women and children lived. Even if Wilmanns was right to argue that this careful provision for the treatment of the sick in a legionary fortress erred on the side of caution and an overcapacity of beds and services, it was also one of the perks of joining the army, since such assistance was not always forthcoming to the civilian.[67]

A variety of personnel attended to the hospitals and the medical needs of the army and navy, including their animals. A legion would have had several doctors, possibly one for each detachment (*vexillatio*), while each regiment of auxiliaries, mounted or unmounted, had a doctor of its own. Similar arrangements were in place in Rome for the household troops, the police (the urban cohorts) and the fire brigade. Several naval doctors mention the ship on which they served, but it is unclear whether this means that each ship had its own doctor or that the trireme named was the flagship of a small flotilla.[68] Responsibility for the running of the legionary hospital fell upon one or two non-medical administrative officers – one such was next transferred to take charge of the camp jail.[69] Two doctors, one with the urban cohorts stationed at Lyons and the other with the elite household cavalry, are recorded as 'camp doctor'; that this was a title given also to the senior doctor in a legionary fortress elsewhere is possible, but far from proven.[70] At the other end of the military hierarchy were bandagers, drug dispensers, vets and recruits learning their speciality.[71]

What rank the doctors (*medici*) themselves held is complicated and controversial. All were technically free from the standard military fatigue duties, and all were also eligible for a higher rate of pay. Naval doctors seem regularly to have been paid at double the rate for a crewman, and pay and a half or double pay may also have been given to the 'soldier doctors'.[72] To judge from the scanty evidence, these may have been enlisted men, perhaps gaining their training and experience in the army itself. At the same time, there were others who called themselves '*medici ordinarii*', a title that implies membership of the *ordo* of centurions, with a pay level of at least ten times that of the ranker.[73]

The difficulty may be resolved by assuming that some doctors joined up for a time, having had a civilian career to which, later, they might wish to return. They were not bound by the usual terms of enlistment for twenty or twenty-five years, and frequently came from families of a higher status and education than those of the average soldier. Marcus Valerius Longinus, a doctor in the Seventh Legion, had already been made a member of the city council at his home town of Drobeta (Turnu Severin, Romania) when he died at the age of twenty-three.[74] Numisius, who appealed to the Emperor Caracalla over the potential loss of his tax immunity at home while he was on service with the Second Adiutrix Legion, was clearly already a man of wealth and was expected by the emperor to return to civilian practice.[75] The flowery dedication in Greek set up to Asclepius, Hygieia and Panacea within the legionary fortress of Chester (England), and possibly within the hospital itself, by doctor Antiochus bespeaks a very high level of literary education.[76] Men like him or Callimorphus, the doctor–historian of the Parthian wars of

185

the 160s, were in social terms far above the average soldier, and would have fitted well into the order of the centurions, who frequently retired into the ranks of civic councillors or government administrators.[77]

A spell in the army, even if for only a few years, would have its attractions. It might bring a provincial physician into contact with some of the leading figures in the Roman Empire, as well as enabling him to see something of the wider world. This was another mechanism whereby doctors with Greek names came to travel even further away from their homes than usual. Antiochus and Hermogenes served in Chester, Marcus Aurelius [Habr]ocomas even further north at Binchester (Durham), Claudius Hymnus at Vindonissa (Switzerland) and Flavius Onesiphorus at Lambaesis. Marcus Rubrius Zosimus, from Ostia, the port of Rome, erected a votive altar in the fort at Obernburg (Germany) to Apollo, Asclepius, Salus and Fortuna, in thanks for their help in curing his commanding officer.[78]

What survives of the written or archaeological evidence for military surgery suggests that Zosimus and his like did not deserve the reproaches of Galen for lack of enterprise. In his view they squandered the opportunity to dissect the corpses of dead Germans left on the battlefield in the campaigns of Marcus Aurelius in the 170s, with the result that their knowledge of the body was no better than that of a cook.[79] But if the instruments found at Neuss

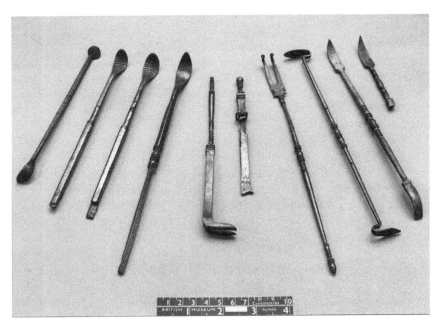

Figure 12.2 The instruments of a Roman lithotomist, comprising specialised scoops, knives, forceps and hooks. Believed to come from near Rome. Museum of Classical Archaeology, Cambridge.

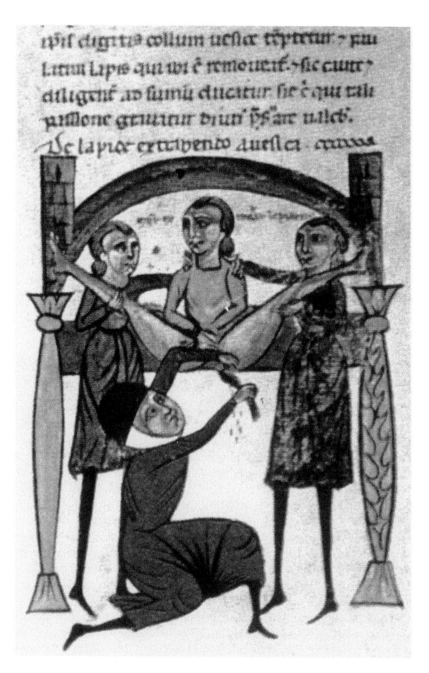

Figure 12.3 An operation for bladder stone recommended by Celsus, *On Medicine* 7, 26, as depicted in a mediaeval manuscript of surgery. Rome, Biblioteca Casanatense, Ms. 1382, fol. 25.

or at Bingen, a German town with military links, are in any way typical of an army surgeon, they imply a wide range of operations and of specialised tools with which to perform them.[80] The so-called Dioclean spoon and the 'glove-stretcher' were commended by Paul of Aegina for use in removing the heads of arrows and even larger projectiles. The technique of extracting small arrowheads by making a counter-opening and then gently pulling the offending object through it is also described by Celsus.[81] Plutarch, writing around AD 90, records a similar case of a small fishbone extracted from the throat in this way, although the patient subsequently died, almost certainly from infection.[82] That military surgery continued to develop in step with the development of new weapons is clear from the chapter devoted to missile injuries in the sixth century by Paul of Aegina, who reports several operations previously unrecorded in our sources.[83]

Celsus and Galen also detail ways to treat wounds from sword cuts and thrusts, whether received on the battlefield or in the arena by the gladiators whom Galen attended. Swift action was essential to replace intestines left hanging out of a wound; cleaning, stitching and firm bandaging to hold the wound together might work if the intestines themselves had not been damaged. Plutarch records a successful case of this sort handled by Cleanthes in the civil wars of the early 40s BC.[84] A century after Plutarch, Galen disliked midline incisions in such cases, because of the difficulty of stitching and the likelihood of complications if the thread was weak, comments that earned him an exaggerated and misleading headline in a modern surgical journal as 'the Father of Catgut Sutures'.[85] He also expected the average surgeon to be able to perform careful surgery on the eye or on fistulae, and to deal with a variety of wounds and ulcers, as well as with hernias and aneurysms.[86] He himself could do better than that – witness his successful removal of a suppurating breastbone of a slave belonging to a popular playwright.[87] He may not have been alone in his aspirations or abilities with the knife. The description of surgical procedures in the contemporary treatise *Introduction to Medicine*, which passes under his name, confirms that, in theory at least, others contemplated similarly complex operations.[88] Archaeological finds suggest that many practitioners possessed a basic surgical kit of a few scalpels, hooks, probes, forceps and bone levers, and some specialists owned far more than this.[89] In 257–8 a surgeon at Rimini, no plutocratic metropolis, had over 150 instruments, many displaying subtle differences from others of the same type, which implies a high degree of specialisation and expertise.[90]

Although all surgical authors recommend the utmost attention to stemming haemorrhages, avoiding inflammation and promoting the agglutination of the wound, they were not always successful in avoiding unpleasant consequences and death. Galen claims that sixteen of the gladiatorial troupe paid for by the high priest of Asia died in the care of his predecessor, whereas he had only two fatalities during his first spell as their doctor and, when reappointed, even fewer.[91] Common operations such as cutting for the stone, extracting or crushing a diseased uvula and removing rotting teeth would always have been attended with some danger of wound infection, although swabbing a wound with wine or oil would have reduced that risk.[92] But cauterisation would have left nasty scars, and a patient who had been cut for the stone in the manner recommended by Celsus, and his successors for centuries after, might also have had to put up with pain and infection if the incision in the perineum failed to heal entirely.[93] That some doctors specialised in the treatment of fistulae is also an indication that such ulcerations could be chronic and long lasting.[94]

In some instances it might even be necessary to amputate a limb, preferably, argued Celsus, by a circular cut which allowed for primary closure of the wound.[95] The lost limb might be replaced by an artificial one. The local carpenter could easily make a crutch or a peg-leg, but other substitutes would require somewhat greater expertise. One soldier is said to have had an iron hand made to replace one lost in battle, while a skeleton from Capua, S. Italy, was buried about 300 BC with an artificial leg made of bronze over a wooden core. Fitting neatly around the stump of the thigh, it stretched from knee to ankle, but had no movable joints.[96] Other artificial limbs are known from N. European graves from the early mediaeval period, suggesting a continuity with Roman practice.[97]

Although no surviving treatise from the Roman period is devoted exclusively to surgery and we have only fragments from the writings of such expert surgeons as Heliodorus and Antyllus, enough remains from the sections on surgery in general surveys of medicine, from Celsus, Galen and the pseudo-Galenic *Introduction* to the Late Antique encyclopedists, to show that the advances made by the Hellenistic surgeons of Alexandria were maintained well down into Late Antiquity.[98] Ionicus of Sardes, who taught in Alexandria around 380, had a great reputation as a surgeon, and high hopes were entertained of the Alexandrian surgeon who arrived at Carthage in the early fifth century to treat St Augustine's friend Innocentius for his fistula. A century later the bishop–historian John of Ephesus describes how one of his colleagues, the presbyter Aaron, had suffered from serious ulceration, 'gangrene', in the genital area. 'The physicians' excised the diseased flesh, applied plasters and bandages and inserted a lead tube to allow him to pass water. Aaron lived for a further eighteen years.[99]

The soldiers in the Roman army would have benefited from these improvements in general surgery as well as from the extra attention devoted to their medical needs by the provision of hospitals, doctors and medical attendants. They enjoyed these advantages not only because of their importance in fighting the enemy and preserving the boundaries of the Empire, but also because the survival of individual emperors depended on the loyalty and well-being of their troops.[100] As the army itself changed in the Late Empire and came to rely more and more on local levies supported by a major mobile striking force controlled from the centre, the military hospitals also declined in importance along with the forts and fortresses. Vegetius, writing his military textbook in the fourth century, still mentions fortress hospitals and the duties of their medical superintendents, but devotes more space to temporary encampments.[101] The epigraphic record also ends at this point, so that we are left uninformed about the medical consequences of the transition from one military system to another. What is clear, however, is that the level of detailed sophistication achieved by the Roman army medical services in the first three centuries of the Christian era was not reached again in Europe until the seventeenth or eighteenth century.

13

THE RISE OF METHODISM

When, around AD 70, the Elder Pliny surveyed the development of medicine in his *Natural History*, he composed a devastating indictment of his fellow Romans and their Greek doctors. As we have seen, he saw the transplantation of Greek medicine to Rome as an index of moral decline, the triumph of luxury over old Roman virtues.[1] Now, blown along by every passing fancy, his fellow citizens put their faith in healers who offered novelty rather than sound prospects of health. Cold-water cures were succeeded by astrological dietetics as the fashionable therapy of the day and this, in turn, by cold baths.[2] Each healer put forward his own pet theory in order to gain patients. Most notorious of all in Pliny's eyes was Thessalus of Tralles, the Methodist whose memorial among the select graves on the Appian Way bore the epithet *iatronikes*, 'champion physician'. Whether in public or at the bedside, confrontation took over from co-operation, disagreement from shared diagnosis, and public morality collapsed along with private health.[3]

Pliny's rhetoric had a basis in reality: the expanding population of the capital allowed a ready market for any and all medical theories and practices. Democriteans, Asclepiadeans, Pneumatists, Hippocratics and Empiricists vied for attention with Tiberius Claudius Menecrates, who proclaimed his own creation of a 'clear and logical sect', and with Leonides of Alexandria, whose soubriquet, the 'Episynthetic', implied that he was bringing together all that was best in others' teaching.[4]

But by concentrating on individuals and their failings, and by implying a constant instability, Pliny's account obscures the rise to prominence of widespread medical groupings, or sects, with long-lasting traditions, especially the Methodists.[5] His denunciation of Thessalus, allied to the disdain of others for various features of Methodism and its practitioners, has had a lasting effect. By contrast with Hippocratism, and its claim to go back to the great age of Greece, Methodism is often viewed as an upstart, a Roman parvenu, born in a society that knew little and cared less about proper medicine.

This chapter's reassessment of the most important Roman contribution to medicine will take the arguments of the Methodists themselves seriously. It will suggest that their major theories were the result of a reasoned response to a new situation, namely the sheer size of the city of Rome, and a dissatisfaction with both the Hippocratic and the Empiricist approaches to diagnosis. They offered a new epistemology of medicine as an ongoing process of knowledge, based on an evident correlation between observations and a small range of possible underlying conditions. Although their opponents accused them of doctrinaire adherence to a fixed system that failed to consider the individual patient, their therapeutic practices did allow for a considerable degree of latitude, and several of their treatments differed only slightly from those of their adversaries.

Methodism, so called because of its claim to follow a uniquely successful *method* of healing, was arguably the dominant medical theory throughout the Roman world for at least three centuries, despite Galen's somewhat slighting reference to it as 'the third sect'.[6] Although its origins can be located among Greek-speaking doctors in Rome and Italy, and although both Pliny and Galen imply that it became successful only by appealing to the lowest and less sophisticated groups there, its influence stretched across the Empire. At Alexandria in the 150s, Julian, a pupil of Apollonides of Cyprus, was composing his forty-eight books (of lectures?) on the Hippocratic *Aphorisms* as well as his *Philo*, a large exposition of Methodist doctrine.[7] Galen's rival as an imperial physician in the Rome of the 170s, Statilius Attalus, was a Methodist who belonged to the same family from Asia Minor as Statilius Crito.[8] Attalus' teacher, Soranus, although he had had experience of Rome, viewed it disparagingly from the perspective of a leading physician of Asia Minor and a native of Ephesus, one of the most wealthy, vibrant and cultured cities in the entire ancient world.[9] His contemporary, Marcus Modius Asiaticus, 'Champion of the Method' and 'Methodist doctor', gazes out from his beautifully carved bust with all the *hauteur* of a leading intellectual at Smyrna (Izmir, W. Turkey), the neighbour and rival of Ephesus in matters cultural as well as political.[10] Methodism was bilingual. Of the major surviving monuments of Methodism, the huge treatise on *Chronic and Acute Diseases* by the North African Caelius Aurelianus was written in Latin, Soranus' *Gynaecology* in Greek. It was also long lasting, flourishing in N. Africa in Late Antiquity with Caelius and influencing early mediaeval medicine in the West to a far greater extent than Galenic Hippocratism.

The origins and general doctrines of Methodism remain controversial, largely because, apart from Soranus and Caelius, no large-scale treatise written by a Methodist has come down to us. As a consequence, the early Methodists on the whole speak only through their detractors, even ones so courteous as Celsus. The advantages of their system of medicine are minimised, not least through being placed in an aridly intellectual environment. Even if modern scholars no longer repeat the facile denunciations of Methodism put forward by Pliny and Galen, they have not entirely freed themselves from these old assertions of its weaknesses. In trying to defend Methodism they have often unwittingly fallen into the trap of fighting on a battlefield already determined by its opponents.[11] Yet, as this chapter will show, the Methodists, once allowed to speak for themselves, present a system of therapeutics that is far from philosophically naive, and that relates neatly to the problems and consequences of medical practice in an urban environment.[12] What Galen saw as evidence of uncertainty and confusion, they considered matters of indifference when treating the patient; much of what he thought essential in a physician they regarded as peripheral in the struggle against disease. Moreover, the desire of Methodism's opponents to tar all its members with the same brush obscures historical developments within Methodism. Even apparently neutral lists, for example, of the succession of leaders of the sect turn out on closer inspection to be untrustworthy, both because of what they leave out and because of their tendency to create a neat line of authority that is intended to carry weight because of a direct succession of distinguished names going back to the founder. Differences and hesitations are smoothed out to suggest a tight coherence that, in reality, was never there. This chapter thus seeks to rehabilitate Methodism by attempting to see it through the eyes of its own adherents over two centuries or more.

The ancient doxography of Methodism tells a simple story: as in a biblical genealogy, name follows name in an apparent succession. 'Themison of Laodicea began the sect, taking his cue from the rational Asclepiades; Thessalus of Tralles completed it; then followed Mnaseas, Dionysius ...'[13] But this apparently unbroken sequence of masters and pupils is intended to give the authority of age to the views of modern Methodists far more than to present a history of Methodism.[14] Not only does it suggest an unchanging body of doctrine, shared by all Methodists, but it appears to skate over difficulties of chronology and geography. If Asclepiades was already dead by 91 BC, as some have thought, the gap between him and Thessalus, whose triumphs in Rome are securely located in the 50s and 60s, cannot be bridged by one man, Themison, especially if he was a direct pupil of Asclepiades.[15] Even on a chronology that puts Asclepiades' main activity forty years or more later the gap between Themison and Thessalus is still uncomfortably wide. Second, Cornelius Celsus, our best contemporary evidence for first-century Methodism, appears to dissociate Themison from what the Methodists of his own day believed, even though they claimed him as their founder and the authority for their doctrines.[16] Celsus himself never mentions Thessalus by name, either because he was writing just before Thessalus became prominent or because he did not wish to be seen to indulge in a polemic with him. Certainly, his references to modern Methodism imply that it was already flourishing even before Thessalus came on the scene. Thessalus himself was notoriously self-assertive, preaching against all other doctrines but his own, and there is little doubt that he introduced changes to what Themison had taught.[17] Indeed, Galen, our single most informative source for early Methodism, takes Thessalus as the object of his attack against Methodism and Methodists ('Thessalian asses') in general. Although he admits that

Themison's ideas were at the root of Thessalian Methodism, especially the doctrine of commonalities, he qualifies this admission by attributing far-reaching changes to Thessalus. In this way he can treat Methodism as something created effectively *de novo* by Thessalus and thus associate all later Methodists, including his competitors, with the bombast and bluster of a man he saw as a great charlatan.[18] The humbler author of the *Introduction to Medicine* offers a similar, if less polemical, schema: Themison broke with Asclepiades to found the Methodist sect, but it was Thessalus who brought it to perfection. But neither Galen's rhetorical strategy nor the anonymous author's apparent precision offers a solid basis for granting (or denying) Thessalus the role of the founder of Methodism, or for choosing between him and Themison.[19]

This debate over founding fathers can be placed within the broader context of the influence of Asclepiades of Bithynia in advocating a mechanistic, corpuscular theory of medicine (see p. 172). His followers spread over the Roman world, from the Rhone valley in S. Gaul to Tarsus in S.E. Turkey.[20] Some doctors well into the third or fourth century were still claiming to be followers of Asclepiades, although by then little Cibyra, in eastern Pamphylia (S. Turkey), where the Asclepiadean doctor Aurelius Varianus Pantauchus was commemorated, was hardly in the forefront of progress.[21] But in the last years of the Roman Republic and the first years of the Empire the intellectual and social importance of Asclepiades' adherents was considerable. M. Artorius was a court doctor to Augustus in 23 BC; Laecanius Arius of Tarsus the friend and mentor of Dioscorides, as well as being himself a celebrated writer on pharmacology.[22] Julius Bassus, Niceratus, Petronius Musa, Diodotus and Sextius Niger, whom Dioscorides condemns in the preface to his *Materia medica* for their reluctance to test the herbs they described, were all respectable writers on pharmacology, and on much else.[23] They shared with Asclepiades a belief in a material world made up of particles as opposed to the elements posited by the Aristotelians and Stoics. In this they may have been akin to the Democritean doctor Philo of Hyampolis, introduced as an interlocutor by Plutarch, who attributed thirst to changes in the shape of the relevant 'channels' ('pores') of the body.[24] There are also links with the corpuscular philosophy of the Epicureans, best exemplified in the discussion of plague in Lucretius' poem *On the Nature of Things*.[25]

It is against this philosophical and medical background that one must set Themison and his ideas. According to Celsus and Pliny, it was towards the end of his life that Themison, an immigrant to Rome from Laodicea in Syria, diverged somewhat from the teachings of his master Asclepiades, but neither author makes the nature of that divergence totally clear.[26] It involved both a shift of clinical emphasis and a theoretical readjustment.[27] Themison declared that good medicine was effective practice, no more, no less; there was no need for complex nosological classifications (though nosology and close observation of symptoms were essential), still less for any investigation into the hidden causes of disease.[28] But empirical observation by itself was not enough. What was required was the understanding that all diseases shared some general and plainly visible characteristics, 'commonalities', and that once these were recognised the choice of treatment followed easily. An examination of the patient would provide a good indication of the appropriate commonality. There was no need of repeated observation, logical demonstration or anatomical investigation:[29] the patient's condition itself gave an objective and immediate pointer to its classification. To go further and investigate precisely what caused these commonalities, as a Hippocratic might want to do, was irrelevant; to hunt for past cases comparable in every detail, as Empiricists advocated, was time consuming and, in the absence of any principle that would direct the search, merely random.

In Themison's view there were three major categories of disease, based on 'stricture', 'looseness' or an intermediate, mixed state. Asclepiades had used similar formulations, but the theoretical shift made by Themison was to extend Asclepiades' view of disease as primarily dependent on the size and organisation of corpuscles to one in which the fault could lie equally with the corpuscles and with the pores through which they flowed. Sometimes the corpuscles were too big, at others the channels were too small; in either case, the result was the same, stricture.[30] At the same time, he divided up diseases according to whether they were acute or chronic, the first being largely the result of stricture, the latter of looseness. Although the distinction is implicit in much earlier writing, it was Themison, according to Caelius Aurelianus, who was the first to write a treatise with this explicit organisation.[31] Early Methodists also divided the treatment of all diseases according to three common and universal stages: an initial increase, a middle period when the level of the disease was constant, and a final stage in which it diminished.[32] Themison may also have been among the first, if not *the* first, to have stressed the importance of the *diatritos*, each three-day period, as marking a significant stage in the treatment.[33]

Themison's doctrines were open to attack on a variety of counts. Celsus accepted that they might have some medical usefulness, but derided them because they appeared to abolish what was, in his eyes, the crucial element in medical practice, the encounter between doctor and patient, which led to an understanding of, and therapy for, the sick individual. More than once Celsus draws a distinction between medicine in a *valetudinarium* or a big city practice, and the activity of the true doctor, able to diagnose and to prescribe for the ills of each patient. He acknowledges that, faced with many sufferers at one time, attention to general common features may be all that the doctor can offer, but, equally, he makes it clear that this is not the course that he himself would choose. Better, he thinks, to pay more attention to fewer patients, and have a potentially lower income, than to treat all and sundry with a therapy that might not be targeted precisely.[34] Nonetheless, from the perspective of the patient, a Methodist physician who offered a swift diagnosis and a treatment that might work as well as any other could have many advantages over an expensive competitor who took his time in reaching any conclusion. Even Celsus was prepared to admit that if one was not already acquainted with the individual condition of the patient, proceeding by commonalities was sensible – but it was far better to have a friend as a doctor than a stranger.[35]

How coherent early Methodism was as a system of medicine is difficult to determine. There were certainly debates about the meaning of terms such as 'fluid' (did it refer to the fluid state of the whole body or of a part; was it to be judged by all bodily secretions or by a few?), but theoretical differences may have had little effect on practice.[36] Similarly, Galen's gleeful denunciation of Methodist inconsistency in talking indiscriminately about 'diseases' and 'affections' demonstrates merely that they had no place in their system for what to him was a fundamental distinction.[37] In his turn, too, Thessalus exaggerated the differences between himself, Themison and other Asclepiadeans by his rhetorical claims to be the founder of his own sect and to be creating a novel type of medicine. His behaviour emphasised his singularity. He was accompanied by crowds wherever he went; he was the correspondent of the Emperor Nero; and he denounced with enthusiasm the follies of all the physicians who had preceded him.[38]

How he developed Themison's ideas is unclear in the fog created by Galen's scorn and his own propaganda. His origins, in the wealthy town of Tralles in Asia Minor, famous for its woollen industry, were turned against him by Galen to imply that he came from a humble family of workers in wool, traditionally a job fit only for women. Thessalus could thus be convicted of effeminacy, and his followers likewise.[39] Their intellectual stupidity was compounded in Galen's eyes by their low social and moral status. Their claim to be able to teach the whole of medicine in just six months to any who might want to learn, slaves, ex-slaves or those who could afford nothing better, seemed further proof of their lack of education and sense of social responsibility.[40]

Galen's satirical picture of Themison's horror at the subsequent transformation of his commonalities by Thessalus suggests that it was Thessalus who developed this central notion of Methodism in a variety of ways.[41] These commonalities became more and more subdivided: those concerned with dietetics were distinguished from those to do with surgery; the surgical divided into abnormalities on the outside of the body – a thorn, for instance, to be removed by extraction – and those on the inside. The latter were further subdivided into those where there was an abnormality of place, for example a sprain or fracture, to be cured by repositioning; of size, such as a tumour or excrescence, to be removed by opening or extraction; and of insufficiency, for example a fistula or ulcer, which needed to be filled. A fifth surgical commonality, the prophylactic, dealt with poisons.[42] Similar types of wounds demanded similar treatment; all those which failed to scar, for instance, required the removal of whatever prevented scarring.[43] In dietetics, the commonalities were subdivided into active and passive according to whether they induced a flux and merely flowed.[44] Once the indications or signs of these commonalities had been grasped, treatment followed a common route without deviation. But different parts of the body might require different treatments: inflammations of the hand or foot were dry diseases; those of the mouth or eyes were mixed. Variations in dosage depended not on the individuality of each patient but on the intensity of the disease, which might vary with the season, the age of the patient or the stage of the disease.[45] In this way the Methodists gained a flexibility of treatment without having to resort to the – to them impossible – task of discovering the specific natural condition of the individual patient and the degree to which any illness diverged from that norm. At the same time, by claiming that a common collocation of symptoms required an identical form of treatment they reduced the range of potential therapies to manageable proportions. The result at times might come very close to the treatment advocated by a Hippocratic physician such as Rufus for the same condition, although the route whereby that decision was reached might be very different. The Methodist stressed a commonality of symptoms; his competitor proceeded from a perception of the individual make-up of the patient that required restoration.[46]

A second innovation that may be attributed to Thessalus is the notion of '*metasynkrisis*', the modification of the pores of the body, whether in illness or in the process of recovery through the application of drugs. It is this process that requires closest attention during treatment, and which, in turn, permits the modification of the treatment in accordance with the particular visible common condition.[47] The fixed plan of treatment proposed by the Empiricists or the Hippocratics, which, once decided upon, should be followed throughout the illness, is thus avoided by the Methodists, who preferred instead to modify it as appeared best to them. Apparently opposed methods may thus be used consecutively if that is what the common conditions suggest.[48] Galen has great fun with this idea, and particularly with Thessalus' insistence that the patient should be kept without food for the first *diatritos* – that is, until the third day. The idea that the patient can be first starved and then stuffed strikes him as stupid, a perversion of method, and in his own dealings with Methodists he delights in pointing out the folly and even dangers of adhering to such a rule.[49] But the notion of the *diatritos* as a general guideline is far from foolish. It breaks down the management of a condition into time periods that are long enough to show some change, or absence of it, while not being so extended as to allow potentially serious developments to take hold. It forms a balance between constant attendance and a Hippocratic doctrine of critical days that might impose many days or even weeks between important changes that required careful attention from the doctor. On the Hippocratic scheme, observing these crises should merely confirm the truths of a diagnosis already made and of a pattern of treatment already decided upon; the Methodist *diatritos* requires a constant process of

197

observation and decision. Both procedures can be accused of a certain degree of inflexibility, but it is far from clear that the Methodists' *diatritos* put their patients in greater danger than the belief of their opponents that, once made, the diagnosis of the cause of a disease imposed a course of treatment that stood in no need of modification.

Galen's objections to the Methodists are also epistemological.[50] Their claim that their commonalities are self-evident he derides as simplistic as well as inconsistent, for there are debates within Methodism as to which commonality is responsible for this or that condition, or whether a particular disease manifesting itself in one part of the body is in fact affecting the whole body.[51] But while such arguments might seem shocking to their opponents, Methodists such as Soranus and Caelius could dismiss them as peripheral or irrelevant to treatment. To them it made little difference whether one part alone was diseased or it merely manifested the signs of illness to a greater extent than others; many of their drugs, although they were generally applied directly to the affected part, did not change their active power when they were applied elsewhere or affected only the point of application.[52] A similar attitude was taken by Methodists towards definitions. For Galen the inability of Methodists to arrive at a clear and certain definition of a disease was a mark of failure, yet no one reading the careful descriptions of diseases in Caelius Aurelianus, who based himself often explicitly on Soranus, could fail to note the similarity between them and what other authors from a variety of sects put forward.[53]

The key to this divergence lies in the underlying attitude to the acquisition of knowledge. For Galen, and for many others in the Hippocratic tradition, medicine was a science, a firm constellation of acquired data and principles; for the Methodists, although they were prepared to use the word 'science', it was more a process of understanding, open to modification in accordance with sensory phenomena.[54] Their science was provisional, although in practice they were prepared to follow some doctrines and procedures, and to accept some chains of cause and effect. In this, compared with Empiricists, they could be considered dogmatists, for they did invoke reasoning. Yet at the same time they refused to grant total certainty to that reasoning, giving priority to the indications from clearly visible phenomena that obviated the need for a logical analysis.[55] It is this provisionality that made them, as the philosopher Sextus Empiricus noted, suitable companions for Sceptical philosophers, and which, at the same time, infuriated those who demanded certainty or who saw inconsistencies between what Methodists claimed to believe and their, at times more rigid, practice.[56] In his frequent polemics with Methodists Galen condemned their adherence to tenets that might be inappropriate in an individual case, and he scornfully derided their efforts to treat all instances of the same disease in the same way, like those who wished to fit the same shoe to every foot. Their philosophical defences struck him as naive and foolish, and, most notably in the first two books of his own *Method of Healing*, he had little difficulty in pointing out what seemed to him to be gross errors in logic. But the Methodists could in turn argue that from their viewpoint Galen's own recommendations were oversophisticated, overlong and largely irrelevant to what was most needed, the effective treatment of the diseased patient.

That Galen was distorting the ideas of Methodism for his own polemical purposes is clear from what survives of Methodist writings, particularly those of Soranus of Ephesus. Although Galen elsewhere admits that there had been changes in Methodism over the years, especially with Menemachus, Olympicus and Soranus at the end of the first century, when indulging his passion for controversy he takes the Methodism of Thessalus as normative.[57] He can thus convict his opponents of slavish adherence to erroneous and outmoded doctrines when they agree with Thessalus, and of inconsistency when they do not. The one Methodist for whom Galen retained any respect was Soranus – and rightly so, to judge from what remains of his writings.[58]

Few details are preserved of the life and career of Soranus.[59] The entry in the Byzantine Suda lexicon gives his parents' names and his place of birth, Ephesus, and states that he lived in Rome under Trajan and Hadrian – that is, in the first quarter of the second century. That he knew Rome is clear from a reference to the practice of venesection there in cases of pleurisy and from his disparaging comment on the reasons for the prevalence of bow-legged children in Rome: they are encouraged to walk too early on the paved and unyielding streets; the water is extremely cold; and their mothers take far less care of their children than do the Greeks.[60] Other passing remarks suggest an acquaintance with Caria, Crete and Egypt: a stay in Alexandria for his medical education would be appropriate – other young men from Asia Minor, including Galen, made that journey – and account for his anatomical knowledge.[61] A later report, by Marcellus of Bordeaux, claims that he settled in Aquitaine, S.W. France, to care for 200 people suffering from a contagious skin disease. But Marcellus' source is unknown, and may be as untrustworthy as the even later stories that link Soranus with Queen Cleopatra as a specialist in cosmetics.[62]

His writings ranged widely, from works on philosophy, grammar and etymology to specialised medical tracts on bandaging, semen, clystering or the commonalities. Alongside general treatises on surgery (of which a section on fractures survives) or hygiene, he also wrote a series of biographies of earlier physicians and their writings, of which the extant *Life of Hippocrates According to Soranus* may be one.[63] His historical interests can also be seen in the careful recording of the opinions of earlier writers as preserved by Caelius Aurelianus in his own treatises on *Acute and Chronic Diseases*.[64] Caelius was avowedly drawing on a large work of the same name by Soranus, for he cites him frequently and in a manner that shows that he was consulting him in the Greek original. How closely he followed Soranus is more controversial. Most scholars now allow Caelius a certain degree of independent thought while accepting that the general outlines and organisation of his work mirror that of Soranus. He made a redaction, not a translation, of Soranus, although in the first book of *Acute Diseases*, which is the only one concerned with a single disease, phrenitis, he may have stayed closer to the Greek original than elsewhere.[65]

But it is for his *Gynaecology*, or *The Diseases of Women*, that Soranus is, and was, most renowned.[66] Not least because, except for the short gynaecological texts in the Hippocratic Corpus and the enigmatic chapters of Metrodora, it is the only treatise on the subject that has come down to us from the classical period.[67] Galen dealt with specific gynaecological topics, especially in his *On Seed*, *On the Formation of the Foetus* and *On the Anatomy of the Womb*, but from a restricted and very theoretical point of view. Later authors, most notably the encyclopaedist Aetius, Caelius Aurelianus in the fragments of his *Gynaecology* and the influential Mustio/Moschion, have preserved a few more details of ancient practice, but they are for the most part heavily dependent on Soranus.[68] Without Soranus, then, we should be almost totally ignorant about ancient childbirth and obstetrics, compelled to create a narrative from scattered finds of instruments, such as vaginal specula, and passing comments on abortion, child-rearing and the dangers of letting a male doctor anywhere near the female members of the household.[69]

Soranus begins his book with a sketch of the ideal midwife – literate, sharp-witted, hardworking and robust (because she has to bear a 'double burden' of both mother and child). She must have a good memory and be sound in both mind and limb; neat and tidy, and, so some recommend, with long thin fingers and short nails to avoid damaging the womb on any internal examination. This ideal, he implies, is not always achieved, and he draws a distinction between an accomplished midwife, satisfactorily skilled in all aspects of practical obstetrics, and her superior, who knows all necessary theory as well as wider aspects of medicine, surgery and pharmacology. He refuses to be drawn on the ideal age for the midwife or whether she should herself have had children. Vigour and sympathy are not confined to any one group, and it is far better to look for moral qualities, honesty, sobriety, tact and an abhorrence of greed and superstition – and also of wool-working, for this makes her hands rough.[70]

Soranus' recommendations raise two major questions immediately: how far do they correspond to the reality of midwives in the ancient world? And what was the relationship of the midwife to Soranus and similar male doctors? Inscriptions record the names of many women who are called '*obstetrix*', '*medica*' or their Greek equivalents, but, as in the Greek world of the Hippocratic Corpus (see p. 102), deciding the precise meaning of these overlapping terms is impossible.[71] Not every *obstetrix* will have confined her attentions to pregnancy and childbirth; nor will every female doctor have treated only women and young children. The social standing and education of Antiochis of Tlos, the correspondent of Heraclides of Tarentum honoured for her medical services by her native town of Tlos in Lycia, will have been vastly superior to those of Hygia, a freedwoman *obstetrix* in the household of Marcella, a relative of the Emperor Augustus, or of Restituta, who set up a monument in Rome to her husband and teacher, Ti. Claudius Alcimus.[72] The tombstone of Valeria Berecunda proclaimed that she was the 'first medical midwife of her precinct' within Rome, an advertising slogan rather than an official position; others, more humble still, have left no memorial at all.[73] The women who attended the wife of Flavius Boethus possessed enough knowledge and experience to gain the respect of Galen when he was finally called in to treat her for what at first appeared to be an incomplete spontaneous abortion. That he would have been so respectful of the barmaid-cum-midwife who assisted at the birth of the great philosopher and sophist Ablabius is less easy to believe.[74] The gulf between the servants of a senatorial household and the average citizen, let alone his wife or daughter, was enormous. Yet the midwife–barmaid, breaking off from her other activities to be present at a birth, may well represent the norm in most communities in the ancient world.[75]

Sometimes the midwife may have picked up her knowledge from attending births with other women and being part of 'women's networks of knowledge'. But the constituents of this knowledge are entirely lost to us, along with much of the learned gynaecological tradition, and it would be foolish to assume any greater precision and accuracy than is visible in our surviving male sources. The wide range of answers to queries on conception and the possible length of pregnancy, themes that had an importance well beyond narrowly medical circles, does not encourage belief in the superior accuracy of any group's notions, male or female.[76]

That is not to say that male writers such as Soranus and Galen did not regard the midwife as subordinate to the doctor. According to Soranus, she might attend to the actual birth, but under the supervision of the doctor, who takes over as soon as things become difficult.[77] Galen's descriptions of his gynaecological cases naturally place him clearly in charge. Soranus' sources, from Euryphon of Cnidus in the fifth century, through Diocles and Herophilus, to other Methodists such as Dionysius and Mnaseas, are resolutely male, and the implication of his prescriptions for the ideal midwife is that she should be as like a male doctor as possible. Even believing that there were specific women's diseases differing in nature from those affecting men did not entail accepting also that the treatment of such diseases should be left in the hands of women.[78] General treatises on hygiene and recipe collections, written by men, included sections on amenorrhoea as well as on baldness, and uterine problems as well as those of the penis. A theoretical acquaintance with the female body is universally assumed in male treatises, and there is little doubt that some doctors gained their knowledge also from practice.[79] But it is unlikely that many devoted all, or even most of, their time to midwifery. C. Julius Epianax and Heliconias from the Greek island of Paros, who called themselves 'maioi' when making a dedication to the goddess of childbirth, were probably relatives responsible for the baby's nurture.[80]

201

But to restrict female healers solely to gynaecology and the diseases of children (and even to discuss them largely in the context of Roman gynaecology) is misleading.[81] A woman such as Restituta or Aurelia Alexandria Zosime, of Adada in Pisidia, who had gained her expertise from a husband or father, would have had a similar training to that of most males. The garrulous Glycon, a Pergamene doctor of the first or second century, praised his late wife Panthea because she had increased the shared glory of medicine and, though a woman, was not his inferior in the medical art. Antiochis of Tlos, the correspondent of Heraclides of Tarentum, was commemorated by the people of Tlos with a statue for her achievements.[82] The wife of C. Julius Vettianus, recorded on her tombstone as a 'woman doctor', bore the supremely appropriate name Empeiria, 'Experience'.[83] Metilia Donata, a female doctor at Lyons who helped to set up a public building or monument there out of her own money in the first or second century, would not have been a lady to be trifled with.[84] There are even hints in the archaeological evidence that some women may have practised surgery.[85] Soranus' subordination of female healers to their male colleagues, and his apparent restriction of their activities to midwifery, thus underestimates both their possible range and their quality, echoing the standard male assessment of the female body as an inferior version of that of the male.[86]

The four books of Soranus' treatise divide neatly into two: the first pair dealing with the natural physiology of women and the normal processes of conception, pregnancy and birth; the latter with abnormal physiology and pathology, to be treated by diet and, in the last book, by surgery and drugs. He shows himself well informed on the whole about female anatomy, although he denies the existence of the hymen and traces the path of a 'seminal canal' from around the ovaries to the neck of the bladder.[87] He is apparently familiar with a wide range of problems associated with pregnancy and the early months of life, from pica, swelling of the ankles and spontaneous abortion to swollen breasts, teething and the risks of employing a wetnurse with a liking for drink.[88] There can be little doubt that he had had experience of most of what he describes, for his errors are, to modern eyes, remarkably few. His recommendations may conflict at times with strict Methodism.[89] Although proclaiming the Methodist line that inflammation demands the same therapy no matter what its cause or organ, Soranus modifies this principle by pointing out that the type and site of inflammation may entail specific choices between therapies in order to gain the best results.[90] Similarly, bleeding to relieve constriction and release the blood held back by a failure to menstruate is not always wise, for sometimes it does more harm than good and weakens the patient.[91] Menstruation, contrary to what Herophilus thought, is always harmful to health, even if its problems are mainly noticeable only among women more sensitive to pain. Women who no longer menstruate are often in robust health, and premenstrual girls are no less healthy in general than their older sisters, which suggests that menstruation contributes not so much to general health as to procreation.[92] This accords with the general assumption throughout this treatise (and generally in Greek and Roman society) that the main function of a woman was to bear children and that one of the duties of the woman's physician was to enable her to do this as efficiently as possible. Hence Soranus' view that a girl should remain a virgin until the onset of menstruation, around 14, for this was the natural indication that her body was ready for procreation. Earlier defloration might cause difficulties, but so might too long a delay, for the neck of the womb tended to become flabby because of the absence of sexual activity, 'as happens also with male sexual organs'.[93]

But Soranus is aware that the natural processes of conception, birth and early growth (whether it is the mother or, as he recommends to his wealthy readers, the wetnurse who breastfeeds the baby) do not always go well. Conception might be difficult, and the consequences of birth fatal to both mother and child. Difficult labour or a miscarriage can result in haemorrhage or paralysis, while the continuing discharge of female semen or blood from the uterus is a common hazard, along with uterine prolapse.[94] The mind might be affected also. 'Satyriasis', a desire for constant intercourse, leads to 'a certain alienation of mind and the casting off of all shame' because of the sympathetic relationship of the uterus with the meninges of the brain.[95] 'Hysterical suffocation', akin to epilepsy or apoplexy and the 'aphonia caused by worms', is defined as an obstruction of the breathing leading to an inability to speak and even to collapse. It is often associated with miscarriages or long widowhood and the ending of the reproductive period, all of which can bring about constriction. Soranus' advice in such cases is to use gentle poultices, sitz-baths, even reading aloud, followed by a more active regime. But he rejects many of the remedies found elsewhere in our sources – sexual intercourse, ice-cold water, forcing air into the vagina with a blacksmith's bellows, substances to provoke vigorous sneezing, the clanging of plates ('likely to give even the healthy a headache') or any of the noxious substances burned beneath or forced into the uterus to induce it to move from its choking position. His words on these procedures are wise: 'the uterus does not emerge like a wild animal from its lair, attracted by sweet-smelling odours or driven away by the stench'.[96]

The physician has also to cope with the potential problem of a difficult birth, either because the child has lain in an unusual position in the womb or because of a stillbirth. Sometimes all that is required is simple manipulation to ensure that the child is nicely positioned in the birth canal; sometimes oiled hooks may be needed to help draw the child downwards.[97] But sometimes, alas, more drastic measures are required that will involve the death of the child. Soranus' instructions for the use of the embryotome or for the best way to crush the skull of a hydrocephalic foetus to extract it dead or dying are coupled with warnings that any rough or careless traction on the living foetus

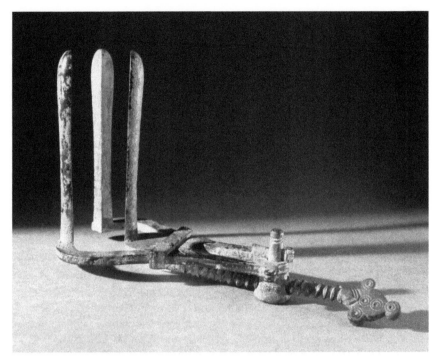

Figure 13.1 A tri-valve vaginal speculum of Roman date, found in the modern Lebanon. London, Science Museum. Photo © Science Museum/Science & Society Picture Library.

may result in horrendous injuries and, very likely, death.[98] Such a difficult birth will also inevitably damage the uterus, and the physician should deal with this as quickly as possible in order to secure the life of the mother.

The impression that one gets from the *Gynaecology* is of a learned, thoughtful and caring Methodist. What remains of his other writings, especially in Caelius Aurelianus, amply confirms this impression. Soranus warns against dangerous operations where other methods are available – laryngotomy for quinsy or Praxagoras' purging intervention to remove intestinal obstruction – as well as what he calls superstition, wild beast skin for hydrophobia, human blood in epilepsy, or using a left hand to pull down the head when the foetus is in a foot presentation, 'because that is the way to lift up serpents'.[99] But he is quite prepared to prescribe an amulet if the patient thought she would be helped by it, and to make recommendations that we might think superstitious, banning red from the sickroom of a patient suffering from haemorrhage, yellow from that of the jaundiced, although he provides an explanation in terms of contemporary science (harmful emanations) or psychology (a reminder of the condition that has confined the patient to the sickroom).[100] He continues the Methodist tradition of detailed attention to chronic conditions, offering careful advice on the treatment of paralysis by physiotherapy, strong jets of water and swimming, even if an inflated bladder is needed to give buoyancy.[101] His treatment of mental diseases combines a similar pragmatism with humane concern. It is better to agree at first with the delusions of a madman and then gradually bring him round to accept the true situation than to attempt to convince him immediately of his folly and to deny any reality to his perceptions.[102] Like Themison and Asclepiades, he attended to all aspects of convalescence, recommending, to exercise the mind, reading, games and even attendance at plays – comedy is good for the depressed, tragedy for the merely foolish. Treatments that are likely to harm the patient must be avoided at all costs: abandoning a sufferer from 'elephantiasis' to exile or banishment is foreign to the humanity of medicine.[103]

Soranus' therapeutics and his application of his Methodist theories to his patients have impressed many medical writers over the centuries. His cautious and humane conservatism, a conservatism that does not rule out drastic measures when they are necessary, stands in opposition to the picture given by the opponents of Methodism. Rashness, obscurity and illogicality are claimed by Galen, and others, to be the hallmarks of their doctrine and practice. On the one hand so simple that even a village idiot could master it, on the other hand so complex that no group of Methodists could ever agree on anything, Methodism was easily dismissed by its adversaries as an aberration or a fraud. Even those, like Celsus, who were less hostile to it on grounds of theory still complained that its practitioners lacked the subtlety of diagnostic and prescriptive reasoning to be able to view each patient as an individual requiring individual care and individual treatment. Yet to the Methodists their ability to see beyond the individual and to grasp the commonalities was something to be proud of. It enabled them to work easily in the great cities of Rome or Ephesus, and to offer assistance quickly without the long rigmarole of diagnosis or searching in past case histories. Their therapeutics, it has already been suggested, encompassed a good deal of flexibility, and in practical terms they may not have been too far from their opponents in what they diagnosed and prescribed.[104] Galen has no qualms about using recipes created by Methodists like Soranus or Mnaseas, or by those followers of Asclepiades criticised by Dioscorides, who was himself trained in that tradition. Soranus in his writings shows what Methodists could do, although few perhaps possessed all his qualities as a physician. Many leading Romans, from the emperors and their families downwards, employed Methodists to treat them, and it would be unwise to dismiss their choice as foolish or as a mere insurance policy to secure a range of treatments, any of which might work, be less painful or take less time. In the first two centuries of the Roman Empire there flourished a veritable marketplace of medicine, with learning and showmanship, practical expertise and eloquence on all sides – Pneumatists, Dogmatists, Methodists or Hippocratics. The wealthy or the leisured who made the choice might, like the author and politician Seneca, be as well acquainted with medical theory as any doctor. There is no reason to agree with Galen's oft-repeated complaint that such patients, by choosing the Methodists and other boors, quacks and conmen like them, were demonstrating the degeneracy of their age and bringing about the decline of true medicine.[105] Galen's prejudices held the field for centuries: they need no longer carry weight with us today.

14

HUMORAL ALTERNATIVES

The hostility of their enemies has rendered the reconstruction of the ideas and opinions of the Methodists difficult, but there can be little doubt as to the extent of their success and importance in the first and second centuries of the Roman Empire. The achievements of their rivals who favoured humoral theories are even more difficult to establish, for precisely the opposite reason. The suffocating friendship of Galen has tended to subsume all who agreed with him under the banner of Hippocrates and to imply that all were united in resisting the novelties of the Methodists and the Empiricists. Differences are downplayed, and Galen's precursors are rarely allowed to speak for them-selves, even to be contradicted. Galen's egocentric rhetoric disguises his debts to his teachers, and developments within Hippocratism, so that it is often difficult to gain a comprehensive picture of what later medical writers called the Dogmatist viewpoint. Historians have until recently had to make do with a meagre collection of fragments in Greek and a handful of treatises, but the rediscovery of more writings of Rufus of Ephesus in Arabic translation, as well as others by Galen himself, has allowed a better understanding of Galen's place within the humoral tradition. He no longer appears so isolated as he claimed to be, and several of his striking medical methodologies can be seen to have been inherited from his teachers or from his immediate predecessors. At the same time, a clearer picture emerges of the ways in which doctors who did not believe in corpuscular theories but in humours applied them to medicine.

Among the most influential rivals of the Methodists of the first and second centuries were the Pneumatists, so called because they placed great emphasis on *pneuma*, or spirit, as the controlling factor in health and disease.[1] A passage pre-served only in later translations of a work by Galen reveals that their founder, Athenaeus of Attaleia (S.W. Turkey), was a pupil of a certain Posidonius.[2] If this is the famous Stoic philosopher and scientist Posidonius of Apamea, and if Galen meant that Athenaeus actually sat at his feet (neither hypothesis is entirely proven), the sect would have been founded in the last century BC, and perhaps as early as 60 BC.[3] But neither Pliny nor Celsus refers to it, and, where dates can be assigned with confidence to its most famous adherents, none can be shown to have flourished before the middle years of the first century AD. On this argument from silence, Athenaeus will have lived in the early years of the Roman Empire, and his adherence to the doctrines of Posidonius will have resulted from his reading, not his attendance at philosophical lectures.[4]

Athenaeus' opinions were a mixture of Stoicism and Hellenistic dogmatic, or Hippocratic, medicine. He rejected the atomistic views of Asclepiades in favour of a cosmos of matter acted upon by hot and cold (the more active qualities), and by wet and dry (the more passive qualities), and held together by *pneuma*, a refined airy element.[5] He eagerly explored parallels between the microcosm of the body and the macrocosm. Just as a living being could not exist without taking in *pneuma*, so too the universe was a living entity imbued with all-permeating *pneuma*. Changes in the body's *pneuma* both brought about and at the same time indicated changes in the body's overall mixture and its properties, which produced illness when out of balance. The heart was the seat both of the governing *pneuma* and of the body's innate heat, and was continually provided by the lungs with a fresh supply of cooling *pneuma* drawn in from outside.[6] Hence, Athenaeus paid particular attention to the environment, including the seasons, the layout of towns and the design of houses, as a contribution to maintaining good *pneuma* and a healthy balance in the body.[7]

He wrote on a great variety of subjects, from the provision of a good water supply to embryology, dietetics and the best method of taking and interpreting the pulse.[8] His most important work was his *Boethemata, Helpful Advice*, in at least thirty books, which was praised by Galen as the best general medical treatise by a modern author.[9] Both here and in his more specialised clinical writings, he often began from a clear and simple definition of the disease before adding details and qualifications to provide a more nuanced picture.[10] Although, in Galen's opinion, Athenaeus was not always right, he had at least the great merit of reporting the views of his predecessors accurately. Such respect for those who had gone before him was only to be expected from a physician who recommended the universal study of medicine and its history, not just for practical reasons, but because it was an intellectual pursuit, the equal of philosophy, which allowed one the pleasure of communing with great minds of the past.[11]

His followers included two major writers on medicine, Claudius Agathinus and Archigenes of Apamea. Agathinus, from Sparta, adopted material from Empiricist and Methodist sources, as well as what he had learned from Athenaeus. His surviving fragments deal, among other things, with pulsation and with fevers, a topic on which he was singled out for approbation by Galen.[12] Given the Roman passion for baths, it is hardly surprising that Agathinus devoted much space to the health aspects of bathing.[13] His comments on this topic have a curiously modern (or at least Victorian) ring at times.[14]

In his opinion, although they could relieve tiredness and help digestion in the short term, warm baths were for wimps, those afraid of cold water or a brisk rubdown. Whereas cold baths were of enormous benefit, even for those who thought little about their health, as they toned the body, sharpened the senses and preserved a good complexion even into old age, warm baths made one flabby, pale, weak and unable to digest properly. Agathinus contrasted the vigour of the barbarians who frequently plunged their children into cold water with the modern habit of bathing small children in warm water, largely because their nurses were glad to see their charges fall into a stupor and not disturb them during the night. Agathinus preferred to give his son a brisk rub before bed, since he was aware that warm baths might bring on epileptiform attacks and worse.

Cold baths, as opposed to warm, could be taken at any time of the year, provided that the water was not too icy, muddy or otherwise dirty. Sea water was particularly good, as the salt gave it an added edge. Best of all was a mixture of cold baths and exercise, taken a little while after dinner. One should undress in the open, out of the wind, but if one was too afraid of the cold one should begin with some exercises or a brisk walk or run while half-undressed. A brisk rubdown by a slave wearing cloth gloves (but taking care to avoid burns from the rough joins of the gloves) should precede the first dip. This should be relatively short and be followed by a short walk. The second dip should be longer, possibly involving some swimming, but one should leave the bath before becoming too cold. In the third dip one should put one's head and upper thorax under a cold spring of water or, if there was none at hand, scoop up handfuls of cold water over one's head. Then comes a rubdown and a scraping-off of the oil with a reasonably sharp strigil, and one feels all the better for it, especially on a hot and sweaty day. Agathinus himself liked to take a bath in the evening, as it then gave him a good night's sleep. The only drawback of a cold bath was that any water getting into the ears might damage the channels there, and one should try and protect them as far as possible.

In this passage sound advice is mixed with personal experience, and the toughness of the barbarian contrasted with the effeminacy of the Romans. Above all, both here and in other fragments, Agathinus emphasises moderation, the best guide of all, and the need to attend to the patient's fears and preferences, especially if he or she was afraid of stronger medicine.

One of Agathinus' most distinguished pupils was Archigenes of Apamea in Syria, who is said to have lived in the time of Trajan, around AD 100, and to have died at the age of sixty-three.[15] He wrote at great length on the pulse, and, although Galen found his exposition of the eight different qualities of the pulse far too subtle to be helpful, some of the names he used to describe the various types of pulse – for instance the double hammer, the mouse-tail or the gazelle-like pulse – are well chosen.[16] His therapeutics show a similar concern with precise differentiation, for example of the types of pain, sleeplessness or mineral baths. He also wrote a large work on pathology; an even larger collection of letters, in eleven books, in which he assembled his advice for his friends; and books on fevers, symptomatology, surgery and nosology. Finally, the two books of his *Drugs Listed by Type* were cited extensively by Galen in his own pharmacological writings, frequently word for word.[17] His remedies included amulets as well as herbal and mineral drugs, although what proportion of these was entirely of his own devising is obscured by his reluctance to name his sources.[18] Despite his frequent criticisms, Galen derived more information and effective treatments from Archigenes than from any other author of the Roman period, with the exception of Rufus of Ephesus.

Archigenes' interest in nosology is mirrored also in the treatise on *Chronic and Acute Diseases* by Aretaeus of Cappadocia. When and where Aretaeus wrote is unclear. The older view, based on the absence of his name from the pages of Galen, was that the two authors were roughly contemporary, both active in the second half of the second century. Galen's silence was thus explained on the grounds either of ignorance or of a reluctance to acknowledge contemporaries or near-contemporaries from whom he had taken much of his material. More recently, following the redating of Athenaeus and other Pneumatists, Aretaeus too has been relocated a century or so earlier, to around AD 50.[19] Aretaeus himself makes no reference to authors of the Roman period in his surviving writings, although clearly influenced by Pneumatist and Stoic doctrines, and quotations taken from his writings are either much later or raise problems of their own. The author of a treatise on fevers that is attributed to Alexander of Aphrodisias (late second century) mentions a work by him devoted to prophylaxis, but this pseudonymous author's own date is far from assured.[20] Two further references, both by Galen, have more significant consequences for Aretaeus' date and for Galen's veracity. Discussing 'elephantiasis', Aretaeus told a charming story of a sufferer, abandoned in the wilderness by his friends, who was then unexpectedly cured by drinking wine from a barrel in which a viper had drowned.[21] An identical story was narrated by Galen in one of his early works, but without giving any source or date.[22] Thirty years later, in the 190s, Galen repeated the story, but this time he claimed that he had had personal experience of the incident in his youth in Asia Minor.[23] If Galen's second version is correct, the case occurred in the 140s or 150s, and fixes Aretaeus' lifetime around then. Alternatively, and perhaps more plausibly, with the passing of time a story that Galen had once read or heard became one in which he was a participant. His source could still be Aretaeus or another author on whom they both drew, but Galen's testimony is then of less value for dating Aretaeus. But the earlier Aretaeus is placed, the more the silence of the omnivorous Galen requires explanation.

Although Aretaeus wrote on surgery and a treatise specifically on fevers, all that has come down to us is his four books *On the Causes and Symptoms of Acute and Chronic Diseases* and the parallel set of four on their cures.[24] They are written in a highly stylised Hippocratic Greek dialect, full of allusions to the Hippocratic Corpus, and were long considered by doctors to offer the finest nosological studies to survive from Antiquity.[25] They combine detailed and precise observation with a clear, well-structured exposition. Each disease is described carefully and systematically: first, the site of the illness, including relevant anatomical information; then, the meaning of the name; the symptoms; and the causes, especially with regard to the age and sex of the patient and the season of the year. The therapies advocated by Aretaeus are typically Hippocratic: diet, simples, venesection and cupping, with surgery recommended only rarely. His descriptions of diseases, for instance of epilepsy, syncope or diabetes, are classics of their kind, combining acute observation, accurate description and clear exposition.[26] In his account of asthma (or 'orthopnoea, because the patient wants to stand and breathe upright'), Aretaeus notes the prevalence of childhood asthma and its frequent disappearance in adolescence.[27] But if it continues into adulthood, especially among men, it can be extremely dangerous. Its cause, he believes, is a cooling and moistening of the *pneuma*, to be avoided or corrected by warmth. This explains why those engaged in jobs that involve heat, lime burners, workers in bronze or iron and furnacemen at the baths, can survive much longer than the average asthmatic, even when they too suffer from shortness of breath. (The fact that this explanation is wrong in modern terms should not obscure his correct differentiation between what we might term congenital asthma and dyspnoea brought on by exposure to harmful fumes.) Aretaeus describes the onset of an asthma attack with graphic clarity: the tightness in the chest, the reddening of the cheeks, the bulging eyes, the desperate attempt to stand and find fresh air, as if what was already in the room might not be enough. He compares the attack to that of epilepsy, noting the asthmatic's cold sweats and foaming at the mouth. Gradually the asthma goes away, the body relaxes and there is a profound sense of relief – until the next time, for sufferers always carry about with them the 'symbols', mementos, of their condition.

Aretaeus' division into acute and chronic diseases is also found in an anonymous work written in the first or second century with a more overtly didactic intent. It is clearly organised, setting out the opinions on a range of diseases held by distinguished physicians, mainly of the fourth and third centuries BC.[28] Its author's interest in disease causation and therapy is shared with the somewhat later writer of the Anonymus Londinensis papyrus himself, who in his final section puts forward ideas that could be called 'Pneumatist'.[29] But the fluidity of Pneumatist doctrines and the obvious tendency towards eclecticism manifested, among others, by Agathinus and Archigenes place difficulties in the way of any clear estimate of the extent and influence of Pneumatism. Indeed, one may have considerable doubts about its very existence as a sect in any strong sense of the word.[30] Its most famous adherents have links with Rome, but Aretaeus' place of writing is unknown and Anonymus Londinensis (if he is to be considered a Pneumatist) was writing in Egypt.[31] The subsequent rise of Galenic Hippocratism easily subsumed many of its ideas and therapies, and obscured the place that it had gained in the early imperial centuries as an alternative to Methodism.

Pneumatists, Methodists and Empiricists were in agreement on one thing: that Hippocrates and the writings that circulated under his name were worthy of great attention and respect. It is true that scurrilous stories were in circulation, alleging that Hippocrates had derived his medicine by copying down the treatments recorded on the cure tablets around the walls of the Asclepieion of Cos, or, even worse, that he had deliberately burned down the archive, presumably in order to prevent others challenging his superiority.[32] But in general the 'founder of our profession', as Scribonius Largus called him, was regarded favourably.[33] Far more papyri of texts from the Hippocratic Corpus survive from Graeco-Roman Egypt than of any other medical author.[34] References to Hippocrates and the Corpus are found in the work of writers of all kinds, from the philosopher Demetrius Lacon in the first century BC to the grandiloquent epigrammatist Glycon of Pergamum and the theologian Clement of Alexandria three centuries later.[35] More tangible representations of the great physician were likewise numerous, both public and private. The island of Cos issued coins bearing his image, and a beautiful mosaic from a Roman-period house there depicts him in conversation with Asclepius (see Figure 4.3). At Ostia, the port city of Rome, his portrait bust – now, alas, sadly battered – was placed in the family tomb of the (royal?) physician, Demetrius.[36] At distant Tomi, on the shores of the Black Sea, the tombstone of one of its sons, Kladaios, proudly announced that he had practised the art of his divine master, Hippocrates.[37] On Corcyra, a grateful pupil recorded his thanks to his dead teacher Theagenes in an epitaph replete with Hippocratic allusions.[38] Memorials of other doctors around the Roman Empire proclaimed the Hippocratic ancestry of their profession by writing the word for doctor in Ionic, even if the rest of the inscription was in the normal '*koine*' ('common') dialect.[39] Since, as we have already seen, some medical men, most notably Aretaeus (see p. 210), took to writing their own books entirely in Hippocratic Greek, it is difficult to decide whether some of the later texts in the Hippocratic Corpus were gathered in accidentally or were intended as imitations, pastiches or forgeries.[40]

Scholars provided these often obscure writings with appropriate exegeses. Basing himself on Hellenistic predecessors, Erotian dedicated his Hippocratic glossary, equipped with parallels from poets as well as physicians, to a court doctor, Andromachus, in the hope that this would encourage others to take an interest in the Corpus as literature and to compare their own knowledge with that of Hippocrates.[41] The antiquarian Aulus Gellius, around 160, did not hesitate to include a passage from *Nutriment* as one of his miscellaneous topics for erudite discussion.[42] He had found it best explained by the commentator Sabinus, who was later characterised by Galen as the most thorough expositor of Hippocrates, even if inclined to attempt to explain everything, including the inexplicable.[43] There was also a general belief that Hippocrates was the founder of the theory of the four humours and the author of *The Nature of Man*. Anonymus Londinensis reacted sharply to the alternative Aristotelian view of Hippocrates by interposing his own quotation from that text as proof of what Hippocrates had really believed.[44] Agreement on the Hippocratic authorship of some treatises led to disputes about the authenticity of other writings that could not easily be made to conform. Erotian's comment in his preface to the effect that *Prorrhetic* 2 was not by Hippocrates is the earliest extant reference to such a debate, but he is unlikely to have been the first to raise the question.[45] Around 120 an otherwise unknown Artemidorus Capito brought out an edition of Hippocrates that was well regarded by the Emperor Hadrian.[46] Building on the work of his coeval and relative Dioscorides (not the celebrated pharmacologist), Artemidorus produced a large edition in many book-rolls, incorporating in its margins variant readings and textual observations by Alexandrian scholars. Although it was not strictly a commentary, Artemidorus discussed within it the authenticity of certain treatises, or parts of treatises, rejecting, for example, the last part of *Regimen in Acute Diseases* and dividing up the *Epidemics* among various authors. He made many stylistic changes – far too many, thought Galen – in an attempt to return the texts to their original Ionic dialect. Galen regarded the editions of Dioscorides and Artemidorus as standard in his own day, and it is likely, although far from certain, that their work lies at the base of the manuscript tradition of the Hippocratic Corpus as we have it today.[47] Others attempted to emulate them, including Rufus of Samaria, a Jew who had moved to Rome about 150 and who collected together the variant readings and interpretations suggested by earlier scholars to produce his own edition of the *Epidemics*. According to Galen's heavily biased account, it was an unoriginal and uncritical ragbag of information taken from Rufus' own large library, although Galen himself did not scruple to draw on it for his reports about the textual preferences of earlier scholars.[48]

How this abundance of Hippocratic material was actually used is more difficult to determine. The huge commentary, forty-eight books long, on Hippocrates' *Aphorisms*, by Julian the Methodist interpreted many of its sentences in a very different manner from that of the Hippocratic Sabinus.[49] Galen's general approval of the latter's work is qualified by his listing of errors and misunderstandings, which, like many of Galen's criticisms of other commentators, may mean little more than that Sabinus was starting from a different standpoint from Galen. Similarly, Galen's complaints that, in his own day, few people followed the teachings of Hippocrates, especially on prognosis, are called into question by the existence of groups such as the Pneumatists, whose medicine, although differing in several important ways from his own, regularly cited Hippocratic precedent.[50] Their interpretations of Hippocrates, even if derided by Galen, were not foolish. Indeed, much of the evidence proposed by Galen for what Hippocrates himself had believed in, most notably the primacy of anatomy and the tripartite division of the body's systems, has very little basis in the Hippocratic Corpus itself, and is far more a wishful creation of Galen's to serve his own purposes than an accurate representation of this great figure from the past.[51]

A more balanced picture of Hippocratism in the Roman period may be gained from the writings of one of the most influential medical writers of Antiquity (and one of the few to gain Galen's seal of approval), Rufus of Ephesus. As with other medical figures, there are conflicting dates for his life. The Suda lexicon makes him a contemporary of Statilius Crito in the time of Trajan – that is, around AD 100. However, Servilius Damocrates, the author of a pharmacological poem, who is known from Pliny to have been active around AD 50, mentions a pharmacologist Rufus as if he were already famous.[52] But there were other doctors or medical authors with this name at this time, including a pharmacologist, Menius Rufus, and it is far from clear that Damocrates' doctor is, in fact, the prolific Rufus of Ephesus.[53]

Like Soranus, Rufus spent time in Egypt, probably studying at Alexandria, for his comments about the general health of the country and specific diseases, such as the Guinea worm, seem to depend on personal observation. His other references to his patients or to what he has seen all relate to S. Asia Minor, and there is no evidence that he ever visited Rome.[54]

What remains of his writings in Greek, whether in their original form or in later quotations, gives only an idea of his enormous range.[55] They include works on therapeutics, *On Gout*, *On Diseases of the Bladder and Kidneys* and *On Satyriasis and Gonorrhoea*, as well as one on anatomical nomenclature for those beginning medical study – 'for the smith, the cobbler, and the carpenter first learn the words for metal, tools and such like. Why should it be any different in more noble arts?'[56] His short treatise *Medical Questions*, advising a doctor on how best to gain information from a patient by means of questions, offers a rare glimpse into the bedside skills of an ancient doctor.[57] There are tantalising fragments of a long botanical poem, in four books of hexameters, and of his views on plague, which may include a very early reference to plague buboes.[58] Other works survive only in translation: *On Gout* in Latin, *On Jaundice* in Latin and Arabic and some of his case histories in Arabic. Even more, however, are known from citations in the medical encyclopedias of Late Antiquity or in Arabic medical writers, for whom Rufus was second only to Galen as an authority.[59]

What is most striking about Rufus' writings as we have them is that theoretical discussion and argument are almost entirely absent.[60] His commitment to the theory of the four humours is justified by the results of his therapies rather than by physiological exposition. The basis of Rufus' medicine can be briefly stated: we are not naturally all the same; we differ very greatly from one another. Hence the need to discover the individuality of each patient by every possible means. A patient's illness could be deduced simply from its external manifestations, but this should be a mere preliminary, for true therapy consists in fitting the remedy exactly to the patient. This takes considerable time and effort, and may involve questions about all aspects of his or her life, from food and drink to habits and dreams. Even when the doctor has found out what is wrong and can foresee the likely outcome, he must ensure that the treatment

214

is adapted precisely to the patient, for 'no substance is so constant in its actions that the physician can place it in a single category'.[61]

Although Galen applauded his profound knowledge of the Hippocratic Corpus and referred several times to Rufus as a commentator on Hippocrates, it is not certain whether he wrote formal commentaries or merely discussed particular passages in the course of other works.[62] But Rufus' 'deep affection for the man and his art' did not mean that he could see no progress beyond Hippocrates.[63] His treatise *On Melancholy*, considered by Galen the best work on the subject before his own, developed the brief sketch in *The Nature of Man* into a detailed exposition of the therapeutic consequences of an excess or deficiency of that mysterious humour.[64] Similarly, the final section of *Medical Questions* is an extension, not a criticism, of Hippocrates' views in *Airs, Waters and Places*. Rufus argues that local circumstances are likely to provide local remedies as well as local diseases, and hence talking with the natives of an area will often lead to discoveries of great value.[65]

Throughout Rufus adopts a pragmatic rather than a confrontational approach. Criticism of others is muted or avoided. He regrets that internal anatomy was better taught 'in the old days' when one could use humans, but contents himself with recommending the dissection of animals closest to man and the demonstration of surface anatomy on a slave.[66] Although most of his treatises are addressed to his fellow doctors, Arabic authors have preserved a large number of quotations from what was a substantial and comprehensive manual of self-help, *For the Layman*, or, as some authors translated its title, *For Those Who Have No Doctor to Hand*.[67] It covered a wide range of diseases, from headache and failing eyesight to kidney and bladder problems, and gave advice for health as well as for sickness, for prophylactic dietetics was a Hippocratic speciality.[68] Rufus also considered groups in society whose particular needs were not always addressed in medical writings – travellers, the elderly and the very young (with very sound advice on child care and paediatrics, on what the wetnurse should be able to deal with herself and when she must call in a doctor).[69] He wrote a specific tract *On Buying Slaves*, in which he reported his examination of a slave with a congenital skull defect and warned against the risks of buying a slave with a suppurating discharge from the ear: this portended serious harm to the slave and a loss of investment to his owner.[70] His sympathies with the sick are clear from his comments on those with sexual dysfunctions or with chronic conditions, where his stress on what is needed to eliminate their cause in each individual is the closest he comes to an attack on the Methodists.[71]

It is the misfortune of Rufus to have fallen under the shadow of Galen, who, while eloquent about his opponents' beliefs, is far more reticent about the amount he appropriated from those with whom he agreed. His general approval scarcely allows us to appreciate all that Rufus did to earn him the admiration of the Arabs. The material that has survived the filtration process of the centuries emphasises his practicality as a physician in his dealings with patients of all kinds. Yet the learning that lay behind all this can be glimpsed only faintly in his advice in *Medical Questions* or the references (not all of them necessarily his own) he provides to explicate anatomical terminology in *On the Names of Bodily Parts*. Enough remains, however, to show his great strengths as a clinical observer and to make us regret the loss of so great a proportion of his writings.

The long shadow of Galen, ever critical of the failings of others, has also obscured the liveliness of medical debates and developments in the second century of our era. This was economically and intellectually the high point of Greek culture in the Roman world. Cities such as Ephesus and Smyrna engaged in expensive rivalry to sponsor the largest and most beautiful temples, the most imposing monuments or the most spectacular games. These now often included, as well as athletics, musical and poetic competitions. At Ephesus, during the two days of the Great Festival of Asclepius, there were even annual contests in medicine and surgery between doctors. The results, in four categories, were inscribed permanently on stone.[72] 'Museums', 'Halls of the Muses', sprang up in imitation of that of Alexandria, providing places where intellectuals of all kinds, from poets and physicians to government officials, might meet together.[73] The prose writers of the age are among the glories of Ancient Greek literature: the moralist biographer Plutarch and the satirist Lucian, historians such as Arrian or Cassius Dio, orators such as Dio Chrysostom or Aelius Aristides and philosophers such as Alexander of Aphrodisias or the Sceptical physician Sextus Empiricus.[74] Medical men participated eagerly in this cultural world. The doctor Heraclitus of Rhodiapolis (S.W. Turkey), 'the Homer of medical poetry', made a triumphant circuit of the famous cities of the Greek East, receiving, in return for copies of his works on medicine and philosophy, honours from the Alexandrians, the Rhodians, the Athenians, the Athenian Areopagus, the Epicureans at Athens and the Sacred Thymelic Synod (a universal theatrical guild). Some of his wealth he used to support the games in honour of Asclepius at his native town.[75] Dr Hermogenes wrote a two-volume history of Smyrna, his home town, several books on the early civic foundations of Europe and Asia, a tract on Homer's birthplace and another on his wisdom, as well as seventy-seven volumes on medicine.[76] At Roman Corinth, Dr Thrasippus was mourned as second to none among the Greeks for his medicine and his poetry, while only an early death prevented the young Dr Barbas of Gangra in Pontus (N.E. Turkey) from gaining a magnificent reputation for his learning and for his medicine in Imperial Rome.[77]

This outburst of creative energy also encompassed the writing of works on medicine proper. There were treatises of every kind, from question and answer textbooks, such as *Medical Definitions*, and short guides, such as the *Introduction to Medicine*, to the massive book on types of fevers in which the (to us unknown) author had set out at length every possible type and combination. Galen, in a *tour de force*, reduced it to a simple summary of a few lines.[78]

Copies of the forty or so books of medicine (in verse), *Chironides* (*The Daughters of Chiron*), by Marcellus of Side were placed in Rome's libraries at the behest of two emperors, Hadrian and Antoninus Pius.[79] Philosophically inclined Greeks and Romans debated whether what was contained in the womb was a living creature or how the foetus came into possession of a soul, while others, more practical, could peruse the large works on drugs by Asclepiades the Pharmacologist.[80] There was a ready market for copies of medical writings, at least in the big cities: Galen came across in Sandalmakers St, the home of the booksellers in Rome, two men disputing the authenticity of a treatise, *The Doctor*, that had been sold under the name of Galen. One was trying to prove to the other that he had bought a forgery, as the style was not that of the great man.[81] Galen's reaction to this wholesale piracy of his writings veered from high-minded disdain (never signing his writings and despising fame as of no use to the dead and a hindrance to the living), through resignation (expecting his works to be treated like an orphan child among drunkards), to a passionate concern that his reputation should not be besmirched by errors and confusion spread by others writing under his name.[82]

Galen's own comments and criticisms allow us to examine two strands in these medical debates. He was conscious that he belonged to a tradition of Hippocratic exegesis, even if he mostly deigned to mention his relatively recent predecessors only when he disagreed with them.[83] Their interpretation took on a variety of literary forms. Galen's own teacher at Smyrna, Pelops, wrote a short *Introduction to Hippocrates*, but their most common method of explaining what Hippocrates had meant was by the commentary-lecture.[84] Some teachers, such as Lycus of Macedon, arranged for the publication of their lectures in a large number of book-rolls; the commentaries of others, such as those of Quintus, could be reconstructed only from the often divergent testimony of former pupils. Others, such as Numisianus or Pelops, never got round to arranging for the publication of their lecture notes, which remained in the hands of their negligent heirs.[85] Discovering what a distinguished teacher had taught, Galen found, was far from easy. The pupils of Quintus, as well as providing telling vignettes of their master's at times eccentric habits, developed his Hippocratism in many different ways. Aeficianus was a Stoic (or a Pneumatist?), Martialis (or Martianus) was a leading Erasistratean in Rome, Satyrus and Lycus (that 'bastard of the Hippocratic sect') leaned more towards the Empiricists.[86] To decide which interpretation was properly that of their master was almost impossible, and it is hardly surprising that Quintus failed to satisfy Galen's austere credentials for Hippocratic accuracy. Yet this apparent deviation from the true Hippocratic doctrine, far from deserving condemnation, is better understood as an indication of intellectual vigour and interest by doctors wishing to develop ideas that they believed had stood the test of time.

How these doctors themselves applied their Hippocratism is more difficult to determine in detail, especially since they speak largely only through the mouth of their strongest critic, Galen, but what remains of two very different Hippocratic commentaries shows both learning and intelligence equal to his. The author of a commentary on the *Oath*, ascribed to Galen, combines quotations from some rare poetry with erudite discussion of the origins of medicine. A doctor from Pergamum, and perhaps a teacher of Galen, he uses the attributes of the cult statue of Asclepius at Pergamum to exemplify the qualities of the ideal doctor – modesty, foresight, learning, intelligence, stability, careful observation and constant awareness. The stories about Hippocrates show how much he exemplified these qualities, not least because he was determined to secure the future of true medicine, endangered by the gradual disappearance of the family of Asclepius, by committing it to writing.[87]

If this commentary displays the elegance and learning typical of the age, another author, Sabinus, reinterprets Hippocratic notions of the effects of the environment in a Roman imperial context. In a few fragments preserved in a later encyclopaedia, Sabinus not only talks about the healthiness or unhealthiness of places in general and about the advantages of a south-facing, sunlit house, but expatiates at some length upon the best way of planning a city.[88] His ideal city has straight streets oriented north–south and east–west, without obstructions, and with clear straight roads leading into them from the suburbs. Gentle winds can thus sweep through the city almost unnoticed, clearing away the smoke and fumes, while the sun can reach every house, no matter what its orientation. By contrast, if the streets are narrow or winding the winds are constantly causing turbulence as they meet obstructions and are forced to change direction. There is a veritable battle of the winds, and the poor pedestrian feels as if he is being tossed at sea. Instead of carrying fresh air throughout the city and driving the bad air out, the winds go where they can, spreading foul air as much as removing it. Similarly, the sunlight never penetrates in some areas, so that any exhalation, *anathumiasis*, cannot be dispersed. The air becomes thick and hard to breathe. This, says Sabinus, is true for a city on a plain. One built on a hill, however, is much better off without straight streets, for the wind blows foul air straight up to the higher ground. With crooked streets, the higher ground is much better ventilated. There is a sociological point at issue here, clarified by a passage in Galen alluding to Pergamum: it was the wealthier classes who lived 'up the hill' rather than in the crowded streets below. Sabinus' advice keeps their dwellings sweet smelling, insulated, one might say, from the noxious odours of the lower town.[89]

Sabinus and Galen, as well as Rufus, Athenaeus of Attaleia and Antyllus, who made similar observations on urban pollution, were writing in the same recognisably Hippocratic tradition of meteorological medicine.[90] Some of Galen's observations come from his commentary on the Hippocratic *Airs, Waters and Places*, and it is tempting to trace other doctors' interest in town planning back to that treatise, whose purpose was to instruct the travelling doctor on how to tell at first glance from the situation of a town just what diseases were likely to be found there.[91] But Sabinus goes well beyond what

218

is said there, and in a way that seems to owe little to Roman example. His discussion is a reminder that there were intelligent Hippocratics before Galen and that public health was not discovered by the Romans.

A second development already underway before Galen came on the scene was the revival of anatomy at the turn of the century 'in the time of our grandfathers'.[92] This claim must be treated with care. It is true that Sabinus, according to Galen, had known little or no anatomy when he wrote his Hippocratic commentaries around AD 100, a major defect in his attempts to explicate the Hippocratic Corpus. But Rufus earnestly recommended the study of anatomy (see p. 214), and Soranus seems to have derived some benefit from his anatomical studies in the 70s or 80s, even if he did not regard them as useful in actual medical practice (see p. 199).

Galen gave the credit for the revival of anatomy to Marinus, a physician and teacher at Alexandria who was active in the first decades of the second century.[93] He was a Hippocratic, for Galen twice mentions his exposition of passages in Hippocrates' *Aphorisms*, probably in a commentary, and praises him for showing that, in a passage in *Epidemics* 2, Hippocrates' anatomy was fundamentally correct.[94] All that remains of Marinus' major work on anatomy are the section headings of each book as they were recorded by Galen. It was a very large work indeed, consisting of twenty books, dealing with the whole body and devoting considerable space to describing the anatomy of the veins and the muscles.[95] It is also very likely that in it Marinus described at length just how one should carry out practical dissection, furnishing a model for Galen's later *Anatomical Procedures*.[96] But Marinus, in Galen's eyes, was more than a skilled dissector; he was also an effective propagandist for anatomy, transmitting this interest to his pupils, such as Quintus in Rome and Numisianus in Alexandria. The latter's writings were lost in a fire after his death, but his reputation as an anatomist was such that it induced Galen to travel to Corinth and then on to Alexandria to seek him out as a mentor. Unfortunately, by the time he arrived the great man had just died, and Galen was refused access to his books and papers by his son, himself an anatomist.[97] Marinus' other student, Quintus, inherited Marinus' notes on his anatomies of apes and other animals, but apart from enthusing his own students with a passion for anatomy, he seems to have made very little of them.[98]

What is clear from these scattered records of past pedagogues is that anatomy was already in vogue in Rome when Galen arrived there in AD 162. Martianus (or Martialis) the Erasistratean was enjoying a great reputation among younger doctors as the finest anatomist of his age, especially for his two books on *Dissections*. Galen thought him an incompetent charlatan, ever willing to pick a quarrel despite his more than seventy years, and he directed against him not only three books on Erasistratus' anatomy but also a massive treatise in six books on the anatomy of Hippocrates.[99]

But Galen's real *bête noire* was Lycus of Macedon, who had arrived in Rome a few years before him and whose writings on Hippocrates and on anatomy must have presented him with stiff competition. Certainly Galen dealt with the Hippocratic heretic Lycus even more severely than he did with Julian the Methodist, rarely letting slip an opportunity to criticise his errors. Nonetheless, Galen at one point thought enough of his main tract on anatomy to make his own abridgment of it in two books. Lycus' treatise was no casual summary, but fully nineteen books long. Although it mainly covered the same ground as Marinus, it went beyond him in one important respect.[100] Whereas Marinus had dealt with the womb, the testicles and the male and female urogenitary systems in a single book, Lycus devoted a total of six books to them, including a whole book given over to the anatomy of the womb and, perhaps more surprisingly, three books on foetal anatomy. Book 16 reported on the anatomy of a uterus containing a dead foetus, Book 17 on the anatomy of a living foetus and Book 18 on the anatomy of a dead foetus. Unless these are all records of animal dissections, they show that Lycus carried out some postmortem dissection on a pregnant woman and, what is perhaps even more important, that this was part of a systematic programme of anatomical investigation, arguably superior to the little treatise *On the Anatomy of the Womb* that Galen himself had composed while still a student at Pergamum in the late 140s.[101] Further evidence for Lycus' vivisections and post-mortem dissections may be provided by his division of the anatomy of the lungs in Books 6 and 7 according to whether the subject was alive or dead.[102]

Lycus' success as an anatomist in Rome may explain the bitterness with which the young Galen, newly arrived there in 162, endeavoured to obliterate memories of his recently dead predecessor. Not only had Galen to face challenges from respectable physicians who believed that Lycus had surpassed all other anatomists and that there was little more to be added to what he had done, but he had also to establish his own reputation, which he did by giving public displays of anatomy and by publishing books with titles such as *What Lycus Never Knew about Dissection*. Whenever Galen appeared at the Temple of Peace by the Forum, the meeting place of Roman intellectuals, he was constantly urged to prove his case by dissection, not by argument, as first one question and then another was tossed at him.[103] His claim that he had answered all his detractors magnificently should not be allowed to obscure the fact that Galen was not the only doctor in Rome with the combination of interests in anatomy and Hippocrates that he liked to portray as largely, if not uniquely, his own. His skills as a self-publicist, the vigour of his rhetoric, the range of his learning and the super-abundance of his literary productions (mostly dictated to shorthand writers rather than composed at the desk) impressed succeeding generations to such an extent that it is now difficult to envisage Galen save on his own terms. The triumphs of his later years, as an imperial physician and an authoritative philosopher, get in the way of placing the young Galen within a context of contemporary medicine and culture. His debts to others are concealed behind a facade of independent certainty.

Yet, as this chapter has shown, they were substantial, if rarely acknowledged, and allow us to situate him within developments already begun rather than instituted solely by him.

15

THE LIFE AND CAREER OF GALEN

Galen of Pergamum is a pivotal figure in the history of Western medicine. Just as the creation of the Hippocratic Corpus in the early Hellenistic period gave a new shape to Greek medicine by establishing a bloc of material against which others could react, favourably or unfavourably, so, 400 years later, Galen by his own example and his writings imposed upon later learned physicians an idea of what medicine was (and, equally important, what it was not) that lasted for more than a millennium. As we saw in the previous chapter, many of his views were not unique to him, but the forceful way in which he developed them and decried others, his frequent claims for the superiority of this or that technique or intellectual methodology, and the sheer power and prolixity of his writings impressed a Galenic stamp on subsequent medicine in Byzantium, the Middle East and the mediaeval West.[1]

Galen was born in August or September 129 into a wealthy family at Pergamum (Bergama, W. Turkey).[2] The city was then at the height of its prosperity: stoas, temples and magnificent houses were being built in the town itself, while, outside the walls, a huge temple to the god Asclepius was being refurbished with the support of the Roman emperor himself.[3] Galen's family profited directly from this building activity. His great-grandfather was a land surveyor, his grandfather and his father, Nicon, both rich architects with several landed estates.[4] The deep affection Galen displays for his father contrasts with his comments on his mother, whose wild, emotional outbursts, abusing her husband and biting the servants for the slightest mistake, Galen recorded with distaste.[5] Nicon was a man of great culture, an expert in geometry and astronomy as well as in architecture, who carried out experiments on his crops and wines to improve their quality.[6] It is tantalising that not one but two architects of this name are recorded from Pergamum at this period, both of whom composed complicated 'isopsephic' inscriptions for public places, in which all the letters are given numerical equivalents and in which the sum total of each line must be the same. That of Iulius Nicodemus, 'called Nicon the younger', graced a colonnade in the marketplace; that of Aelius Nicon a base for a statue of a satyr. Where a second poem by Aelius, in honour of the sun, was located is unclear, but it too was visible to the public.

This author's technical delight in putting into verse descriptions of the cube, sphere and cylinder and of the organisation of the universe certainly fits with what Galen says about his father, and makes Aelius on balance a more likely candidate than Iulius. But, whichever man was Galen's father, both had obtained Roman citizenship, and Galen must thus have been a Roman citizen also, although he never explicitly refers to this fact.[7]

Nicon's influence on Galen was enormous. Not only did he offer him an example of morality and intellectual rigour, but he guided his career from the very cradle. Galen was brought up speaking the best Greek, and Nicon not only chose his teachers but even accompanied him to the lectures on philosophy that he heard at Pergamum when he was fourteen.[8] It will have been Nicon who taught him to make little wooden carts as toys and encouraged him to work day and night at his studies. The story, preserved in Arabic, that his fellow pupils were baffled and annoyed by Galen, who never had time to play and joke with them, rings true, as does his withering response that he preferred knowledge to play and that such childish pleasures were therefore obnoxious to him.[9] Above all, it was as a result of a dream (or dreams) sent by Asclepius to Nicon that the sixteen-year-old Galen was turned towards the study of medicine.[10] Nicon's death, three years later, besides providing Galen with a substantial independent income, affected him deeply. He left Pergamum for further study at Smyrna and, after a fruitless visit to Corinth, at Alexandria, and he was not to return for almost a decade.[11]

Of the details of his medical studies, with Aeschrion, Satyrus, Stratonicus and Aeficianus at Pergamum, with Pelops (and Philippus) at Smyrna, and with a variety of lecturers at Alexandria, we know relatively little, save that most of his teachers could be described as Hippocratics and professed an interest in anatomy.[12] It was for the latter in particular that he travelled to Alexandria, although his disdainful description of what he found there, the food, the climate, the natives and the quality of teaching, scarcely explains why he should have chosen to spend four, five or even six years there. The high reputation of the city, 'the foundation of health for all men' as a later geographical writer called it, and the fact that most of his teachers had themselves studied there will have attracted him. But neither they nor the cachet of having attended lectures there need have detained him for long if the reality was as dire as he makes out.[13] He found Alexandrian lecturers on Hippocrates tedious, pedantic or just plain wrong, and, to judge from his surviving writings, he seems never to have set foot in the famous Library or Museum. More tempting for a man with an observant eye, whether of the fighting habits of the weasel or Egyptian methods of water-cooling, was the opportunity afforded by the great entrepôt of Alexandria to converse with shippers from all over the Mediterranean world and beyond, and to learn from them about astronomical navigation as well as about the rare drugs and minerals they were carrying.[14] He may also have been instructed in the very latest of Alexandrian surgical techniques, since it was as a surgeon to the gladiatorial troupe owned by the high priest that he gained his first job on his return to Pergamum in autumn 157. He had been away a long time.

The significance of Galen's education cannot be overestimated, since it established, to his ever-repeated satisfaction, the basic principles of proper medicine as he understood it. But his education was unusual in various ways. In the first place, Galen was a wealthy latecomer to medicine. There were humbler doctors who died at a younger age than Galen was when he embarked on an educational odyssey that was both longer and geographically more extensive than any other known to us.[15] Parallels can be found for doctors studying medicine with local physicians and travelling further afield to a more prestigious town, especially if, like Galen, they came from the well-to-do sections of society in Asia Minor.[16] But it is the length of time that Galen spent before entering upon his actual practice, and specifically at Alexandria, that is without precedent as far as our evidence goes.

Galen's was also an extremely bookish education. He would have been well suited to a career as a professional sophist, a public intellectual such as Polemo of Laodicea or Herodes Atticus, demonstrating in public his skills as a man of learning and his Greek style. On the other hand, he may have had in prospect merely the life of a cultivated gentleman dividing his time between his estates and the busy round of city theatres, clubs and polite conversation, where the ability to recognise quotations from long-dead poets or to allude gracefully to the dining habits of the ancient Athenians would ensure a welcome at the dinner table of the good and great.[17] At Ephesus, and probably elsewhere, doctors joined with other intellectuals in a Museum, and official decisions on their tax privileges placed them in the same context as sophists, grammarians and philosophers.[18] All of them had enjoyed an education based on the ancient classics, on Homer and the dramatists, on Thucydides, Plato, the Attic orators and on other authors less familiar today. Although Galen was well capable of competing in these intellectual games – his books include expositions of obscure colloquialisms in Attic comedy and an answer to the question of whether one could be a grammarian and a critic at the same time – he was no pedant. He despised those who devoted their time entirely to a passion for etymology, and he tried to steer a middle course between those always itching for novelty and those who would not utter a word unless it had been spoken five hundred years earlier by Demosthenes. He preferred clarity to linguistic fashion or hyperexactitude, writing a tract, in six books, against those who condemn others for verbal solecisms.[19] His Greek style bears out his claims, although it is marred by prolixity and constant repetitions, especially in those works that were taken down from an oral presentation. In *On Problematical Movements*, for example, one topic leads on to another in a rushing sequence that ends so abruptly with chapter 10 that some manuscripts divide the work into two separate books.[20] But his own enthusiasm for books – as already noted, his own library was enormous and his own rate of production astounding[21] – led him to elevate a knowledge of the literature to a far higher level of importance than others less fortunate than him would have done or than was always appropriate. The would-be patient in search of a doctor is told that if a personal recommendation is not forthcoming he should interrogate possible candidates at length on their understanding of the theories of the great doctors of the past (advice that demands from the patient as substantial an acquaintance with the relevant medical literature as from the doctor).[22] This book learning Galen uses as a weapon against his competitors: he is a better Hippocratic than they because he can interpret the words of the master through a more precise understanding of Hippocratic language. It is an argument that would appeal to intellectual tastes in an age of intellectuals and serve to raise Galen above the snotty-nosed cobblers, dyers, carpenters and tax collectors whom he saw as his competitors.[23] Equally, it was liable to lead to pedantic textualism in the hands of doctors less practically gifted than Galen.

Such learning was essential first and foremost, in Galen's eyes, in order to understand the greatest medical authority of them all, Hippocrates. This commitment to Hippocrates he had derived from his teachers, yet one may wonder whether any of them went as far as he did in the process of self-identification with Hippocrates.[24] When Galen discusses medical ethics, it is with the practical Hippocrates of the *Epidemics* and the *Letters* in mind, saving Greece and despising Persian gold.[25] He finds proof in the Hippocratic Corpus that the great man had carried out anatomy (although he had never found time to write up all his discoveries), and Plato's passing comments are used to demonstrate Hippocrates' logical and philosophical interests. It is not only that Galen found within the Hippocratic Corpus evidence to justify and approve what he himself wished to do; he also imposed on his hero theories, beliefs and practices that he is unlikely to have shared.[26] Some of these notions he undoubtedly gained from his own teachers: the pre-eminence of *The Nature of Man*, the theory of the four humours, the importance of prognosis and a holistic approach to an individualist therapy. But Galen may have gone far beyond them in his creation of an unerring Hippocrates in his own image.

He did this throughout his writings, but principally by means of a series of commentaries that occupied him on and off for twenty years or more, from the mid-170s at least until the early 190s. In all he commented on seventeen treatises, some of which, like *Prorrhetic*, were, in his view, not entirely by the hand of the master.[27] His avowed aim was to make clear to intelligent readers just what Hippocrates had meant in his writings, without necessarily entering into long discussions of the truth or error of each passage.[28] Often he achieves this aim, explaining clearly, if not always succinctly, what the Hippocratic Greek had meant, linking it to his own and others' clinical experiences, and even occasionally admitting the impossibility of making sense of what were little more than jottings without a context. But, inevitably, his good intentions were sometimes cast aside in the pursuit of intellectual hares. The later commentaries on the *Epidemics* discuss variant readings and questions of authenticity; a few lines of Hippocrates may extend into a wholesale

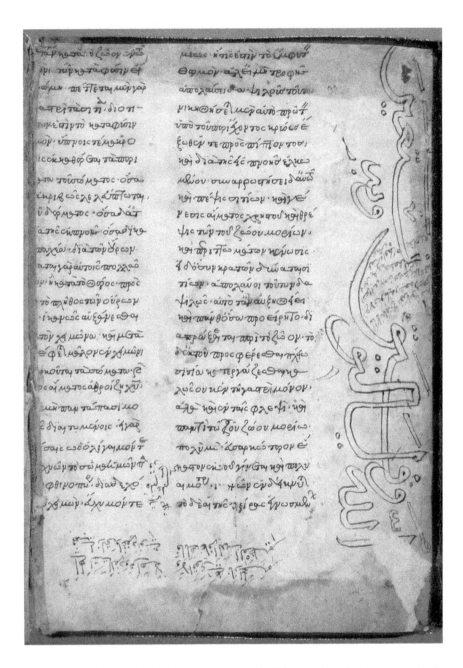

Figure 15.1 A fragment of Galen's commentary on the Hippocratic *Aphorisms*, written in the Near East (Cyprus?) in the thirteenth or fourteenth century, and preserved in an Arabic Gospel book. St Petersburg, Institute of Oriental Studies, C 263.

discussion on contemporary medical themes; and commentators who disagree with Galen are roundly controverted, sometimes at length. Here is scholarship, but at times it detracts from the educational purposes for which he wrote his commentaries.

Questions of good and bad medical practice inevitably enter in, as Galen endeavours to make sense of obscure passages. Galen is convinced of the didactic aim of the Hippocratic texts he selects for comment, culminating in the *Aphorisms*, which he sees as the summation of all accumulated Hippocratic knowledge.[29] The brief aphoristic form expresses succinctly and, more importantly, memorably the essential truths of Hippocratic doctrine, to which he himself is utterly committed. But it is not always clear what these truths are or were. The meaning of the words in the Corpus may be disputed, or they may not correspond entirely to the facts of everyday practice half a millennium later. Galen's response to the first problem is to collect lists of everyday words from prose writers and playwrights contemporary with Hippocrates, and particularly comic writers such as Aristophanes, to determine what everyday words meant at the time, for a playwright whose jokes could not be understood by the audience would be a poor writer indeed.[30] Elsewhere, he supports the general interpretation of his teachers with an abundance of vituperative scholarship that proves, to his satisfaction, that no other view is possible.[31] The second problem he resolves by dividing up the Hippocratic Corpus according to various degrees of authenticity.[32] Although he cites most of the texts in it in his *Hippocratic Glossary*, some of them, and indeed some sections of them, do not come from the pen of Hippocrates himself.[33] Instead, they are productions by other members of his family, such as Thessalus and Polybus, or by pupils, like modern undergraduates, not always accurate in their recollections of their master. Others reflect something of the Hippocratic spirit, even if, like *Prorrhetic* and *Ancient Medicine*, they also contain a great deal that is at variance with what Galen considers true Hippocratic doctrine.[34] The more error Galen detects in a treatise, the more likely it is not to have been written by Hippocrates, and hence it can be excluded from his medical purview.[35] Thus Galen the scholar–physician creates a picture of an unerring Hippocrates that, in turn, justifies and inspires Galen. The self-identification of hero-worshipper with hero is almost complete.

The other major strand in Galen's intellectual formation was a commitment to philosophy. As we have already seen, the intertwining of medicine and philosophy went back many centuries, and Galen's philosophical interests find contemporary parallels in the Sceptical doctor Sextus the Empiricist and the well-travelled Heraclitus of Rhodiapolis.[36] Galen's philosophical writings extend over the whole of his adult life. *On Medical Experience* was a product of his student days at Smyrna; *On My Own Opinions*, his last work, was written almost sixty years later.[37] They also cover a remarkably wide range of themes and approaches. Galen could deliver short moralising sermons on how to profit from one's enemies or avoid excessive grief, as well as write technically sophisticated studies of the logic of propositions.[38] Above all, he was convinced that no one could be a proper physician without philosophy, although he was prepared to accept that one might be an extremely good physician without ever realising that one was also a philosopher. As ever, Galen claimed Hippocratic authority and precedent for his views. Effective medical practice required both logic in the making of a diagnosis and ethics in one's relationship with patients, whether or not one was aware of this while carrying out treatment.[39]

His studies as a young man at Pergamum with philosophers from the four major sects, Stoic, Platonist, Aristotelian and Epicurean, not only gave him a detailed knowledge of their conflicting doctrines but also produced a deep uncertainty, from which he was rescued only by a consideration of the eternal truths of mathematics and geometry.[40] Henceforth, till the end of his long life, he was convinced of the futility of many of the questions hotly debated among the philosophical schools – the eternity of the world, the nature of the deity, the existence of worlds beyond our own – since the evidence on either side fell far short even of plausibility, let alone certainty.[41] Instead, he devoted himself to what he termed 'scientific demonstration', the application of logical thought and evidential proof. His most extensive treatise on this theme, *On Demonstration*, survives only in a few scattered fragments, and we have only the titles of his many shorter writings attacking a variety of dogmas of the individual philosophical schools, but his *Introduction to Logic* and his *On Ambiguities in Speech* are enough to show his impressive expertise.[42] The Arabs credited him with the discovery of the so-called fourth figure of the syllogism, although it might be more properly considered an extension of earlier logic rather than a totally new development.[43]

His own philosophy was avowedly eclectic, for he regarded it as a mark of weakness to commit oneself unequivocally to the doctrines of any one sect (like the Christians and Jews, whose adherence to their sacred texts and belief in miracles he found extraordinarily naive), and he encouraged all his hearers to think for themselves.[44] His methodology was simple: one should begin with 'obvious phenomena' or matters on which there was general agreement and proceed to draw conclusions logically from them. In this way, by beginning in concord and with agreed definitions of terms, one might be able to bring one's adversary along towards an agreed conclusion that was 'firm', 'certain' and 'precise', especially if, as Galen regularly did, one proceeded by impeccably accurate logical steps. The weakness of this approach, however, resides in the nature of the premises from which it begins, which are often neither as obvious nor as universally agreed as they appeared to Galen.[45]

Galen's eclecticism manifested itself in his view of the universe and of the microcosm of the body. In his concepts he is most indebted to Aristotle, especially for his theory of elements, qualities and mixtures within an ordered cosmos.[46] His view of the faculties, the body's capacities to perform its normal functions, each deriving from a specific combination of elements and qualities at the most basic level (a nice anticipation of modern notions of DNA and the structure of proteins), can only be understood against the background of Aristotelian physics. But his language and his understanding of the body are heavily Platonic, dependent especially on the *Timaeus*, which, Galen believed, contained medical doctrines consonant with those of his medical hero Hippocrates. He rejected the unitary soul of Aristotle and the Stoics in favour of Plato's tripartite soul, but he was even more scathing about those who denied the very existence of a soul (although he refused to commit himself on its nature) or who refused to admit that what went on in the body had a direct effect on psychic behaviour.[47] Similarly, he believed passionately in the existence of a divine creator (although without pretending to have knowledge of the divine essence) and in the purposeful organisation of the natural world, producing arguments in favour of teleology that are arguably superior to those of Aristotle.[48]

His philosophy and his medicine interact throughout his life. The opening books of the *Method of Healing* are an exercise in logic applied to the basic concepts of medicine, and his diagnostic procedures are models of careful and accurate argument.[49] In turn, his anatomical discoveries provide solid support both for Aristotle's notion of a purposeful creator in *On the Use of Parts of the Body* and for Plato's tripartite bodily system in *On the Opinions of Hippocrates and Plato*. Galen's books on causation, a favourite topic among Stoics and Aristotelians, are at once important contributions to philosophical discourse and practical guides for the thinking doctor.[50] His discussions on the role of experience within medicine have been given a wider significance by a modern scholar as challenging reflections on the nature of science as a whole.[51] In another area of ancient philosophy, his ideas on ethics and psychology both draw on and contribute to his experience and understanding of cases of madness, anger, grief and even the naughtiness of children, some of whom 'seem to be born naughty'.[52] The behaviour of animals can also throw light on human behaviour. To attempt to divide his philosophy from his medicine is impossible, even when considering his day-to-day activities. Not only did Galen associate with philosophers, such as Arria, the female Platonist, and benefit from their ideas, but he welcomed them to his anatomical displays and even to the bedside, and wrote treatises at their request.[53] Whatever the failings of his philosophical arguments over his long life – and there are many examples of inconsistency, evasion and hectoring bluster – Galen also triumphantly showed the importance of the physician thinking about his work, his patient and his moral universe.

But it was not philosophy that gained Galen his first major recognition on his return to Pergamum in 157 but his knowledge of surgery and, one might also suspect, his family connections with some of the wealthy citizens of Pergamum and the province of Asia.[54] He was retained by the high priest to look after his official troupe of gladiators that performed in the arena at the major festivals.[55] Gladiatorial combats were a highly popular form of entertainment among the Greeks of the Roman Empire; Pergamum itself had a magnificent amphitheatre. But gladiators, especially good fighters, were becoming expensive items, for those who were responsible for the great festivals could no longer rely on large numbers of captured slaves and prisoners to make up their numbers.[56] Galen's duty was to keep his gladiators alive, and not only in the immediate aftermath of their appearance in the arena. He attended to their diet, cleaned and stitched up their wounds, principally to their thighs, arms and buttocks (which would produce much blood, but not necessarily lasting damage), and oversaw their general health.[57] He claims that under his supervision only two gladiators died in his first period in office, compared with the sixteen lost by his predecessor, and he was thus re-engaged by the next high priest, seven-and-a-half months later, and by his three successors.[58]

He also treated other patients at Pergamum, but precise details are lacking. In summer 162, however, he left Pergamum for Rome, his reputation already established, even though he believed that he had not yet fully learned all the methods of the doctors in the region. It is not clear whether he went directly to Rome or, somewhat less likely, took the opportunity to leave the direct route for visits to interesting sources of rare drugs.[59] Although it was perhaps inevitable that a man of such talent, wealth and ambition should seek to make a career at the very heart of the Empire, there is a passing hint that there was a more pressing reason for his move. His implication that the ending of a *stasis* at Pergamum made it easier to contemplate a return home in 165 or 166 suggests that he, as a member of the governing class at Pergamum, had been on the wrong side in one of the local political squabbles that affected even the most prosperous of Asian cities.[60]

Whatever the reason for his departure, once in Rome Galen set about making a name for himself by public anatomical displays and by openly disputing with leading physicians. But it is also worthy of note that his first important patient, his old philosophy teacher Eudemus, believed that Galen had come to Rome to establish his reputation as a philosopher, not a physician. His cure of Eudemus, in winter 162–3, also serves as a reminder that Galen was no friendless alien in a hostile Rome.[61] Old acquaintances, like Epigenes and Teuthras, were already in Rome before him, and his links with Eudemus brought him immediately into contact with leading senators and members of the imperial household. Consuls such as Sergius Paullus and Flavius Boethus asked him for writings or sponsored his debates, the emperor's uncle and son-in-law attended his anatomical demonstrations, both in public and, when hostility to Galen brought these showpieces to an end, in private.[62] The city prefect, C. Aufidius Victorinus, was the dedicatee of a short tract on Hippocratic diet, while the wealthy and respectable L. Martius, cured by Galen of melancholy, declared that Galen spoke like an oracle 'from a golden tripod'.[63] It is no wonder that his name came to be touted about as a possible doctor to the emperor, or that others less gifted, less fortunate but no less ambitious should be roused to anger at Galen's success and at the unscrupulous and provocative ways in which he announced his superiority. In his turn, Galen portrays himself as victim, not villain, constantly beset by opponents seeking to gain advantage by flattery and pandering to the gross desires of the wealthy. He draws a parallel between his own situation and that of the great Hippocratic Quintus, driven out of Rome by hostile competitors, and, even more dreadful, that of a young provincial murdered because of his talents. It is this incessant hostility that he blames for his decision in summer 166 suddenly to sell up and slip away secretly to Campania, Sicily, and thence home to Pergamum.[64] At the end of his life, he gave another reason for his flight, the desire to avoid the plague (probably of smallpox) in Rome. Such a motive, however prudent, might be thought cowardly or worse in a doctor, if true. But it is possible that Galen is mistaken, for if the Antonine plague was indeed brought back from Persia by the returning army of the Emperor Lucius Verus it could not have attacked Rome until several months after Galen's departure. Similarly, Galen's return journey undoubtedly brought him to regions where the epidemic was already raging without apparent hope of a human cure.[65]

What Galen did once he returned home is obscure. He himself says only that he 'did the usual things', presumably writing and treating patients, and perhaps travelling to Lycia and Cyprus in search of rare mineral drugs.[66] Towards the end of 168 he received a summons to attend the Emperors Marcus Aurelius and Lucius Verus in N. Italy as they prepared to go on campaign against the German tribes who had crossed the central Danube and invaded the Empire. Scarcely had he joined them than the emperors left abruptly to avoid the plague. Within a few days at most, Verus died suddenly, and Marcus Aurelius and his immediate entourage returned to Rome for the state funeral.[67] Galen was not with them, and it was several months before he and part of the army arrived back in Rome.[68] As one of a corps of imperial physicians, Galen was expected to accompany Marcus Aurelius when he set out again on campaign with the army later in the year, but, for the second time in his life, Galen's career was changed by divine intervention. His 'ancestral god' Asclepius appeared and forbade him to go. The pious Marcus had little choice but to agree.[69] The less than courageous Galen was given instead the task of looking after the health of his heir apparent, the young Commodus. It was no easy job, as the prince and his court wandered around palaces in Italy and the young man, when he fell ill, displayed all the petulance and self-will that he was to show, a decade or more later, as sole emperor.[70]

From this point on, biographical details become still harder to fix chronologically. Galen's life was centred on the court and on Rome, on writing and on treating innumerable patients, rich and poor, slave and free, from those anxious about being assassinated by Commodus to athletes injured in the training ring.[71] He claims never to have charged patients a fee – although that did not preclude the acceptance of substantial gifts from grateful patients – and never to have taken any payment from his students, such as Glaucon or Epigenes, who accompanied him to the bedside along with friends and colleagues.[72] How many students he had and who they were is obscured by the fact that he addressed his comments and his books to 'lovers of medicine' as well as to actual practitioners. It is ironic that the only man we know of who claimed actually to have studied with him turned out to be a Syrian quack with a talent for conjuring. Galen's anger is directed as much at his presumption as at his charlatanry.[73]

Except for a visit to Pergamum in the 190s, of uncertain duration, Galen remained in Rome or nearby as one of the court doctors at least into the first decade of the third century.[74] But to write his biography for these years is almost impossible, for he refers only very occasionally to wider events. His praise for the fortitude of the slaves of Perennis when tortured to reveal the details of his conspiracy against the Emperor Commodus in 185 can hardly have been made public until after the death of Commodus at the end of 192.[75] This was a difficult period for Galen also. Patients and patrons disappeared in what he termed the worst reign in recorded history, and it is not surprising that he left Rome in 191–2 for an apparent retirement in his Campanian villa. His *Avoiding Distress* is an almost audible cry of relief after the murder of the tyrant.[76] His *Public Pronouncements in the Reign of Pertinax*, alas now lost, suggests that he remained in Rome throughout the turbulent events of late 192–3, and that he accepted the claim of the victorious Septimius Severus to be avenging the murdered Emperor Pertinax and restoring good government.[77] The last datable incident mentioned in any of the surviving treatises is a reference in *On Theriac, for Piso* to an accident that took place during the Secular Games of 204.[78] But very few of his cases reported in his later writings can be given even an approximate dating, and there is also the likelihood that, as he grew older, the boundary between what he had once read and what he himself had done became blurred.[79] His numerous cross-references do allow a rough chronology of his writings to be drawn up, pointing, for instance, to a renewal of interest in pharmacology in the 190s, but this is complicated both by his possible additions and reworkings and by his self-proclaimed consistency. With one exception, the order of the formation of the organs in the foetus, he claims never to have changed his mind on any major doctrine from his teens onwards, and hence, although one can point to inconsistencies and slight changes of emphasis at times, a developmental approach to understanding Galen and to dating his treatises is not very fruitful.[80] The same ideas, and often the same wording, can appear years apart. Galen decided to write the last eight books of the big *Method of Healing* twenty years or more after he had broken off the project following the death of its original dedicatee, yet one would be pressed to discover discrepancies even of style between the two parts.[81]

232

When Galen died is open to dispute. The brief entry in the Byzantine lexicon, the Suda, puts his death at the age of seventy – that is, in 199–200 – but a strong tradition in Arabic authors, possibly reflected also in Byzantine chronographers, has him dying aged eighty-seven – that is, in 216–17 – having spent seventeen years as a student and seventy as a practitioner. Although the circumstances of his death according to these authors, at Perama in Egypt while on a pilgrimage to Jerusalem, is the stuff of legend, the date can be supported from both within and without the Galenic Corpus.[82] The Arabic biographers drew on a comment by Alexander (of Aphrodisias?) that Galen had wasted eighty years of his life in coming to the conclusion that he was ignorant, a clear reference to the second chapter of *On My Own Opinions*, where Galen admits his inability to assent to any conclusion about some of the standard topics that divided the philosophical schools.[83] Furthermore, fitting the large number of tracts, some of them several books long, known to have been composed by Galen after the death of Commodus into a period of, at most, eight years presents difficulties, even for so prolific a writer. This problem is eased somewhat once it is clear that, save for the death date given by the Suda, there are no strong grounds for doubting the authenticity of *On Theriac, for Piso*, a work which cannot have been written before 204 and perhaps not before 207.[84] Language, style and content bespeak an author whose career, age and attitudes mirror those of Galen precisely. The case for extending Galen's life into the third century is thus overwhelming.

It is all too easy in evaluating Galen's career to accept at face value his own view of himself or the compliments paid him by others as mediated through his writings. His report that the Emperor Marcus Aurelius praised him as a true gentleman, 'the first among doctors and the only philosopher among philosophers', needs to be balanced against the absence of any reference to Galen in Marcus' *Meditations*.[85] Likewise, against his own story of his meeting with Herodes Atticus must be set the silence of Aulus Gellius or Philostratus, both writers well acquainted with Herodes and his circle.[86] Even some of his autobiographical details may require qualification. Galen's case histories are artfully presented to show his own abilities and the failings of others, and, occasionally, to link his own actions with those of great names from the past. One may suspect that the differences between Galen and his colleagues are here sharpened to make a good story and to put on display the philanthropic, philosophical and medically infallible Galen. He is rarely if ever wrong: when patients such as Theagenes the Cynic die it is as a result of their perverse refusal to follow Galen's advice or of circumstances that would have caused Galen to modify his prescription had he been made aware of them in time.[87]

But this does not mean that the search for the real Galen should be abandoned as hopeless, for at least two factors can help to put his self-portrait into perspective. First, so abundant is the evidence provided by Galen's writings that the alert reader can often read between the lines to gain a different understanding of events. As we have already seen, the Methodists were neither as naive nor as incompetent as he made them out to be, and in his devotion to Hippocrates and in his passion for anatomy he had had precursors, not all of them entirely congenial to him.

Second, inscriptions and the writings of Greek authors such as Plutarch or Lucian provide a context in which to set his career. They indicate beyond any doubt that his rise to prominence was similar to that of other imperial physicians, including his colleague and competitor the Methodist Statilius Attalus. They show that there were other young men from wealthy families in Asia Minor who studied at Alexandria and came to play leading roles in their communities and to establish links with the provincial, or even senatorial, aristocracy.[88] Despite his long residence in Rome, Galen's world, like theirs, remained the world of the Greek East. His favourite authors were the Greek Classics, and, although he clearly knew Latin, his reliance on Latin writers was minimal at best.[89] He thought of himself as a Greek first rather than a Roman, and, as *Avoiding Distress* reveals, he remained in touch for many years with friends back in Pergamum.[90] It is telling that, with one exception, 'with us', 'in our past', 'at home' and similar phrases refer to Pergamum and Classical Greece rather than to Italy and the city of Rome, where he spent the major part of his life.[91] Like many an exile, he referred back nostalgically to the sights, sounds and smells of his original home: to the sweetness of honey grown on a hill just off the coast road, the noise of the Pergamum hunt as they set out in search of their quarry on a crisp winter morning or the taste of local wine from the hill of Tmolus, superior even to the Falernian that he came to know for the first time in Italy.[92] Only towards the end of his life does Galen become more Roman, praising the public benefactions of the 'greatest of emperors', Severus and Caracalla, who reigned together from 198 to 211, the water supply of Rome and Trajan's road-building programme in Italy.[93] Typically, the last example is noted only as a parallel for what he himself believed he was doing in medicine, restoring what had once been good and realigning it for the greater benefit of mankind.

Such personal details allow us to form an intimate picture of Galen that can be compared only with that of Cicero or Seneca among figures from Classical Antiquity. Combative, opinionated, pedantic, long-winded, even unscrupulous, are all adjectives that can readily be applied to him, yet there are also times when he appears eirenic, open-minded, practical, succinct and generous. His philosophy is far from other-worldly, and his use of empirical evidence often gives the lie to many later accusations of empty theorising. Yet the sheer size of his surviving writings and the very forceful way in which they are expressed encourage his audience to follow him in his conclusions, and, more subtly, to treat much of what he says as typical of ancient doctors as a whole. The historian should be more cautious, for Galen's whole career, from cradle to grave, was very different from that of most practitioners, few of whom ever came to Rome, let alone became an imperial physician, as he was well aware.[94]

Of the extent of Galen's success there can be no doubt, even if we dismiss as exaggerated his portrayal of himself as the humble provincial making good in the metropolis; after all, he began his ascent of the ladder of fortune several rungs above the majority of his competitors. But his many references to distinguished patients, such as the wife of the consul Boethus or Diodorus, the grammarian who collapsed while teaching in the forum, can hardly have been invented, even if Galen chose to include them more because of the cachet they gave him than because of the complexity or medical interest of their cases.[95] The sheer number of patients mentioned in his writings also confirms that he had a considerable practice, sometimes even by correspondence.[96] Wealthy sufferers from eye diseases wrote to him for advice from Spain, Gaul, Asia Minor, Thrace and elsewhere, and, having received his diagnosis and his recipe for the so-called 'Holy bitter drug', commended him to their friends.[97]

Evidence for the respect in which he was held by others at the end of his life is unusually varied in nature. Athenaeus of Naucratis included him among his 'sophists at dinner' as a man who had produced more works on philosophy and medicine than any before him, although the opinions on wines and breads that are put into Galen's mouth are likely to be Athenaeus' own invention rather than citations from lost works of Galen.[98] The Aristotelian philosopher Alexander of Aphrodisias composed at least two treatises against him, and, although he thought little of him as a philosopher, he included Galen alongside Plato and Aristotle as examples of what it meant to be 'a man of repute'.[99] Around 210, a group of Christians in Rome led by Theodotus the shoemaker paid such respect to Galen's criticisms of their faith as ethically exemplary but philosophically naive that they modified their beliefs in ways that later Christians considered heretical.[100] Another theologian, the great Origen, writing around 240, seems to allude to Galen as an anatomist who could explain precisely why Providence had made each part of the body for its particular purpose.[101] The geographical spread of knowledge of Galen's writings is particularly noteworthy. Within a generation or so of his death his *On the Opinions of Hippocrates and Plato* was being copied in Upper Egypt and Gargilius Martialis, a retired army officer who died in 260 at Auzia (modern Morocco), could cite him as an authority in thirteen chapters of his short Latin handbook on *Medicines from Vegetables and Fruits*.[102] Such swift success in so many different subjects and in so many different regions can be demonstrated for very few other ancient authors. Galen was not exaggerating unduly his own impact on his contemporaries.

16

GALENIC MEDICINE

Galen's injunctions on the correct way to practise medicine are ubiquitous. They range in length from a few lines to whole books, and are directed to patients and doctors of greater maturity and experience as well as to those embarking on a medical career. Their message, that one should follow Galen's advice and example as a Hippocratic physician, is constantly reinforced by instances of his successful intervention or of the failure of others. Time and again he emphasised that it was not enough simply to have read the right books and have gained a theoretical understanding of medicine; this must be supplemented by practical expertise, which reinforced, and was in turn reinforced by, philosophy. Indeed, his sympathies at times were far more with the approach of the Empiricists, with their store of practical information, than with those who put forward theories, however intellectually exciting, based on little or no acquaintance with the facts of medical life.[1] Galen strove for a unified art of medicine, in which the effective treatment of the sick depended on a profound understanding of the body coupled with a broad acquaintance with all types of therapy. Although he acknowledged the existence of specialists, particularly in big cities such as Rome and Ephesus, the practitioners for whom he wrote were of necessity generalists and were required to know how all the constituent parts of the medical art came together.[2]

At the base of Galen's medicine lay his conviction of the supreme importance of anatomy. An ignorant incision could easily result in the death of the patient, and a misunderstanding of the pathways of the nerves could delay or frustrate a cure.[3] But considerations of medical prudence and practical utility were only part of Galen's justification for anatomy. In his opinion, only through dissection could one gain a proper understanding of the organisation and workings of the body, in sickness and in health. To this end, he wrote a variety of treatises on anatomical themes, ranging from short elementary tracts on bones, nerves, veins, arteries and muscles to a big manual of dissection, *Anatomical Procedures*.[4] He repeated his conclusions in two other large treatises aimed at showing the value of anatomy for philosophers interested in the human body. In *On the Use of Parts* he discussed his discoveries in Aristotelian terms, whereas in *On the Opinions of Hippocrates and Plato* he defended Plato's ideas on physiology and psychology against the Stoics.[5] Both here and in his discussions elsewhere on the *Timaeus* he argued that Plato was well acquainted with contemporary medical theory, even if few scholars today would agree with him that Plato's teleological anatomy depended on the teachings of Hippocrates.[6]

But no amount of book learning or theoretical understanding could replace actual dissection for fixing in one's mind all the details of the human body.[7] Practice, and still more practice, was essential. The failure of an 'excellent Empiricist' to save the life of a schoolboy who had been jabbed in the arm by a sharp stylus is turned by Galen into a cautionary tale of how, even if one had read everything available on anatomy, one might not fully understand the tiny details of the nervous system that only dissection could reveal. Even then, one might have to repeat the process several times before one had really grasped all that was thereby revealed.[8]

How one should perform a dissection was specified at length in *Anatomical Procedures* and in two other treatises, now lost in Greek but known in Arabic, that dealt with the practical details of dissection and vivisection.[9] Galen was well aware that it was impossible to carry out systematic dissections on human bodies; gazing at a skeleton or at the surface anatomy of a slave was all that was done even in the best medical schools.[10] But that should not prevent one from taking advantage of what chance had placed in one's way – a corpse stripped bare when the tomb in which it lay had been opened to view by a flood, an executed criminal hanging on a gibbet or the bodies of dead Germans that littered the battlefield after one of the victories of Marcus Aurelius.[11] The wise practitioner would also profit from the cases brought to him to gain experience of the internal organisation of the body.

Above all, one could experiment on animals, both living and dead. Galen was conscious of the problem of extrapolating from animals to human beings, often warning his audience about drawing rash conclusions solely from animal dissections, but he could do little else, even if it led him into errors at times.[12] His human womb has cotyledons like that of a ruminant; his thyroid cartilage is that of a pig; and his belief that the left kidney was lower in the body than the right is true of apes, but not humans.[13] However, animal dissection also had advantages, not least in allowing experimentation on living bodies as well as dead. The sudden cessation of the loud squeals of a pig when the free passage of nerves along the spinal cord was interrupted by ligation or cutting could not fail to have a powerful effect on the audience. Although he also recommended sheep and goats as good subjects for public dissections, Galen preferred to use monkeys, such as the Barbary ape, on the grounds that they most resembled man.[14] But the look of pain on the face of a monkey being vivisected might be too much to bear, and sheep, pigs and goats could serve just as well at times.[15] Galen seems to have taken advantage of whatever came his way. On one occasion he even managed to obtain from the emperor's cook the heart of an elephant, which he began to dissect in order to see whether there was a bone in the middle. Finding a bony structure there, he concluded that such huge beasts did indeed have a bone in the heart. He was not to know that in elderly elephants the fibrous triangles separating the aorta and the ventricles often ossify and give the impression of a bone.[16]

His daily dissections, some at first in public, not only gave him the necessary dexterity for his surgical interventions but also enabled him to go beyond what the Alexandrians and his immediate predecessors had done.[17] His descriptions of many of the bones of the body would be acceptable today, and his errors in his reports of the heart and vascular system are far more the result of working with animals and of mistaken interpretation than of incompetent dissection. His studies of the nerves and muscles are remarkably accurate, especially given that they were performed without modern aids and involved at times structures that are hard to see with the naked eye. He made important discoveries concerning the ducts of the sublingual glands, the Achilles tendon (although his description more closely resembles the tendon in monkeys) and the muscles of the face. He was prepared to change his views if presented with new anatomical evidence. The muscles that flex the first joint of each finger and toe, the *musculi interossei*, were for a long while unknown to him, but were described at length in books from the mid-160s onwards, *On the Anatomy of Muscles*, *On the Use of Parts* and *Anatomical Procedures*.[18] His descriptions of the nerves are particularly impressive. In a complex and difficult series of experiments he traced the pathways of the nerves from inside the brain and down the spinal cord, identifying in the process the recurrent laryngeal nerve and establishing the relationship between the intercostal muscles and nerves in producing the voice.[19] It is a substantial list of discoveries, comparable in extent, as far as we can tell, only with those made much earlier by Herophilus and Erasistratus.[20]

Galen used his anatomical experiments to find solutions to many problems posed by his predecessors.[21] So, for example, he refuted Asclepiades' ideas on the functions of the bladder and ureters by a series of dissections that proved that urine flowed in one direction only.[22] This tradition of anatomical demonstration he traced back to Hellenistic times, if not to Hippocrates himself.[23] He repeated Erasistratus' experiments on blood flow, inserting a cannula into an artery to see whether pulsation continued beyond the cannula, and what happened if the artery was ligated.[24] He vivisected the heart and lungs to see the beating of the heart and arteries and to investigate what would happen if one constricted the heart.[25] His erroneous conclusion that the pulse itself was a movement contained within the coats of the arteries, not the result of blood forced by the heart into the arteries, may be excused by the difficulty of performing such an experiment without the help of modern technology.[26]

These dissections confirmed Galen in his view that the body consisted anatomically of three near-separate systems. Whether they developed simultaneously from the very first stages of the foetus or whether the heart or, as he came to believe at the end of his life, the liver was formed first was a difficult question, even when investigated by careful dissection along the lines pioneered by Aristotle.[27] But Galen rejected the Aristotelian and Stoic view of the primacy of the heart as the seat of the controlling power of the body, insisting time and again that the results of his dissections proved that Plato was right to believe that the liver, the heart and the brain were the origins of three parallel systems, each of which had a different function.[28]

The liver was responsible for nutrition. In the liver 'digested' or 'concocted' food received from the stomach and intestines was turned into nutritious blood, which was then transported within the veins to provide the essential nutriment for all the body.[29] Every living being, plants as well as animals, was provided by the Creator with the four 'natural faculties' of attraction, assimilation, excretion and growth. Each part of the body had thus the potentiality, as a result of its elemental organisation, to feed on this nutritious blood, to assimilate whatever it needed to grow and to function, and to excrete potentially harmful residues that it no longer needed.[30] The body was a living universe, responding to changes and actively seeking whatever it needed in order to exist and to function. Galen's vitalist approach thus contrasted with the mechanistic understanding of the body proposed by Erasistratus and Asclepiades, in which, for instance, the excretion of residues through the kidney and bladder did not require any active participation from the organs themselves but only obedience to the laws of physics.[31]

The nutritious venous blood, produced in the flesh of the liver, was attracted into the various parts of the body as each required.[32] Some of the venous blood that reached the right side of the heart then passed through perforations in the intraventricular septum to the left side, where it joined refined air, *pneuma*, coming from the lungs via the pulmonary vein. Galen was aware that the pulmonary artery carried blood from the heart to the lungs and that some of this blood returned in the pulmonary vein, but he seems to have regarded this means of transit as secondary to that via the septum.[33] He may have been strengthened in this belief by his discovery that in the foetus there is a direct connection between the two sides of the heart via the *ductus arteriosus* and the *foramen ovale*, which closes at birth, and by his correct observation of pittings within the actual septum. It would have been simple for Galen to conclude that one connection replaced the other after birth, although he himself never states this.[34] Similarly, although he accepted Erasistratus' view that the arterial and venous systems were linked by invisible capillaries, he considered that they allowed only for the transfer of a small amount of nutritious venous blood and *pneuma* between the two systems, and were fully opened only in unusual or abnormal circumstances.[35] Although Galen provided much of the anatomical data on which, fifteen centuries later, William Harvey was to base his theory of the circulation of the blood, Galen's own discoveries in no way entailed that conclusion, and they could be easily explained by his own physiological theories.[36] Given his conviction of the separate functions of his three systems, Galen was hardly likely to have searched diligently for a means to unify only two of the three into a single circulation of the blood.

According to Galen, the mixture of blood and *pneuma* in the left side of the heart was then further concocted by the heat of the heart to produce a thinner, red blood that then flowed within the arteries to energise or vivify the body by its 'vital spirit'.[37] That the arteries contained blood was the theme of another of his anatomical demonstrations, designed to confute the Erasistrateans, who thought that they contained only *pneuma*.[38] As with venous blood, a small proportion of this arterial blood was passed on, to be refined further in a vascular network at the base of the brain to produce a 'psychic *pneuma*' that circulated in the ventricles of the brain and throughout the nervous system.[39] Also nourished by air breathed in through the nostrils (shown by the speed at which people died if their air supply was cut off), this 'psychic *pneuma*' was responsible for consciousness, sensation and voluntary movement.[40]

Galen claimed that this tripartite physiological system, which was both demonstrable anatomically and based on the discoveries of the Alexandrians, had many advantages. It refuted the view of Aristotle and the Stoics, who posited a single controlling organ, while at the same time it still preserved the unity of the individual being. It linked body and soul together, explaining how and why physical changes in the body could alter one's mental balance and behaviour, and vice versa. Basing himself on the theory of the four humours as expressed in *The Nature of Man*, Galen accepted nine possible mixtures or, as later Latinate interpreters called them, temperaments: one an exact balance of the four Aristotelian primary qualities – hot, cold, wet and dry – the others with a predominance of one or two qualities, which indicated a predisposition to certain types of illness rather than being in themselves unhealthy. Every individual had his or her natural mixture, and it was this that the good physician sought to restore by his therapies.[41]

This mixture determined not only one's physical well-being and susceptibility to certain illnesses but also one's mental state.[42] Later Galenists developed this notion still further so that today terms such as 'phlegmatic' or 'sanguine' are applied to behaviour or attitude rather than to physical condition.[43] This link between body and mind also explained certain movements that at first sight seemed neither ultimately involuntary (like breathing) nor completely voluntary (like speech). Sometimes, like a tic or an inability to control the movements of the tongue, this was the result of physical weakness; at others, like the erection of the penis or yawning, the brain had been stimulated by external phenomena to thoughts and imaginings that had physical consequences.[44]

Above all, Galen's anatomical experiments proved the wisdom and foresight of the Creator or of Nature (for Galen in his account of the body used these terms indiscriminately along with 'God').[45] Whether one considered the eye of an insect, the trunk of an elephant or that supreme masterpiece the human hand, one could not help but conclude that everything had been designed for a purpose, as Plato and Aristotle had seen long before.[46] Each part, even the smallest, was constructed with its proper function in mind, with a precise balance of elements, qualities or humours that allowed it to do what it had to do and that if altered resulted in some functional impairment. Those, like the Jews and Christians, who believed in miracles and in a god who could change the order of the universe at a whim, failed to recognise the supreme majesty and thoughtfulness of divine creation.[47] It is no coincidence that Galen called the final book of his great work on teleological anatomy, *On the Use of Parts*, an epode, a hymn to the purposeful Creator or Nature.[48]

Galen's description of the body takes the male as the norm. Woman is a rational being – that is, one capable of acquiring knowledge (an interesting definition) – but is in every activity and mode of learning inferior to man. The female is, indeed, the weaker sex, with a body colder than the male and adapted by nature for childbearing and to fit the character of the soul that inhabits it.[49] There is hence no need for women to have beards, since they do not possess the august character of males and require less protection from the cold because they usually stay indoors.[50] There are women's diseases, but these are related to the female reproductive organs and functions, when they are not the result of the natural imperfection of the female body compared with the male.[51] This predisposition to ill health differentiates female from male, and influences the sort of remedies that should be used. Women should be treated more gently than men, not because they are female *tout court* but because they share the same position on the spectrum of hardness and softness as children, eunuchs and men who are passionately addicted to the baths. They are as far removed from Galen's average man as he is from tough peasants and sailors, and, like all other patients, they must be given treatments appropriate to their physical make-up.[52] Galen's attitude to women is thus complex. Although it may appear at times patronising, it did not necessarily involve a dismissal of women for being women: Galen had no difficulty in accepting the information provided to him by female medical attendants.[53] But there were limits: it is still Galen, the male doctor, who diagnoses and prescribes, and his friendship with Arria the philosopher is a rare contrast to his general contempt for ladies of luxury, liable to flee at the mere sniff of the pungent hair dye of Asian peasant girls, and to his ambivalent reaction to the imperious Annia Faustina, a royal relative.[54] Male superiority was, for Galen, simply a fact of nature.

Galen's understanding of the body directly benefited his therapy by revealing links that might otherwise have passed unnoticed. When the Syrian sophist Pausanias lost all sensation in three fingers after a fall from a chariot, it was Galen's knowledge of the pathways of the nerves that enabled him to diagnose and treat him successfully.[55] He could explain why delirious sufferers from fever might continue to act as if they were doing their normal jobs – a schoolteacher expound a poem by Sappho or Bacchylides, an orator perform a test piece, a mathematician solve problems – or behave in a manner that was totally unfamiliar (such as a respectable citizen mouthing abuse and obscenities).[56] That the mind or soul could be affected by changes in the body was in his view universally accepted, no matter what view on the nature of the soul might be held.[57]

But just as fever or an excess of alcohol had an effect on the mind, so in turn mental perturbation had physical effects on the body. The idea that one's emotions affected one's physical state had long been familiar in literature, at least since the sixth century BC, when Sappho described the effects of gazing on one's beloved – a hot flush, drumming in the ears, sweating, trembling and pallor of the face.[58] Two centuries later, the comic poet Philemon was uttering a commonplace when he told his audience that 'Grief has brought madness and many incurable diseases to many people'.[59] But, although Galen claimed that understanding the effects of the emotions was not difficult, he also depicted himself as unusual in taking over these popular notions into his clinical practice and in providing them with a medical explanation.

Stress diseases became a speciality of Galen's. He claimed Hippocratic precedent for this, and, in the final book of his commentary on *Epidemics* 6, he recorded a series of cases of individuals who had fallen ill or died as a result of mental disturbance – grief at a family death or loss of property, and fear of the future or of the emperor's wrath.[60] In another case, baffled by the inability of his young patient to recover, he diagnosed from signs of stress that the boy had been eating food surreptitiously – and then went on to show where he had hidden the forbidden food and how it had been brought to him by his doting mother.[61] In a repetition of a famous diagnosis, ascribed to Erasistratus among others, Galen discovered that the wife of Justus was in love with a leading actor of the day. But Galen added his own twist to the story, deriding those who believed in lovesickness as a specific condition and emphasising that the physical symptoms of his lovesick patient were no different from those of any other person suffering from stress.[62]

In his treatment of mind–body problems Galen also extended the role of the doctor into areas that others would certainly have disputed. He accepted the continuum between doctor and philosopher that Aristotle had posited, but it was now the doctor who intervened in matters of morality, over which philosophers had traditionally claimed jurisdiction. It was not enough for the doctor to act the candid friend and to point out the consequences that might ensue from the passions and errors of the soul – a task for which Galen considered himself well qualified from his daily reading and rereading of the so-called *Golden Words* of Pythagoras.[63] He could now offer medical advice that would remove or mitigate them and restore moral as well as physical well-being – and the example of his own imperturbability after the loss of so much in the fire of 192 confirmed, as his old friend acknowledged, that he practised what he preached.[64]

Galen's claim to understand the workings of the human body better than his competitors was only one of the ways in which he advertised his superiority. His book learning, his powerful rhetoric and his logic also contributed to the impression of omnicompetence that he sought to make on potential patients. There were other factors that were medically more relevant. He deliberately cultivated an authoritative bedside manner when visiting patients or treating them in public or in his own house, even if he did not always follow in every detail his own recommendations for appropriate medical behaviour. His ideal doctor should strive for the mean between boorishness and over-weening hauteur, dressing and choosing his tone of voice and language to suit his patient – intemperate jokes, baffling technicalities and slovenly grammar should all be avoided. One should select the best time and manner to arrive at the bedside, for nothing would be more likely to cause annoyance than barging in on a sleeping patient with clumping feet and an over-loud voice. Personal appearance mattered – clean clothes, neat nails, well-trimmed hair cut in a conservative fashion and a pleasant freshness, unlike Quintus, who once visited a rich patient while smelling of drink, or the unfortunate doctor from Asia whose naturally smelly armpits put patients off.[65] Many of Galen's recommendations find parallels in the Hippocratic *Precepts*, *Decorum* and *Testament of Hippocrates*, and also respond to contemporary criticisms of doctors with flashy instruments and high-flown rhetoric or, at the other extreme, uncouth behaviour and shabby clothing.[66]

Above all, over and over again Galen stressed the importance of gaining the patient's confidence in the battle against disease, although he reshaped the Hippocratic triangle of doctor, patient and illness to ensure the doctor's dominance.[67] This was best achieved through the art of prognosis as laid down by Hippocrates. Alas, although Galen himself believed this knowledge to be easily attainable, few of his contemporaries practised it, at least to a level that satisfied his standards. As a result, when he himself made a successful prognosis he was regarded in amazement as a miracle-worker.[68] While we might suspect that such an appellation was not unwelcome to Galen, especially if it brought in patients, he took pains to dissociate himself from any suggestion of soothsaying or indulging in the magic arts, emphasising instead the logical basis of his procedures and the ignorance of his opponents.[69]

Fundamental to any prognosis was observation, using all one's senses to understand both the patient's individuality and any abnormalities in his or her condition. Even when one allows for a substantial element of rhetoric and self-praise in the construction of his exemplary case histories, there can be little doubt that Galen was a brilliant observer, whether of physical changes in the body or of objects in the sickroom, a jar of hyssop on a windowsill or a rough pillow on a truckle bed. He listened carefully to patients, their friends or other medical attendants, for, even if he came to disagree with what they believed, their information could be crucial in helping to form a diagnosis.[70] He often examined the patient's faeces, paying special attention to their colour, smell and consistency, and urine, noting any unusual colours, turbulence or clouds in it, since they offered significant information on the weakness or failure of organs deep in the body.[71] So, for example, diabetes, which he saw only rarely, he attributed to a failure of the kidneys to retain or transform fluid.[72] Taking the pulse he also considered extremely helpful, for its condition was often a very accurate guide to changes elsewhere in the body, although, as we have seen, Galen saw the pulse itself as a movement within the coats of the arteries, not as a result of the pumping action of the heart. Building on Hellenistic pulse doctrine, such as is found also in the little pulse treatise by his near-contemporary Marcellinus, Galen attempted to correlate the different types of pulses with certain diseases (and vice versa).[73] He employed a variety of categories, such as speed, rhythm and tension, as well as a series of metaphorical descriptions (taken over from predecessors such as Herophilus and Aristoxenus) for what he found, for example the gazelle pulse, the mouse-tail pulse, the ant-like pulse or the double-hammer pulse (rightly seen by him as indicating a life-threatening condition).[74] Typically, Galen declares that his own superiority is the result of having attained through long practice a 'most sensitive touch' that allowed him to feel the various stages in the dilation and contraction of an artery.[75] Equally typical is his desire for precision and clarity, which, he suggests, would best be gained by expressing the ratios between pulse beats in musical, as well as verbal, terms.[76]

Having made his observations and gathered as much information as he could, Galen then proceeded to a diagnosis and forecast. His usual method was to employ logic to establish a differential diagnosis, classifying the patient's condition with ever-increasing precision until he could identify what was wrong and assign it a cause.[77] He was aware of the ambiguity inherent in the word 'cause', and followed Athenaeus and the Stoics in differentiating between initial (or procatarctic) causes, preceding causes and containing causes. The first group originated outside the body, such as a blow or bad food, the second were bodily predispositions and the last were the immediate causes of present effects, as when the tightening of the choroid membrane loosens the pupil of the eye.[78] Once a diagnosis had been established and the chain of causation identified, one could select an appropriate treatment to restore the functional or humoral imbalance. At the same time, one could predict the course and future outcome of the illness with confidence.[79] One need not have to worry at every change in the body and constantly alter the proposed therapy because an 'accurate' and 'certain' prognosis (two favourite words of Galen's) would have already revealed what would happen and the doctor would have taken account of that in his initial prescription.[80] By following the method of prognosis carefully one would never fail – or, if one did, the fault did not lie with the physician. Sometimes the patient disobeyed orders or failed, even on occasions deliberately, to tell the truth in the consultation with the doctor. Sometimes, events beyond the doctor's control or an unfortunate intervention by servants or friends led to changes that could not have been predicted earlier.[81] Theagenes the Cynic would have lived had he not been persuaded by the Methodists to disregard Galen's advice – Galen's stage management of the death-bed scene to cause maximum loss of face for his fellow imperial doctor, Attalus, also shows his ruthlessness in exploiting a situation to his best advantage.[82] Credit for success thus rested with Galen, and with those who followed him; responsibility for failure with others.

This aura of infallibility was deliberately promoted by Galen, who was almost pathologically concerned at all times to protect his reputation. He went to great lengths to ensure not only that his books were read and his theories understood in the way that he had intended, but also that treatises or practitioners masquerading under a Galenic title could be easily exposed as frauds.[83] A Syrian doctor offering a dubious remedy for toothache that he claimed to have obtained from Galen himself was apprehended by Galen in Rome and handed over for punishment by the civic authorities.[84] Since the man's cure involved a conjuring trick rather than the administration of a drug, it is not easy to see why he should have been punished, and we may suspect that Galen's friendship with a prefect of the city may have had more to do with it than strict legal liability.[85]

The art of prognosis allowed treatment to proceed on an individual basis. Although Galen recognised groups of symptoms as constituting diseases, these offered only general indications of what was wrong, and every patient suffering from, say, apoplexy or dropsy had an individual balance that needed to be restored.[86] Galen constantly attacked the Methodists for attempting to treat all those suffering from a given condition alike, for, as he put it, one shoe does not fit all feet.[87] He wrote relatively few tracts dealing with diseases as such (that on marasmus is a rare exception), preferring instead to look at the ways in which each part of the body functioned or failed to function and to examine the symptoms and processes of illness.[88] Again following Hippocratic precedent, particularly in the *Epidemics*, *Prognostic* and *Aphorisms*, he divided an illness into various stages, concentrating in particular on the crises and critical days that determined whether a patient recovered or not.[89] His observations often correspond to modern clinical data. For example, he noted the aura that often preceded an epileptic attack, describing in detail a case of a thirteen-year-old boy that can be identified as Jacksonian epilepsy.[90] He rightly acknowledged the greater frequency of apoplexy or stroke in the elderly, emphasising the rarity and seriousness of such attacks among the under-forties and the decreasing likelihood of recovery with each successive stroke.[91] There are adumbrations of modern ideas in his ingenious recommendation that a person suffering from headache might benefit from applying a live electric eel to the head to dull the pain, since a fisherman who had accidentally stabbed his metal trident into such a fish would lose all sensation in his hand or arm.[92]

Therapy followed on from observation and diagnosis, and here too Galen professed a universal mastery. Descriptions of his surgical cases are rare, in part because he never completed his proposed work on surgery.[93] Nonetheless, there is ample evidence that he was adept with the knife, even if he implies in *On Examining the Physician* that such operations were the province of the surgeon, not the doctor.[94] To remove the suppurating breastbone from the slave of Marullus the mime-writer was no easy task. Gymnastic trainers in Rome and in its port city of Ostia regularly referred patients to him with complicated dislocations.[95] His commentaries on the Hippocratic *Fractures* and *Joints* provide further evidence for his competence in surgery and of his training in the Alexandrian tradition.[96]

But surgical intervention was the treatment of last resort, with one major exception. Galen was strongly in favour of letting blood from a vein as a regular part of therapeutics. In this he adopted a stance at variance with many of his competitors, most notably the Erasistrateans. When Galen first came to Rome in the 160s he was attacked by them for his support for phlebotomy, a procedure they believed to have been condemned utterly by Erasistratus. Galen's response was to argue that they had misunderstood their texts of Erasistratus and that if one read them carefully one would find that even he had advocated this procedure at times. When he returned to Rome for his second stay he found that the Roman Erasistrateans had been so far convinced by his arguments that they were now enthusiastic phlebotomists, bleeding all and sundry with scant concern for whether it was appropriate or not. He felt impelled to write another treatise, again expounding Erasistratus, but this time emphasising the contraindications.[97] Only those who were sufficiently strong to withstand bleeding – and this excluded the elderly or very young – should be given this treatment, whose use should be considered against the wider background of the season of the year, the type of condition and the availability of alternative therapies. After all, the best physician was the one most capable of treating surgical conditions by means other than the knife, and particularly by diet and drugs.[98]

Diet, for Galen, was more than just food and drink, and encompassed one's whole lifestyle, including exercise, sleep and environment. While it was in one sense true that one was what one ate – those who consumed the flesh of asses, lions or even camels became like them[99] – it was diet in the widest sense that determined whether one's healthy state turned into the preternatural one of illness. It was only to be expected that wealthy Roman women fell ill and were unable to stand even the slightest of restraints, since their life was entirely one of luxury.[100] At the other extreme, Galen saw nothing incongruous in both writing sympathetically of peasants in Asia Minor forced for lack of anything better to eat horse and donkey meat and, in more than one passage, dismissing them as asses, thoroughly brutish in their nature.[101] As Galen himself remembered from a youthful excursion into the backwoods of modern Turkey, the rough porridge that was the only food available brought on flatulence, constipation and headaches, and even the natives admitted that it was hard to digest.[102] One had only to look at the hard skin of the scrawny Egyptians to realise the consequences of a diet of salt fish, snails, beans, lentils and pulses, supplemented by the flesh of vipers, camels and donkeys and washed down with thin wine and barley beer. By contrast, there were few cases of skin disease among the Germans or the Mysians, and almost none at all among the milk-drinking Scythians.[103]

If eating the wrong sort of food produced illness, it was also true that health could be maintained, and often restored, by an appropriate eating plan. Galen devoted several large treatises to foodstuffs and their role in health, and hence it is not surprising to find him as one of the interlocutors in Athenaeus' *Sophists at Dinner*.[104] But whereas Athenaeus' speakers are interested mainly in the history of food, capping each other's learned quotations from Attic comedy or oratory, Galen, while not disdaining the occasional learned quotation, looked more to its medical value. He offers a comprehensive survey of the foods available in his own time, adding many details from his own observations: the quince tarts exported from Spain to Rome, the ingenious ways in which Egyptian peasants clarified and kept cool the water they had taken from the Nile, and the morning honeydew, 'Zeus' rain', that covered shrubs and trees in the hills behind Pergamum in summer.[105] The district's local honey was, for Galen, unsurpassed, even if also unsung. Near the village of Britton a rocky outcrop produced a honey of exquisite sweetness, but too much of it induced vomiting. He knew another bank where the wild thyme grew, a hillock to the left of the road from Pergamum to Elea, which produced scented honey far surpassing that of Thasos or Hymettus.[106] He noted the various types of cereals that he saw growing in Asia Minor and northern Greece, as well as a veritable catalogue of Mediterranean wines, although he himself preferred those from near Pergamum, from Titacaza, Aegeae, Perperene and the hill of Tmolus.[107] One should not forget that his father had owned a vineyard and experimented to see how best the life of a vintage could be prolonged.[108]

Galen tried to relate the properties of foods to the four humours and their various constituent qualities. Some foods were heating, others cooling, moistening or drying; some thickened the humours, others thinned them, making them easier to excrete and thus acting as a sort of slimming aid. Galen's listings and his placing of foods according to their digestibility, strength and suitability for human beings differ little from those of other ancient writers on food.[109] White meat, poultry and fish were far easier to digest than red meat; white wines more suitable for the sick than strong reds. Pork was the meat most easily digested, since it was most like human flesh, witness the habit of rascally innkeepers in serving up human flesh as part of a pork stew.[110] The sick should be initially given soups, especially barley broth, and gradually returned to their normal diet.[111] Most of Galen's recommendations would meet with the approval of a modern dietician, with one major exception. He placed an almost total ban on fresh fruit, which he considered a frequent cause of illness. His father had warned him of the dangers of eating such fruit, but he had once been led astray by his friends into eating a lot of fresh fruit in autumn. The result was an acute illness. The next year, taking fruit only in moderation, he remained free from illness, but after his father's death the pains returned, until, aged 28, he decided to abandon all fruit save for small amounts of figs and grapes. Others, like his fellow citizen Protas, who fell ill after eating unripe apples and pears, had similar stories to tell, and the difficulties of keeping fruit in a warm climate should not be underestimated. It thus came as no surprise to Galen that Asian peasants fed apples to their pigs.[112]

In his advocacy of physical exercise, Galen follows the same policy of moderation. His heroes were Telephus the grammarian, who lived almost to 100, and Dr Antiochus, who daily walked the half-mile or so from his house to the Roman forum and continued to visit his patients on foot or, if they resided further off, in a litter or chariot, until he was well past eighty.[113] Their example showed what benefits could be gained by an active lifestyle, in moderation. For professional athletes Galen had little but contempt, convinced that their passion for training in order to attain peak fitness was counterproductive. How much better to indulge in intellectual pursuits than sweat and struggle in the gymnasium! Galen's quotations from the Athenian playwright Euripides shows that the contempt of the intellectual for the hearty has very ancient roots.[114] But Galen had no objection to watching such physical activity, allowing patients to go to wrestling matches, and the theatre, as part of their convalescence if this would help in their recovery.[115] But if one wished to exercise oneself Galen recommended using a small medicine ball to tone up the body.[116]

Galen says remarkably little about bathing, traditionally part of the lifestyle of every Roman. Moralists might denounce the evils of bathing, and even its partisans might acknowledge that, along with wine and sex, 'bathing ruins our bodies'.[117] But it also made life worth living, as both literary texts and the archaeological remains of large thermal complexes from all over the ancient world abundantly testify.[118] As part of the therapeutic process, Galen does occasionally recommend bathing, especially in mineral springs such as the Aquae Albulae near Rome, but he is very cautious about its effects.[119] Too much bathing renders the flesh soft, white and flabby, and produces the sort of moist diseases that are found in women. Moderation is again his watchword.[120]

If dietetics failed, Galen usually turned next to drugs, seeking to regulate disorder by using a drug of opposite quality or action to restore the body's original balance. But to do this properly one needed to know why and how a particular drug worked. Galen accepted that, often, the Empiricists' practice of employing in similar cases a drug already proven effective was likely to work, but when faced with an unknown patient and an uncertain condition to rely merely on past cases was to trust to luck rather than judgment. The true doctor not only tailored his medicaments to the individual patient (unlike the Methodists with their commonalities), but also knew why one drug was likely to work better than another.[121]

In making this claim, Galen was, as far as we can tell, going beyond earlier writers and combining the diverse approaches of Dioscorides and Scribonius Largus within a specifically medical framework.[122] He studied carefully the properties of drugs (predominantly simples, rather than compounds), and he related them closely to the elemental qualities that he found within the body and in his Aristotelian physical universe. Most drugs, he concluded, acted on the body through one or more of the four primary qualities, hot, cold, wet and dry, but there was a further class of drugs whose activity could not easily be assigned by investigation to any one or to any pair of the qualities but whose efficacy had been shown by long experience.[123] These drugs Galen believed worked through their 'total substance', their individual components mixing together in such a way as to produce a new and more effective combination.[124] Most of Galen's 'strongest' drugs, including purgatives, poisons and near-poisons, fell into this category, which offered a way of accounting for many drugs that had long been used empirically. Unlike drugs with qualities that counteracted the excess or deficiency of the same qualities in the

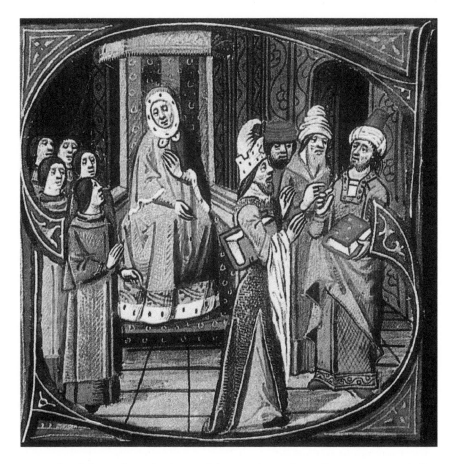

Figure 16.1 Galen explains the theory of drugs to his students. His opponents, including Asclepiades, Archigenes and Erasistratus, are less enthusiastic. Dresden, Sächsische Landesbibliothek, Db 93, fol. 390r.

patient, these drugs operated directly on the part affected through some affinity with it. A phlegmagogue, for instance, attracted phlegm, a cholagogue excessive bile, and expelled it from the body swiftly and effectively.[125]

Galen's theory of drugs thus brought together two separate aspects of pharmacology. On the one hand, in treatises like *On the Properties of Simples* he investigated how and why individual substances worked as they did. On the other, in his two huge treatises *On the Composition of Drugs* he examined their suitability in treatment from two complementary perspectives, that of the part of the body affected and that of the types of drug available.[126] The same recipe could thus be discussed both as a remedy for headache and as an example of a plaster, pill or lotion, while its individual components were analysed theoretically elsewhere. Galen did not see these as distinct methodologies. Rather, they all formed part of a single overall conception of therapeutics and of a project that occupied him for more than half a century. His early treatise on *Drugs*, lost in the fire at the Temple of Peace in 192, was subsequently rewritten and expanded enormously, yet it is also striking how deftly Galen was able to interrupt his work on pharmacology and then take it up again, sometimes decades later, without major inconsistencies.[127]

Evaluating the thousands of pages of his writings on pharmacology is an immense task. But modern research has succeeded in establishing at least the outlines of his vast output.[128] It is now clear that well over half of the recipes he cites are taken directly, and often verbatim, from a small range of intermediate sources, Dioscorides and a body of writers on pharmacology active in the previous century – Heras of Cappadocia, Servilius Damocrates, Asclepiades the Pharmacist, Statilius Crito, Archigenes and the two Andromachi, doctors respectively to Nero and Trajan.[129] But Galen by no means always reproduced what they said without comment. He frequently corrected a recipe or introduced an alternative that he thought superior, either from another source or of his own invention – Galen's so-called *Hiera* ('Holy Drug'), a bitter purgative recommended for almost anything from headache to period pains, was far more familiar to doctors in early mediaeval Europe than any of his medical treatises.[130]

And Galen would not be Galen if he had not added his own individual touches to the information he received from others. Time and again he insisted that what he was doing was bringing an appropriate 'method', 'argument' or 'reasoning' to a familiar subject that had for too long been handled empirically.[131] His theoretical innovation did not end here, for he expressed his dissatisfaction with a model that, like Dioscorides, described the working of drugs in terms solely of possessing the property of acting in a particular way. This formulation was both ambiguous and unhelpful, for it was not precise enough to account for the different results that might be obtained by giving, for instance, one purgative rather than another, and it appeared to take little account of the patient to whom it was given. A Hippocratic doctor wishing to choose a treatment appropriate to the individual sufferer required a more profound understanding of drug action than the bald statement that, for instance, scammony removes bile.

One solution to this problem put forward by Galen was to classify the action of drugs into four main categories or grades of intensity, weak, obvious, strong and massive, each of which was subdivided further into three: small, moderate and substantial.[132] At one end of the spectrum were substances so powerful that the slightest of applications resulted in the immediate destruction of the part or the death of the patient – some caustics and poisons, for example. At the other were simple herbs whose action was almost totally imperceptible, to be used in cases where extreme delicacy or precision of treatment was required. Other substances could be located along this spectrum according to the intensity of their qualitative action.

But to categorise in this way the properties of all, or even most, drugs was no small task, as Galen himself admitted. In his investigation of 475 botanical simples, he provided detailed grades for only one-third, 161.[133] But correlating the intensity of drug action with the patient's condition was even harder. There was no instrumentation that would allow even the rough precision demanded by Galen's schema for classifying drugs, let alone patients. Not surprisingly perhaps, Galen put forward over the years a variety of apparently conflicting suggestions. Writing in the 160s, in the first part of the *Method of Healing*, he asserted that there might be fifteen different degrees of a dry distemper, each requiring one of fifteen different degrees of moistening.[134] Thirty years later, in his *Art of Medicine*, he proposed that if a particular part was ten times hotter than normal and seven times drier it should require a remedy ten times colder and seven times moister than the norm.[135] It is not easy to see how either formulation fits with the twelve categories of drug action that he adopted in his studies of simples and which formed the basis for later Galenic pharmacology, particularly in the Islamic world.

But Galen was far from being purely a theoretician. Indeed, the most striking feature of his pharmacology is his insistence on empirical observation and on securing the widest range of alternative therapies, either through books or through talking with others. At some point in the 160s Galen heard of a doctor in the backwoods of Bithynia (N.W. Turkey) who had discovered a herb that could thin blood to such an extent that it could dissolve any clot. Having found the man and learned of the drug, Galen, somewhat unsportingly one might think, handed him over to the authorities, who subjected him to torture. When he revealed that this was a herb found in profusion and that he had experimented with it on humans, he was hauled off to execution lest he start an epidemic of murder. Galen, of course, maintained a judicious silence about what he had learned, while accusing his rivals of heedlessly including in their books potentially deadly information.[136]

His collection of recipes was, he believed, before the fire of 192 the best in the world. Two major collections had been passed on to him, some recipes he devised for himself and others he obtained by exchanging some of his rarities for those of others.[137] His acquisition of the actual drugs around the Mediterranean was equally wide-ranging. He interviewed shippers at Alexandria, he bargained with a camel driver for his load of medicaments, he visited the Dead Sea and the coast of Lycia in search of rare minerals that he might stock up on to use for the rest of his life, and, as a friend of the superintendent, he was permitted to go down a mine on Cyprus to obtain copper ores.[138] In 168, on his way to Italy, he called in at the island of Lemnos in order to obtain some seals of the famous Lemnian earth.[139] By mischance or geographical ignorance, he landed on the wrong side of the island and had to wait for another twenty years or more before he could return. This time he was more fortunate, arriving just after the ceremony in which the priestess of Diana blessed the hill from which the earth was extracted. Never one to miss an opportunity of bulk buying, Galen bought 20,000 of these medicinal seals, stamped with the image of Diana, which he used successfully to treat wounds and as emetics against poisoning by the 'sea-hare' mollusc or by blister-beetles.

In Rome he knew where to find the sellers of viper flesh or of a special type of thin cord for ligatures, imported from Gaul and sold just off the Via Sacra that led from the Temple of Rome to the main Forum.[140] As one of the emperor's doctors he had the run of the palace stores, where baskets of rare herbs, sent by imperial rootcutters from that botanical Eden Crete, were stored sometimes for decades.[141] It was here that he found a whole cinnamon bush, seven feet tall, that had been brought in fifty years before, when theriac, a complicated antidote originally ascribed to Mithridates VI, was in fashion and when the Emperor Marcus Aurelius used to take a small daily dose as a sort of tonic.[142] In all he had to hand some eighty pounds of theriac, more cinnamon than could be found in all the Roman pharmacies put together, and many other choice ingredients, all destroyed in the fire of 192.[143] When Septimius Severus became emperor in 193 and asked Galen to prepare him some theriac, the more modern ingredients were found to be somewhat less effective. This did not deter those who wished to copy the imperial example, and at least, so Galen noted, by taking the common good as their aim the new emperors had turned a secret of the *cognoscenti* into a remedy accessible to all.[144]

Galen frequently emphasised the absolute necessity of obtaining a detailed, first-hand acquaintance with drugs.[145] Only in this way could one detect the tricks of unscrupulous dealers who passed off inferior products as genuine Hymettian honey or Laodicean spikenard, stuffed the stems of their plants with useless substances and filled the bottom of their drug baskets with weeds or simply earth.[146] Away from the big city, a country doctor, unable to afford a wide range of drugs and requiring a small selection that he could easily take with him on his journeys, was well advised to rely on what was available locally, supplemented by windfalls, literally and metaphorically.[147] Even in Rome, a sound knowledge of the humble plants and herbs growing in the woods and fields just beyond the city gates would prove both profitable and beneficial to one's patients, even if some of the more snobbishly wealthy disdained to be treated with a cheap local drug.[148] Then, according to Galen, what the doctor needed to know was how to add the harmless spices, perfumes and the like that would push up the price while not destroying the drug's effectiveness.[149]

Galen's pharmacological writings thus display his typical combination of intelligent reasoning, detailed observation and empirical testing along-side a passionate urge to correct the mistakes of others and to demonstrate his own superiority. He saw his therapeutics, the healing of the sick, as the culmination of a range of other skills, in logic, argument, understanding and experiment. His ideal doctor, as represented by Hippocrates, combines reason and experience, book learning and personal skills, anatomical knowl-edge and speculation about the natural world in general, intuition and sound judgment.[150] Although Galen's orotundity, his pedantry, his desire to have his own cake and eat it, and his constant insistence on his own superiority may jar on us, as they did on some of his Byzantine readers, enough remains in his writings to show how he came to acquire so swiftly the reputation of being a great and effective doctor.[151] Galen is an impressive and challenging figure, and it is only too easy to succumb to his powerful rhetoric – or to be repelled by his constant self-praise and tendentious arguments. A survey of the activities of other practitioners, such as we shall now attempt, is essential to gaining a balanced perspective, not only on Galen but also on the whole medical world of the Roman Empire.

17

ALL SORTS AND CONDITIONS OF
(MAINLY) MEN

It is essential, when considering the roles and social position of the providers of healing in the ancient world, to be careful about assuming that they formed a coherent group whose status, reputation and ideology can be clearly determined.[1] It is true that some ancient authors talked about a 'profession of medicine' and sought to lay down universal standards of behaviour, but the context in which they made these demands suggests that they were frequently disregarded, not least because many of the institutions that today support the notion of a medical profession were entirely absent.[2] Similarly, even the broadest of definitions of a doctor, as a person who offered to treat illness for money, does not allow for the fact that he or she might be carrying on other profitable activities at the same time, or might have switched to medicine from a totally different occupation.[3] Even distinguishing terms such as 'high' and 'low', 'formal' and 'informal' medicine cannot entirely capture a historical situation in which the predominant feature is the fluidity of all defining boundaries. Indeed, rather than employ a succession of dichotomies demarcating good healers from bad, professional from amateur, religious from secular, in an attempt to define what an ancient doctor was and did, one might more appropriately adopt the metaphor of a series of overlapping spectra, on which can be mapped the great diversity of data concerning the wealth, status, education, ideology and methods of the practitioners of healing in Antiquity, particularly in the first three centuries of the Christian era. That there were lines of demarcation between those who were called, or who called themselves, 'doctors', *iatroi* or *medici*, and those who were not, is beyond doubt. But where those lines were drawn was a matter of individual choice and of individual context, as we shall see. Galen's view of who should be a doctor, and what he or she ought to be able to do, differed substantially from that of Thessalus of Tralles, and the perspective of both of these metropolitan practitioners would in turn differ from that of a patient or a doctor in Britain, the Nile Valley or the mountains of central Asia Minor. Besides, the title of doctor in no way guaranteed competence.[4] As the Alexandrian Jew Philo put it around AD 50:

> In medicine there are those who know almost everything there is to know about treating affections, diseases and ailments, yet who can give no account of them, whether accurate or even plausible. On the other hand there are those who are marvellous expositors of the signs, causes and therapies that make up the art of medicine, but who are hopeless at treating the sick and contribute not a jot to their recovery.[5]

One major reason for this fluidity is undoubtedly the absence of any legal criterion setting out who could or could not be called a doctor. Although the law, particularly in Rome, defined certain medical practices as unlawful – poisoning, giving love potions and performing castration – it did not at first say who was a doctor.[6] Even when it did, the ruling of the lawyer Ulpian acknowledged the principal difficulty. In offering his opinion as to who was entitled to sue for fees as a medical practitioner, he allowed specialists in the treatment of ears, fistulae and teeth, as well as midwives 'who have apparently shown a knowledge of medicine'. But he drew the line at those who used incantations, imprecations and exorcisms, 'even though some have claimed to have received benefits from them'.[7] He defined a *medicus* as someone who used physical methods to treat his patients, while at the same time he was forced to acknowledge that healing could be achieved by other means, and that the line might be drawn differently by those who concentrated on the result, not the means, of intervention.

Only in two respects, taxation and civic salaries, do we find traces of a system of public examination that would help to differentiate between approved and non-approved healers. The appointment of a civic doctor by a town council, common in the Hellenistic world as we have seen, allowed potential patients the opportunity to investigate their future physician, and the honorary decrees often given at the conclusion of a civic contract could be regarded as a testimonial for distinguished services rendered. But there will have been many other healers who neither performed so well before the town councillors nor even applied for such a post.

Tax privileges applied across a much wider range of practitioners. A fragmentary decree from the 30s BC records the granting of a certain degree of tax immunity and exemption from military call-up and billeting to all doctors in the Roman Empire. This was not a totally new idea, even if its extension to the whole Roman Empire may have been: it confirmed a practice widespread among the Hellenistic cities and familiar from surviving honorary decrees.[8] Its universal application may also be compared with the grant of citizenship to all doctors working in the city of Rome made by Julius Caesar about fifteen years earlier and later confirmed by his heir, Augustus.[9] This was a considerable privilege, for it carried a new and superior legal status as well as freedom from public obligations (liturgies) in the doctor's native town.[10] It must have been regulated in some way, but how and by whom is unclear. Evidence from Roman Egypt suggests that it was necessary to make a declaration before a magistrate that one was a doctor, probably accompanied by some form of testimonial, in order to obtain the appropriate tax privileges. The criteria may have been easily fulfilled. In 142 a local doctor, Psasnis, appeared before the governor of Egypt to protest against his fellow villagers' illegal imposition of duties from which he was exempt as a doctor. The governor's response was cutting: they had possibly found his treatments useless. However, if he returned to his local region and made the appropriate declaration his immunity would be restored.[11] Tax immunity, it would seem, was no guarantee of competence.

But one man's immunity is also another's extra burden, and this universal freedom was restricted by a decision of the Emperor Antoninus Pius, probably in the early 140s, who allowed a maximum of five, seven or ten immune doctors, depending on the size and rank of the city.[12] The choice was made by the town council, made up of laymen and potential patients – not until the creation of the super-elite College of Physicians in Rome in 358 is there a legal reference to any selection made by fellow doctors alone.[13] A further series of decisions followed from then on, setting out the criteria on which councils were to base their choice, 'sound morals and expertise in the art', and warning against yielding to fear or favour.[14] This creation of a 'select group entitled to the benefits given to doctors' must have left out others who were almost equally capable, particularly if, as seems likely, Pius intended to enlarge considerably the number of those now compelled to undertake liturgies. Some privileges may still have remained to those who were excluded, for the law codes show a constant struggle by these lesser individuals over the next four centuries to retain what little was left to them, while their better-connected confrères, the city physicians and court doctors, gained ever-greater honours and authority.[15]

But the law was not the only means of defining who was or was not a doctor. From at least the first century onwards, there were 'colleges', confraternities or clubs, sometimes exclusively of doctors, but sometimes formed in conjunction with other groups, such as teachers. At Rome and at Ephesus their clubhouse was a substantial building adorned with statues and plaques recording honorary decrees.[16] Some of their activities were purely social or religious: attending an annual banquet, guarding the tombs of former members or sacrificing to Asclepius.[17] At Smyrna, the doctors contributed in large part to the (re)building of the lighthouse.[18] But other activities had a more medical character. At Ephesus, the walls of the 'Hall of the Muses' were adorned with the records of the victors in the medical contests held annually over the two days of the great festival of Asclepius.[19] At least two of those named as winners or officials are known to have held civic magistracies and priesthoods, and similar wealth can be assumed for several other leading doctors of the city.[20] But whether only the rich were accepted into the college, or whether, as in mediaeval Florence, any healer could join, is an open question. When in AD 7 the *plethos* of doctors at Alexandria came together to honour with a statue Caius Proculeius Themison the *archiatros*, we cannot tell for certain if this group included all the surgeons, the masseurs and the other healers who thronged the small streets of the city or was a more restricted body.[21] Although one might suspect that only the educated and successful would join such a group, it is possible that the rich and powerful constituted its leadership and that the inherent bias of the epigraphic evidence towards the wealthy has robbed us of information on its lesser members. Certainly in Rome a wide variety of medical craftsmen participated in the Quinquatrus, a festival in honour of Minerva that lasted from 19 to 23 March each year, when weavers, fullers, dyers, cobblers, doctors, teachers, painters and engravers marched together in procession round the city.[22]

This public assertion of membership of an occupational group helped to define who was a *medicus*, at least for those who watched the processions or read the results of the medical contests, but it did not prevent others outside

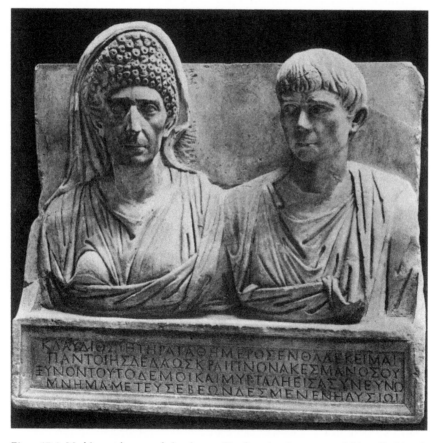

Figure 17.1 Marble tombstone of the doctor Claudius Agathemerus and his wife Myrtale (ANMichaelis.155), Rome, *c*.AD 100. Ashmolean Museum, University of Oxford.

257

this group from offering healing or from calling themselves or being called *medici*. We have already met Galen's quack from Syria, the wandering healing prophets of Palestine, the snake-handling Marsi and their even more exotic equivalents, the Psylli and Nasamones.[23] At Athens, a medicine man, 'one of those who put snakes on display', came to a gruesome end when, in a display before his fellow professionals, he could not immediately rinse his mouth of the asp poison he had just sucked from a bite on his arm because his water jug had overturned. Suppuration and physical disintegration set in, and he died in agony two days later.[24] Others pursued less dangerous specialisms, under a variety of titles. In Egypt and the Levant there were doctors specialising in circumcisions – in Egypt the 'circumcision doctor' became an official post after the 120s.[25] Elea in S. Italy, with its *pholeon* (a quasi-religious organisation) of doctors that looked back to the philosopher Parmenides, was also home in the Early Empire to a 'doctor–prophet'.[26] Nor should one forget the travelling healer, wandering from fair to fair with a limited range of drugs, or the oculists of Britain and the N.W. provinces, whose sets of surgical instruments suggest that their expertise extended beyond the treatment of eye diseases with salves.[27] A listing of some of the names who are credited in Galen's drug books with particular recipes gives a neat indication of the variety of occupations that might be concerned with human health: Achillas the eye-coucher; Antonius the drug dealer; Apollonius the pharmacist; Axius, doctor in the British fleet; Celer the centurion; Diogas the trainer; Euschemus the eunuch; Flavius the boxer; Orion the groom; Pharnaces the Persian rootcutter; Philoxenus the school master; and Simmias the crowd-puller (or mountebank).[28]

Another name on Galen's list, Aquillia Secundilla, who had a favourite recipe against lumbago, serves as a reminder of the importance of domestic medicine, and of women's roles in it.[29] Her Roman name also suggests that she belonged to a level of society in which one might take an intellectual interest in medicine without ever descending to practice, save perhaps on one's immediate household. Many distinguished authors from the Roman Imperial period wrote at length about medicine, and expected their readers to share that interest. Cornelius Celsus, as we have seen, composed his eight books *On Medicine* as part of a wide-ranging encyclopaedia of *Arts and Sciences* for the instruction of his fellow gentlemen. The Greek moralist Plutarch of Chaeronea, around 110, had the interlocutors in his *Table Talk* discuss a variety of medical topics from anatomy to new diseases.[30] Fifty years later, Aulus Gellius, recalling youthful debates in the Athens of Herodes Atticus, regarded it as disgraceful for a man of education to be unaware of the distinction between veins and arteries.[31] This was a mistake that would hardly have been made by the senators, ex-consuls and imperial relatives who attended Galen's anatomical displays or came with him to the bedside of the sick, and who later demanded from him copies of his lectures.[32] The orator Apuleius, on trial for sorcery around 140, produced a string of medical arguments,

258

citing Plato, Aristotle and Theophrastus on epilepsy, to show that his accusers, unlike the learned judge, were mere country bumpkins, only too capable of mistaking medicine for magic.[33] L. Annaeus Seneca (d. 65), tutor to the Emperor Nero, displays in his writings such a command of medicine that he convinced a nineteenth-century medical historian that he must have also been an experienced medical practitioner.[34] Seneca's knowledge, however, is more likely to have come from books and from his own struggles with asthma and ill health under the guidance of his physician ('whose constant attentions have turned him from hireling into friend') or in the gymnasium as he tried to carry out the instructions of his unforgiving trainers.[35]

The existence of such learned lay men and women, which is presupposed by Galen in his treatise on how to choose the best physician, is a characteristic that marks off Greek and Roman medicine from that of many other societies.[36] But it should not be allowed to obscure one important fact. The practitioners of the healing arts rarely came from the highest levels of society. Seneca's honeyed praise of his doctor shows the low expectations he originally had of him, while Cicero's eulogy of medicine as a 'liberal and well-bred art', even if it is his own and not taken from a Greek author, is subtly qualified by its context. It is, indeed, a noble art, but only by comparison with the work of tax collectors, carpenters, cooks and dancers: it ranks below oratory, politics and estate agriculture, and is suitable only for those of 'an appropriate social class'.[37] Cicero, of course, was not among them. This disdain lasted a long while. The ex-consul and historian Cassius Dio regarded the attempt of Gellius Maximus, the son of an imperial doctor, to become emperor in 219 as the culminating proof of the decadence of society.[38]

Such an opinion was only to be expected in a society that placed considerable value on *otium*, the leisured independence of the land-owning gentleman. Hence the delight that Galen took at being addressed as a 'gentleman' by his grateful patient, the Emperor Marcus Aurelius, for this was an acknowledgment of his social position as well as of his independence of thought. In this way the emperor elevated Galen above the average doctor, who, it is clear, was on the social level of an artisan, possessing neither wealth nor importance.[39] Galen's attempt in his *Exhortation to Medicine* to include lawyers alongside doctors in his circle of superior practitioners, 'whose art does not fail them even as they grow old', is a piece of special pleading, for doctors in general were neither as wealthy nor as politically and socially prominent as lawyers.[40] In the many small towns and villages of Roman Egypt the doctor, when not exempt, paid roughly the same amount in taxes as the village carpenter, and he rarely figured among the elite of the large towns.[41]

A similar pattern of social status can be recognised in another type of source with a wider geographical distribution – astrological handbooks. Their authors offer long lists of occupations associated together under the same star or planet. Under the protection of Mercury, for instance, they placed doctors, lawyers, teachers, grammarians, rhetors, architects, priests, prophets, astronomers, dream interpreters, sculptors, weavers, musicians and wandering magi, many of whom processed together in Rome at the Quinquatrus.[42] By themselves these listings reveal little, but when taken with other comments by their authors they enable us to be a little more precise about where in society one might find a doctor. For Vettius Valens, a contemporary of Galen, doctors were intelligent but fickle, learned but addicted to novelty and foreign travel (*xeniteia*). They were numbered among the providers of luxury – perfumiers, goldsmiths and sword-dancers – and it took little for them to join the even less respectable classes, the travelling salesmen, the mountebanks, the money-changers, the counterfeiters, the coiners and the forgers.[43] Two hundred years later, there is little that separates the doctor from the cook, the corpse-washer and the undertaker. The *medicus* leads a moderate life: he is a member of the middle class, but only precariously so. He is always in danger of poverty and of descending to the level of snake-charmers, sellers of poisons and inveterate liars. According to Firmicus Maternus, writing in the fourth century, it takes only the tiniest change in the position of a star at birth to determine whether one becomes famous, a leading politician, a judge or the like, or merely a doctor, a surgeon, a soldier or a gladiator.[44] Only a very few doctors are likely to join the lawyers and administrators in amassing great wealth and influence. This select few will be entrusted with legations from their own cities to the emperors; they will enjoy the friendship of kings; but they will pay for it. After much toilsome and tedious travel, they will come to a violent end through offending their monarch.[45]

Firmicus' heavenly map of the doctor's career finds close parallels among the inscriptions of doctors from the first three centuries of the Roman Empire. At the very top of the pyramid were those who served the emperor and his immediate family, or the leading members of the court, the Senate and the imperial bureaucracy. Although in the first century many were originally non-citizens who gained citizenship through their service at court or in Rome, they often came from respectable families in the Greek world or from Marseilles, that outpost of Greek culture beyond the Alps.[46] Direct access to the emperor meant, or was assumed to mean, direct access to power and its fruits – wealth, prestige and patronage. Honours and money were heaped on Antonius Musa for his cold-water cure of Augustus in the crisis of 23 BC, and the island of Samos hailed him as its benefactor even after his fall from favour for failing to cure Augustus' nephew and chosen successor, C. Claudius Marcellus.[47] But proximity to the emperor also attracted hostility. Pliny the Elder's denunciation of the leading doctors of Rome is a powerful indictment of lustful greed. He derides Arruntius, Charmis, Crinas and Alcon for their huge fees, even though they spent them on public works, rebuilding a city wall or erecting a beautiful temple. Eudemus and Vettius Valens are accused of an even worse crime, adultery with their royal patients.[48] The jokes of satirists, Greek as well as Latin, about the propensity of doctors to have sex with their female patients, and to murder their husbands to cover up their

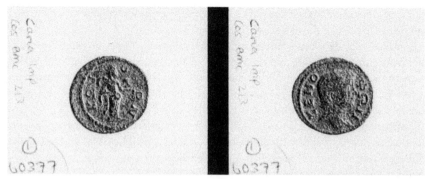

Figure 17.2 A bronze coin struck by the island of Cos around AD 50. The obverse shows the head of C. Stertinius Xenophon, doctor to the Emperor Claudius (see below), along with the name Xenophon. On the reverse, the goddess Hygieia feeds the sacred snake of Asclepius. British Museum, Reg. No. 1850,1128.56. © The Trustees of the British Museum.

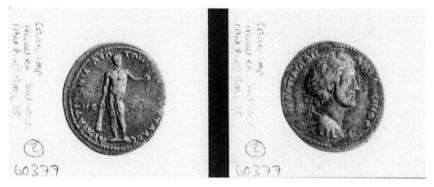

Figure 17.3 A bronze coin struck by the city of Heraclea Salbace between 150 and 161 to commemorate a gift to its Youth Association by the Methodist Statilius Attalus, Galen's colleague and rival at the Roman court (see p. 258). The obverse shows the head of the future Emperor Marcus Aurelius, the reverse Hercules and his club. British Museum, Reg. No. 1844,0425.184. © The Trustees of the British Museum.

affairs, are here given a historical context.[49] Every sudden death in the imperial household was attended with rumours of poisoning, whether justified or not. The death of the Emperor Claudius in AD 54 was widely attributed to the wiles of a female herbalist-cum-poisoner, Lucusta, assisted by the emperor's chief physician, C. StertiniusXenophon.[50]

Xenophon, a member of a wealthy family from Cos that claimed descent from both Hercules and Asclepius, exemplifies the new elite physician. Immensely rich – his city practice alone allegedly brought him in 500,000 sesterces annually[51] – he was employed in imperial service for at least fifteen years. He accompanied the Emperor Claudius on his expedition to Britain in AD 43, for which he received military decorations appropriate to his (honorary) titles as centurion and 'Superintendent of the Engineers' (*praefectus fabrum*). Ten years later his ministrations preserved Claudius in a serious illness. He also acted as one of the emperor's Greek secretaries, and was publicly numbered among the 'friends and councillors' of both Claudius and Nero. On Cos both coins and a large number of inscriptions to him and his family commemorated his benefactions to his native island – heading an embassy to secure its freedom from Roman tribute, among other things, and serving as priest for life of the imperial cult. His devotion to Asclepius was evinced by his priesthood at the great shrine and, above all, by the new buildings he erected there, a library, a small temple and bath houses with improved plumbing.[52]

Fifty years later another imperial doctor, Statilius Crito, followed a similar career. A member of a wealthy family from the small town of Heraclea Salbace in Caria (central Turkey), Crito moved to Rome, where he became doctor to the Emperor Trajan about AD 100. He was famous as a historian, writing in Greek his 'Gothic wars', a record of Trajan's campaigns north of the Danube in what is now Hungary and Romania. More remains today of his writings on pharmacology, for which he drew in part on a treatise on cosmetics ascribed, almost certainly wrongly, to the greatest beauty of her age, Queen Cleopatra of Egypt.[53] He too received honours and offices: he became an imperial procurator, at least in rank, and when he retired to his native region he was honoured with numerous priesthoods. He was a benefactor of both Heraclea and the metropolis of Ephesus, where the 'doctors who sacrifice to their ancestor Asclepius and to the emperors' erected a grateful memorial to him.[54] He was a member of a prolific medical family at Heraclea, at least one of whom (his great-nephew?), Statilius Attalus, also entered imperial service in the 150s and was a prominent benefactor of his native city.[55] A younger contemporary of Attalus as an imperial doctor, L. Gellius Maximus, also became a government procurator and gave generously to his home town of Antioch in Pisidia.[56]

Men like this, in close relationship with the emperor, acted as a conduit for the aspirations of their family and their cities. They were on easy terms with senators, they stayed on visits in the best houses in town and they were perceived to possess power and influence, although whether it was their medical or their social skills that attracted the notice of the emperor in the first place can never be known.[57] Even those a little lower down the social scale might benefit from a relationship with the emperor, however remote. Calpurnius Asclepiades, a doctor from Prusa (N.W. Turkey), obtained citizenship from Trajan for himself, his parents and his four brothers, as well as a nice sinecure as one of the assistants to the magistrates at elections both in Rome and in Asia Minor.[58] How patronage might work is revealed both by Calpurnius' boast that his 'learning and morals had gained the approval of very distinguished men' and by the anxious letters of the younger Pliny following his illness in 98.[59] Pliny first asked the new Emperor Trajan for citizenship for his masseur, an Egyptian called Harpocras, the ex-slave of an Egyptian woman.

262

Scarcely had his request been granted when Pliny discovered that Roman citizenship should be conferred on Egyptians only if they were already citizens of Alexandria. Pliny's apology and further request for Alexandrian citizenship met with a somewhat grudging response from the emperor: the whole procedure was most unusual, but since he had already granted Harpocras Roman citizenship he saw no alternative but to allow the petition. Within a few months Pliny was back with a further request for citizenship, this time for several relatives of his Greek doctor, Marinus.[60]

Harpocras, as a mere masseur and a non-citizen of Alexandria, was socially inferior to the many physicians who came from medical families in the Greek East with deep roots in their locality, such as the Statilii at Heraclea in Caria, the Philalethae at Men Karou or the Acilii of Claudiopolis. At least three generations of the family of Moschianus served as civic physicians at Thyateira (Asia Minor).[61] As local worthies, they contributed to shrines and festivals, became civic magistrates, went on embassies and participated generously in the cultural life of their communities.[62] It is hardly surprising that men such as this might occasionally marry into other wealthy families with links to the court and the Roman administration, or that a local bigwig might allow his son to take up medicine as a career, like Lucius, a member of a moderately wealthy family from Maeonia in Lydia, who died while studying with a local doctor, Tatianus.[63] Had he lived longer than nineteen years, he might have ventured further afield, like the young men from similar families who travelled hundreds of miles for their medical education, moving from Tieium on the Black Sea to Smyrna, or from Pergamum and Adada in Phrygia to Alexandria.[64] But these were the elite of their profession, and one should not forget there were many poorer healers in the Greek-speaking world – witness the requests to Galen to provide alternative ingredients for his recipes that might be more easily obtainable and at a cheaper price, and his gifts of books and instruments to those less well off than himself.[65] Such practitioners will have travelled only a short distance for their education, if at all. Most of them will have learned their skills from other members of their family, a father, a master, even a husband, or they may have been self-taught.

This pattern of status in Asia Minor differs markedly from that of Rome, Italy and, although the evidence is far less in quantity, the Latin-speaking provinces. Here remarkably few *medici* are recorded on inscriptions as holding municipal offices, priesthoods and the like. Only one doctor, C. Julius Rogatianus, from Sufetula in Africa, is named as a magistrate, and there are no recorded holders of priestly office, except for a dozen or so *seviri Augustales*, officials in a cult of emperor-worship largely managed by ex-slaves.[66] Very few doctors appear to belong to families with long connections with a particular town: indeed, the great majority bear names indicating an immigrant origin. A rough estimate suggests that 90 per cent of doctors named on inscriptions in the first century of the Roman Empire had Greek names, and the percentage was still over 60 per cent two centuries later.[67] In the city of Rome itself in this period more than 90 per cent of the names of doctors are Greek, and only in N. Africa does the number of non-Greek names equal the number of Greek.[68] A similar preponderance of Greek names is to be found on the several hundred so-called oculists' stamps discovered in Gaul, Britain and Germany.[69]

A second, related, discrepancy between the East and West is the much higher proportion in the West of doctors, of both sexes, who are slaves or ex-slaves. This very obvious divergence may in part be explained by differences in the so-called epigraphic habit: more public decrees are known from the Greek East, and Rome in particular had many burial sites associated with the households of the emperors or wealthy senators. Most of the vast array of slaves and ex-slaves within these households were looked after by doctors who were themselves of similar status, organised into 'decuries', groups of ten, as with other occupations within the household. There were both male and female medical personnel, some of them bred and trained for that purpose within the imperial palace.[70]

But these factors alone cannot account for these marked differences between the East and West, especially when they are confirmed by our literary evidence. Even if one views cautiously Galen's assertion that Rome acted as a magnet for incompetent provincial doctors from the Greek East (as well as for a few with greater talent), the doctors in Seneca's writings and in Pliny's letters are all foreigners. The satirist Juvenal's inclusion of the doctor, along

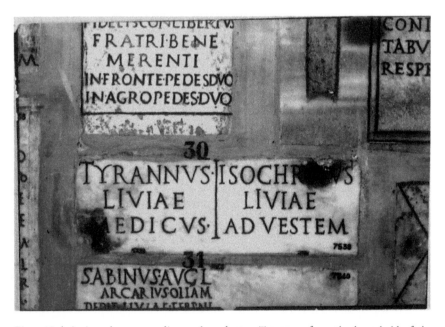

Figure 17.4 A tiny plaque recording a slave doctor, Tyrannus, from the household of the Empress Livia in Rome. *CIL* 6, 3985. Courtesy of the Vatican Museums.

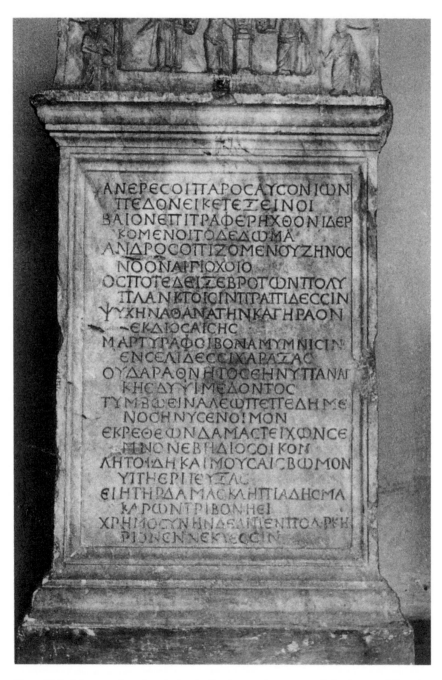

Figure 17.5 A long, verbose inscription in Greek verse in memory of the doctor–philosopher Asclepiades (fl. AD 300). *IG* 14, 1424. Courtesy of the Vatican Museums.

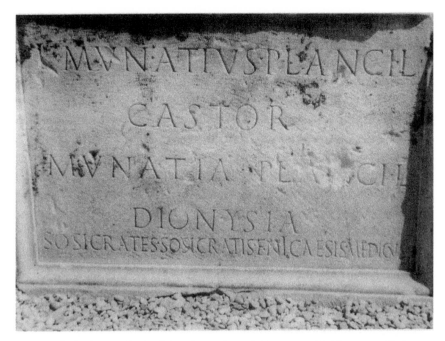

Figure 17.6 Tombstone of a Greek immigrant doctor in Rome, *c.*AD 20. The name of Sosicrates,
son of Sosicrates, of Nicaea, is squeezed onto the bottom of a tomb inscription
recording two ex-slaves of the Munatius family. Rome, Museo delle Terme.

with the masseur, the teacher, the painter, the fortune-teller, the magician
and the tightrope-walker, as the typical profession of the 'hungry Greekling',
is not wide of the mark.[71] This perception that medicine was in some way
foreign, carried out often by immigrants, ex-slaves or transitory practitioners,
must have contributed to the relative absence of doctors holding public office
in the West, even if few observers took their dislike to the extent that Cato
and Pliny did. The modern British experience with doctors coming from
Africa, India and Pakistan (or with dentists from S. Africa) provides a useful
insight into these ancient attitudes, even without the complications of being
treated by slaves and ex-slaves. It suggests that the process of assimilation
could take a considerable time, and that stereotypes would continue to define
attitudes for several generations.

That is not to say that doctors in the West could not make money; one
of the attractions of Rome and Italy was the possibility of finding wealthier
patients than in a small town in central Asia Minor. The mausoleum of the
Greek doctor Patron and his family in Rome was decorated with beautiful
frescoes in the very latest style of the Augustan age.[72] The recent discovery of
the house of a physician at Rimini bespeaks a fair degree of wealth, while the
so-called house of the surgeon at Pompeii, although not as lavish as some in
the town, is in no way the home of a pauper.[73] That Trimalchio-like figure,

266

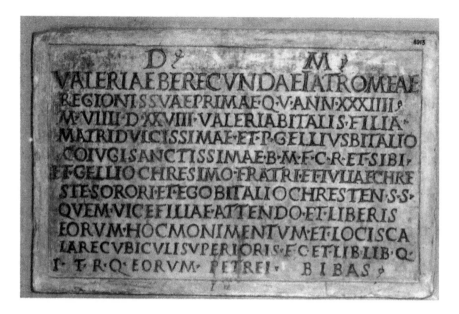

Figure 17.7 The tombstone of Valeria Berecunda, 'the first midwife of her region', who died aged 34. *CIL* 6, 9477. Rome, courtesy of the Vatican Museums.

the ex-slave P. Decimius Merula Eros, 'clinician, oculist, and surgeon', paid 2,000 *sestertii* (HS) for the office of *sevir*, and donated 30,000 HS for statues at the temple of Hercules at Assisi and 37,000 for paving roads, as well as leaving 800,000 HS at his death. He was made to pay for his ambition too: the 50,000 HS he gave for his freedom was well above the contemporary norm of 2,000 HS.[74] At Beneventum in the second century the son of a Greek immigrant (possibly himself a doctor) became a civic doctor and made enough money to rank as a knight. But it was his son, almost certainly not a doctor, who became a local magistrate and a benefactor of his fellow citizens.[75]

There were other constraints on making money, not least that of competition. Galen's world is filled with a multiplicity of healers, clustering round the bedside of the sick to offer their independent advice.[76] They are ubiquitous in the epigraphic record. A doctor from Nicaea in Bithynia was buried at tiny Perrhaebia in Thessaly, 'having wandered much over land and sea', unlike Zeuxippus, honoured by the equally small town of Cyparissus as 'an excellent citizen in the tradition of his ancestors, and still continuing to practise'. In the mountains of the Abruzzi, Q. Peticius L.f. Chirurgus prepared a tomb for himself and his family, while at Ameria in Umbria an ex-slave, almost certainly of a doctor, bore the medical name of Hippocrates, freedman of Zeuxis.[77] It is true that it was wiser for an unlucky vine-dresser who had sliced off the top of his finger to come into town to find a surgeon than to wait for one to appear on his rounds, and many wealthy travellers would find it useful to take along their own doctor in their entourage.[78] But doctors were to be found even in tiny places such as Daldis in Asia Minor or Tithorea in S. Greece, derided as an apology for a town by the traveller Pausanias because of its decaying public buildings and its reliance for its water supply on a spring at the foot of the hill.[79] A middling town such as Pompeii may have had almost a surfeit of practitioners, even if not all the twenty-five or so houses with medical instruments were occupied by doctors, and neighbouring towns like Sorrento and Stabiae, recommended by Galen as a good place for those suffering from phthisis, also had their own healers.[80] There was a living to be made in medicine, but one needed access to wealthy patients to profit substantially.

Questions of wealth and status also depend on the starting point of the comparison. We may suppose that most healers found patients, whose attitude depended in large part on whether after treatment they considered themselves cured or in some way improved. But even that consideration would be determined in part by one's initial expectation of a cure, one's appreciation of the abilities, or claims to ability, of the individual healer and the existence of alternatives. All these might vary considerably. Many medical conditions were difficult, if not impossible, to treat with any degree of success, and both those who offered and those who received therapy may have adjusted their hopes accordingly. Similarly, even if the average doctor was not a plutocrat, particularly in a small town, he might be better off than the majority of the population. Between fifteen and twenty-seven of the ninety-seven doctors recorded in the Egyptian papyri from the first two centuries AD had gained Roman citizenship even before the universal grant of citizenship by Caracalla in 212; and many of those who did not possess it do not fall into the lowest category of tax-payers, and appear to be well regarded in their own community.[81] One must also bear in mind that expectations and attitudes would also vary from place to place. The tombstone of the doctor Fadianus Bubbal, portrayed at Caesarea in Mauretania wearing a rough tunic and brandishing a cleaver around AD 200, is far less elegant than the beautiful bust of the Methodist M. Modius Asiaticus at Smyrna or that of the Roman doctor Claudius Agathemerus and his wife two centuries earlier.[82] But these aesthetic judgments merely point to the gulf between provincial and metropolitan conceptions of wealth and beauty. In his own community, Fadianus was relatively unusual in having a sculptured tombstone at all, which suggests that he enjoyed at least moderate riches.

An excellent example of the importance of the local perspective in determining attitudes is found on a gravestone from the island of Cythera, off the southern tip of Greece. A young man would have enjoyed a glorious career, his epitaph declared, had he not been struck down after his medical studies at Boiae on the facing mainland and then at the somewhat larger Sparta.[83] Boiae was hardly more than a village, and Sparta, despite Archagathus and Leonides, scarcely a prestigious medical centre. But a move to the mainland

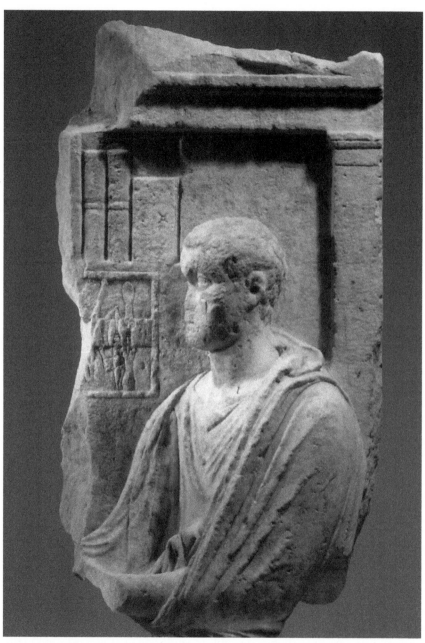

Figure 17.8 A doctor's memorial from Roman Asia Minor. This beautiful tombstone was made in Attica around 375 BC. Four hundred years or so later it was re-used to commemorate an unknown doctor from Asia Minor by carving representations of an open box of medical instruments and of book-rolls. Freiburg im Breisgau, Museum of Classical Archaeology.

and then to the big town of Sparta would have been as challenging to this young islander, and hopefully as rewarding, as the migrations of Galen to more renowned centres of medical instruction.

This enormous variety of practitioners in their wealth, status and education renders problematical any generalisation about their therapeutic methodologies and procedures. What a travelling doctor could do was inevitably limited by the drugs and instruments he had at his disposal, and by the time he could spare before moving on. 'Whoever can cure the sick while on the move?' wondered Seneca, disapprovingly, for 'travel doesn't make a man a doctor'.[84] By contrast, a doctor resident in one town could turn his house into a surgery or a cottage hospital, where the sick might spend several days under the watchful eye of the doctor and his assistants.[85] There were various opportunities for such a man to gain patients or social prestige. Some doctors were retained by the associations of young men, 'ephebes', at Athens and possibly elsewhere.[86] Others accompanied formal civic processions to the shrine of the oracle at Claros and, from time to time, provided medical services to the large crowds assembled for a major festival or the Olympic Games.[87] Others gave public lectures, at times to the bewilderment of their audience.[88] In Spain some doctors may have had contracts with large-scale mining companies to attend to the health of their workmen.[89]

From at least the fourth century BC in Greece doctors were called upon to examine slaves for sale, and their successors in Rome were similarly used to look for signs of epilepsy or a suppurating ear.[90] In Roman Egypt 'public physicians' acted, either alone or in concert, to certify death or injury to the local police authority. They also wrote out the ancient equivalent of sick notes. In AD 316 two 'public doctors' of Oxyrhynchus were sent to examine, at his own request, a member of the governor's staff, and to confirm that he was ill.[91] Whether they were alone entitled to make forensic reports or certify that a person was too ill or infirm to fulfil his tax obligations and whether this system applied outside Egypt are questions impossible to determine with certainty.[92]

Amid this abundance of information one thing stands out. The practice of medicine was a public art. Despite Hippocratic injunctions to secrecy and the existence of 'secret' remedies and techniques, the sick were frequently treated in public, in the midst of eager onlookers. St Luke was reflecting reality when he often set the stories of healing in the *Acts of the Apostles* in the street, just outside a temple or in a house filled with people. There are numerous witnesses, who tell the stories to others, who come flocking in their turn to see the new wonder-worker and to touch the hem of his garment.[93] The doctor's surgery, like a barber's shop or a cobbler's workshop, acts as a meeting place; it is indeed an *ergasterion*, a 'workshop', filled with servants, slaves, customers and possibly the doctor's family all around.[94] In the marketplace prospective patients stood gawping as a doctor showed off his instruments and ministered to the sick, and some might even engage him in animated conversation.[95]

The doctor–craftsman must, like other artisans, expect to perform in front of spectators, not all of whom can stand the sight of a bloody operation.[96] Indeed, it might be wiser at times to tell a lie about postponing the operation to another day, and then act in secret, particularly if the patient is likely to be frightened or ashamed to reveal his buttocks or genitals to an inquisitive crowd. But, even then, it might prove impossible to get rid of everyone from the room, and all the doctor can then do is to whisper to the patient that he will try his best to keep things hidden from their prying eyes.[97] In such a public arena, manner was likely to matter as much as content, announcing what one was doing almost as much as the actual result.[98]

It is not surprising, then, to find that the tombstones of some doctors proudly depict him in action or indicate his profession by a set of medical instruments.[99] One grave-relief from Roman Ostia has the doctor reading in front of his book cabinet.[100] But the extent and nature of medical literacy are hard to determine. Galen, ever keen to stress the importance of book learning, demanded that his fellow practitioners should know the major tenets of a chain of great physicians, from Hippocrates down to Asclepiades of Bithynia.[101] Whether they (or their patients) could consult all these writings in the original is doubtful, despite the existence of a flourishing trade in medical books in Rome. It is likely that most relied on summaries, often produced in question and answer form, that set out the views of great doctors on particular diseases and their treatment.[102] Other authors composed their *Introductions to Medicine* in the form of short definitions of terms, sometimes referring expressly to the views of earlier doctors, followed by brief indications of an appropriate therapy. The same definitions can be found over the centuries, in a variety of forms, in texts of different doctrinal orientation, and in Latin as well as in Greek. But, although this might suggest coherence, they were combined in many different ways, and there might be substantial variations of content even between versions of what purported to be one and the same work.[103] Nor should it be assumed automatically that masters and pupils, even if proclaiming adherence to one medical creed, always understood it in the same way. There was no effective means of securing doctrinal compliance, and, as we have seen with the Methodists and with the Hippocratics before Galen, different emphases might develop over the years, so that the characteristics of a shared belief might alter between generations and between authors. Nor did the ascription of a work to a famous physician of the past in any way guarantee that the doctrines found in it corresponded to those of its alleged author, as Galen found on more than one occasion.[104] The so-called letter of Diocles to King Antigonus (which is also ascribed to Hippocrates and addressed in its various forms to King Antiochus, Ptolemy and even to Maecenas, the friend of the Emperor Augustus) divides the diseases of the body into four groups, depending on the head, the chest, the belly and the bladder.[105] Although the author accepts the Hippocratic notion that aligns different diseases with each season of the year and believes in the four

271

major humours (although he does not use that word), he divides blood into 'sweet' and 'bitter' serums, and his correlation of the predominant humours with the seasons does not correspond to that of *The Nature of Man* or to Galen's schema. Even to call such an author Hippocratic demands courage; to identify him with the historical Diocles, with whom he shares only an interest in dietetics, requires a major leap of faith.

If there were considerable differences of interpretation over medical theory, medical practice presented even larger variations. It was not only that the healer might be confronted by a wide range of diseases. Galen's list of the conditions he expected the good doctor to be able to treat by drugs and diet ranges from gout to migraine, and from a stroke to the coughing up of blood. It is impressively long, particularly if it represents his minimum requirements for competence.[106] It also largely corresponds to what is found in Celsus and in the short, pseudo-Galenic *Introduction to Medicine*. But how a healer chose to act varied from individual to individual. Some, particularly in the big cities, might specialise in one type of complaint; others offered cures for all ills. Galen regularly emphasised the unity of medicine in all its parts, and expected his doctor to be as familiar with drugs and surgery as he was with diet. His contemporary, the pseudonymous author of the *Introduction to Medicine*, likewise included a good deal of information about some, at times complex, surgery.[107] But, like Scribonius Largus' insistence that the doctor must have a substantial knowledge of drugs and their workings, this plea for surgery also implies that this speciality was in fact being left to others more adroit or more daring. If an individual's prudence suggested that he should not attempt a particular procedure, his caution did not attract universal criticism. The argument of one of the earliest Erasistrateans, Strato, that one should refrain from venesection because of the difficulty of distinguishing between veins and arteries and because patients might die of fright at the thought of being bled would have been accepted by many, doctors as well as patients.[108]

But there were other differences in medical practice that depended far less on prudential considerations than on a conviction that certain beliefs and methods should not be included within medicine. In 162–3 Galen himself came under attack for practising in a manner contrary to proper medicine. A leading Erasistratean in Rome accused him of resorting to magic in forecasting the future course of the illness of his old teacher, the philosopher Eudemus. Predictions like this, he alleged, could only have been made through some form of divination – watching the flight of birds, inspecting the entrails of sacrifices, noting chance occurrences or casting horoscopes. Galen's angry response was to state that he had never come across in Rome a prophet who had made a correct prediction, and that he had never tried one elsewhere so could hardly be accused of copying their methods. Furthermore, his own prognoses were made on the basis of observation and rational calculation, not by acting as a prophet, an augur or an astrologer who sought to predict the future without allowing for changing circumstances.[109] When he chose to refer to the heavens, it was not to calculate the positions of the stars at the onset of illness, but, like Hippocrates, to use astronomy as an aid to understanding the changes in the weather that were so important in causing disease. Those who acted otherwise were foolish. Bird-diviners might argue amongst themselves and produce learned tomes and many witnesses to the truth of their predictions, but their methods, according to Galen, were fallible in the extreme, more suited to explaining the astronomical poem of Aratus than contributing to medicine. When they were right, it was for reasons other than they supposed: fine days, whether forecast from the flight of birds or from some other indication, were always likely to be healthier than wet, as Hippocrates had stated centuries before.[110]

But, even in Galen's writings, the line between drawing acceptable and unacceptable conclusions from the positions of the stars was a very narrow one. He repeated, apparently without qualms, a recipe against rabies that had to be concocted 'after the rise of the Dog-star, when the sun has moved into Leo and the Moon reached its eighteenth day'.[111] There were methodological similarities also between medicine and astrology that favoured their co-operation. The astronomer–astrologer Ptolemy, mentioned favourably by his contemporary Galen, used medicine as a model of a conjectural art akin to astrology and considered the supreme merit of Egyptian astrologers to be that they had united the two arts.[112] In his turn, in Book 3 of *On Critical Days* Galen showed himself to be very well acquainted with the technicalities of astrology, the houses of the planets, the decans and so on, and expected his readers to be familiar with them too.[113] He also allowed that many of the observations of Egyptian astrologers had turned out be true, especially when they discussed the influence of the moon, while his comments on the effects of beneficent or malign planets at birth do not suggest hostility to the concept. But he rejected decisively any suggestion that what he himself was doing was astrology, and he expressed considerable doubt about the ability of Egyptian astronomers to predict the course of a disease solely through the configuration of the heavens, although he accepted that many people believed they could.[114] He admitted the validity of what the astrologers had seen and calculated, but he then offered a different interpretation of what it all meant. What determined health and illness was not the constantly altering positions of the stars in the zodiac and their influence on the individual, but the changes within the atmosphere that resulted from these changes in the heavens. To deny this fact was to fly in the face of experience, like any 'cheapjack sophist'.[115]

But Galen was fighting an uphill battle. Belief in the abilities of Egyptian astrologers to forecast health and disease was widespread, even if one regards as artistically exaggerated the claim of the satirist Juvenal, writing around AD 110, that when she fell ill the rich Roman woman would not eat or drink except at the moment prescribed by Petosiris, the celebrated Egyptian founder of astrology.[116] Many surviving texts of ancient astrology have a medical component, usually sections on when best to bleed or take a drug, whether a disease will last for a long time or be quickly cured, and, in particular, whether a disease will prove fatal or not.[117] A new papyrus fragment from Egypt, from the fourth century, contains a leaf of an iatromathematical treatise dealing with magical herbs, amulets and precious stones, as well as instructions on treating wounds in accordance with the position of the zodiac.[118] Its emphasis on the potency of herbs and stones at a particular conjunction suggests that its author said little about another common astrological theory that allotted each part of the body to a particular zodiacal sign: Cancer was responsible for the breast, Pisces the feet and so on.[119]

Nor was every medical man as opposed to medical astrology as Galen and the Methodists. The grave epigram of a wealthy doctor from Naples, Decimus Servilius Apollonius, a 'scion of Epaphus' – that is, an Egyptian – ended with the comment that he had died at ninety-three, 'as I was wont to predict'. Medical astrology was also profitable. Crinas of Marseilles, according to Pliny, made his great fortune by using astrological almanacs to prescribe remedies at the most appropriate time.[120]

Medical astrology penetrated even into the Galenic Corpus, albeit in the form of a short pseudonymous treatise on *Prognostics from Taking to One's Bed*, possibly of Egyptian origin. It shows how to use the astral conjunctions at the time that the patient takes to his or her bed, not only to predict whether a disease will be cured or not, but also to diagnose the cause of the condition: 'If someone takes to his bed when the Moon is in Cancer when Saturn is either conjoined, in opposition or in the square, the disease will be caused by bathing or by getting cold ... warm remedies will prove useful.'[121] Its author appeals to the Stoic justification for astrology as part of a divinely ordered universe, as well as to earlier doctors, not least Diocles, who made their prognoses by taking account of the passage of the moon.[122] He even includes an otherwise unattested quotation from Hippocrates to the effect that doctors who do not practise physiognomy are condemned to ignorance and bewilderment. That this praise of physiognomy is absent from the Hippocratic Corpus as we have it is not unexpected.[123] But the author then makes an even more extravagant claim, asserting that physiognomy, the art of interpreting character from the lineaments of the face, is the most important division of astrology, and thus that, a fortiori, this warm endorsement of physiognomy must apply also to astrology. Galen, although accepting the value of the physiognomical observations in *Epidemics* 2, 5–6, and acknowledging the link between physical appearance and underlying constitution, knows nothing of this exaltation of medical astrology by his hero, and would doubtless have sought to explain it away if he had.[124] It is ironic, then, that at least one of the mediaeval Latin *Prognostics of Galen* is influenced by this type of predictive astrology.[125]

The methodological parallels between predictions based on bodily humours and those based on the stars were indeed close. Both doctor and astrologer appealed to the facts of experience, and both relied on an expert's complicated interpretation of data that were visible to all – the movement of the planets and bodily fluids. The Hippocratic doctrine of critical days closely resembles the astrologer's belief in climacterics, specific times, even hours and days, that were of crucial significance in determining the outcome of illness, and it is no coincidence that Galen's longest discussion of the medical value of astrology comes in his exposition of the principles behind the notion of critical days.[126] Galen's claims that medical astrology was far too crude to allow for the inevitable variations in events or in individuals could easily be countered by the astrologer's insistence that a truly accurate prediction could be achieved only by the highly skilled expert with an exact knowledge of the individual. Indeed, it was precisely the acceptance by Galen of the factual basis behind some of the theories of the astrologers that allowed medical astrology to become the stock in trade of the educated Galenist physician in Late Antiquity and the Middle Ages. By disputing the interpretation of the astrologer's observations of heavenly phenomena, not their accuracy, Galen offered, albeit unwittingly, a way to reconcile astrology and medicine.[127]

He had far stronger objections to number mysticism and magical pharmacy, which lacked any scientific basis at all in his estimation. That anyone should call one number Athena and another Apollo and attribute medical value to them he considered bizarre. There was no reason in his view why in treating hebdomadal fevers one should introduce the seven Pleiads, the seven stars of the Great and Little Bear, and even seven-gated Thebes: one might as well, he thought, toss in the seven mouths of the Nile, which were at least real, whereas all astronomers and philosophers had long proved that no constellation had only seven stars.[128]

Galen's attitude to magical pharmacy was similarly robust. He distinguished between appropriate and inappropriate remedies on three broad criteria. He rejected, on the whole, all those that involved excreta, 'Dreckapotheke', although he was well aware that so learned a pharmacologist as Asclepiades the Pharmacist (fl. AD 90) had written a great deal on the therapeutic virtues of dung.[129] Asclepiades' eminence may have saved him from Galen's wrath, unlike Xenocrates of Aphrodisias (fl. AD 70), whom he denounced for employing abominably filthy remedies, such as sweat, menses, and human bones and flesh (although even Xenocrates deplored straightforward cannibalism), as well as parts of elephants and horses from the Upper Nile, and allegedly even the basilisk.[130] However, many of the recipes in Pliny's *Natural History* are of this type, and Galen's scruples may not have been shared by many or even most other doctors. His second criterion was that of the sources used by the pharmacological writers. Galen dismissed the drug book of Pamphilus as a mixture of old wives' tales and Egyptian wizardry, comparing its author to a herald reading out a list of runaway slaves, unable to identify the items listed even if they were in front of him. Pamphilus had relied on some extremely dubious writings, such as the treatise of Conchlax on snakebite and a pamphlet dedicated to Egyptian Mercury that listed thirty-six herbs, each with its horoscopic sign.[131] Galen's final criterion was that the workings of a drug should be explicable in terms of medicine and physics. This is why he rejected incantations, charms and talismanic amulets, which he thought added nothing to the properties of the drugs themselves.[132] A telling example of where he drew the line comes in an account of an amulet made from green jasper stone and recommended as a help in stomach complaints. According to his source, a large work ascribed to the Egyptian pharaoh and magician Nechepso, it was necessary to carve the stone into an image of a snake with the sun's rays before placing it over the mouth of the stomach.[133] This Galen derided as an unnecessary refinement: he had found it to work perfectly well uncarved. On another occasion a reliable informant told him that an amulet from grape-stone cured snakebite, but Galen considered even this to fall outside 'the use of a true method'; it was no different from employing a blood-red hawk-stone to cure haemorrhoids.[134]

Galen's opposition to the inclusion of such remedies within medicine was shared by many – witness the objections of Scribonius Largus to the use of gladiator's blood and to the quasi-magical advice of Ambrosius of Puteoli.[135] But others clearly disagreed. The treatise on medico-astrological herbal medicine ascribed to Thessalus begins with a preface in which the author, ostensibly a man of wealth and education, describes how his philosophical and medical studies in Alexandria led him to an interest in medical herbs and how he had found in its libraries the astrological-magical tract of Pharaoh Nechepso, which he decided to imitate.[136] Despite Galen's strictures, writers like Pamphilus and Xenocrates enjoyed a considerable following, and their remedies continued to be copied and read for many centuries to come. An acquaintance of Galen owned a book on magical medicine akin, Max Wellmann suggested, to the *Medical, Natural and Antipathetic Remedies* of the second-century author Aelius Promotus.[137] This collection, dedicated to an emperor, possibly Hadrian, includes herbal remedies, including one against catarrh in the lungs that was approved by Trajan for use in the army, as well as amulets and remedies from excreta.[138] Julius Africanus, around 225, giving advice to the military physician on treating wounds and on amputation, recommends, as well as sharp instruments ('less painful than blunt ones'), charms and the placing over the wound of a metal plate bearing magical signs.[139] The *Book of Stones* by the late first-century author Xenocrates of Ephesus, when translated in the ninth century into Arabic, exercised a major influence on Arabic treatises on the uses of precious stones.[140] A similar work probably lies behind the discussions of the medical value of precious stones in the late Greek compilation called the *Kyranides*, which also drew on an earlier miscellany by Marcellus of Side.[141] His near-contemporary Archigenes of Apamea included many medical amulets in a sober work on pharmacology in several books.[142] With such endorsements, it is no wonder that a historian labelled those who objected to the use of amulets to ward off disease mad.[143]

It is clear that magical remedies, spells and chants against disease were widespread, whether one considers the papyrological evidence from Roman

Egypt, literary sources or archaeological finds like the gemstone amulet bearing the image of the healing deity Sarapis and an inscription indicating that the god was a 'faithful source of healing'.[144] However much Galen might inveigh against magic practices, and complain of misrepresentation when he was compared to a sorcerer, those in need of healing took a more liberal view. The sorcerers Elymas and Simon Magus are depicted in Acts as attracting a large clientele eager for their cures, and the Elder Pliny warns against the dubious remedies of the Persian magus Ostanes, while at the same time carefully reporting them in case they should prove effective.[145] No wonder, then, that the historian Ammianus Marcellinus, describing a series of panic prosecutions for sorcery in the late fourth century, deprecated the fact that a man could now be put on trial for using an old-fashioned charm to soothe a pain, which authoritative doctors had long permitted, and that the mere act of wearing a remedy for quartan fever or another disease around one's neck was likely to lead to a capital charge.[146] Only the severest repression could stamp out these practices, and that was rarely tried for long or with sustained success.

The result was a medical pluralism, a mixture of many competing types of healing, with a range as broad as the social status of their practitioners and as the variety of doctrines that they held. A counterargument would contend that this conclusion is misleading in that it underestimates the degree of coherence that did exist among *iatroi* and *medici*. Doctrinal differences within the sects were relatively small; minor changes of emphasis were magnified by unscrupulous opponents, notably Galen, into wholesale dissension. The social gulf that separated a Stertinius Xenophon from a doctor in an Egyptian village was scarcely greater than that between a Harley Street specialist today and a local GP in central Bradford or rural Wales. The world of astrological or magical healing, it might also be suggested, bore as little relevance to the ideas and therapies of the average Greek or Roman doctor as acupuncture, aromatherapy and the astral Galenism of a modern healer in Torquay do to the average doctor in London or Lyons.[147] Despite the increasing presence of alternatives coming in, especially from Egypt and the Near East, Greek learned, rational medicine continued to flourish. It was of men such as Dioscorides, Rufus, Soranus and Galen, confident heirs to a long medical tradition, that ancient Greeks or Romans thought when they used the word 'doctor'. To believe otherwise is to misrepresent what the ancients understood by medicine and to give undue weight to the chance survival of inscriptions and papyri.

Nonetheless, as the evidence assembled in this chapter shows, the existence of a general demarcation between doctors and other purveyors of healing should not obscure the substantial overlap between their styles and methods. Many doctors, even those who ostensibly followed a rigorously rational (or philosophical) approach to medicine, were prepared to accept various theories and methods that did not conform to the rules of Aristotelian or Hippocratic logic. Therapies a Galen might decry could be accepted by a Lycus or a Xenocrates, and certainly by their patients. For instance, despite Galen's vigorous condemnation of the use of gladiator's blood as a remedy for epilepsy, it continued to appear in the medical literature for centuries as 'an excellent and soundly proven remedy', even long after the last gladiator had perished in the arena.[148] Conversely, astrological healers were prepared to appeal to the authority of Hippocrates or the Stoics to explain or justify their own cures.

Moreover, despite attempts by authors such as Scribonius Largus or Galen to set professional standards, the absence of any legal backing left the decision about who was or was not a doctor, or whom one might consult for a cough or a fistula, firmly with the patient. Medical colleges, processions and public displays might offer ways of asserting corporate identity, but personal recommendation or sheer necessity was far more likely to have influenced the choice of a doctor than any of these. This is not to deny entirely that boundaries might exist, or that some therapies, some doctrines, some healers were rejected and excluded even if, as Ulpian remarked, they were considered effective.[149] But the dominant feature of these boundaries is their fluidity. The jokes about becoming a doctor overnight, or switching equally quickly from medicine to undertaking, typify the life of the jobbing craftsman, turning his hand to whatever might make money and, outside the cities, to judge from Egypt, very often combining medicine with smallholding. And indeed, Galen's oft reiterated complaints about the ignorance of Hippocratic medicine among his contemporaries in fact suggests that, for their part, they regarded many of Hippocrates' ideas and practices as unnecessary or superfluous.

Deciding what characteristics to ascribe to the 'average' doctor in the Roman Empire is ultimately a question of perspective. If one takes as a yardstick the high, Hippocratic tradition of medicine as represented by Galen, it is easy to dismiss much of the evidence in this chapter as irrelevant to or unworthy of medicine. But that opinion would not have been shared by the patient seeking help and advice from whatever healer they could find, and looking for effectiveness rather than erudition. The doctor was like other skilled artisans, whose wealth, status and, probably, expertise varied according to the wealth and size of the communities they served. In a metropolis such as Rome or Smyrna there was considerable money to be made from the sophisticated treatment of rich inhabitants, not least the emperor and his court; the perspective of a doctor on Cythera or in Spanish Tarragona was very different indeed.[150]

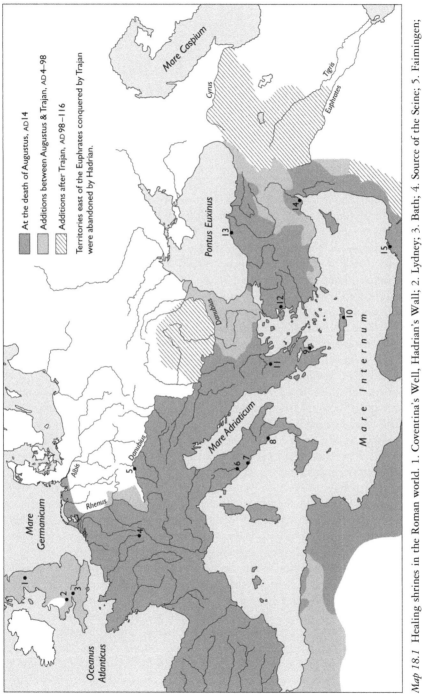

Map 18.1 Healing shrines in the Roman world. 1. Coventina's Well, Hadrian's Wall; 2. Lydney; 3. Bath; 4. Source of the Seine; 5. Faimingen; 6. Rome; 7. Antium; 8. Elea; 9. Epidaurus; 10. Lebena; 11. Tricca; 12. Pergamum; 13. Abonuteichos; 14. Aegeae; 15. Alexandria.

Map legend:
- At the death of Augustus, AD 14
- Additions between Augustus & Trajan, AD 4–98
- Additions after Trajan, AD 98–116
- Territories east of the Euphrates conquered by Trajan were abandoned by Hadrian.

279

18

MEDICINE AND THE RELIGIONS OF
THE ROMAN EMPIRE

The world of the Roman Empire was permeated with the divine to an extent almost unimaginable in a modern secular world.[1] Gods were everywhere, as benign creators or angry avengers, as patrons of cities and occupational groups, even occasionally as distinguished ancestors. The doctor C. Stertinius Xenophon on Cos, for example, proudly proclaimed his descent from both Asclepius and Hercules.[2] Few dared to doubt the existence of gods, although they might well have sought to extend the limits of human self-sufficiency by stressing natural over supernatural causes or, like the Epicureans, denying the gods any direct involvement in human affairs. Conversely, few believed, like Theophrastus' superstitious man, that divine wrath was always likely to strike unless one took the right precautions at every possible opportunity, and that only by consulting the right experts – dream interpreters, prophets, priests, astrologers and the like – could one be reasonably certain of the favourable outcome of any action.[3] But between these two extremes lay a variety of ways in which space could be made for both divine and human agency. While there might be disagreements and uncertainties at times over the boundaries between the two, it would be wrong to see this in a medical context as a conflict between sacred and secular intervention. As we have already seen, the Hippocratic author of *The Sacred Disease* emphasised his own superior piety in acknowledging the divine nature of all creation and in rejecting the exorcists' appeals to the gods to intervene directly in diseases susceptible of an entirely natural explanation.[4] His attitude was shared by many other doctors, not least by the pious Galen, and rules out a simple dichotomy between a secular and a religious approach to health and healing.[5] Nor was it thought in any way incongruous to ask an oracle whether or not one was going to recover, while seeking medical assistance from a secular healer.[6] Yet, as this chapter will show, there were at times differences between the various religions of the Roman Empire in their attitudes towards medicine that had a major impact on the way in which the practice of medicine developed over the centuries.

One common misunderstanding needs to be corrected at the outset. Given the ubiquity of deities as protectors or saviours, it is misleading to talk of 'healing gods' as if they formed a distinct category, for one could direct a prayer for assistance with health problems to any god one wished.[7] The divinity might be purely local, like Coventina, who presided over a spring at Carrawburgh on Hadrian's Wall, or universal, like Apollo.[8] He or she might be endowed with a specifically human form, like Asclepius, or remain an almost anonymous abstraction, like the Most High God, 'a title that almost any honest man could apply with a clear conscience' to any god treated as the supreme being.[9] There were noteworthy regional and chronological differences. The early Romans, unlike the Greeks, placed many of the events, both good and bad, of agricultural life under the tutelage of a specific power responsible solely for that event. Thus they prayed to Blight or the Goddess Fever in an attempt to avert potential catastrophe.[10] When such divinities appear in a Greek context, it is likely to be under Roman influence, whether exerted directly by settlers or merchants, or indirectly.[11] The peoples of the Levant, by contrast, frequently attributed illness to the malignity of demons, who took possession of the individual and needed to be appeased or exorcised to bring about recovery. Although in the New Testament demons are particularly associated with mental conditions, as in the story of the Gadarene swine, most texts from the region make no distinction between physical and mental illness.[12] The demon Barsaphael was believed to give 'those who reside in my hour' migraine headaches, as was the female demon Antaura, mentioned on a tablet found in the Roman military camp at Carnuntum (Austria) and dating from either the late first or the second century. This tablet, containing a short account of the victory of Artemis of the Ephesians over Antaura, was clearly worn as protection against migraine attacks. Versions of the same story can be found in Christianised forms well into the Byzantine period.[13]

The presence of this tablet, written in Greek with some Hebrew words, in a settlement on the Danube points to another feature of religion in the period from 100 BC to AD 300 – the spread of beliefs and cults around the Roman Empire in part facilitated by the polyethnicity of the Roman army. Sometimes this took the form of an introduction of new cults from outside a region, at other times of a merging of the local with an imported equivalent.[14] At Bath, the god of its healing waters, Sul, was equated with Minerva; across the Severn, at Lydney, a dedicator inscribed his plaque to Mars Nodens, another fusion of a Celtic and a Roman divinity.[15] From the third century BC, if not earlier, Asclepius was assimilated to a variety of indigenous healing deities; for example, in Egypt to Imhotep/Imouthes, and in Phoenicia to Eshmun.[16] In the Dolomites, the Venetic god Trumusiatis or Tribusiatis became identified with Apollo, with the rituals and types of dedication at his sacred spring continuing apparently unchanged from the first century BC until the fourth century.[17] Hot springs in particular, or those with an unusual colour, taste or smell, often had their own deities.[18] As a late commentator on Virgil put it, 'there is no such thing as a non-sacred spring'.[19]

Some of these shrines developed a regional or even an empire-wide reputation. A stonemason from Chartres and soldiers on leave, or merely passing through, made their dedications to Sul at peaceful Bath, while the temple of the Dea Sequana at the headwaters of the Seine drew worshippers from all over Gaul and beyond.[20] In 213–15 the Emperor Caracalla, 'who suffered from both visible and hidden diseases of the body as well as those of the mind', went in person to seek help from Apollo Grannus at Faimingen, S. Germany, from Asclepius at Pergamum and from Sarapis at Alexandria.[21] His personal attendance and his lavish gifts, reports the historian Cassius Dio, were no more successful than the prayers, sacrifices and benefactions his servants had previously made on his behalf.

Caracalla's pilgrimage also indicates that some gods were indeed viewed more widely than others as effective protectors and sources of healing.[22] A list would include the Deae Matronae, Mars, Minerva, Diana, Hercules, Men (a Phrygian god, often given the epithet 'he who hears'), the Egyptian gods Isis and Sarapis, and, the big two, Apollo and Asclepius.[23] Although the next few pages deal mainly with Asclepius, the ubiquity of local healing deities and shrines should not be forgotten, nor the protection offered by any divinity to his or her worshippers.[24]

An abundance of coins and inscriptions attests the universality of Asclepius cult in the first three centuries of the Roman Empire, from Lusitania and Hadrian's Wall in the West to Mesopotamia in the East.[25] Temples were established, rebuilt and enlarged, and festivals and games set up in honour of the god. The Asclepieion of Cos underwent a massive reconstruction in the 50s

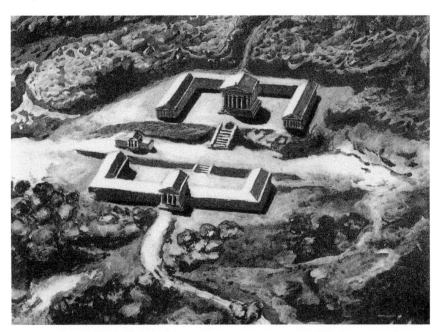

Figure 18.1 The Asclepieion of Cos. A reconstruction by T. Meyer-Steineg.

and 60s, largely at the expense of the imperial doctor Stertinius Xenophon, and was transformed from a collection of individual buildings into an architecturally impressive ensemble.[26] At Lebena on Crete the Asclepieion benefited also at this time from the generosity of the family of Sosarchus, attracting suppliants from N. Africa as well as from the island itself.[27]

Of the history of other major shrines we know little before AD 100, or even later. The temple of Asclepius at Aegeae in Cilicia (S. Turkey) was certainly drawing visitors from a wide area by the end of the first century, although most of our information about it refers to the third or even fourth centuries.[28] At Epidaurus, a major building programme took place in the second century at the expense of a Senator Antoninus, possibly the Emperor Antoninus Pius, who built a bathhouse and a temple of Egyptian Health, Egyptian Asclepius and Egyptian Apollo. Outside the main precinct itself he restored the Colonnade of Cotys, where sufferers might be brought to die or women give birth, since both were forbidden within the sacred area itself.[29] The shrine at Pergamum also began to flourish again in the 80s, but it was the second century that saw the expansion in its size and influence that made it 'the most celebrated healing shrine in the whole Empire'.[30] Here, beginning in the 120s or 130s, a wealthy senator, C. Cuspius Pactumeius Rufinus, supported by the Emperor Hadrian, 'the new Asclepius', embarked on a massive rebuilding programme that transformed the temple complex into one of the wonders of the ancient world.[31] Pergamum was now considered the main home of Asclepius, as Delphi was of Apollo or Ephesus of Artemis, and, as such, a veritable rival of the great temple of Zeus at Olympia.[32] New buildings were erected within the precinct, including a beautiful round temple dedicated to Zeus Asclepius the Saviour and adorned with variegated marbles and niches holding statues.[33] There was a second massive circular building, a small theatre, a library and spacious porticoes, all approached through a monumental entrance: of the Hellenistic temple, only the cult buildings and incubation rooms remained undisturbed.[34] Together with the colonnaded street that stretched for more than a mile from the city to the Asclepieion, the whole complex proclaimed wealth, beauty and power. It attracted tourists as well as the sick, and rapidly became an intellectual as well as a religious centre where one might meet the wife of an Ephesian banker as well as a champion athlete.[35] At its heart was the temple of the god, with its famous statue of the Pergamene Asclepius, and the complex of buildings around the sacred spring and the underground tunnel. Here, as centuries earlier at Epidaurus, the sick would purify themselves before retiring to sleep in the hope of receiving a vision from the god. In the morning they would plan to follow the god's instructions directly or, if the message required interpretation, enlist the help of one of the temple wardens.[36]

What these messages might have been like we can gather both from inscriptions set up at the shrine and from the *Sacred Tales* of Aelius Aristides (117 to after 177).[37] A famous orator, Aristides spent years of chronic ill

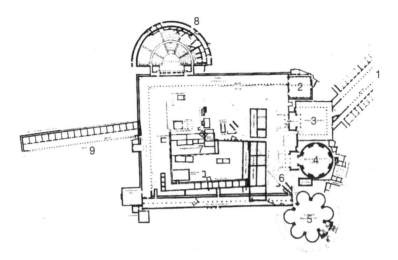

Map 18.2 The shrine of Asclepius at Pergamum in Galen's lifetime. 1 Sacred Way; 2 Library; 3 Ceremonial Gateway; 4 Temple of Asclepius; 5 Round building; 6 Tunnel; 7 Incubation rooms; 8 Theatre; 9 Stoa.

health visiting and staying at various of the shrines of his protecting deity Asclepius and of other gods, such as Sarapis and Apollo. Galen, who saw him in Pergamum, remarked that he had never seen a mind so strong that triumphed over so frail a body.[38] It is no wonder that Aristides' doctors were concerned at his decision to plunge into a raging torrent in mid-winter and suspected that his obedience to the god contributed as much to his ill health as to his recovery.[39]

Aristides' six *Sacred Tales* (*Orations* 47–52) have an apparent immediacy as an account of his struggles with illness, overcome with the aid of Asclepius and other gods.[40] But although based on diaries and papers, they must be viewed with caution, for they are a highly wrought, consciously rhetorical and at times tendentious presentation of the orator's relationship with the god throughout his life.[41] They are a record of divine protection and support, and not just in illness. Aristides' battle with ill health is set alongside his rescue from potential shipwreck, his inspiration to compose his orations and poems, and his successful fight to preserve his tax immunities against the impositions of his fellow citizens, in all of which Aristides believed himself to be guided by the gods, and by Asclepius in particular. Through dreams or by incidents that later turned out to be significant, Aristides was restored to (fitful) health and gained a reputation as the leading public speaker in the Greek world of the day.

His descriptions of his illnesses are long and detailed. Coughs, vomitings, swellings, headaches, pains, intermittent inability to breathe or walk properly, even an attack of the plague in AD 165 are all carefully recorded.[42] His choice of words, and his explanation of some of the causes and cures of his illness, would not be out of place in a Galenic text. Indeed, some of the cures prescribed by the god gain added authority because they can be expressed in familiar medical terminology or correspond to treatments found in contemporary medical writers. But the god's advice on phlebotomy, for instance, also goes beyond what a human doctor might advocate. Far from objecting to being bled several times, Aristides takes pride in the endurance enjoined on him by the god, remarking that no other suppliant has been bled to such an extent by divine command, save for Ischuron, who was 'a particularly unusual case'.[43]

However, Aristides' relationships with his doctors are far from universally hostile: he was not one of those who on principle refused to obey any instructions from a doctor unless they had first been sanctioned by the god.[44] In the plague of 165 many doctors came out from Smyrna to attend to him and his servants as they lay ill in his suburban villa; when the daughter of his foster sister fell ill he immediately sent a doctor to treat her; and Heracleon, described as a companion, was only one of the many doctors who came, out of inquisitiveness or friendship, when Aristides obeyed the god's advice to bathe in the river at Smyrna in mid-winter.[45] On another occasion, when he fell ill on his estate, a doctor was summoned who took at least a day to make his way there through the winter countryside.[46] Even if, on the whole, the doctors' advice is depicted as unhelpful, that did not mean that Aristides rejected it entirely. Galen's teacher, Satyrus, visited Aristides when he was in bed at Pergamum.[47] After examining him, he strongly advised against any more bleedings, recommending instead that a plaster be put over the stomach and abdomen. Aristides refused to disobey the god's command and refrain from venesection, but decided to try Satyrus' plaster, when the time was ripe, since it did not involve any departure from what the god had ordered and he might indeed benefit from it. It did not work; the whole of his face seized up. Aristides sent his foster-father to enquire of the oracle of Apollo at Colophon how he might be cured. Zosimus returned with the news that Asclepius would himself perform the cure. This he did, 'curing my consumption, my catarrh, and my stomach', and even sending a prescription with another member of Aristides' family, unsalted olive oil, to be taken thrice daily.[48] On another occasion, Aristides happily accepted wild greens as prescribed nourishment from his doctor.[49] His foster-father Zosimus was himself skilled in medicine, dying after a fall from his carriage while on the way to treat a sick slave; his skill and his self-sacrifice in the line of duty were alike commended by Aristides.[50]

When the prescriptions of his doctors and those of Asclepius diverged, Aristides believed that he had no choice but to obey the god, even though he might be criticised for credulity or cowardice in the face of the knife or the hot iron.[51] In their turn, Aristides' doctors, even if at first they were doubtful, were brought to accept the overriding power of the god.[52] What the god commanded was paramount, whether the dream in which the orders were given took the form of a riddle that required interpretation or of a consultation and prescription as if in a doctor's surgery. Such dreams and visions could occur anywhere, at home or on a journey, not just when at Pergamum or a similar sanctuary. They might be given before, whilst or after seeking advice from human healers: the manner and the time were determined by the will of the god.

Divine and human healing were thus complementary, and how and when each was to be used was a personal decision. Like the woman with the issue of blood in the Gospels, some turned to the divine when doctors had failed.[53] At Sora, near Rome, about 150 BC, a man 'in despair about his afflictions' vowed a tenth of his property to Hercules if he were to recover; two hundred years later a public slave sacrificed a white heifer to the rustic Bona Dea Felicula, who had restored his eyesight when he had been given up on by his doctors after ten months of treatment.[54] Others, however, may have preferred to go straight to a sanctuary and pray for recovery as a first resort. Prepousa sought the aid of Men Axiottenus for her son as soon as he became ill, because she did not wish to 'waste money on doctors'.[55]

Aristides' devotion to Asclepius should not then be dismissed out of hand as eccentric or as hostile to medicine. It differs only slightly from that of Galen, an avowed 'worshipper of Asclepius', who was equally confident that his whole career had been guided by the god. It was Asclepius who appeared to his father Nicon in a 'clear dream' (that is, one that required no interpretation or mediation) enjoining him to let his son become a doctor, and it was Asclepius' intervention that stopped Galen from going on a potentially dangerous campaign in 169.[56] A dream caused him to rewrite a section on the anatomy and physiology of the eye, which in its original form had left out some difficult description and thus did 'less than justice to that most divine of organs'.[57] Although he was prepared to interpret some dreams simply as indications of a physiological state, on more than one occasion his treatment was influenced by what he had seen in a dream or by what others had had confirmed for them in a vision.[58] Others agreed. A commentator on the Hippocratic *Oath* reported that many people had been cured through dreams and visions sent by Sarapis or Asclepius, at Epidaurus, Cos or Pergamum, his home city, and that 'people in general bear witness to the fact that God has given them the craft of medicine through inspiration in dreams and visions'.[59] The dream-interpreter Artemidorus made a similar comment, going out of his way to emphasise that the gods in healing visions, at Pergamum, Alexandria and elsewhere, offered cures 'entirely in line with proper medicine and in no way alien to medical reasoning'.[60] Grateful patients in Rome and at Cibyra (S.W. Turkey) gave thanks to Asclepius and Hygieia for cures vouchsafed to them through the medium of doctors acting 'according to divine instruction'.[61] A cure by Asclepius of an epileptic was reported by Rufus of Ephesus in the middle of a sober discussion of the possibility that one disease might change into another, although he expressed some doubt as to whether

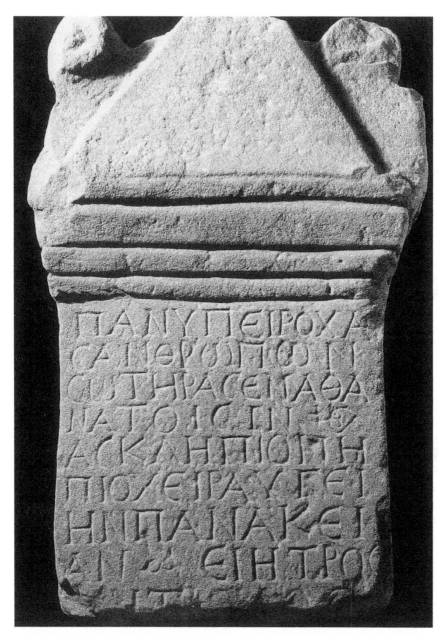

Figure 18.2 A Greek dedication from Chester set up by Antiochus the doctor to 'the all-surpassing saviours of men among the gods, Asclepius, gentle-handed Hygeia and Panakeia', inv. CHEGM: 1968.37. Photo © Cheshire West Museums.

the therapy could be achieved by human intervention alone.[62] Other doctors took a more sceptical view of Asclepius' medical expertise even as they were forced to accept that their patients believed strongly in the possibility of a divine cure.[63]

It is no surprise, then, to find doctors prominent in support for Asclepius, their patron deity.[64] We have already seen that the doctors at Ephesus made annual sacrifices and held games in his honour.[65] The wealthy medical lit-terateur Heraclitus of Rhodiapolis, a priest of Asclepius and Hygieia, erected a temple in their honour, complete with statues, spending lavishly on this and on their games.[66] Elsewhere in Asia Minor shrines of Asclepius were paid for by doctors at Oenoanda in Lycia and at Nysa, further north, in the Maeander Valley.[67] At a small town in Phrygia, Menodorus, a doctor and priest of Asclepius, joined with his son, a priest and magistrate, in providing a new vaulted annexe, two pillars and a new roof for a shrine of Asclepius.[68] The patriarch of a medical dynasty from Thyateira in Asia Minor was pub-licly honoured by his friend Secundus, president of the games of Asclepius.[69] Similar gifts of statues and buildings were made by doctors to other deities, and, while a priesthood of Asclepius might be an entirely appropriate office for a doctor to hold, his profession in no way ruled out priesthoods in other cults.[70] Indeed, in the Greek world of the second century the holding of such public offices, with their opportunities for public benefaction, was expected of any wealthy individual or family. It is thus no coincidence that many of the doctors whose gifts were recorded for posterity come from long-established families or that they were frequently *archiatri*, civic physicians, for a back-ground of wealth would lead almost automatically to such offices, medical as well as religious.[71]

This public show of reverence for the gods, whether expressed in the form of a priestly office or of a contribution to the building or adornment of a shrine, reflects the wealth of the second century and, particularly in the Greek East, the ostentatious habit of carving inscriptions for general view far more than it does any new and widespread upsurge in anxiety or sense of crisis.[72] Indeed, the votive images of bodily parts, in terracotta, marble or even pre-cious metals, that hung around the walls of the shrine, the altars, statues and inscriptional plaques that bore witness to a cure or a divine revelation in a dream, or some other proof that the god had responded, in fact attest a crisis overcome.[73] They mark a personal recovery, and gratitude to the god who had answered one's prayers.[74]

Such concerns about health and illness remained at an individual or family level, with one exception: pestilence. As the Christian writer Lactantius put it, in times of disaster, when the pestilential force of disease hangs over them, all men turn to god.[75] Epidemic disease affecting a whole city called for civic measures, as we have already seen with the plague of Thucydides and the plague that led to the introduction of Asclepius cult into Rome. The health of the city, involving political as well as medical stability, was a matter for all its citizens, and called for action on a civic level that mirrored what the individual might do.[76] When the Antonine plague reached Asia Minor in 165, the response of many towns was to send a delegation to consult various oracles, particularly those at Claros and Didyma, to find out the future outcome and what divinely approved measures might mitigate impending disasters.[77] Like the Roman Senate centuries earlier consulting its religious authorities and the Sibylline Books in times of plague, the authorities at a small town in Lydia turned to the oracle of Apollo. The god's response was to reassure them that the statue of Artemis they had recently set up would 'free them from the man-slaying poisons of plague', once they had destroyed some wax puppets, which, presumably, they had recently found and believed indicated the handiwork of a magician.[78] Another town, Callipolis (near modern Gallipoli, Turkey) was instructed to set up a statue of Apollo 'the warder-off of plague', and to sacrifice to the gods below the earth, carefully sprinkling the pyre with grey sea water. If plague returned – and driving it away was far from easy – Apollo promised to send further instructions.[79]

Another shrine that attracted suppliants from far and wide during the Antonine plague was that at Abonuteichos on the south shore of the Black Sea. Here a cult had been established in the 150s based on an artful combination of Pythagoreanism, Asclepius worship, hymns, choirs and mystery religion. It featured a snake-god, Glycon, who offered oracular advice and healing to all comers. Not only did the oracle send out envoys throughout the Roman Empire warning of impending destruction through fire or plague, but it also distributed wholesale a brief message that would guarantee safety. The single-line message, 'Phoebus the long-tressed the plague cloud shall dispel', was then affixed to house doors to ward off the advent of plague: one example, carved in stone, has been found several hundreds of miles away from Abonuteichos in the ruins of a house at Antioch in Syria.[80] Lucian, our main literary source, jokes that, far from being protected, the inhabitants of houses displaying this message were often the only ones to be affected by the plague. His sceptical, and at times grotesque, account of Glycon, 'the new Asclepius', concentrates on the tricks of the false prophet Alexander and the contradiction between his pious pronouncements and his sordid immorality. Those who flocked to the shrine almost deserved to be cheated: they were, after all, thick and stupid peasants from the backwoods of Paphlagonia.[81] Unlike Lucian, they were unable to see how Alexander linked features of Asclepius cult – the snake and the egg – with other famous contemporary oracles and with the most famous wonder-worker of the century, Apollonius of Tyana.[82] It was, in Lucian's opinion, a giant confidence trick, unworthy of the generals, senators and even rulers who consulted Glycon. The grey-haired doctor Paetus, who applied after Alexander's death to be his successor as interpreter of the god, is condemned as a disgrace to old age and to his profession.[83]

Louis Robert has shown how the success of this new cult, which spread quickly all around the Black Sea, in Asia Minor and along the Danube, can in part be explained by the broader cultural, intellectual and religious context in which it was established.[84] He points out, too, that Lucian directs the full force of his attack against Alexander's claims for prophecy rather than his medicine, making only mild comments on his medical abilities. Lucian merely notes in passing the shrine's claims to heal the sick and raise up the dead, as well as the medical training and expertise of Alexander himself. Alexander had a wide and useful acquaintance with drugs of all kind, and he prescribed diets and other widely recognised therapies. His use of bear grease, far from being an invention of the satirist, would have been standard medical practice for a region in which these animals roamed.[85] With these claims, and with what even Lucian had to acknowledge as brilliant propaganda, it is no wonder that suppliants came in large numbers to the new god, or that many towns in the region for over a century issued coins bearing the image of Glycon the snake-healer.[86]

In cults like that of Glycon or Asclepius the focus is on the future, on the possibility of recovery and the fulfilment of the bargain with the god. If the god wished to intervene and save – and that was the god's decision alone – then the suppliant would reciprocate by a gift, a sacrifice, an altar or some other benefaction. What is mentioned much less often is any belief in the involvement of divinities in bringing about the disease in the first place. The god intervenes to cure where others have failed, and has, on the whole, no concern for past causes of illness. The notion of disease as some form of divine punishment, familiar in the theatre and in later Christian writers, is largely absent from most accounts of pagan cures. Aristides, for example, if he indicates a cause, speaks usually in terms of what he has eaten or the season of the year.

One death, however, allows him to juxtapose divine and secular explanations. Zosimus the doctor had earlier fallen ill while on a journey, and had recovered, somewhat unexpectedly, through being purged with barley gruel and lentils.[87] His recovery, and the means thereof, had been foretold to Aristides in a dream by Asclepius, but the treatment itself would appear to have been devised by a human doctor. Four months later, Zosimus died suddenly while on a visit to a sick slave in mid-winter. Aristides offers three overlapping reasons for his death. The first is simply the winter cold; the second is Zosimus' disobedience in not following Aristides' (and Asclepius') advice to refrain from strenuous outdoor activity and to build up his strength; the third, which was only revealed in a dream later, was that Zosimus had inadvertently touched sacrificial meat intended for the god.[88] The last two explanations, however, are employed by Aristides to account, not for Zosimus' illness, but for his death and for the failure of the god to intervene. Zosimus' decision to go and treat his patient triggered an illness that led to his death, as Asclepius had warned. The responsibility was thus that of Zosimus alone, and, admits Aristides, the combination of bodily weakness and, although Zosimus was not to know it, divine displeasure meant that his death could have happened by any means and at any moment. Aristides consoles himself with the thought that the god's first intervention had allowed him to enjoy fellowship with Zosimus for longer than he might have hoped.

A much closer link between illness and divine displeasure is asserted on a group of inscriptions coming from the uplands of Lydia in Asia Minor and probably dating from the second century.[89] Written in an unpretentious Greek, these texts are addressed to a variety of local deities. They record that an individual has in some way sinned against one or other of these gods and has been punished by some disaster befalling the offender, another member of the family, or even his or her property. The sinner is then brought to confess, makes expiation, warns others and publicly acknowledges the power of the gods. The range of afflictions recorded on these confession texts is not noticeably different from that found elsewhere on votive inscriptions – blindness, madness, diseases of the breasts (a speciality of female divinities), arms and legs. Some of them are chronic, others the result of an accident, for instance a sickle falling on a foot. Confession is the first step to cure: it prevents matters from becoming worse, and it may lead to a cure, although most of these inscriptions say nothing about a favourable outcome. Where they do, the healing involves a priest or priestess performing appropriate rituals and incantations.[90]

The notion of a link between human action, divine punishment and illness, as we have already seen, goes back a long way, to the Homeric poems and to Greek tragedy, and can be found on some of the inscriptions from Epidaurus.[91] What is striking is that, with very few exceptions, all the errors that occasion misfortune can be classified as direct offences against the gods – ritual impurity (wearing unclean clothes, eating forbidden food), failure to fulfil a vow or offer sacrifice, perjury, unjustified cursing, and damage to sanctuaries often by one's animals wandering into a sacred grove in search of food. Even the cases of theft can be subsumed into the category of religious offences. Although other humans may be involved, it is not offences against them that draw down divine judgment, but only transgressions where the gods are directly involved.

How widely shared such attitudes were in the ancient world is a difficult question. Certainly the number of deities involved and the fact that these inscriptions come from more than one site in that area of Asia Minor indicate that we are dealing with at least a regional attitude. Likewise, the parallels with inscriptions found elsewhere suggest that many others believed that perjury or failure to fulfil a vow was likely to result in some divine punishment in the form of illness.[92] But the public confession of one's error as part of the process of propitiation and cure, and its public recording, seems, on the evidence so far available, to have been somewhat restricted.[93]

The link between sin and suffering is a major theme in Jewish writings.[94] The *Book of Job* is a remarkable meditation on the relationship between individual afflictions, including physical suffering, and an all-powerful God.[95] It raises the question of why a pious and god-fearing man should be beset with disasters, and explores the paradox of adherence to a god who may appear to be both remote from his adherents and capricious in his actions. It is Job's friends who argue that suffering is the direct consequence of impiety and error, and that it must be viewed as a punishment or correction by God that cannot be avoided by the wicked, even if they appear to prosper.[96] Job himself rejects this simplistic approach in favour of one that accepts the inscrutable majesty of God and his ultimate justice.

Job's response depends on a firm belief in the unique power of Jahweh, and on the covenant made between God and the Israelites, as described in the early books of the Bible. There are other gods, of the Philistines, the Egyptians and the Babylonians, but to the Jews these were false gods. Their God was supreme, and would guarantee their prosperity as long as they followed his ordinances. Failure to do so was likely to have serious consequences, for the individual and for the Israelites as a whole. At a national level, this could be a plague, a famine or a Babylonian exile; for the individual, it could be illness or death. When King Asa placed his cure solely in the hands of his doctors and did not appeal to the Lord, the swellings in his feet became ever greater and he died.[97] Even the eulogy of the physician by Jesus b. Sirach (c.200 BC) is qualified by his conviction that sin causes disease and that the physician, for all his merits, can only bring about a cure when the sinner has made a proper repentance.[98] Similar beliefs in a link between sin and suffering are presupposed in many New Testament narratives, even if they are apparently rejected by Jesus himself.

But there is a major difference in the concept of sinfulness. Whereas in Greek and Roman polytheism ritual offences against a god provoke retribution, in Jewish monotheism the range of offences is widened to include almost any aspect of one's moral behaviour. The Ten Commandments forbid both physical actions, theft or murder, and inner inclinations, lust and covetousness. The covenant between God and mankind is a covenant of justice and righteousness in all one's activities and beliefs, with the consequence that the possibilities of breaking that covenant become ever greater. To a Jewish believer in religious causes of illness the range of possible sins is multiplied well beyond what the average Greek, or even, as we have seen, Lydian, would have accepted.

The religious bias of our surviving Hebrew texts also emphasises to a greater extent than elsewhere the power of the holy man to heal.[99] In direct communication with God, he can bring healing and even raise the dead to life as a mediator of the supreme omnipotence of God. His healing is effective because it is joined to spiritual authority. Ben Sirach's physician is honoured because of his links with God and because of the role set for him by God. His knowledge extends to areas that were forbidden to others, to healing provided by plants or by the stars and constellations.[100] Such Jewish healers were frequently credited with a knowledge of magic and incantations, some of which were believed to go back to that noted magician King Solomon.[101] While the Rabbinical texts generally speak of healers and healing in the same way as their non-Jewish counterparts, the links that they make with what some might see as magic, as well as their acceptance of healing as a gift from God that might be vouchsafed to prophets as proof of their authority, give a different meaning to the practice of medicine. Religion plays a role in defining what is and is not acceptable as therapy that is considerably greater than in other parts of the Graeco-Roman world.

Christianity, which grew out of Judaism, retained and developed many of its distinctive attitudes towards medicine.[102] The foundation texts of Christianity, the Gospels, describe Jesus very much in terms of a wandering prophet and miracle-worker, proclaiming the need for repentance and confirming his direct relationship with God by acts of healing. Although he preached a spiritual salvation and a heavenly immortality to those who believed in him, Jesus' miracles of bodily healing also figure prominently in all four Gospels. Some involve physical infirmity, like that of the blind man, the paralytic or the woman with the issue of blood; others a variety of mental ailments, which the onlookers and the Gospel writers themselves frequently attributed to demonic possession.[103] The healing of lepers was both the removal of a physical disfigurement and the cleansing of a religious impurity.[104] Jesus' power extended even to raising the dead.[105] Some miracles were performed by Jesus himself in the presence of the sick; in others, like that of the centurion's servant, his pronouncement of future recovery was enough to ensure the well-being of the absent sufferer.[106] This power to heal was also passed on by Jesus to his followers, who were enjoined to go out and heal the sick.[107] Some of their miracles are recorded in *Acts*, where they serve also to confirm the authority of leading members of the new church.[108]

To attempt to define a specifically New Testament attitude towards medicine is fraught with difficulties. It is not only that each of the New Testament writers themselves has his own slightly different perspective and bias, but also that, even when they describe acts of healing, their focus is rarely on their strictly medical components. In Owsei Temkin's words, on the whole the world of Jesus and the world of secular medicine – including Hippocratic medicine – are not congruent.[109] So, for example, when the failures of doctors are noted they are mentioned as background to the events, not as an indication of antagonism towards secular medicine.[110] Indeed, if the traditional identification of Luke as the 'blessed physician' and travelling companion of St Paul is correct, Christianity had, almost from its inception, its own model physician.[111] Besides, as eventually constituted, the New Testament contains a variety of texts that may present in minor details opinions that are not always easy to reconcile with each other. Paul's practical advice to take a little wine for the stomach's sake balances the demand in the *Epistle* of St James that the Christian should rely only on a medicine of faith, prayer, confession and the laying on of hands.[112] At other times, it is possible to detect alternative views even within the same author. Jesus'

293

position on the relationship between sin and disease, a favoured topic in contemporary Rabbinical debates, is set out with great care.[113] Although his interlocutors urge a direct link between sin and disease, Jesus is never represented as accepting that position.[114] Rather, he takes the line that sinfulness is an obstacle to receiving divine healing, and that repentance and faith are both necessary if the sufferer is to be healed – and to remain so. At other times, the healing takes place without any explanation. Whatever has taken place before the healing is thus irrelevant: what matters is the relationship between the individual and the healer, and ultimately between the healer and God, that allows him or her to receive divine healing.

These subtle differences of emphasis at times within and between the individual writers of the New Testament were interpreted by later Christians in a variety of different ways. Some, focusing on sinfulness and the Christian medicine advocated by St James, eschewed all secular medicine, and certainly those parts of it that seemed to be close to magic. Tatian, in the second century, declared the use of drugs to be a form of apostasy from God, warning that a recovery brought about through these secular means was a delusion of the Devil: the demons, who were the true cause of the disease, had decided voluntarily to end their sport and had flown away.[115] If Tatian's point of view is perhaps extreme, there were others who considered that true Christians, by living sinless lives, could avoid disease or at any rate could ensure a cure by prayer and faith. Others, concentrating on the eternal life open to the Christian soul, saw the body as a mere tomb, a transitory habitation of the immortal soul. Physical health was thus irrelevant to the soul's salvation. Indeed, there were some who saw the mortification of the flesh as a proof of their faith, and illness and infirmity as, if not deserved punishment, at least a divine means of testing, strengthening and even rewarding their faith. Non-Christians would have recoiled at the joy of the African bishop Cyprian, who told his flock to welcome the plague of 252 as proof of God's love and mercy, because unbelievers were sent more swiftly to Hell and the just would attain even more speedily their everlasting refreshment.[116] By contrast, many Christians accepted secular healing with gratitude: it was a gift from God, who did not wish mankind to be bereft of help in times of illness. As such, it was part of God's work of creation, to be distinguished sharply from what was offered by pagan magi and exorcists. From Simon Magus onwards, these practitioners were held up as devilish impostors whose wish to belong to the church should be closely scrutinised – and rebuffed.[117]

Amid this multiplicity of attitudes to medicine among Christians of the first three centuries – and one should not forget that there was at this date no 'official' Christian view and no means of securing the adherence of all believers to one, had it existed – one thing is clear. The miracle stories in the New Testament and in the Apocryphal Gospels are not casual insertions. They demonstrate the divine healing power of Jesus and his followers as well as its capacity to attract potential converts. Sufferers flock to Jesus from far and wide; they struggle to get close to experience his healing power for themselves; if they cannot come in person, they send friends or relatives to make contact with him.[118] Stories of healing figure prominently in many of the early missionary accounts.[119] Philip at Samaria drew crowds to watch him perform miracles of healing on those possessed and paralysed.[120] In Judaea Peter's healings at Lydda and Joppa convinced many to become Christians.[121] On Paul's first missionary journey in Asia Minor the crowds at Lystra interpreted his cure of the cripple as proof that he and Barnabas were themselves gods in human form; at Ephesus, handkerchiefs and scarves that had merely been in contact with him were reported to cure the sick.[122]

The Apocryphal Gospels and Acts are full of such miracles, as well as repeating the healing stories from Matthew, Mark and Luke.[123] St John, healing an old woman in a packed theatre, expressly says that his healing miracles will convert those who have come along simply out of curiosity. St Andrew, by his alleged cure of a proconsul and others at Patras in Greece, brings the whole city to accept Christianity.[124] The *Acts of Peter*, probably written around AD 200, records alongside many healing miracles Peter's 'failure' to cure his own paralysed daughter. He first orders her to rise up and walk, 'to convince' the onlookers and 'to increase the faith', but then, since God has ordained her infirmity, Peter orders her to return to her sickness, since she may harm many souls if her body remains healthy.[125] These miracle stories circulated widely in the early church, and may have formed a major part of the church's appeal.[126] The fourth-century ecclesiastical historian Eusebius ends the first book of his history with the conversion of King Abgar after he had been healed of a chronic disease by the apostle Thaddeus. Eusebius, drawing on local stories and citing what is to him a genuine correspondence between Abgar and Christ, emphasises over and over again the cures of Christ, 'made without drugs and herbs', and the subsequent fame that they enjoyed in Judaea and beyond.[127] In Eusebius' own day a bronze statue at Caesarea Philippi was believed to represent the woman with the issue of blood in the act of stretching out her hands to Jesus, and a strange form of mould growing on the statue base was eaten as protection against diseases of all kinds.[128] That the story of Abgar, documents and all, is an invention of the third century, and the statue possibly that of Asclepius and Hygieia, only indicates the strength of the continued belief in Christianity as a religion that offered to heal the body as well as the soul.[129]

Christianity also adopted and extended the Jewish concept of charity and care for one's fellow Jews in ways that overlapped with physical healing.[130] The Jewish scriptures and the Rabbinical commentaries frequently emphasised the charitable duty of all Jews to their fellow believers. This was a communal obligation, very different from the euergetism of the Greeks and Romans, which stressed the individual nature of any public benefaction and confined actual obligations to those affecting one's family and clients. Jewish charity often took the form of a communal chest, from which money might be given to support the poor and needy, or of a hostel where fellow Jews might be housed, fed and looked after as they made their way on pilgrimage to Jerusalem.[131] Later traditions attributed the first such hostel to Abraham, an inventive interpretation of the tamarisk tree that he had planted at Beersheba.[132] By the first century of the Christian era, if not a century earlier, some of these hostels were more than a room in a private house, and were intended to last. That erected by Theodotus, son of Vettenus, in Jerusalem around AD 30 was a substantial building with a wide range of facilities for pilgrims, as well as for religious study.[133]

These Jewish notions of charity had a major influence on early Christianity. Not only were the twelve apostles sent out to cure the sick, raise the dead, cleanse the lepers and cast out demons, but in parables and in direct injunctions Jesus told his followers to feed the hungry and care for those in need.[134] The very early Christians pooled their goods and distributed them among the community as and when required. But as the numbers of those receiving assistance increased, so too did complaints about unfair distribution: the Greeks among the early Christians in Jerusalem thought that Jewish widows were being given preferential treatment. As a result, a system of 'deacons' ('servants', 'distributors') was created to oversee the daily allotment.[135] This system of organised charity was swiftly adopted by other Christian communities around the Mediterranean, and became a prominent feature of the early church.

This organised charity went beyond the Jewish notion of a communal charity chest in three ways. First, it was not confined to members of one religious group, but was extended to all in need, whatever their beliefs. As such it had an important role to play in the evangelical mission of Christianity. Second, the numbers of those involved in the organisation and distribution of charity were substantial. Already by the late second century the church in Rome, which was caring for well over a thousand poor, was being held up as a model for others to follow.[136] In an epidemic at Alexandria in 262, Bishop Dionysius directed a massive relief operation, tending the sick and burying the dead, in sharp contrast, so he alleged, to the pagans, who threw their sick relatives out of the house and left their own dead to lie unburied in the streets, afraid that they would catch the disease.[137]

Third, there was an explicit duty to care for the sick as part of this charitable outreach. Bishop Dionysius was only one of many clerics who enjoined their flock to follow Jesus' teaching in caring for the sick. Polycarp of Smyrna in the early second century thought it a major responsibility of the elders of the church, while the so-called *Apostolic Constitutions*, reflecting practice in Christian communities at the end of that century, expected all bishops to care for the sick, even, so a Roman rulebook suggested, going into private houses to seek them out.[138] By the fourth century the church of Alexandria had a corps of '*parabalani*', strong men equally adept at bringing in the sick, carrying out the dead for burial and battling against angry pagans.[139] A bishop like Cyprian or Gregory Thaumaturgus would, like a father, take into his house those members of his family – and to the Christian all alike were potentially members of the Christian family – who needed help.[140]

It is thus not surprising that in 362 the Emperor Julian, seeking to restore pagan religion, should write to the high priest of the province of Galatia to encourage him to imitate Jews and Christians in their charitable activities. Whereas they had gained adherents by their moral uprightness, their philanthropy to strangers and their concern to give an appropriate burial to even the poorest, pagans rarely gave relief even to fellow pagans. This disgraceful state of affairs, when no Jew went in need, and when the Christians cared not only for their own, but also for pagans, was a reproach to traditional religion. The high priest was ordered to set up several hostels in every town, for the benefit of those in need, pagan and non-pagan alike, and he was offered money for food and wine for distribution among the poor and the stranger.[141] In the words of a later Christian historian, 'he thought he could trick the people by endeavouring to imitate the good works of the Christians, ordering *xenones* and *ptocheia* to be organised'.[142]

Charting the interplay of religion and medicine in the first three centuries of the Roman Empire is a complex task. As we have seen, individual attitudes varied, although few were hostile to the very notion of divine healing, whether obtained through dreams, oracles or simply the bargaining implied in making a vow for one's future health. Conversely, evidence for opposition to, or even disappointment with, secular medicine on the part of those who sought religious healing is also relatively rare. The great majority of the population, one might conclude, had no difficulty in accepting the co-existence, and at times the collaboration, of both types of healing.

Inscriptions, coins, papyri and archaeology show healing shrines built or refurbished throughout the Roman Empire in the first three centuries, more likely the result of the general peace and prosperity, particularly in Asia Minor, the Levant and N. Africa, than of any great surge of interest in, or necessity for, religious healing compared with previous centuries. What they reveal above all is the sheer variety of healing cults and divinities, something that is easily forgotten in a concentration on one or two of the best known, like that of Asclepius or Sarapis. Many cults were local or regional at best, and only a few spread across the Roman Empire. Some of them were associated with a particular place, often a spring; in others, one can see at work a process of convergence with more universal divinities. Some deities, Asclepius and his family above all, can be considered specialists in restoring or perpetuating the well-being of their votaries, but there are many others, for example Mars or Hercules, for whom healing was only a relatively minor part of their activities.

Jewish and Christian sources from the period before AD 300 present an interesting range of contrasts with their pagan contemporaries. It is not only that their monotheism was strongly opposed to the religious pluralism that would accept that a plague could be ended by the introduction of the worship of a new god into a community. Both Jews and Christians debated the relationship between sin and suffering on the basis of a definition of sin that was far more extensive and moralistic than that of pagans. In both religious communities the power to heal was linked closely with the will of God, whether it was seen as something placed on earth by God for the benefit of mankind or, in the case of prophets and apostles, a sign of special favour that gave added religious authority. Particularly among Christians, one consequence was the need to distinguish sharply between true and false prophets, between miracle and magic, and between the intervention of God and his angels, on the one hand, and that of demons on the other.[143]

Finally, healing occupies a leading place in the historical literature of Christianity. The miracles of Jesus and his followers are recorded in detail, and Jesus' instructions to his disciples repeated in episcopal letters and ordinances. Although one should not underestimate the tendency of pagan shrines to exploit their own healing miracles for propaganda purposes, Christians gladly used their charitable and curative gifts as a way of attracting others, along with their promise of eternal salvation. Crowds of curious onlookers flocked to see signs and wonders, and, as both Christians and pagans agreed, Christian kindness and generosity to all in need broke with the conventions that restricted them to one's family and clients, or to an ostentatious benefaction of a temple or a feast to one's fellow citizens.

But, it should be remembered, until the fourth century Christianity was still a persecuted religion, alien to many of the inhabitants of the Roman Empire. Although its missionary zeal sharply increased the numbers of its adherents, the impact of its ideas on the wider community was far less great in the third century than it was later to become. Christian debates and discussions remained largely confined within the Christian community, and were arguably of far less significance to the average Roman or Greek than the many pagan oracles and temples to which the majority of the population resorted in time of need. From another perspective, however, it is precisely in this period that the ideas were formed within the Christian community that were taken for granted in the Later, Christian, Roman Empire and that went on to influence more widely the ways in which medicine was envisaged in Late Antiquity and beyond.

19

MEDICINE IN THE LATER ROMAN EMPIRE

By AD 650 ancient medicine had taken on the form in which it was to dominate the theory and practice of medicine in the Greek East, and subsequently in the Muslim world and the Latin West, for a millennium – namely, Galenism. Learned doctors and other intellectuals were now agreed that the human body, organised anatomically and physiologically into three almost separate systems based on the brain, heart and liver, depended for its health ultimately on a balance between its four constituent humours, blood, bile, black bile and phlegm. This balance varied according to the individual's age and diet (in the broadest sense of the term), the season of the year and the environment, and determined not only physical but also mental well-being. It was a system standing firmly on the twin pillars of observation and logic, and gained added authority from the longevity of the theories on which it was based and from the ease with which it could be co-ordinated with other systems of thought, such as Aristotelianism, Platonism and monotheism. It was not entirely immune to change, although its rhetoric of certainty did not allow for radical developments or more than a circumscribed area of disagreement. Such a theory, backed up by centuries of observations and apparently effective therapies, had deservedly triumphed. The vigorous debates of fifth-century BC Greece or second-century Rome were long gone: arguments over the interpretation of Galen had replaced disputes over alternatives to Galen.[1] How the pluralism of earlier medicine developed into this near-monolithic system and how it interacted with an increasingly desecularised world are the main themes of this chapter.

Any answer to the first question runs into an immediate difficulty. The century and a half that follows the death of Galen is a black hole in the history of medicine. No completely surviving text can be assigned with confidence to this period, except for Gargilius Martialis' book on *Medicines from Fruits and Vegetables* and a strongly Neoplatonist essay, preserved under the name of Galen, on the way in which the foetus receives its soul.[2] Several recipes for both animals and humans, as well as magical tricks and useful hints on everything from archery to surveying, were included by the Greek writer Julius Africanus in his *Tapestries (Cestoi)*, written about 225.[3] A few scattered fragments of

299

veterinary authors such as Theomnestus, writing around 326, and his slightly earlier source, Apsyrtus, remind us of a once-flourishing literature on animal medicine, in Greek as well as in Latin.[4] The inscriptional record of doctors also drops away substantially after the middle of the third century (although the geographically restricted evidence of the papyri continues). There is likewise a diminution in the quantity of literary and historical material available, with the exception of Christian writers, who focus on medical matters only incidentally or in the context of the miracles of saints. But hagiography is an elusive genre, and the modern historian must work hard to win nuggets from even so apparently informative a source as the life of St Gregory Thaumaturgus ('the wonder-worker', c.220–72), bishop of Pontus.[5] Tracking medical developments in this period is thus an act of faith, not of history.

When our information reappears in quantity, from the 340s onwards, the picture that emerges has altered greatly since the second century. The Roman Empire has gained a second capital, Constantinople, and a newly authorised religion, Christianity, and in law, literature and astronomy as well as in medicine the codification of earlier learning has taken over from original thought. Compendia, commentaries, large collections of extracts from earlier authors and short guides to self-help medicine replace the wide-ranging discussions of Galen; systematic anatomical investigation ('Hippocratic butchery', as one Christian author called it) has disappeared;[6] and belief in demons, chants, charms and magical herbs obtrudes into the rationalities of natural philosophy. Although the name of Hippocrates has now come to stand for medicine itself, the Hippocratic physician appears an endangered species in a world increasingly dominated, and divided, by religion.[7] It is a situation that continued at least into the seventh century.

One explanation for this new medical landscape puts the emphasis on social, political and economic changes in society at large. The invasions and civil wars of the middle years of the third century and the first quarter of the fourth disrupted the prosperity of the Empire and its institutions. The response of emperors such as Diocletian (reigned 284–305) and Constantine (reigned 307–37) was to cling more closely to the past for justification, even as they imposed radical changes on society. Although it would be going far too far to see this as a decline, patterns of behaviour and thought, as well as political and social priorities, altered in reaction to altered circumstances. An inhabitant of the new eastern capital, Constantinople, massively enlarged from a town to a megalopolis within a few decades, was bound to have a different outlook from that of an aristocrat in Rome.[8]

Linguistic, cultural, military and political circumstances also combined to break the unity of the Roman Empire. From 364 onwards the two halves of the Empire were ruled by separate, although initially related, emperors and gradually drew apart. The city of Rome progressively lost political importance, even as it asserted its ecclesiastical pre-eminence. By 600 the Latin West, under the impact of a series of barbarian invasions, had split into a number of independently developing kingdoms or regions. Their economic foundations were no longer as strong as those in the East; towns were fewer and their urban institutions weaker. *Medici* can be found, even in areas as remote as the Lleyn peninsula in N. Wales, but they appear in isolation.[9] Learning, where it existed, was mainly under the protection, and for the purposes, of the church: the syntheses of medicine and of anatomy in Books 4 and 11 of the *Etymologies* of Bishop Isidore of Seville (d. 640) were intended to be studied as words, by grammarians.[10] Medical practice thus developed in different ways to cope with different societies.

However, the emphasis of this sociological explanation on change underestimates the continuities and the distorting effect of Galen and the Galenic Corpus. If we did not have the many volumes of the garrulous Pergamene, the pattern of medical life would scarcely seem to alter over the centuries, especially in the Greek half of the Empire. Civic doctors in small towns in Late Antiquity still assert their right to tax immunity in the face of demands from needy tax-payers. Public regulations, extended in 368 to Rome and its new college of doctors, still urge the merits of medical education and emphasise the need for honest practice – and continue to be evaded.[11] Law codes continue to lay down the exact price for a slave trained in medicine, just as if this was the Rome of Augustus.[12] Handbooks, drug collections, guides such as Celsus or Rufus' *For the Layman*, compilations of information from other writers, such as the *Introduction to Medicine*, medical catechisms and summaries are found in both the High and the Later Empire. A belief in the powers of chants, amulets and spells is not confined to Late Antiquity.[13] What was unusual was Galen, with his philosophical disquisitions, his insistence on anatomy and his long-winded theoretical expositions of causes or symptoms. To take Galen as typical, one might argue, results in a historically flawed perspective that plays down the similarities between the centuries and creates the impression of a catastrophic decline the moment Galen disappears from the scene.

To decide between the validity of an approach that stresses the continuities and one that emphasises the differences between the centuries is far from easy. And even if one opts for change, the superiority does not always lie with the authors of the earlier period. Caelius Aurelianus' massive Latin treatise *On Acute and Chronic Diseases*, written around AD 400, is fuller and at times clearer than the similar one of Aretaeus two centuries or more before. Pelagonius, writing his substantial Latin treatise on veterinary medicine at the end of the fourth century, shows no concern about a medical decline: true, while on a journey it might prove difficult to find assistance immediately, and any owner of horses should acquaint himself with at least the basics of horse medicine, but that had always been the case.[14] By contrast, it is more often the information in our non-medical sources that suggests a difference in tone, a reduction in overt speculation, a closing in of horizons, perhaps even a growing split between a tiny elite and the rest of society. A passing comment of the church historian Philostorgius neatly exemplifies this shift. Posidonius, a learned doctor at the end of the fourth century and an expert on mental diseases, was regarded as unusual for maintaining that madness was not the result of attacks by demons but had a physical cause in the imbalance of humours.[15]

This ambiguity in our sources' characterisation of medicine in Late Antiquity was neatly summarised by Owsei Temkin in 1962 when he argued that Byzantine medicine 'represents the formation as well as the continuation of a tradition, broken and unbroken'.[16] In other words, one can detect important changes taking place, even as the participants themselves claim to be maintaining past tradition, and these changes in turn come to be seen as part of that tradition. Very rarely can one point to a specific individual as the agent of change – there is no Herophilus, no Asclepiades, for instance – or to any one decisive moment. Often these developments can be seen only over the long term, by comparison with what went before or as laying the foundations for others yet to come – for example the development of Galenism, the growing split between theory and practice, the role of translation and bilingualism and, above all, the accommodation of medicine to the new institutions of Christianity. All these developments, as we shall see, give the lie to any interpretation of the medicine of Late Antiquity in terms of stagnation and uncomprehending decline. Rather, they show new, and at times vigorous, responses on the part of doctors, of all kinds, to the society around them, even as they assert continuities with their own heritage.

These responses took a variety of forms. For example, the general surveys by the three most substantial Greek medical writers to survive from Late Antiquity, Oribasius of Pergamum (c.325–400), Aetius of Amida (S.E. Turkey, fl. 530) and Paul of Aegina (active in Alexandria c.630), differ substantially from anything found earlier.[17] Celsus and Pliny may have derived most of their material from what they had read, but they imposed on it their own individual emphases and style. By contrast, in the later syntheses extracts from earlier writers are assembled, often verbatim and duly acknowledged, into a coherent mosaic of opinions, ideas and remedies. Comments by the compiler himself are almost non-existent. These encyclopaedias varied greatly in size; Oribasius produced one for his patron, the Emperor Julian, in seventy books, of which over thirty survive, another in nine books for his son Eustathius, one in four books for his friend and biographer Eunapius (340–c.414) and a further single volume (now lost) of Galenic extracts, the fruit of midnight discussion with Julian while on campaign in Gaul c.358.[18] These medical encyclopaedias display learning, elegant organisation and practicality, virtues not to be despised or dismissed in favour of novelty. They are more than mere repertories of the past, valuable though they are for that reason. Paul's Book 6 is by far the most informative (and most practically minded) Greek surgical text extant, covering everything from hernias and fistulae to sprained ankles and varicose veins, and from the removal of missiles from battlefield wounds to the surgical reduction of over-large breasts in a man, 'which bring the reproach of femininity'.[19] Paul's text is also a tribute to an ongoing Alexandrian surgical tradition, in which complicated operations continued to be performed, with apparent success and with a more than local fame, at least until the seventh century. The procedure he recommends for removing a severely damaged rib could well be followed today, while his comments, based on Antyllus, about the dangers involved in an emergency trachaeotomy imply that that operation had been attempted, and may well have succeeded.[20] One can see why the Scottish physician and translator Francis Adams of Banchory should have chosen in the 1820s to embark on a translation of Paul, furnished with an extensive commentary, because of its practical relevance to contemporary therapeutics.[21]

But, at the same time, much was lost in this process of redaction. As these encyclopaedias developed, they became more and more brusque. Alternatives became irrelevant luxuries, and the word of Galen came to dominate over all others. The long citations in Oribasius were often amalgamated, and the names of the different authors omitted or lumped together under that of Galen, to form a coherent and succinct account of a particular topic. Galen's hesitations and qualifications (and even self-contradictions) were edited out, and the practical and empirical side of his work was replaced by the dogmatic. Galen was becoming Galenism.

This process was assisted by Galen's own rhetoric. More than once he had claimed to be perfecting medicine, or to be transmitting what Hippocrates had already completed. Hence it was easy to believe that all medical knowledge was contained in his many volumes, if one did but look closely. 'Hippocrates sowed the seed, Galen reaped the harvest', said one resigned author, with the implication that only unprofitable stubble remained.[22] The sheer size of Galen's achievement was also daunting. Few believed that they could now master the whole of medicine as he had done, and they preferred either to summarise or to concentrate on only one part of the medicine that he had unified.

Nevertheless, the spread of Galenism was neither universal nor immediate. There were still Asclepiadeans in Asia Minor in the fourth century, and Methodists flourished in the Latin world for some time after that.[23] Even among followers of Galen, there were rival interpretations and arguments between pragmatists and rigorists. Alexander of Tralles, writing around 560, contrasted his own willingness to employ a variety of therapies with the reluctance of the book-bound, ineffective and even murderous Galenist to depart from his master's words, even when common sense demanded it. Alexander was no backwoodsman relying on a few books and herbal remedies, but a cosmopolitan Greek, the brother of both the Emperor Justinian's legal adviser and the architect of Hagia Sophia, the greatest church of Byzantium. He had travelled widely, to N. Africa, Italy and further west with the emperor's troops, and he had sought out remedies from peasants, *more galenico*, in

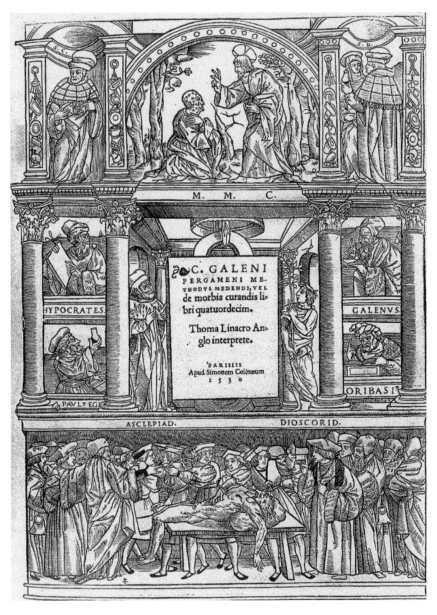

Within the illustration:

M. M. C.

C. GALENI
PERGAMENI ME-
THODVS MEDENDI, VEL
de morbis curandis li-
bri quatuordecim.

Thoma Linacro An-
glo interprete.

PARISIIS
Apud Simonem Colinæum
1530

HYPOCRATES.

GALENVS.

PAVL⁹ EG.

ORIBASI⁹

ASCLEPIAD.   DIOSCORID.

Figure 19.1 The great doctors of Antiquity, Hippocrates, Galen, Paul, Oribasius, Asclepiades and Dioscorides. Frontispiece to Thomas Linacre's Latin version of Galen's *Method of Healing*, Paris, S. de Colines, 1530. The artist depicts the dissection of a human body, perhaps alluding to Galen, although the book itself has nothing to do with anatomy. Courtesy of Wellcome Library, London.

Tuscany, Gaul, Spain and even Armenia. His knowledge of Galen is impressive, and he at times displays a similar spirit of inquiry, even if, as with his store of chants and charms, he is prevented from displaying all that he knows in his writings. How many others shared his independence and combativeness we cannot tell because of the paucity of our sources.[24]

A second important development in Late Antiquity that favoured Galenism was a growing split between theory and practice. The earliest extant reference to medicine being divided in this way dates from around 200, and by 400 it had become a standard feature of all medical textbooks.[25] It was encouraged by the legacy of Galen, whose insistence on the need for a doctor to understand philosophy came to be interpreted as a demand for a preparatory training in logic as well as for a greater theoretical content in medical education. It is thus not surprising, or uncommon, to find in fifth- and sixth-century Alexandria the same man commenting on Aristotle as easily as on Hippocrates. Stephanus of Athens (c.550–c.630), for example, lectured on at least three works by Hippocrates and Galen and four by Aristotle, as well as writing on theology and astronomy.[26]

This increased interest in theory also encouraged the move towards a definition of medicine in terms of specific books. Although Galen himself had commented on various texts of Hippocrates and regarded the *Aphorisms* as essential for any physician, he had laid down no canon of set texts. In contrast, by 500 in Alexandria one can trace not only a syllabus of Hippocratic texts (largely those preferred by Galen), but also the appearance of a Galenic canon, the so-called sixteen books (in reality twenty-four, some being subsumed into larger works).[27] They were read in a specific order and were further explicated by means of formal lectures and commentaries. They offered a coherent and well-structured syllabus, beginning with first principles, as laid down in *On Sects* and the *Art of Medicine*. There followed brief guides to taking the pulse and therapeutics, before the student embarked on more extensive and specialised treatises. In modern terms, he was instructed in anatomy, physiology, pathology and therapeutics, ending possibly with dietetics and hygiene.[28] Although he would be encouraged to read further Galenic treatises, this syllabus in itself provided an overall view of Galenic medicine that was sufficient for many practitioners. It was translated in the early sixth century into Syriac, the vernacular language of the Middle East from Palestine to Persia, and commentaries on it survive in Latin from sixth- or seventh-century Ravenna, the centre of Byzantine administration in N. Italy.[29]

These texts were also abridged for ease of memorisation, thus imparting yet further rigidity to Galenism. Short texts on the four humours or on prognostic added new material, such as the four winds or the three spirits, to Galen's advice and interpretation, and in the so-called Alexandrian summaries, passages might be brought together from the whole Galenic Corpus to produce an impression different from that originally intended by Galen.[30] One such conflation became a leading motif in later Galenist therapeutics:

a brief passing comment on the factors that altered the pulse was combined with a section from a commentary explaining Hippocrates' view of the determinants of health (diet, environment, exertion, sleep, excretions and mental activity) to form a programmatic statement of the aims of the whole art of medicine.[31] From now on, Galenists generally organised their diagnoses and, particularly, their treatments, at the bedside and in their writings, to take account of these 'six non-naturals', a technical term also produced by conflating several Galenic passages.

This process of consolidation of Galenic doctrine, of change within continuity, is neatly exemplified at the end of the fourth century in the career of Magnus of Nisibis (S.E. Turkey), the most famous of the teachers at Alexandria, 'the foundation of health for all men', as a contemporary geographer put it.[32] He was awarded a public lecture theatre by the city of Alexandria (a unique privilege, as far as we know) and dominated the medical life of the city for a generation.[33] So great was his reputation that a poet imagined him descending to Hades to defeat death by argument.[34] His biographer, Eunapius, a friend of Oribasius, claimed that Magnus could persuade those cured by others that they were still ill purely by the force of his oratory. Eunapius drew a contrast between Magnus and his equally eminent colleague Ionicus, an expert in practical medicine, especially in bandaging and surgery, but no speaker.[35] Eunapius' preference is obvious, and it was shared by the many students who flocked to hear Magnus from all over the eastern Mediterranean.[36] A book on urine that survives under the name of Magnus of Emesa (a city not far from Nisibis) may be his. It is avowedly based on scattered incidents and ideas in the Galenic Corpus, selected, organised and worked up into an elegant and effective guide to diagnosis through the urine.[37] It marks also a significant shift, for it transforms uroscopy, which Galen had used as an occasional guide to diagnosis, into an essential element in medical practice. Henceforth, in both the East and West, the urine flask becomes the symbol of the educated physician. There were similar short, comprehensive guides to taking the pulse, such as that by Philaretus (or Philagrius), which extended what Galen had done in his own abridgments of his pulse treatises.[38]

It was not only in the Greek world that there were new developments in Late Antiquity. Throughout N. Africa the fourth and fifth centuries saw an upsurge in learned Latin medicine parallel to that in learned theology – this was, after all, the age of St Augustine. Cassius Felix of Cirta (Constantine, Ksantina, Algeria), 'an adherent of the logical sect', who compiled a medical handbook in 447, drew heavily upon Greek sources, Methodist and Galenist alike, for his synthesis.[39] His older contemporary Caelius Aurelianus (c.420), a doctor from Sicca Veneria (El-Kef, Tunisia), displayed an even wider range of learning in his large nosographical handbook *On Acute and Chronic Diseases*, although it remains unclear whether he was simply translating an earlier Greek Methodist work by Soranus of Ephesus or added substantial material of his own.[40] At the very least, Caelius abridged and possibly reorganised some of his Greek material with care and intelligence.[41] This is Latin learned medicine at its best, as befitted a region in touch with Alexandria.[42]

Caelius' work is far broader in its coverage of diseases and more academic in its approach than similar contemporary productions from Italy and Gaul, which emphasised the need for self-help in a society in which the social and intellectual institutions that had sustained Galenic medicine were rapidly disintegrating. The drug handbook of Marcellus, a highly placed official of the Emperor Theodosius at the end of the fourth century, adds to Scribonius Largus a variety of local Gallic remedies, as well as chants, charms and more popular material, in order to produce a manual of domestic medicine.[43] The differences between this book and the similar handbook of Alexander of Tralles a century later signify two very different worlds. The Greek Alexander added his chants and charms to a Galenic synthesis that derived both stability and effectiveness from its roots in a Hippocratic past. There were constraints on what a doctor could now use in a Christian world, but Alexander was still able to see himself as part of a traditional intellectual community within a confident Eastern Roman Empire.[44] For Marcellus, despite his links with the court and the leading men of Gaul and N. Spain, and despite the presence in Bordeaux of other cultivated doctors like the father of the poet Ausonius, many of the old certainties were disappearing in a new landscape.[45] Although he recommended that *medici* should be summoned in difficult and dangerous cases, Marcellus' readers were, for the most part, expected to rely on themselves; they must, like him, be *empirici*, not as followers of the Greek Empiricist sect, but as experts in what worked. In Marcellus' book the agricultural tradition of Cato reappears just as the civic organisation of Roman Gaul splinters into that of the great mediaeval estates.[46]

The fifth and sixth centuries are also the time when a few older Greek medical texts were turned into Latin. But whereas Caelius and Cassius Felix, like Cornelius Celsus before them, had claimed to reinterpret Greek learning in their own Latin handbooks, these (largely anonymous) translations made no such assertion of originality. When around 570 the wealthy senator Cassiodorus advised the monks of his new foundation at Vivarium (S. Italy) to aid the sick with medicines and the hope they had in God, he commended to the monastery library a few essential medical texts – Gargilius Martialis; some Latin versions of Hippocrates and Galen's *Method of Healing, for Glaucon*; an anonymous compendium; an (illustrated?) Dioscorides; Caelius Aurelius, *On Medicine*; Hippocrates, *On Herbs and Cures*; and a few other books, a meagre harvest from Classical Antiquity.[47] Although at first sight the authors are well known, the names may well hide a variety of suppositious works. Five or six tracts from our Greek Hippocratic Corpus were available in Latin by this date, including *Aphorisms*, *Prognostic* and *Airs, Waters and Places*, but *On Herbs and Cures* is not among them, unless, as some scholars think, it was the title given to a compilation of extracts from *Diet*.[48] Early mediaeval Latin manuscripts transmitted under the heading of Galen's *Method of Healing, for Glaucon*, alongside a translation of its two genuine books, others that were certainly not by Galen, even if within the Galenic tradition.[49] 'Caelius Aurelius' may refer to Caelius Aurelianus, *On Acute and Chronic Diseases* (although the sheer size of this work makes it unlikely), or to a popular compendium on fevers ascribed simply to one Aurelius. Likewise, the treatise of Dioscorides may not be a Latin version of his famous herbal, but the tract *On Feminine Herbs* goes under his name and survives in at least seven manuscripts written before 900.[50] Such short practical works attributed to famous names of the past (or simply anonymous) are characteristic of these early Latin medical manuscripts.

A similar process of translation can be found in the East, where the priest, doctor and diplomat Sergius of Resaena translated the Alexandrian syllabus of Galen into Syriac.[51] His endeavours enabled Syriac authors such as Ahrun and Theodorus to write their own compendia of medicine, and laid the foundations for the (far more extensive and more accurate) translations into Syriac and Arabic made in the ninth century by Hunain ibn Ishaq and his colleagues.[52] In this way Galenism became the basis for formal medicine in the Muslim world, and, through Latin translations of Arabic works from the eleventh century onwards, was transmitted to the learned world of the mediaeval European universities.

Like Sergius, many doctors were bi- or even trilingual, mediating between different religious or political groups as guides, ambassadors or court politicians. Elpidius, a doctor and deacon with connections in S. Gaul, Liguria and Milan, knew Greek well enough to serve on an embassy to Constantinople in 515–17. He later returned to Italy and became doctor to King Theodoric of the Ostrogoths.[53] His physician contemporary Anthimus sent a letter, written in everyday Latin, to 'Theodoric, King of the Franks', giving him advice on diet: lightly boiled fresh hens' eggs, taken with a pinch of salt, are the best food for both sick and healthy.[54] Sergius himself became involved in an obscure theological dispute with his bishop and, as a consequence, was sent by the bishop of Antioch to Rome with a letter for Pope Agapetus. He died at Constantinople in 536 while on his way back, to the delight of the Monophysites, who thought his death in agony fit punishment for 'so lustful and incontinent a heretic'.[55] His contemporary Stephen of Edessa, after a period of service as court doctor to the Sassanian King Kavad I (d. 531), returned to the Roman Empire and his native city, acting as its envoy when it was later besieged by the Sassanians. In the subsequent peace negotiations King Chosroes insisted on the return of his personal physician, Tribunus, from the Byzantine Empire.[56] In the complicated religious and political rivalries between, and within, the Byzantine and Sassanian Empires in the sixth and early seventh centuries doctors played – or were thought by contemporaries to have played – key roles in securing the predominance of one side or another. The Monophysite Christian physician Gabriel of Singara, for example, who was said to have gained influence over the Sassanian monarch Chosroes II through treating Queen Sirin, was notorious for centuries among the Nestorian Christians for his diplomatic double-dealing and for his oppression of their leaders. They consoled themselves with the thought that when challenged in a religious debate before Gabriel in 612 their representatives had stood firm in their adherence to the true faith, despite facing punishment and even death as a result.[57]

This debate, formally organised in Persia but involving Syriac-speaking Christians drawn also from the Eastern Roman Empire, exemplifies the changed role of Christianity over the previous three centuries. From 313 onwards, not only did Christianity cease to be a persecuted religion, but imperial resources and imperial favour were put behind it to an unprecedented degree. By the end of the fourth century, state legislation was increasingly used to forbid, or at least to restrict, non-Christian cults, and questions of Christian orthodoxy, and its opposite, heresy, had become important subjects of imperial policy. The Christian Church adapted to meet this new situation, becoming more structured and more authoritarian. Bishops became more important in politics and in society at large than provincial governors. When plague struck the small town of Myra (S.W. Turkey) in 542, it was to their bishop, Nicholas, that the inhabitants turned. When the local farmers wisely refused to come near the affected town a food shortage followed, and the bishop was almost arrested on the suspicion that he had induced this boycott in order to drive up prices.[58] There was what some historians have called a process of desecularisation, as the claims of the Christian Church extended into areas of life scarcely touched by the older forms of religion.[59] The rest of this chapter will be devoted to exploring the impact on medicine and medical practice in Late Antiquity of this new series of relationships.

It should be understood at the outset that ecclesiastical authorities were not concerned with many aspects of medicine, unless and until they impinged on religious belief. They were not interested in traditional remedies and practices, for example, until, particularly in times of political or religious crisis, their use could seem to support an accusation of heresy or paganism. It then became a matter of importance that to the untutored or the prejudiced the art of prognosis might appear no different from magical astrology, or the recitation of a formula might be equated with the invocation of a pagan deity.[60] When an elderly patient fell seriously ill after having taken a drug once prescribed him for the same condition by a leading physician, he and his friends were at first convinced that the initial success had been obtained by illegal (that is, magical) means. Only when the doctor proved to them that the drug was now less effective because of the patient's age was all threat of punishment lifted.[61]

But, in general, Christians took a benign attitude to medicine. Methodius of Patara (d. *c*.311) even set his dialogue on the Resurrection in the house of a doctor, Aglaophon, and made him one of the chief speakers.[62] The Galenic conception of a wise Creator acting in the interests of mankind and placing herbs and other remedies on the earth to relieve suffering could easily be used to support Christianity itself. Theodoret of Cyrrhus (c.393–466), for example, referred to many medical ideas and cases as proof of the providence of the Christian God.[63] But the most extensive use of medical material occurs in the treatise *On the Nature of Man* by Nemesius, bishop of Emesa around 370, who quoted from or summarised at least fifteen treatises by Galen, including the rare *On Demonstration*. In this first Christian anthropology Nemesius placed his evidence from Galen almost on the same level as that from Scripture: both were necessary in order to understand the place of mankind in God's creation.[64] Galen's strong belief in the wise and benevolent purpose of a Creator, who could easily be equated with the Christian God, will have helped, over the long term, in the acceptance of Galenism.[65] But not all were willing to go quite so far yet. A century after Nemesius, Bishop Isidore of Pelusium drew a careful distinction between Galen's truly excellent medical expertise and his somewhat less successful forays into philosophical theology.[66]

Although certain types of healing, particularly involving divination or exorcism, were viewed with intense suspicion, and their practitioners forbidden baptism, some doctors continued to practise medicine even after being ordained.[67] Bishop Theodotus of Laodicea was famous for his excellence in medicine, both bodily and spiritual.[68] The tombstone of Dionysius, a doctor captured by the Goths in their assault on Rome in the late fifth century, proudly records that he was a priest and had demonstrated his Christian charity by treating his captors.[69] Gerontius, a deacon and doctor, fled to Constantinople from Milan after a disagreement with his bishop, Ambrose, and, through powerful friends, was made bishop of Nicomedia (N.W. Turkey). When the bishop of Constantinople, in response to a letter from Ambrose, tried to depose him the Nicomedians complained strongly, citing his unstinting use of his medical abilities among them.[70] Some medical men, like the martyred Zenobius, priest and doctor of Sidon, even came to be regarded as saints.[71] St Julian of Emesa was a leading citizen of the town, and a skilled physician of both body and soul; St Pantaleon had studied 'the learning of Asclepius, Hippocrates and Galen'; while SS. Cosmas and Damian were 'well acquainted with the tenets of Galen and Hippocrates'.[72] The refusal of the last pair to charge fees was a mark of their Christian charity, not a reproach to their fellow doctors or a sign of amateurism.[73]

Possession of medical skills, however, could be viewed as dangerous by one's opponents in the bitter inter-Christian disputes of the fourth and fifth centuries. Hieracas of Leonton was denounced by the heretic-hunter *par excellence*, Epiphanius of Salamis, as one 'trained in Greek learning, the art of the iatrosophists, magic and astrology'.[74] Aetius, one of the founders of Arianism, learned medicine from Sopolis, a doctor at Antioch, before becoming involved in theological controversy. Gregory of Nyssa, his opponent, called Sopolis a cheat and a ruffian, and Aetius a mere rhetorician; the Arian Philostorgius, by contrast, praised their medical skills and charity towards the poor.[75]

It was attachment to the older gods, however, at least as much as heresy, that increasingly attracted the suspicions of the Christian authorities. The relative tolerance of the first Christian emperors had allowed the pagan healing shrines to continue as before well into the fourth century. Indeed, the shrine of Nodens at Lydney in Gloucestershire seems to have enjoyed its best days in the middle years of that century.[76] But increasingly the large urban temples became the major focus of Christian hostility. At Aegeae, the great temple of Asclepius was razed to the ground in 331, and its columns either removed or reused in the Christian church on the site. Pagans viewed this as an outrage and an insult to the many thousands who had flocked there in search of healing. Not surprisingly, when the Emperor Julian in 363 wished to restore the older cults this was one temple that he attempted to have rebuilt.[77] The great Serapeum of Alexandria, which had been turned into something resembling a fortress of paganism, was destroyed in 391 after a major battle involving the *parabalani*.[78] At nearby Menuthis, the shrine of Isis was converted at this period into the church of St John the Evangelist, but worshippers of Isis continued to visit the town to receive healing and to consult the oracle. In response, the Bishop of Alexandria deliberately fostered (or invented) the cult of the Christian miracle healers, SS. Cyrus and John, whose 'surgery' was deliberately placed opposite that of Isis. Not until 483 was the decision taken to act against the many pagans who were still visiting the temple, and, after another riot, the Christians succeeded in destroying it completely.[79] At Epidaurus and at Pergamum, Christian churches were built by the end of the fourth century on the site of the great temples of Asclepius.[80] The cult images were destroyed, and, at least at Pergamum, all traces of them removed. At the shrine of Glycon at Tomi, worshippers themselves took away the cult statues and hid them carefully underground.[81]

The replacement of pagan healing gods was a gradual process. Bishop Theodoret, in the mid-fifth century, was convinced that Asclepius was still being worshipped in the rural hinterland of his large diocese of Cyrrhus in Syria.[82] At Athens, perhaps as late as 470, the philosopher Proclus was able to enter the next-door shrine of Asclepius, along with a fellow philosopher, and pray for the return to health of a young girl, but the shrine had been demolished by the time Marinus wrote his life of Proclus some fifteen years later.[83] In the early sixth century Caesarius, bishop of Arles, was afraid of a countryside where folk medicine and superstition were rampant, and he viewed even the expensive medicine of the towns as tinged with paganism.[84]

His suspicions, and those of many other zealous Christians, of what Temkin has called the doctors' commitment to a 'religion of Hippocrates' were not entirely misplaced.[85] One can sense the pleasure and relief of Arnobius, writing at the end of the fourth century, that, at long last, doctors of talent were turning to Christianity.[86] But it was a slow process, not

311

least at Alexandria. There the medical teachers and students included many who later became celebrated (or notorious) for their adherence to the older ways. Gregory of Nazianzus, describing the medical education of his brother at Alexandria around 315, was less impressed with Caesarius' intellectual triumphs than with his steadfast adherence to Christianity and the fact that he had refrained from swearing the (pagan) Hippocratic *Oath*.[87] In his *Life of Isidore*, written at the end of the fifth century, the Neoplatonist philosopher Damascius included many leading physicians in his account of the struggles of sympathisers to maintain the old religion in the face of Christian persecution.[88] The paganism of Hesychius and his son Jacobus Psychrestus, a court doctor at Constantinople famous for a new 'refreshing' treatment that reduced stress, embroiled them in political as well as medical controversy.[89] Jacobus' pupil Asclepiodotus of Aphrodisias was renowned for his knowledge of plants and stones as well as for his expertise in theurgy and mysticism, in part the product of a visit to the country of the magi.[90] Eusebius, a doctor at Emesa in Syria, travelled more than thirty miles to find the remains of a fallen star, which he affixed to the wall of a temple of Athena. The stone spoke, and henceforth Eusebius acted as the mouthpiece of the new oracle.[91] Another contemporary, the Alexandrian professor of medicine Gesius, 'whose rhetorical expertise removed all difficulties of exposition', was officially a Christian, but his pagan sympathies were revealed when he protected a pagan philosopher on the run from the emperor.[92] When he doubted the miraculous nature of the cures of SS. Cyrus and John, pointing out that this one could be traced back to Hippocrates and that to Galen, he was afflicted with a disease no mortal doctor could cure. Only after a full and contrite confession of his impiety, so Christians boasted, did he recover, through the divine powers of the saints whom he had ridiculed.[93] Little wonder that Bishop Procopius of Gaza, who was familiar with Gesius and his circle, explained the biblical story of the death of King Asa by blaming the King's doctors for using chants and similar mumbo-jumbo.[94] Asa's death was fit punishment for one who should have set an example to his subjects.

For pagans and Christians alike the ability to heal validated their religious message and the special nature of the healer's relationship with the divine. The author of the life of St Theodore of Sykeon, in sixth-century Galatia, includes the saint's healing miracles as merely one of the ways in which the divine power granted to him was manifested in action.[95] But there are also important differences between the representations of the pagan and the Christian healer. Damascius' stories of his wonder-working doctors and philosophers emphasise his heroes' wisdom and learning (*mathemata*), the product of a long and difficult education. By contrast, Christian lives of the saints, modelled on the miracles in the Gospels, often stressed the ordinariness of the saint and the immense power of simple faith in Christ.

By the end of the fourth century, accounts of healing miracles, particularly those effected with the aid of relics of the saints, become plentiful.[96] Bishop

Victricius (*c*.330–*c*.407), welcoming the arrival of a holy relic to Rouen, produced a long list of cures wrought by the saints to explain to his flock the reasons for his delight at his new acquisition.[97] St Augustine (354–430) was somewhat more reserved. Although he gladly acknowledged the validity of miracles from Italy and N. Africa, to him these cures by holy oil, relics or baptism were marks of special providence, and hence rare, a qualification lost on his flock, who brought children to baptism to regain physical health, applied the eucharistic host to a child's closed eyelids, and wore the four Gospels as amulets to ward off disease.[98]

In Christian hagiography, occasional comments on the expensive failures of secular doctors over a long period serve to highlight the power of Christianity as invested in the saint rather than to attack secular medicine. Few authors were as bitter as the writer of the *Miracles of St. Artemius*, who provides a very detailed account of the failings of the medical practitioners and institutions of Constantinople in the early years of the seventh century.[99] For the most part, when hagiographers mention medical details, such as the successful insertion by a surgeon of a drainage tube to relieve a painful condition, it is simply to add colour and authenticity to their narrative.[100]

The medicine of Galen and the medicine of Christianity were, for the most part, regarded as complementary: medical skills and herbs came from God, and were to be valued as such, but a total reliance on human intervention unaided by prayer and faith in God was foolish and unspiritual.[101] Conversely, although some clerics, such as Nicetas, bishop of Remesiana, and Caesarius of Arles, warned their flocks against trusting in secular medicine, and particularly in chants and charms, and advised them to follow only the Christian medicine advocated in the *Epistle* of St James, they were in a minority.[102] Most religious writers, while allowing the possibility of cures by faith and prayer alone, took the view that such austerity, like asceticism, was something suitable only for super-Christians, monks and the like – and perhaps not even for them.[103] Diadochus of Photike, who wrote his *On Spiritual Knowledge* in N. Greece around 480, had his doubts. Even ascetics, when surrounded by other people in towns or in monastic communities, cannot always maintain the perfect charity towards others that is necessary for faith healing to work. Indeed, to boast in public that one has not needed a doctor for years is a sign that one has succumbed to the devil's temptation to pride. But out in the desert it is a different story. The solitary hermit can draw near to the Lord, who heals all kinds of sickness, and can thereby gain that true dispassion that waits joyfully for death as the gateway to a truer life.[104]

Others preferred to preach Christ as the healer of the soul rather than the body. This metaphor is found everywhere in sermons and treatises, in pastoral letters and religious poetry.[105] Mostly it is a passing allusion, but sometimes the image is worked out at length. Christ is the *archiater*, the chief physician, purging, applying remedies or extirpating sin with the equivalent of cautery and the knife.[106] The agonies of temptation, such as those of disease, can be

313

removed only if one comes to the 'surgery' of Christ, whose healing is both assured and free.

But the Church's overriding concern for the eternal salvation of the soul rather than for the maintenance of the transitory body did not imply a disregard for the obligations to others laid down in the New Testament.[107] With the legalisation of Christianity in the fourth century, the Christian duty of care for the sick and needy became ever more visible, expressed in bricks and mortar in a new architectural form – the 'hospital'. Both the date of the first such buildings and the specific circumstances that lay behind their erection remain obscure, but there is no doubt that the origins of the Christian 'hospital' are to be sought in the Greek-speaking world of the eastern Mediterranean rather than in Italy.[108] Bishop Leontius of Antioch (344–58) founded a number of hostels, *xenodokeia* or *xenones*, in the city (S.E. Turkey), as well as one at Daphne, a fashionable spa nearby.[109] Between 357 and 377, Eustathius of Sebastia (N. Turkey) had built a 'poorhouse' (*ptochotropheion*) where those who were 'crippled with disease' could find succour.[110] At the same time, St Basil erected outside the walls of Caesarea (S. Turkey) 'almost a new city', where the sick, the leprous, the poor and the stranger could be cared for, and receive some medical assistance.[111] The defensive tone of the letter in which he justified his decision implies that he faced a certain amount of opposition.[112] That he was concerned with public order as well as charity is also suggested by the assertion of his friend Gregory of Nazianzus that Basil had been moved by the sight of large numbers of lepers, half-dying of ulcers and sores, who forced themselves in desperation into churches and shrines.[113] By the end of the century similar institutions are recorded in Constantinople (there called 'sick-houses', *nosokomeia*), and they were common enough to form the basis for an extended metaphor in a bishop's letter.[114] Such buildings were erected somewhat later in Rome and the Latin West, the first of them, that of Fabiola in Rome around 397 and that of Pammachius at Ostia a few years later, being set up under Eastern influence and example.[115] St Augustine, early in the fifth century, records the construction of a similar hostel at Hippo (N. Africa).[116] But only a few are known from N. Italy, and even fewer from beyond the Alps, a reflection of the economic and social dislocation of the fifth and sixth centuries there rather than the paucity of surviving sources.[117]

It is almost impossible, alas, to trace their geographical distribution over time, certainly outside major towns, but there are indications that the fifth century saw a proliferation of such institutions. When in 404 the bishop of Constantinople, John Chrysostom, was sent into exile to the small town of Cucusus in Armenia, his journey was one of constant suffering, aggravated by a lack of medical facilities. Racked with fever and stomach pains, he found care, attention and sympathy only once, in a suburban inn at Caesarea, where he could at last sleep in a bed, eat decent food and drink clean water. Cucusus itself was little better, for this settlement, in John's view, lacked any pretension to civilisation and suffered from a chronic shortage of doctors, drugs and other necessities.[118] By contrast, from the middle years of the fifth century onwards, hospitals, *xenodokeia*, are ubiquitous in the East. Church law codes in Syriac repeatedly enjoined the provision of hospitals in the local community, even if they were no more than a room off the courtyard of a church or monastery.[119] They are found even in remote spots.[120] To the legislators they were a necessary form of public charity, manifestations of Christian concern for those in need. By 500, for example, the town of Edessa (S.E. Turkey) had two or three such institutions, all of them small, in a community of perhaps 8,000–10,000 souls. In an emergency, as in the famine of 500–1 and the ensuing plague outbreaks, they were supplemented by beds set up in public colonnades to house sufferers who had flocked from the countryside in search of aid.[121]

As time went on these hospitals became ever larger and more complex. Ephesus in 420 had one with seventy beds; Jerusalem in 550 one with 200 beds; that of St Sampson in Constantinople may have been larger still.[122] Signs of specialisation also appear. By 500 Edessa had a hospital for women, and by 600 some big hospitals at Antioch and Constantinople were divided into male and female wards.[123] The anonymous author of the *Miracles of St. Artemius* shows that by 640 surgery was being carried out at St Sampson's, and that a specific section of the hospital was set aside for those suffering from eye diseases.[124] Physicians were in attendance at a variety of hospitals – in 570 at Oxyrhynchus in Egypt one medical family even ran its own small hospital – and there can be no doubt that some of these institutions provided treatment as well as nursing care for the sick.[125]

Yet to seek here a purely medical hospital is a work of supererogation. Many of the smaller *xenodokeia* would have offered little more than a place to lay one's head, rest and eat. Monks, ex-army officers, even the occasional civilian administrator are far more prominent in the actual running of these hospitals than physicians.[126] Financial rather than medical problems are the pressing concern of the ecclesiastical codes, which stress again and again the importance of the head's moral rectitude and administrative ability.[127] Both would be needed to cope with the complexity of grain distributions to those in need or with an institution that consisted of a leper house, a hostel and a home for the sick.[128] To chart a passage in these hospitals from religious care to medical cure is equally illusory. Caring and curing were never far apart, and, as we have repeatedly seen, medical knowledge was not confined to doctors. The variety of names used for these institutions – hospice, hostel, poorhouse, sick-house, orphanage, home for the elderly, hospital – indicates a variety of overlapping, and at times competing, aims within the overall ideology of shelter and Christian charity. Some institutions may have specialised in one type of inmate – transient pilgrims, for example, particularly in Rome, Constantinople and the Holy Land – but often this exclusivity was confined to their title. Early Christian hospitals promoted a combination of charitable activities, not just one.

There were also non-medical considerations to be borne in mind. The Statutes of the theological school of Nisibis (S.E. Turkey) laid down in 476 that sick students were to be cared for in their own cells by their cellmates, a neat form of domestic medicine.[129] Seventy-five years later a hospital, *xeno-dokeion*, was erected near the school with a grant from the King of Persia, and provided with every necessity.[130] It was built not only to shift the time-consuming burden of care from students to an official, but also to protect sick students from being 'plundered and dishonoured' when they went into town in search of more sophisticated assistance. The head of the school himself was to visit the sick three times a day.[131] The Statutes of 590 placed responsibility for the administration of the hospital and for the welfare of its inmates on a 'steward', chosen for his probity and efficiency. He was not a doctor – indeed the same Statutes evince a distinct suspicion of secular medicine. Theology students were forbidden to associate with physicians, 'for the crafts of the world are unworthy to be read with the books of holiness in one light', and those who did were only allowed to continue with their theological studies if they were of good character and actual natives of Nisibis.[132] Theological, social, pragmatic and charitable reasons thus combined to create a hospital without doctors, but it is never suggested that its treatment was ineffective or inferior.[133] Elsewhere, some institutions, both sacred and secular, took a similar line, while others, no less sacred, appointed a doctor to attend their hospital.

The most notable characteristic of the hospital of early Christianity was thus its variety – of form, size, organisation and purpose. But all were united within an overall religious framework of care, compassion and charity.

Medicine in the Later Roman Empire thus bears a very different stamp from what had gone before, with new forms of learning and new institutions. Some developments take place within medicine, while others reflect the need to reach an accommodation with a newly dominant Christianity, which had its own priorities and aspirations. One example suffices to show the result of this intermingling. Earlier collections of *Medical* and *Scientific Questions*, a genre going back at least to Aristotle, have no counterpart to a question attributed to the theologian and bishop Athanasius: 'Should a man flee from plague if, as was possible, it was sent by the wrath of God?' The answer neatly combines the theological with the medical. Flight is acceptable if the plague has a purely natural cause, in the filth and overcrowding of towns or in the polluted air; but divine retribution will seek out the sinner, even in the desert, and thus flight may well prove vain.[134]

Above all, both Christianity and learned medicine come in Late Antiquity to be defined in relation to a fixed series of books, a canon of orthodoxy. The fluid beliefs of the early Christians and the variety of stories about Christ on which they drew were replaced by our New Testament and a whole series of creeds and conciliar decisions. In medicine, the process was more protracted and more informal, although no less effective. Alternatives to Galenism gradually disappeared from academic medicine, replaced by Galenic commentaries and summaries or ideologically neutral handbooks of practical medicine. There was scope for new ideas, as in theology, but that scope was restricted to what could be derived from the canonical base of the Galenic Corpus. Oribasius' massive encyclopaedia of extracts, for instance, contains little or nothing that did not agree with, or could not be easily reconciled with, Galen. Those who practised or who wrote about medicine within this framework of ideas found it neither constraining nor irksome. Many of the problems that had troubled earlier generations had apparently now been resolved, and the successes of Galen and the other writers they drew on only confirmed the validity of what they themselves were doing. They saw past authority as supportive, not burdensome, as they went out to meet their patients. It is only later historians who lament the transition from the variegated medical world of Galen's day to the monochrome certainties of Galenism.

20

CONCLUSION

This book has covered the whole span of medicine in Greek and Roman Antiquity, from its earliest written records until the seventh century of the Christian era. It has taken a broad view of what medicine was and how it was practised, trying above all to set it within a context of other developments in ancient society. Such a project could be extended almost indefinitely in a whole series of volumes, but this study has chosen to emphasise three aspects of ancient medicine that provide complementary reasons why one should take an interest in the medical world of so distant a past: its place in the development of Western medicine in general; its continuing influence on modern preconceptions about health and healing; and the diversity of ancient medical practice.

The theories of Antiquity formed the very foundation of Western medicine for centuries, even if they were eventually rejected. On this interpretation of the importance of ancient medicine the crucial moment comes very early in the story, as a result of the interaction of medical practice with the new philosophical ideas of the sixth and fifth centuries BC. To the novel form of medicine that developed then were added a more subtle understanding of dietetics in the fifth and fourth century and of human anatomy in the third, with its repercussions for surgery. As a result of wars and conquest the medicine of the Greek-speaking world of the Aegean was successfully transplanted to the Hellenistic world of Egypt and the Levant, and, with even more momentous consequences, to Rome and its Empire. Such medicine, compared with what is known, for example, of Egyptian or Babylonian medicine, can be characterised as progressive, even if authors like Galen saw all progress as ultimately finite and largely achieved by their own day.[1] Galen is an ambiguous figure: prodigiously learned and a remarkably talented observer and anatomist, he left a legacy that variously inspired, daunted and constricted his successors. After him, mediaeval learned physicians, writing in Greek, Syriac, Arabic, Latin or Hebrew, strove to synthesise what they knew of ancient medicine and to harmonise its contradictions, confident from their own experience that it provided an effective way of understanding health and disease and of curing patients. Many mediaeval institutions, such as hospitals, civic physicians and collegiate associations, can also be traced back to an origin in Late Antiquity,

318

if not earlier. When, in the medical Renaissance of the fifteenth and early sixteenth centuries, the writings of the ancient Greeks were rediscovered by humanist scholars and read again in their original Greek in Western Europe for the first time for a thousand years, the belief was widespread that, through this return to the very springs of medicine, the accretions of later error and uncertainty could be purged away.

But after this high point in the early 1540s, the influence of Greek and Roman writings within modern medicine began to diminish. Doctors and surgeons set out to emancipate themselves from the perceived tyranny of the ancients by appeals to their own experience and to more modern theories. Galen's authority was challenged and overthrown, first in anatomy, then in physiology and finally in therapeutics. The more protean Hippocrates survived, but it was as the author of observations and of the *Oath*, not as the giver of clinical precepts, a medical Moses, that he continued to be honoured.[2] The conviction, still strong in the 1820s, that the ancient authors contained much valuable information on diagnosis and therapy was severely shaken by new developments in chemistry and physiology.[3] By 1860 ancient medicine was something that could be left definitively in the hands of philologists and antiquarians. Those who wished to derive practical benefit for the present from the theories and practices of the Classical past were viewed as cranks or worse.[4] The obituary of Alexander Kavvadias, the son of the excavator of Epidaurus and a distinguished endocrinologist who in the 1920s and 1930s championed a neo-Hippocratic holism, refers slightingly to his wealthy foreign patients and his association with Colonel De Basil's Ballet Russe.[5] Galenism, as Yunani (Greek) medicine, may still endure today as a living learned tradition in the Muslim world and be investigated with the help of the latest technology and scientific experimentation, but Western biomedical science has no longer any need of its ancient past.[6]

Nonetheless, even if it does not contribute directly to the latest scientific developments, ancient medicine has framed our Western medical tradition and continues to do so in many different ways.[7] Patients in darkest Finchley have been shown to assimilate the latest discoveries of modern medicine best if these can be placed within a context of ideas of individual balance and the environment that derive directly from the Greeks. A similar study, also in London, has revealed a continued belief in the six non-naturals as the prime determinants of health, although the technical term itself was never used.[8] Patients, of course, can be dismissed as more traditional in their outlook than their doctors, and easily lured away from hi-tech therapies by the siren song of holistic medicine. But, more recently, many doctors too have come to appreciate anew some of Galen's methodologies in studying foodstuffs, anatomy and the sick patient.[9] In the 1990s a best-selling and academically respectable study of child psychology argued strongly that Galen's theory of the four temperaments and his somatic model of interaction between mind and body offered a better way of understanding psychological development than Freudianism and its successor theories.[10]

Other features of the Greek and Roman medical legacy pass almost unnoticed because they are taken for granted in our Western medicine. The notion that diseases operate through cause and effect in natural ways, without intervention from outside the natural world, and that these can be investigated and identified stands at the very centre of modern medicine. As a recent newspaper headline put it, 'missing proof of cause and effect makes doctors sceptical'.[11] There is also a widespread expectation that a doctor or surgeon should be a thinking individual, not just content to repeat prescriptions or practices because the textbook says so. Our belief in argument and proof alone as the determinants of medical science goes back to the ancient Greeks and Romans. Although public debates in the forum or agora over the latest scientific discovery have disappeared (or relocated to the radio phone-in or TV studio), modern medical journals attest the continued supremacy of debate and discussion as part of the ongoing process of medical development. 'Secret' remedies and discoveries not open to refutation or application by others are considered no part of medical science.

Claims for the autonomy of medicine also go back in a direct line to the Hippocratic Corpus. Even if, as in the past, the limits of that autonomy have to be negotiated with government and public, there is still an acceptance of the need for medical independence. Although many scholars no longer believe in the image of the Hippocratic physician created by Emile Littré in his monumental nineteenth-century edition of the Hippocratic Corpus, his emphasis on the doctor's freedom from religious prejudice (via *The Sacred Disease*), unnecessary speculation (via *Ancient Medicine*) and outside interference in his relationship with his patient (via the *Oath*) still resonates today. The belief that, in some way or other, the Hippocratic *Oath* encapsulates the overriding principles of medical ethics remains as strong as ever, even as individual sentences or sections in it are consigned to the dustbin of history.[12] The aims of medical teaching are still recognisably akin to those advocated by Galen and Scribonius Largus; and the probing fingers of medical students on a ward round are no different from those satirised by Martial nineteen hundred years ago.[13]

Powerful as these arguments are to justify an interest in the history of medicine in Antiquity, this appeal to an understanding of the roots of Western medicine carries with it a danger: that ancient medicine may be studied only for its contribution to something superior – modernity. This is not to decry the attempt to discover how we came to be where we are: that is both a valuable and a challenging question to pose, and an answer may be found in these pages. But it is not the only question.

This book has taken a different tack. It has tried to look at the practice of medicine in Greece and Rome not simply as a contribution towards the Western medical tradition, but also in its own right, as something rooted in time and space within Greek and Roman society. It has reacted strongly against taking the medicine of Hippocrates and Galen as if it were necessarily dominant or superior to any other available in the past, and it has endeavoured to redress the balance by introducing many less familiar figures and by delaying the introduction of some well-known texts, authors and episodes into the story. It is, in one sense, the first anti-Galenic history of ancient medicine.

From this perspective, what is most striking about ancient medicine is its diversity. A reading of the medical doxography in Anonymus Londinensis, alongside the Hippocratic Corpus as a whole, demonstrates that one cannot speak easily of a single tradition of Greek medicine even in the time of Hippocrates himself. The most cursory reading of Galen shows that in his day uniformity still remained no more than a distant hope. This diversity was not confined to the realm of ideas. More than in most societies, medicine in ancient Greece and Rome was open to influences of all kinds and could be studied, and indeed practised, by many who did not think of themselves as doctors. Aulus Gellius regarded it as a social as well as an intellectual solecism not to know the difference between veins and arteries.[14] The discussions of lay authors such as Gellius, to say nothing of the encyclopaedias of Cornelius Celsus and the Elder Pliny, are more informative on many aspects of medicine, and especially surgery, than many surviving treatises by medical practitioners. Indeed, this book has relied on these non-medical sources to such an extent that the division between them and strictly medical sources has been almost abolished.

The same diversity is visible in the variety of those offering healing – exorcists, drug sellers, magicians and midwives, as well as *iatroi* and *medici*. However much individual writers might pontificate about a unified medical profession, this was at best an aspiration. In the absence of any formal, legal and enforceable definitions of what medicine was, it is hardly surprising that ancient medicine operated in an open market. Medical ethics was concerned less with the well-being of the patient (and certainly with what we might term today moral dilemmas) than with defending one's reputation and livelihood from competitors. The boundaries of acceptability between the various types of healers were constantly shifting: one individual's acceptance of chants and charms might arouse the derision of another, and, over time, therapies fell in and out of fashion. The coming of Christianity only added to this complexity of relationships, especially from 320 onwards, as it endeavoured to ensure the overall conformity of society with the ideals enunciated in the Gospels. But rather than think in terms of a constant or entrenched opposition between medicine and religion – for many doctors, like Galen himself, were firmly committed to a belief in God or Gods – one should view their interaction as a process of negotiation, of defining and redefining their separate spheres of action.

Considerations of change and development also involve questions of historical perspective, both temporal and geographical. Rather than make sweeping statements linking together information five hundred years or more apart, this book has paid close attention to chronology, not only to avoid anachronisms but also to allow some less familiar combinations of evidence. By teasing out strands within the Hippocratic Corpus, for example, even if only on rough chronological grounds, one can place individual treatises against different historical backgrounds. Tracts such as *Decorum* and *Precepts* illustrate changes taking place within the Hellenistic world, not in Greece in the lifetime of Hippocrates. Conversely, a work such as the pseudo-Aristotelian *Problems*, also of Hellenistic date, shows the growing influence of Hippocratism more clearly than any strictly medical text that survives.

A sense of place is also essential, whether that is a healing shrine on Hadrian's Wall or an Egyptian village, Boiae or Cucusus, Ephesus or Constantinople. The fact that the great majority of our evidence comes from the major cities, most notably Rome, has distorted our perceptions of what medicine was like in Antiquity for most people. We get only the occasional glimpse of the travelling physician, the local farmer-cum-healer, the barmaid turned midwife. The medicine of the countryside, with its knowledge of local plants and herbs, appears fitfully across the centuries. Urban literature implies an abundance of healers, of all kinds, within the small towns of the ancient world, and contrasts it with their near-absence once one moves into the countryside, where self-help or the ministrations of a fellow traveller is all that is available.[15] Where the truth lies is far from easy to determine, but one should beware a stereotype that takes the plutocratic physician in Rome as a typical healer.

There are other absences from the historical record. Galen's suffocating friendship has left us knowing far less about the predecessors with whom he agreed than about his opponents. The balance can be redressed in part by introducing fragmentary authors, some unfamiliar even to the most dedicated specialist, in order to counteract Galen's self-projected image of himself as a lone figure fighting for truth in the midst of ignorance. Methodists, other Hippocratics and the elusive Pneumatists are thereby given a fairer hearing. But often the fault does not lie with any individual from the past. The tendency, evident above all in Late Antiquity, to view medicine in terms of a knowledge of certain books means that our understanding of those areas of medicine that are difficult, if not impossible, to put into words is limited. Surgery is far less well represented than physic, although the number and variety of surgical instruments found in hoards such as those at Bingen, Vindonissa and, most recently, Rimini confirm the evidence of Celsus and Paul of Aegina that some surgeons at least had attained a level of competence and sophistication hardly reached again until the nineteenth century.

But the largest lacuna is that engulfing women healers. Most, if not all, of our surviving medical texts, even on gynaecological topics, are written by men for men, and, as this history itself has done, subsume the treatment of women under that of men. When women do appear, they are more often attending at a birth or treating its related gynaecological problems than providing more general therapy. This certainly underplays their role in dealing with other feminine disorders, let alone in the wider provision of health care for men as well as children, but we cannot know exactly how. To talk about women's networks of information, hypothetical creations of historical gossamer, or about a medicine for women by women may give comfort to modern feminists, but neither corresponds to the ancient evidence nor sheds real light on the extent and viability of domestic medicine. Most diseases would have been first diagnosed and treated in the home, but by whom is far from clear. The agricultural medicine ('*Hausvatermedizin*'), such as we find in Cato, is addressed in the first instance to the male head of the household. But Xenophon, writing his treatise on household management in the fourth century BC, places responsibility for the health of the servants firmly among the duties of a wife, alongside checking the household accounts and ensuring that stored provisions do not go mouldy. Similarly, the Roman author Columella recommends that the wife of the farm bailiff should look after the health of the slaves, a worthwhile task that would only serve to increase goodwill, respect and better work.[16] Scattered references to 'wise women' and to remedies by wealthy women such as Antiochis of Tlos and Aquilia Secundilla, 'ladies of the manor', extend our knowledge of female involvement in everyday medicine. They are likely to be closer to the truth than heroic studies of Hagnodike, the alleged pupil of Herophilus, or Phaenarete, the midwife mother of Socrates, which have revealed far more about the prejudices of their authors, in Antiquity as well as in the present, than about historical reality.[17]

Above all, this book has tried to give a sense of the excitement of ancient medicine, what it must have been like to have seen Hippocrates at the bedside of a patient, Erasistratus experimenting, Asclepiades or Thessalus holding forth, or Galen dissecting a pig. Our own knowledge of modern medicine works against any easy acceptance of the theories of Soranus or Galen, however powerful their rhetoric. Yet to read a work like *Airs, Waters and Places* or any of the *Epidemics*, to question the patient with Rufus, face the difficulties of childbirth with Soranus, or listen to Galen as he expounds his achievements in prognosis or dissection is to get some idea, albeit dim, of their impact on contemporaries.

It was an impact that was re-experienced over the centuries by those hearing or reading their message for the first time as the discovery or rediscovery of ancient medical texts, sometimes in the original Greek, sometimes through translations into Syriac, Arabic, Hebrew or Latin, enthused and inspired some of their readers to emulation. Crucial developments in anatomy, botany and clinical medicine, or simply in thinking about the place of medicine in the natural world, have been traced back directly to encounters with the distant medical past.[18] Indeed, the two most effective challenges to Galenic medicine and physiology were made by men steeped in classical learning. Andreas Vesalius (1514–64), who edited Galen's anatomical treatises for the 1541 Juntine Latin edition, put into practice in his dissections of human bodies the methodologies that Galen himself had advocated but had been unable to follow. His ridicule of Galen in his *De humani corporis fabrica* (1543) for relying on animals was, as contemporaries did not hesitate to point out, monstrously unfair and ungenerous to an author from whom he took over so much.[19] William Harvey's discovery of the circulation of the blood in animals, published in 1628, was made possible only by his deep acquaintance with the methods, theories and logic of a classical comparative anatomist, Aristotle.[20] That ancient ideas could have retained for so long their power to provoke and to stimulate – and with such effect – is a further reason why they deserve attention.

But the history of medicine is more than the history of medical ideas. It is also the record of men and women striving to come to terms with illness, whether as sufferer or as healer. Here, simply because we need to deploy a wide range of sources in order to create a narrative, there is the opportunity to engage with many individuals from the past and hear their voices. It is not only in Galen that one finds a character from Antiquity who reveals, consciously or unconsciously, much about himself, his beliefs and his prejudices. There are many others whose careers or experiences can enrich any account – the pompous Decimius Merula, the much-travelled Democedes of Croton, the ever-inquisitive Erasistratus or Scantia Redempta, the Christian doctor from fourth-century Capua, 'a woman beyond compare ... the very mistress of discretion ... and her husband's partner in healing as well as in life'.[21] We can sympathise with the torments of Seneca as a patient, and accompany the ailing and elderly John Chrysostom on his journey across Asia Minor into exile. We may wonder at the faith (some might say the hypochondria) of Aelius Aristides, as well as at the fortitude of those prepared to undergo the extirpation of a breast cancer by means of cautery and the knife. Palaeopathology too can reveal the painful and even fatal consequences of accidents or bad diet, to complement the descriptions of illness in medical handbooks. And one can contemplate the difference in status and lifestyle between Demetrius, the keeper of theriac for the Emperor Marcus Aurelius, and Thyrsus, a slave doctor commemorated on a tiny funeral plaque in Rome.[22]

To look at the history of medicine in Antiquity, as this book has tried to do, as a history of individuals in a past society facing, and often overcoming, ill health allows us to see that medicine in its context and to appreciate it on its own terms. It is an account that supplements, but does not abandon, the more heroic chronicle of medical progress as an accumulation of skills, ideas and practices over the centuries from Early Greece to the triumph of Galenism. In so doing, it reinterprets historiographically two of the most famous sayings from the Hippocratic Corpus. Not only does it recognise the long (and often halting) development of the art of medicine, but it also endeavours to give an appropriate weight to the three elements involved in any medical practice, the healer, the patient and the illness. The legacy of Antiquity is still with us.

NOTES

1 SOURCES AND SCOPE

1 By deliberately choosing in this chapter to cite evidence drawn from across the centuries, I am also hinting at some long-term continuities, particularly in conditions of practice.

2 Scribonius Largus, *Drug Recipes* 122; Alexander of Tralles, *Handbook* 1, 15; 1, 565 Puschmann. Varro (*On Agriculture* 2, 10, 10) claims that an ability to read is essential for a rural farmer-cum-vet, but how far his 'one ought' was obeyed is unclear. The very late Latin author, Muscio (*Gynaecology* pr., ed. Rose), expects that 'ill-educated midwives' will have his simple book read out to them by better-educated women.

3 Temkin 1977: 144–6; Yunis 2003. On the consequences of literacy and the sporadic survival of records for the historian, cf. Clanchy 1993.

4 Lloyd 1983: 119–26; Arnott 1997: 249–77; Arnott *et al.* 2003. Cf. [Hippocrates], *Epidemics* 5, 28: V, 227 L. For trepanation in early Rome, see Germanà and Fornaciari 1993; and for early Britain, see *The Times*, 21 August 2002: 8.

5 [Hippocrates], *The Sacred Disease* 1, 10–46: VI, 354–64 L.; Justinian, *Digest* 50, 13, 1, 3 (from Ulpian). Some idea of their charms and incantations can be gained from H. D. Betz 1992; Önnerfors 1993.

6 Paribeni and Romanelli 1914: 60, no. 49, probably around 50 BC.

7 Majno 1975; Krug 1985: 70–103; R. Jackson 1988; Marganne 1998. Note also the use of artistic evidence in Verbanck-Piérard (1998) and for ancient medical conditions by Grmek and Gourevitch (1998).

8 Marganne 1981: esp. nos. 9–19, for potsherds.

9 Soranus of Ephesus, *Life of Hippocrates* 3–4. And nothing remains of another Soranus, the Cilician, regarded as second only to Hippocrates by a doctor in Late Antiquity, Suda s.v. Soranus, S. 851; IV, 407 Adler.

10 Dorotheus, Phlegon, *Marvellous Stories* = *FGrH* II B 74, fr. 36, 6; Olympus, Plutarch, *Antony* 82 = *FGrH* II B 198 with Scarborough 2012.

11 Galen, *Against Julian* 1: 18A, 248; Apuleius, fr. 14; cf. Harrison 2000: 13, 25.

12 Some temple libraries in Egypt housed collections of medical books; Galen, 13, 776 (from Heras, first century AD); Reizenstein 1904: 121, n. 6 (a recipe 'originally in Egyptian letters' for arthritis); Reymond 1976; Thompson 1988: 208–11. (The libraries at the Asclepieia at Cos and Pergamum probably housed religious literature or belles lettres rather than medical texts.) Cf. Scribonius Largus, *Drug Recipes* 97, for a recipe placed (by imperial order?) in 'public libraries', and Galen, *Avoiding Distress* 21, for copies of his works placed in public libraries. In general, see L. Robert 1969: 178–85; Casson 2001; W. A. Johnson and Parker 2009; and for the new Galenic evidence, Nicholls 2011.

13 *ILS* 8971. His father, Ti. Julius Celsus, consul in AD 92, was related to many of the great dynastic families of Asia Minor.

14 Hillert 1990: 155–8, no. 29 (a clearer photo is in McCann 1978: pl. 174–5); Meyerhof 1929: 84.

15 Menecrates, *IG* 14, 1759; Galen, 2, 215–17: tr. C. Singer 1956: 1–2; 19, 17: tr. P. N. Singer 1997: 7.

16 For handbooks, see Andorlini 1999.

17 Galen, 5, 48: tr. P. N. Singer 1997: 123; cf. *On Examining the Physician* 5: *CMG* Suppl. Or. 4, 68.

18 Rosenthal 1975: 35. The existence of such a philosophical manuscript at this date is far from proven.

19 'Interest' need not mean solely for their medical value: a book might be preserved as a symbol of age and authority, a link with a distant past. For a different approach to the question of survival, see Netz 2011.

20 Galen, *Commentary on Epidemics VI*: *CMG* 5, 10, 2, 2, 495; *Avoiding Distress* 6, 14–22, 31–7. The extent of his losses is detailed in the recently recovered *Avoiding Distress*, ed. Boudon-Millot *et al.* 2010: tr. Nutton 2012a. Some were never recovered; others, like *On Prognosis*, survived unbeknown to him.

21 *Plinii Secundi Iunioris qui feruntur de Medicina Libri tres*, *CML* 3; for the variant versions of the *Physica*, see Sabbah *et al.* 1987: 127–9; Fischer 2000b: 43–5. For medical digests, see Fischer 2000a.

22 See pp. 169–70, 180–1 here.

23 See pp. 307–8 here and Garofalo and Roselli 2003. Even this material may have been geographically restricted: for example, manuscripts of the Galenic and Hippocratic translations and of the Ravenna commentators do not appear to have circulated much further than the Po Valley. For examples of Greek medical writings surviving also in Latin quotations, see Fischer 2001, 2012.

24 Nutton 1984a: 1; Temkin 1991.

25 See pp. 199–201, 178–80 here; for the latter treatise, see Wilberding 2011.

26 The most accessible list of Galenic treatises recovered from mediaeval translations is given in the 1965 reprint of Kühn's edition of Galen's *Opera Omnia*, Hildesheim: G. Olms, vol. XX, pp. LV–LXII, supplemented by Nutton 2002a; Boudon-Millot 2007; Hankinson 2008. For Rufus, see pp. 213–16 here.

27 Gerstinger 1970; Collins 2000: 39–50.

28 Bergsträsser 1925: 38–9, 17. Fragments of the former remain in Arabic, but the latter is now entirely lost.

29 See p. 215 here. Substantial quotations remain in Arabic texts, albeit under a variety of titles.

30 Thorndike 1946; Nutton 2002a.

31 Nutton 2011: 4–30.

32 For a brief general survey, see Nutton 1993d: 15–28.

33 This is, of course, not the same as saying that any book was consulted frequently, if at all, over the last five hundred years: many ancient medical texts, even in the Hippocratic Corpus, slumbered unread for generations, and it is not uncommon today to find a printed edition with its pages still unopened.

34 The piecemeal nature of ancient book production and publication means that it is unwise to assume *a priori* that any ancient medical writer had access to (let alone read) all of the material we have today, or to a large part of what was written in his lifetime. Paradoxically, modern scholars may be better informed about texts within the Hippocratic Corpus than were ancient doctors.

35 Kudlien 1971. This complaint continues to be echoed by those who search for an identification of the disease; see pp. 22–3 here.

36 Procopius, *Wars* 2, 22–3; Bratton 1981; Little 2007; Horden 2008: XIV, 134–60.

37 [Joshua the Stylite], *Chronicle* 41–3; Segal 1970: 147–8.

38 Isocrates, *Aeginetan Speech* 24–9. Note also the general opinion that by attending diligently to the sick man his adopted son was likely himself to catch the disease. For a range of interpretations of disease in both medical and non-medical sources, see Lloyd 2003.

39 Weyh 1911–12: 46. For the conjunction of human and animal medicine, see Epicharmus, frags DK 23 B 10 and 60; J. N. Adams 1995; Bliquez 1994: 96. For doctors going on a circuit from their base, cf. Justinian, *Digest* 27, 1, 6, 2 (*c.*230 AD) on 'socalled circuit doctors'. Professor Peter Warren tells me that Cretan dentists today still make circuits by car to visit patients in the remoter villages. For the negative connotations of a 'sedentary' doctor, see Magdelaine 2007.

40 For the problems of authorship in the Hippocratic Corpus, see pp. 60–1 here; Meyer (-Steineg) (1909: 30–2) devotes three pages out of more than 350 to a dubious biography.

41 Künzl 1982, 2002; R. Jackson 1990a; Bliquez 1994; Grigorova 2000; Evershed *et al.* 2004; De Carolis 2009.

42 *I. Ephesos* 1161–9, 4101.

43 *I. Ephesos* 622, 1677.

44 *MAMA* VI 373; Caracci 1964: 93 and pl. 4. In general, Gummerus (1932) and Samama (2003) offer useful collections of inscriptions.

45 Jouanna 1999: 370–2.

46 Most accessible in Gummerus 1932; Figure 17.4 here.

47 See p. 76 here.

48 Galen, 14, 31: 988.

49 Harrauer 1987: 88–100; Hirt 1996.

50 Tibiletti 1979: 133–4 (originally P. Ross. Georg. III. 2).

51 Marganne 1981; Andorlini 1995, 1997, 2001, 2004, 2009; Parsons 2007; Hanson 2010.

52 Collins 2000: 36–8; Leith 2006. Stückelberger (1994: 74–94) gives the wider context.

53 H. D. Betz 1992; Keyser 1997: 175–98.

54 Till 1951; F. Hoffmann, forthcoming.

55 Reymond 1976; Opsomer and Halleux 1991.

56 Cf. Conrad *et al.* 1995: 1–6; French 1994: ix–xx.

57 The discovery of medical instruments in a grave from Stanway near Colchester (S.E. England) datable to the years around AD 43 not only places the owner as a healer associated with a noble or royal household in pre-conquest Britain, but also suggests that he could carry out some complicated surgery and was also in touch with similar healers across the Channel (see R. Jackson 1997).

58 Justinian, *Code* 6, 43, 3, 1; 7, 7, 1 (of AD 530 and 531).

59 Cf. the provocative comment by the eminent physiologist Gustav Born (2002: 238):

> It is surely no accident that natural science germinated only twice in human history: for the first time in Athenian Greece, where it did not survive; and for the second time in post-Reformation Europe, where it did. Both times it happened in societies which began to permit freedom of thought and communication.

60 This view is clearly articulated in Longrigg (1993a, 1997); for a considerable modification of this view, see van der Eijk (2005b: 8–14, 2011), discussing recent developments.

61 One might aptly compare the generally favourable attitude of scholars towards the medical Renaissance of the first half of the sixteenth century and lack of interest in the far less familiar developments that followed in the next half-century.

62 [Hippocrates], *Airs, Waters and Places* 16 and 23–4: II, 62–6; 82–92 L. Although the author here uses 'Europeans' more often than 'Greeks', there is little doubt that he has the mainland or island Greeks most in mind.

63 Lucian, *Hired Scholars*. For the background, see Bowersock 1965, 1969.
64 The longest and most detailed accounts of post-Erasistratean Greek medicine remain those written by historians of medicine and science three-quarters of a century or more ago (Neuburger 1910; Thorndike 1923). The tradition is continued by Prioreschi (1996a).
65 See pp. 164–9 here.
66 Hahn 1991; Beagon 1992.
67 One might also note the absurdity of assuming that all doctors in the Western half of the Roman Empire regularly conversed in Greek with their (often monoglot) patients.
68 King 2002; Cantor 2002.
69 W. D. Smith 1979: 31–44.
70 King (2001) provides a very brief and succinct survey based on an anthropological approach to healing.
71 Sigerist 1951–61; von Staden 1997a.

2 PATTERNS OF DISEASE

1 But, conversely, the relatively restricted range of movement of the population might mean that a voyage of a few hundred miles at most would expose an individual to new, and thus more dangerous, pathogens. Cf. Grmek 1979.
2 For trade with the East, see Raschke 1978; Pigulewskaja 1969; for Britain, see Plutarch, *On the Cessation of Oracles* 18: 419E–F.
3 R. G. Collingwood and R. P. Wright (1967) *The Roman Inscriptions of Britain*, I, *Inscriptions on Stone*, Oxford: Clarendon Press, nos. 1337, 1463 (Spain); 1778 (Syria); 1872 (Dacia); 758 (Commagene); 1065, 1171 (Palmyra).
4 Horden and Purcell (2000) draw attention to the fact that many islands, like Aegina, because of the variety of sources of income provided by the sea, might support a much greater population than an equivalent land area.
5 Bagnall and Frier 1994; Corvisier *et al.* 2001. Parsons (2007: 12) estimates that Oxyrhynchus, a regional capital, had 20,000 inhabitants at its largest extent.
6 For the difficulties in estimating population decline in even a relatively well-documented period, compare Brunt (1971) with Morley (2001).
7 Rathbone (1990: 114–19) suggests sporadic outbreaks with a mortality of 20–30 per cent. Scheidel (2002: 162–6) is far more cautious.
8 This assessment of the population is based on Brunt 1971: 221, 259–61; Kolb 1984: 80–4; Rich and Wallace-Hadrill 1991; Parkin 1992; Bagnall and Frier 1994: 173–8; Scheidel 2001a, 2002.
9 Galen, 14, 624: *CMG* 5, 8, 2, 92–3, undoubtedly an exaggeration when applied to his native Pergamum as a whole, but valid for the local elite.
10 Cato, *For His Son*, Marcus fr. 1 = Pliny, *Natural History* 29, 7, 14.
11 Galen, 6, 552: tr. Powell 2003: 69; 6, 755; 783; 14, 17.
12 Wenskus 1990.
13 Horden and Purcell (2000) stress that 'self-sufficiency' should not be interpreted in the strong sense that each farm produced only to fulfil its own needs; it aimed also at an exchange of surpluses within a localised microeconomy.
14 Garnsey and Whittaker 1983; Garnsey 1988, 1999.
15 Gregory of Nazianzus, *Oration* 43, 34–5, cited in Garnsey 1988: 22.
16 Hesiod, *Works and Days*, line 243; West 1978: 106–7, 218.
17 Galen, 6, 518, 523, 551: tr. Powell 2003: 54–6, 551–2; 749. At 6, 686 (tr. Powell 2003: 125) he believes that a malnourished peasant wetnurse could transmit her sores and ulcers to the child she was suckling.
18 Procopius, *Wars* 6, 20, 18–33.

19 Galen, 2. 55; *Life of St. Nicolas of Sion* I, 40; II, 243–4 Anrich; Forbes and Foxhall 1995: 69–86.

20 Cf. Galen, 6, 605, 620, 665: tr. Powell 2003: 91, 97, 116; 6, 686, for the regular dearth of food in early spring.

21 Parkin 1992; Frier 2000: 787–816; Scheidel 2001a, 2001b.

22 Grmek 1989: 2–4; Sallares 2002; Scheidel 2002. Dobson (1997), from a much better-documented period, stresses the difference in patterns of health and disease even between neighbouring villages.

23 For malaria, see pp. 32–3 here; Tifernum, Pliny, *Letters* 5, 6, 6 and 46. For cities, see Scheidel 2002: 166–71; Edwards and Woolf 2003; King 2005: 12–96; Parsons 2007: 180–2.

24 Parkin 2003: 36–56.

25 Suder 1988; Demand 1994. By contrast, women played little part in such dangerous occupations as soldiering and mining.

26 Soranus, *Gynaecology* 4, 2–3; Gourevitch 1984a: 158–68.

27 Galen, 19, 104, 107 (explaining Hippocratic terms); Herophilus, fr. 247 von Staden; Soranus, *Gynaecology* 4, 9–12. Caesarean section was unknown in Antiquity, despite the story that the term derives from the birth of Julius Caesar and the association of his name with 'caesus', 'cut'. No source reports this linkage until Isidore of Seville (AD 600) in his *Etymologies* 9, 3, 12; the name Caesar was already in his family (Pliny, *Natural History* 8, 9, 47), and, as Isidore also suggests, it is more likely to be connected with 'caesaries', 'hair', as a nickname given to a child born already with a full head of hair. Caesar's mother lived for many years after his birth, and none of his biographers or contemporaries mention this remarkable entrance into life. See Gourevitch 2004.

28 Soranus (*Gynaecology* 2, 6) gives without comment instructions to the midwife or doctor as to which children are worth rearing. How frequent exposure was is debatable; cf. Eyben 1980–1; W. V. Harris 1994. Its appearance in literary compositions, from the story of Oedipus onwards to later Greek novels (not forgetting the biblical account of Moses), made for striking scenes of recognition (or its opposite) but can give no indication of whether this was a normal practice. Roman and probably Greek law required the father to take a positive decision to rear a child. Even if the ninety-seven bodies of small babies found at Yewden, Bucks. (Eyers 2011) come from a brothel, the number is still remarkable.

29 Leven 1998; Graumann (2000) is more sanguine.

30 Thucydides, *History* 2, 47–54, 58; 3, 87. Longrigg 1980, 1998: 125–6; Carmichael 1993: 934–7. The abundance of alternative suggestions, ranging from poisoning and toxic shock syndrome to viral diseases, or a combination of diseases, continues. That typhoid was present is clear from Papagrigorakis *et al.* (2006), but doubts still remain as to whether this was the cause of the plague; cf. Shapiro *et al.* 2006. The problems raised by Thucydides' evidence were already clear to Galen (7, 290; 850–4; 18A, 729).

31 P. Potter 1989: 9–19; Grmek in Jouanna 2000: lxxvi–xc; Graumann 2000.

32 For the tablets, see pp. 109–11 here. Similar caveats apply to Christian miracle stories, pp. 294–5, 313 here.

33 *Leviticus* 13, 47–59; 14, 33–53.

34 Useful surveys are given by Roberts and Manchester (1998) and Aufderheide and Rodriguez-Martin (1998). For an overview of skeletal finds from one region, see Breitwieser 1998: 105–39; Roberts and Cox 2003: 107–63.

35 Grmek (1989) offers a series of interesting studies of particular diseases. There is much valuable material in Sallares 1991; Kiple 1993; Gourevitch 2001b. A different approach is taken by Touwaide (1999: 793–803), analysing the diseases recorded by the pharmacological writer Dioscorides. J. M. André (2006: 59–331) painstakingly lists the literary reference to diseases in Latin sources.

36 Plato, *Timaeus* 82A–84C. Aristotle's opinions of the decay of old age (*On Youth and Old Age* 5: 469b; *Metaphysics* 4, 1: 379a–b) also depend on a belief in the recalcitrance of matter (cf. *Metaphysics* 8, 5: 1045a; *On the Heavens* 1, 12 and 2, 6: 283b, 286b) but develop in a different way.

37 [Hippocrates], *Prorrhetic* 2, 11: IX, 32 L.; *Coan Prognostics* 30, 502: IX, 700 L. Cf. Roberts and Cox 2003: 113–14.

38 Galen, *On Unnatural Tumours* 7, 705–32; cf. also 11, 139; 9, 693; 6, 814.

39 Galen, 10, 976–9; 17B, 688; 18A, 59–61.

40 Celsus, *On Medicine* 5, 28; Brunner 1977.

41 Galen, *On Marasmus* 7, 666–704; Theoharides 1971; Niebyl 1971. In general, see Parkin 2003: 36–56.

42 Pliny, *Natural History* 25, 9–10, 27; 26, 67. Cf. Phlegon of Tralles, *The Long-lived*, ed. Jacoby, *FGrH* II B 257, fr. 37; Lucian, *The Long-lived*.

43 Galen, 6, 332–3: tr. R. M. Green 1951: 202.

44 Plague in the narrow sense of bubonic plague (or its closely related manifestations pneumonic and septicaemic plague), the result of infection by *Yersinia pestis*, does not appear with any certainty until the sixth century, with the plague of Justinian, after which it remained endemic for several more centuries mainly in the Near East. In what follows, I use the word 'plague' to translate '*lues*', '*pestis*' or '*loimos*', without implying any equation with bubonic plague.

45 Sallares 1991: 253; Sherman 2006; Little 2007, 2011; Horden 2008: XIV, 134–60.

46 Orosius, *History* 4, 2, 2. A list of plagues in Rome is given by Duncan-Jones (1996: 110–11), who rightly points out that local annalists, from whom derives much of our information concerning Rome, may not have been in a position to know the wider picture.

47 Tacitus, *Annals* 16, 13; Cassius Dio, *History* 53, 33, 4; 54, 1, 2; Suetonius, *Nero* 39.

48 Thucydides, *History* 2, 48; 54. Pausanias (*Description of Greece* 10, 11, 5) mentions that the Peloponnesian town of Cleonae was among those affected.

49 Livy, *History* 4, 26, 5; 4, 30, 8. Livy also notes outbreaks in 433 and 432 BC (*History* 4, 25, 4; 4, 25, 6).

50 Gilliam 1961; Ebbell 1967: 53–9; Littmann and Littmann 1973; Duncan-Jones 1996; C. Bruun (2007) provides a good overview of the debate. There is earlier evidence for smallpox in a few Egyptian mummies.

51 *Historia Augusta, Verus* 2, 7; 8, 1, 1–2; Ammianus Marcellinus, *History* 23, 6, 24, both locating the origin of the disease in the vapours in a cavern opened up by the sacrilegious destruction of a sacred statue. The combination of religious and non-religious explanation is piquant. Ammianus talks of the deadly vapours coming out of the naphtha wells (ibid. 23, 6, 16), comparing them with other famous exhalations of deadly fumes.

52 Galen, 4, 788: tr. P. N. Singer 1997: 60. Cf. Cassius Dio, *History* 72, 4, 13, 4.

53 Cyprian, *On Mortality* 14; Oxyrhynchus Papyrus 3817; Orosius, *History* 7, 21, 5; Zonaras, *Annals* 12, 21; Zosimus, *New History* 1, 26, 2; 27, 3.

54 Rufus' mention of buboes (cited by Oribasius, *Medical Collections* 44, 17) may indicate an earlier outbreak in Libya, Egypt and Syria in the first century BC. Recent discoveries in the DNA of victims appear to show that the plague of Justinian was caused by *Yersinia pestis* – see Cule 1975: 141–55; Bratton 1981; Conrad 1981: 83–119; Horden 2008: XIV, 134–60; Little 2007, 2011.

55 Ammianus, *History* 19, 4, 1.

56 Diodorus, *History* 13, 86, 2; 14, 70, 4–71; and 14, 76, 2.

57 Livy, *History* 25, 26, 7 ('a common problem outside a city in autumn'); 37, 23, 2; Polybius, *History* 1, 19, 1.

58 Granius Licinianus, *Histories* 21–2F.

59 A report from Vindolanda (N. England) early in the first century AD shows that ten out of the thirty-one unfit auxiliaries in the First Cohort of Tungrians were suffering from

'blear-eye'; fifteen others were sick and six wounded; Bowman and Thomas 1991: 69; Marichal 1994.

60 Herodian, *History* 6, 6, 2.

61 Kiple 1993: 606–8, 676–9, 1080–4.

62 Not that these passed unnoticed in Antiquity. Sallust (*Jugurthine War* 44) criticised a lazy commander who never moved his troops from one encampment to another until forced by lack of fodder or by the smell. By contrast, in the permanent camps and forts of the imperial period attention was paid to an adequate water supply, including to the latrines, although Galen (*Commentary on Nature of Man* 2, 4: 15, 119) alludes to a case of mass illness in a camp through bad water.

63 Three hundred years later the historian Procopius ascribed a similar military failure in the same region to the same cause. The siege of Theodosiopolis in 561 had to be abandoned because many of the Roman troops brought from Thrace had gone down with various fevers, unable to bear the hot, dry climate and their stifling tents (Procopius, *Wars* 2, 19, 31–2). Julianus Africanus (*Cestoi*, pp. 61, 67 Vieillefond), around 225, gives advice on how a doctor might prevent heatstroke and exhaustion in an army, and (p. 68) how one might start a plague in the enemy's camp.

64 By 'thickening' Herodian may be thinking in terms of humours to explain, for example, leathery skin.

65 The gulf would be even wider if one took into consideration explanations, mainly found in texts from Near Eastern and Christian sources, in terms of demons or dragons. Contrast Longrigg (1992: 21–44) with Horden (1992 = 2008: XIV, 45–76).

66 Cf. Plutarch, *On the Cessation of Oracles* 18: 419F; major changes in the atmosphere 'often poison the air with pestilential sicknesses'.

67 [Hippocrates], *The Nature of Man* 9: 6, 54 L.; cf. Galen, *Commentary on Hippocrates' On the Nature of Man* 2, 3–4 = 15, 119–22.

68 In general, see Leven 1993; Nutton 2000a.

69 Even in public health, ideas of contagion and pollution often carry with them religious connotations as well (cf. Horden 2000 = 2008: III, 17–40).

70 Nutton 1983; Holman 2001: 159, citing Gregory of Nazianzus, *Oration* 14, 27, who rejects the view of some that plague can be transmitted from person to person, but attributes it to common factors in the air or water.

71 Nutton 2000a.

72 Nutton 1998, 2000a.

73 Galen, 6, 722–3: tr. Powell 2003: 6, 58; 140–1: tr. R. M. Green 1951: 35; cf. 6, 795. Juvenal, *Satires* 5, 103–6; Hobson 2009.

74 Bodel 2000.

75 Nutton 2000b.

76 Jarcho 1975–6; J. H. Phillips 1984; Borca 2000.

77 For the Subura, see Juvenal, *Satires* 11, 51; Galen, *Commentary on Airs, Waters and Places* (information from Prof. G. Strohmaier): Wulf-Rheidt 1998. Two mediaeval authors claim to have located the house of Galen: Gibril ibn Bakhtishu' around 700 (Strohmaier 1981: 187); and, five hundred years later, Theodore Doukas Laskaris (*Letters*, pp. 106–8 Festa).

78 Galen, 4, 497: tr. Furley and Wilkie 1984: 114–17; 7, 109; 8, 72: tr. Siegel 1976: 44. Scribes, 3, 776: tr. May 1968: 473.

79 Lucretius, *On the Nature of Things* 6, 808–17; Lucan, *Pharsalia* 4, 298; Pliny, *Natural History* 33, 40, 122; cf. 34, 50, 167; Strabo, *Geography* 12, 3, 40. The pale complexion of miners may have been caused by hookworm disease, ankylostomiasis (cf. G. S. Martin 1922).

80 'A grim place', Xenophon, *Memoirs* 3, 6, 12; Waldron and Wells 1979; Hong *et al.* 1994, 1996; for the Wadi Faynan, see Mattingly 2011: 167–99.

81 *CIL* 22, 7, 334.
82 Cato, *On Agriculture*; Varro, *On Agriculture* 1, 16, 4, with Boscherini 1993a; Celsus, *On Medicine* 1, 35, for 'sickplaces', *valetudinaria*.
83 Plato, *Laws* 4, 720c–e. Whether Plato was describing a real or an ideal situation is disputed (cf. Kudlien 1968a; Joly 1969), but in either case Plato implies that such discrimination would be uncontentious.
84 E.g. *CIL* 6, 3984, 8904; *IGUR* 30; for surgeons, see *CIL* 6, 3982b; for oculists, see 3986, 3987. Note also female slave 'obstetricians', *CIL* 6, 4457, 4458; and 'sickplaces', *valetudinaria*, *CIL* 6, 9084, 9085, 33917.
85 Cicero, *Letters to Atticus* 15, 13; *Letters to His Friends* 16, 4 and 9, for favourite slaves.
86 Plato, *Laws* 11, 916a; Rufus, cited in Rosenthal 1975: 204; Apuleius, *Apology* 45; Pliny, *Natural History* 32, 47, 135; Bosworth 2002: 350–3. For possible legal redress if a sold slave turned out to be too ill to work, see n. 102.
87 Temkin's (1977: 419–71) is a classic exposition. The Greek and Latin terminology for 'disease', 'affection', 'ailment', etc. was never agreed or precise.
88 [Aristotle], *Problems* 7, 4: 886b.
89 Deichgräber 1965: 308–13.
90 Meinecke 1927 remains a useful collection of primary sources. See also Grmek 1989: 177–97.
91 Galen, *On Medical Terminology*: German tr. by Meyerhof and Schacht 1930–1.
92 In many instances only the palaeopathological identification of material will prove beyond doubt the existence in Antiquity of a modern disease; conversely, the identification of modern diseases through DNA analysis does not prove that the Ancients thought of that disease in a modern category (or even as a disease at all).
93 For the seasonality of major killer diseases, see Shaw 1996; Scheidel 2002: 25–51.
94 For tapeworms, see Kiple 1993: 1035–6; for ascarides, see ibid. 603–4; for Guinea worms, see Rufus, *Medical Questions* 12, with Gärtner's (1962) commentary, *CMG* Suppl. 4, 100–1.
95 Touwaide 1999: 798.
96 Pliny, *Natural History* 26, 2, 2–3, 6, noting that it brought in its wake specialists from Egypt claiming to cure it.
97 Dzierzykray-Rogalski 1980; Grmek 1989: 198–209; Manchester 1992; Roberts *et al.* 2002.
98 Especially in *Leviticus* 13 and 14; Lieber 2000.
99 Democritus, fr. 300, 10–11 = DK II, pp. 215–16.
100 Pliny, *Natural History* 26, 3, 5 (but not connecting it directly with any of Pompey's expeditions in the East); Plutarch, *Table Talk* 8, 9: 731B. Celsus (*On Medicine* 3, 25) says that in his day, the early first century, it was infrequent in Italy, although very familiar elsewhere.
101 Strato, according to Rufus of Ephesus, quoted by Oribasius, *Medical Collections* 45, 11; Archagathus, Caelius Aurelianus, *Chronic Diseases* 4, 1, 7.
102 Sudhoff 1929. The immediate context of the phrase in this and other papyri, between 'sacred disease' and 'weals', seems to exclude the meaning of 'legal charge', although the words 'without any touch' can also be applied to property. The phrase is found also in sale documents outside Egypt (Feissel *et al.* 1997: 11–12, 17). If 'the sacred disease' recurred within six months the slave could be returned and the price refunded.
103 Aretaeus, *On Chronic Diseases* 2, 13; Caelius Aurelianus, *Chronic Diseases* 4, 13. In general, see Kudlien 1986b; Grmek 1989: 152–76, 198–204; Kiple 1993: 834–9; Roberts *et al.* 2002.
104 E.g. *Mark* 1, 40–2 (= *Matthew* 8, 3; *Luke* 5, 12–14); *Mark* 1, 40 (= *Matthew* 8, 2); *Luke* 17, 12. Later legends of Christian healings of historical personages, such as King Abgar of Edessa (Segal 1970: 72), the leprous daughter of Constantine II or, at a much

later date, even Constantine I, only added to the sense of the importance of this disease in God's plan for the world. O. Betz (1986) nicely links the Old and New Testament narratives with a discussion of the Talmudic commentaries; Gläser 1986; Pilch (2000: 39–54) uses leprosy as a test case to show the difficulty of reconciling ancient and modern medical definitions of the disease, and to stress the importance of the context of the various narratives. For palaeopathology, see Manchester 1992.

105 Kiple 1993: 1088–92.

106 Celsus devotes a very long chapter (*On Medicine* 7, 26) to bladder stones; the operation is illustrated, from a mediaeval ms., in Figure 12.3 here.

107 Doctors specialising in the treatment of fistulae are allowed the legal privileges given to doctors in general (Justinian, *Digest* 50, 13, 1, 3).

108 Holcomb 1941; Oriel 1973a, 1973b; Rothschild and Rothschild 1977; Grmek 1989: 133–51; Kiple 1993: 756–63, 1025–35; Aufderheide and Rodriguez-Martin 1998: 169–70, 288–9; Sherman 2006.

109 The treponeme of syphilis is reported from the Hellenistic necropolis of Metapontum in S. Italy (Carter 1998: 531–3) and from a fourth-century AD cemetery at Costebelle (S. France) (Palfi *et al.* 2000). But the remarkable spread of the infection in 1493 suggests that the population had not previously been exposed to venereal syphilis to any great extent.

110 Aretaeus, *On Chronic Diseases* 2, 12.

111 Roberts and Cox 2003: 145–50, 153–7.

112 [Hippocrates], *Joints* 41: IV, 178–80 L.; for the Colles fracture, see ibid. 27: IV, 138 L.

113 Dasen 1993; Grmek and Gourevitch 1998.

114 Porter and Rousseau (1998), quoting from an eighteenth-century English translation of Lucian, *The Triumphs of Gout*.

115 Galen, *On Examining the Physician* 14, 5: *CMG* Suppl. Or. 4, 137. For eye diseases in general, Hirschberg 1982 (a translation from the German of 1899) remains fundamental. Cf. also *L'Année Epigraphique* 1994: 840, and, for a graphic description in a letter from a sufferer from trachoma, Papiri della Società italiana I 4, 299.

116 Feugère *et al.* 1985. The texts are: Celsus, *On Medicine* 7, 7, 13–14; Antyllus (second century AD), quoted by Rhazes, *Kitab al-Hawi* II, 343–5; Paul, *Seven Books* 6, 21.

117 R. Jackson 1996; Voinot 1999, 1999–2000.

118 Temkin 1971; Wohlers 1999. Two recent studies of the whole treatise have very different aims: Laskaris 2002; Lo Presti 2008.

119 For the *ephialtes*, related also to the sexual *incubus*, see Paul, *Seven Books* 3, 13–17, Metzger 2011; for the slave, see Galen, 8, 226–7.

120 I *Samuel* 16, 14–16; 21, 13–15; Rydén (1981: 106–13) looks at the Christian tradition, as does Laharie (1991). Dols (1992), despite its title, offers a detailed study of the relationship of prophecy and madness in pre-Islamic society. For the melancholy genius ([Aristotle], *Problems* 30, 6), see Pigeaud 1988; van der Eijk 2005b: 279–98. Klibansky *et al.* (1964) and Arikha (2007) cover both Antiquity and later history.

121 For early epic, note the madness of Ajax in the *Sack of Troy*, fr. 1 Davies; for tragedy, Euripides' *Bacchae* is paradigmatic, and see Padel 1995; for Latin poetry, see Hershkowitz 1998. Major studies of mental diseases include Simon 1978; Pigeaud 1981, 1987a; S. W. Jackson 1986; W.V. Harris, forthcoming.

122 Stol 1993; *Matthew* 8, 16: 28–34.

123 For an opposition of medical and non-medical beliefs, see Philostorgius, *Ecclesiastical History* 8, 10. Hippocratic ideas on mental illness are surveyed by Simon 1978; for Rufus, see p. 215 here; for Galen, see pp. 240–3 here. Heiberg (1927) is still useful for its information on post-Hippocratic mental diseases. Von Staden (2000: 79–116) explores some of the consequences of Hellenistic anatomical discoveries for an understanding of mental functioning.

124 Recent surveys of the history of malaria in Antiquity are: Bruce-Chwatt and de Zulueta 1980; Grmek 1989: 245–83; Burke 1996; Sallares 2002.

125 The classic account of W. H. S. Jones (1907), which built on the recent medical discoveries of Sir Ronald Ross and which gave Jones for the rest of his life, and beyond, the soubriquet of 'Malaria Jones', was wrong in using malaria to explain the decline of Greece from 430 BC onwards, but his insights certainly apply to later periods. Celli (1933), the work of a distinguished malariologist, is still worth reading, although his conclusions, like those of Jones, have been considerably refined by modern studies (cf. Sallares 2002: 13–42; Sallares *et al.* 2004).

126 Respectively, Herodotus, *History* 2, 95, 1 and Tacitus, *Annals* 15, 43; [Aristotle], *Problems* 1, 19: 861b; Vitruvius, *On Architecture* 1, 4, 11–12; and Strabo, *Geography* 5, 1, 7. For seasonal mortality, see Scheidel 1994; Shaw 1996.

127 Pliny (*Natural History* 3, 5, 59) says that there were once twenty-five cities there, and that (3, 5, 70) in Latium as a whole fifty-three cities had disappeared by his day. For Cethegus, see Livy, *History, Summaries* 46. In general, see Sallares 2002: 103–15, 168–91, building on Dobson 1997.

128 Brunt (1971: 618–24) emphasises also the co-existence of malarial and non-malarial areas of the Campagna in the Republican period. Evidence for major (new?) *Falciparum* infestation in the mid-fifth century at Lugnano in the middle Tiber valley shows the gradual spread of the disease inland (Sallares 2002: 66–9). For Egypt, see Scheidel 2002: 75–93.

129 Nriagu 1983; Kiple 1993: 820–7.

130 See notes 79–80 above.

131 Nicander, *Antidotes* 1, 600; Paul, *Seven Books* 3, 43.

132 Vitruvius, *On Architecture* 8, 3; 8, 6, 10–11.

133 Eisinger 1982: 284–8.

134 For dentistry and dental problems, see Hoffmann-Axthelm 1985; Aufderheide and Rodriguez-Martin 1998: 393–412. By contrast, for Egyptian evidence for atherosclerosis after a high meat diet, see David 2010.

135 Galen, 6, 498–9: tr. Powell 2003: 46–7; cf. 507: tr. Powell 2003: 50, for Galen's views on the eating habits of peasants in Cyprus.

136 Galen, 6, 596–8: tr. Powell 2003: 87–8; cf. 6, 602–4: tr. Powell 2003: 89–91; 11, 367–8.

137 Tacitus, *Annals* 12, 66; 13, 15; Suetonius, *Claudius* 44. Grmek (1989: 210–45) links the Pythagorean ban on beans with the possible consequences of favismus.

138 Andorlini and Marcone 2004: 158.

139 Pliny, *Natural History* 29, 8, 18. In Roman law, although a suit could be brought under a law against damaging property, the lex Aquilia, for killing one's slave or a member of one's family, the family had no such redress against the doctor if the deceased was the independent head of the household. The only legal ruling suggesting that a free, independent citizen could claim even for damages for medical injury under this law (Justinian, *Digest* 9, 2, 13, pr.), of about AD 210, is universally suspected of being a much later interpolation (see Below 1953: 108–34). Furthermore, the laws against malpractice, as opposed to deliberate poisoning and the supplying of love philtres, would, as often today, have been difficult to enforce.

140 *CIL* 3, 3355.

141 *ILS* 9441; *Carmina Latina Epigraphica* 94.

142 *L'Année Epigraphique* 1952: 16.

143 Von Staden 1990: 85–93; Erasistratus, fr. 285 Garofalo.

144 Recognised, too, by many patients. The parents of a young boy who died after having had serious problems almost since birth, including the amputation of his left foot by 'friends of his father', blamed Fate for his affliction (Klitsch 1976; Grmek 1989: 196).

145 Galen (6, 311: tr. R. M. Green 1951: 189) thought only a coward would choose to continue living with chronic pain. One can only imagine the pain of surgical intervention with little or no anaesthetic (see [Hippocrates], *The Physician* 5: IX, 210 L.; Cavenale 2001).

146 [Hippocrates], *Diseases* I: VI, 150–2 L.; contrast *Art* 8, 6 and 13, 1: VI, 14 and 26 L., defending the principle of non-intervention in such cases.

147 Galen, 11, 344; 18A, 80.

148 *Mark* 5, 26 = *Luke* 8, 43; Roesch 1984: 290.

149 *IG* 5, 1, 1119; cf. *CIL* 2, 4314.

150 *CIL* 6, 68.

151 Augustine, *City of God* 22, 8. The stories in the later *Miracles of St. Artemius* offer many insights into the consequences of illness.

152 For Bethesda, see *John* 6, 1–9; for Rome, see Suetonius, *Claudius* 25, 2.

153 For Seneca, see Migliorini 1997: 21–94; for Aristides, see pp. 284–8 here.

154 Bodson 1991; Grmek 1991.

155 Plutarch, *Table Talk* 8, 9: 731B–734D (written about AD 110).

3 BEFORE HIPPOCRATES

1 Frölich 1879. He had ancient predecessors in this. [Plutarch] (*On Homer* 200–11) finds evidence for all the principles of modern medicine within the Homeric poems, and Galen wrote a (lost) discussion of medicine in Homer (see Kudlien 1965). The Byzantine scholar Eustathius (*Commentary on Homer* 1, 1, 41) believed that Homer's description of the plague was a restatement in verse of modern medical ideas. Apollo's arrows were the sun's rays, heating and putrefying the plain about Mt Ida, from which arose noxious vapours; animals died before men because they were more susceptible. When the climate changed and the sun became less hot, the plague ended.

2 Homer, *Iliad* 11, 514–15. The second line was condemned as 'unHomeric' by some Alexandrian scholars precisely because it detracted from the praise of the doctor. For the contortions of later Greek commentators in trying to explain why only Machaon is mentioned at this point, see Erbse 1974: 222–3.

3 Frölich 1879: 58–9; Saunders 1999; Salazar 2000: 126–58. Cf. also the illustrations of wounding scenes on Greek vases (Geroulanos and Bridler 1994). Detailed surveys of medicine in the Homeric poems are by Lorenz (1976) and Laser (1983).

4 Homer, *Iliad* 4, 219; 2, 730–1. In one of the sequels to the Homeric poems, the *Little Iliad*, Machaon is killed in battle by Eurypylus (fr. 1, ed. M. Davies 1988). In general, see Cordes 1994: 12–18.

5 Homer, *Iliad* 11, 518 (the same words are applied to Asclepius at 4, 194); 11, 506.

6 Homer, *Iliad* 4, 193–218. The word '*pharmakon*' used here covers both healing drugs (*Iliad* 4, 190; 11, 846; 13, 392; *Odyssey* 4, 230; 10, 287, 302; 11, 741; 22, 94), magical potions (*Odyssey* 10, 290, 317, 392) and poison (*Odyssey* 1, 261; 2, 329).

7 At Homer, *Odyssey* 19, 455–8 Odysseus' uncles use incantations to staunch the flow of blood (Renehan 1992: 1–4).

8 Arctinus, fr. 1, ed. M. Davies 1988, written probably in the sixth century, but depending in outline on earlier traditions.

9 The scholiasts (Erbse 1974: 223), having found two of the three (later) main divisions of medicine, are then exercised by the absence of the third, dietetics; Byzantine authors go further and wonder why Homer should concentrate on the practical, since it is the 'theoretical' that is the most important.

10 Homer, *Iliad* 5, 401; 901.

11 Cf. also Homer, *Odyssey* 5, 394–8; for the simile of a father, ill following the assaults of a 'loathsome *daimon*', and then cured by the gods.

12 Holmes 2010: 41–8, 79–83. Professor van der Eijk drew my attention to a parallel with Babylonia, where it is the seer–doctor, *asipu*, not the *asu*, doctor, who first advises on the appropriate action.

13 Homer, *Iliad* 1, 8–474. Cf. the summoning of the Cretan seer Epimenides to 'purify' Athens after the conspiracy of Cylon (Aristotle, *Constitution of Athens* 1; Diogenes Laertius, *Lives*, dating it around 596–5 BC; Plato, *Laws* 642d, dating it to 500 BC, when there was some form of epidemic; and Thucydides, *History* 2, 47, 4, reporting that in the plague of Athens the consultation of oracles and seers proved worthless).

14 There is an ambiguity in Homer's wording. Although Achilles' words could mean that Apollo acted in response to someone else's (that is, Chryses') vow, the more natural explanation is that he was angry because of a broken vow made to him.

15 E.g. *Leviticus* 26, 25; *Deuteronomy* 28, 27; I *Samuel* 5, 9; 6, 19; van der Toorn 1985.

16 Shilts 1987; Grmek 1990.

17 Homer, *Iliad* 21, 483–4; 24, 605–7; *Odyssey* 9, 411.

18 Homer, *Iliad* 2, 716–25. This does not, of course, preclude a belief that the encounter with the snake was also divinely planned (cf. p. 51 here).

19 Hesiod, *Works and Days* 100–4; 238–45.

20 Aristophanes, fr. 322, ed. Kassel-Austin, probably from his *Heroes*. Cf. Cordes 1994: 51–9.

21 Kudlien 1967; Lloyd 1990: 14–38.

22 Homer, *Odyssey* 17, 383–6.

23 Nutton 1990a: 1–2; Edel 1976; Zaccagnini 1983; Durand 1988: 543–84; Massar (2005: 37) draws attention to the contract of a doctor with the ruler and city of Idalion *c*.500 BC.

24 Ventris and Chadwick 1973: 547; PYEq 146.

25 Herodotus, *History* 3, 129–37; Griffiths 1987. Onasilas and his brothers, hired around 490 BC by king Stasikypros and the Cypriot town of Idalion to treat wounded soldiers, were paid a silver talent, in the form of land, and Onasilas had the usufruct of two other properties (van Effenterre and Ruze 1994: 131–7).

26 Ctesias, *Histories*, *FGrH* III C 688, F 14 Jacoby.

27 Bardinet 1995; Nunn 1996; Westendorf 1999; Kolta and Schwazmann-Schafhauser 2000.

28 Homer, *Odyssey* 4, 219–32.

29 Laser 1983: 119–24; Laskaris 1999.

30 Von Staden 1989: 16.

31 Marganne 1993.

32 Goltz 1974; J. R. Harris 1971: 112–37; von Staden 1989: 1–22, with Ritner 1989.

33 The tradition of the ubiquity of healers in Egypt carries on through Antiquity (cf. Fulgentius, p. 9 Helm; Historia Augusta, *Forty Tyrants* 7, 4; 8, 3). Herodotus' claim that they believed all diseases were produced by food and that they regularly used cathartics (*History* 2, 77) is more accurate.

34 Isocrates, *Busiris* 22, giving the lie to Longrigg's claim (1993a: 1) that the Greeks nowhere recognised a debt to Egypt. Certainly authors of the Roman period – Pliny (*Natural History* 7, 56, 196) and, after him, the author of the commentary on the Hippocratic *Oath* (fr. 1: pp. 56, 59 Rosenthal) – report that some people believed in an Egyptian origin for medicine.

35 Pritchett (1993: 237), a passionate defender of Herodotus' general veracity, acknowledges the problem. It is easiest to assume that Herodotus, who may have seen strangers talking to the sick lying outside their houses on beds in the street, was misled by his informant as to what was going on. For other possible explanations, see Worthington 2009: 55.

36 Geller 2010: 125–7.

37 Archaeological evidence, although highly informative about drugs, techniques and diseases, cannot entirely replace literary evidence. For the Mycenean background, see Laser 1983; Arnott 1996, 1997.

38 Cf. the discussions on the relationship between Greek and oriental science conducted in *Isis* (83, 1992, 554–607) between D. Pingree, G. E. R. Lloyd, H. von Staden and M. Bernal, and in *History of Science* (31, 1993, 227–87; 32, 1994, 445–68) between Bernal and R. Palter.

39 There are correlations in Greek medicine with Egyptian birth prognoses, and with some techniques of setting fractures and using cautery, but none of these could not be explained by the nature of the subject or by coincidence; parallels with Babylonian techniques are even slighter.

40 Burkert 1992; West 1997. It is also probable that Greek astronomy owes a great deal to the Babylonians.

41 Diodorus, *History* 1, 25. Burkert (1992: 75–9) also proposes a Babylonian origin for a cult title for Apollo on the Aegaean island of Anaphe.

42 Steuer and Saunders 1959; Biggs 1969; Geller 2001–2, 2007, 2009, 2010: 140–53 (for parallels in prognosis); Geller and Finkel 2002.

43 Nunn 1996: 165–78; Finkel 2000; Scurlock 2006. Cf. also van der Toorn 1985: 56–93.

44 Anonymus Londinensis col. IX 37: p. 51 tr. Jones. For this author, see p. 72 here.

45 The Greeks may well have considered the 'ethnic' aspect of his medicine unimportant.

46 There may have been other Egyptian doctors who knew Greek earlier but they have left no trace. His name, however, is non-Egyptian.

47 Steuer and Saunders 1959.

48 Lloyd 1987, 1990: 135–45; Longrigg 1993a.

49 This arrangement in the form of 'disagreements', while useful for classification and memory, may overemphasise the confrontational aspects of these theories, and there are many texts in the Hippocratic Corpus that prefer juxtaposition to confrontation.

50 [Hippocrates], *Regimen in Acute Diseases* 1: II, 224 L.

51 Goltz 1974; Geller 2001–2, 2010: 118–19, 123, noting also differences between pre- and post-700 Babylonian medicine.

52 For the Uruk tablets, see Geller 2010: 141–60. Lloyd (1979: 226–67) argued for the democratic ethos of Greek science; a better context might be one of 'broad oligarchic' legal debates and public discussions. Even Thersites has his say among the Homeric chiefs.

53 Xenophon, *Memoirs* 4, 2.

54 See p. 63 here.

55 We know what Tatian (*Against the Greeks* 21) thought of it around AD 160: it was 'extremely stupid'.

56 Either because this had become the 'normal' language of scientific discourse or because they wished for an audience or for patients in the larger and wealthier Ionic-speaking communities (cf. van der Eijk 1997b: 99–100).

57 An imaginary modern counterpart would be the writing of medical texbooks in the language of Robert Burns as a mark of the importance of eighteenth- and nineteenth-century Scottish medical schools. For the later use of Ionic, cf. Alexis, fr. 146 Kassel-Austin; Lucian, *How to Write History* 16, 24–5; Deichgräber 1971; Roselli 2005; for tombstones, see *Bulletin épigraphique* 75, 1962, n. 374.

58 See p. 38 here.

59 Longrigg 1993a: 46; Lloyd 1991: 417–34; Holmes 2010: 86–7. The Hippocratic author of *Regimen* explicitly uses parallels from the wider world to indicate the body's processes and to 'see the invisible through the visible' (1, 11–24: VI, 486–96 L.).

60 For the career of Democedes of Croton, a celebrated physician from S. Italy, see p. 63 here; Michler 2003.

61 Empedocles, DK B 6 = 12 Inwood, with the context A 32 = 6, pp. 172–5 Inwood.

62 Anonymus Londinensis 14–20. For the significance of the omission of Hippocrates from this list of believers in some form of elemental balance, see pp. 58–9 here; for Philistion and Menecrates, see, further, pp. 72, 82, 116–17 here.

63 Grmek (1989: 210–44) suggested a connection with a rare genetic allergy to beans known as favism and particularly common today in S. Italy and Sicily, the home of many Pythagoreans.

64 Fabbri and Trotta 1989; on medical prophets, see Holmes 2010: 80. For Oulios/ Ouliades, see p. 356, n. 41 here: it cannot be entirely excluded that Ouliades is a patronymic, occurring in alternate generations, although the number of Ouli-oi makes this unlikely. The building itself is of Hellenistic date, not the fifth century, and a certain amount of doubt still remains about the relationship of the bust and statues to the actual building.

65 Longrigg 1993b: 29–34. Diogenes Laertius, *Lives* 8, 57; 61; 67; 69 = DK 31 A, 1 = pp. 155–8 Inwood. Such stories, of course, are good evidence for what later generations believed him to have been, and for their acceptance of the congruity of these interests.

66 Diogenes Laertius, *Lives* 8, 62 and 59; DK 31 B 111, 112 = fr. 15, 1 Inwood. The promise of healing '*pharmaka*' is followed by claims that the pupil will be able to control the weather and 'bring back from Hades the strength of a dead man', which suggests a combination of interests removed from those of the author of *The Sacred Disease* but not necessarily to be discounted as unusual for that reason.

67 Diogenes Laertius, *Lives* 8, 77; DK 31 A 1 (600 lines long) = p. 161 Inwood; cf. A 2 = p. 161 Inwood. However, their authenticity is far from assured.

68 [Hippocrates], *Ancient Medicine* 20, 1: I, 620 L. (DK 31 A 71 = p. 187 Inwood), but the precise meaning of both words is hard to determine (see Vegetti 1998a). For Empedoclean influences in the Hippocratic Corpus, see Jouanna 1961.

69 Kingsley 1995, although not all of his speculative combinations are securely based. Plato (*Republic* 426b) saw incantations as a typical part of the doctor's armament against illness, along with drugs, cutting and burning.

70 Martin and Primavesi (1999: 114–21) remain agnostic on the question whether *On Nature* and *Purifications* form one poem or two. Scholarly opinion is now tending to accept these apparent inconcinnities and to reject a strict separation between the religious and scientific elements in the poem(s) (see C. Osborne 1987; Inwood 2001: 8–21).

71 Empedocles, DK 31 B 6, 98, 96 = fr. 12, 98, 62 Inwood; A 78a = p. 191 Inwood.

72 Empedocles, DK 31 B 84 = fr. 103 Inwood; A 86 = pp. 195–7 Inwood.

73 Empedocles, DK 31 A 76–7 = pp. 190–1 Inwood.

74 Empedocles, DK 31 A 81, 85 = pp. 193–5 Inwood.

75 Aristotle, *On the Generation of Animals* 777a7–12, on Empedocles, DK 31 B 68 = fr. 73 Inwood, although the text itself is far from certain.

76 Longrigg 1985: 277–87.

77 Longrigg 1993a: 48–50.

78 Aetius, *On the Opinions of the Philosophers* 5, 30, 1 = Alcmaeon, DK 24 B 4. It is not entirely clear whether Alcmaeon saw deficiency or surfeit as a direct cause of or as the catalyst for the changes of heat and cold.

79 Cf. Archytas, DK 47 B3; for the continuation of the political metaphor in later medical writing, see, for example, [Hippocrates], *Breaths* 15: 6, 114 L.; Menecrates, cited by Anonymus Londinensis 19, 22.

80 Theophrastus, *On the Senses* 25–6 = Alcmaeon, DK 24 A 5.

81 Chalcidius, *Commentary on the Timaeus* 246 = DK 24 A 10; Lloyd 1991: 164–78; Longrigg 1993a: 59–60.

82 Galen, 5, 281–3: *CMG* 5, 4, 1, 2, 164–8. The reference (19, 495) to Diogenes' belief in the importance of bodily (humoral?) colour as a diagnostic tool comes in a pseudo-Galenic tract, *On Humours*. The recipes (12, 686; 13, 313) could come from another Diogenes.

83 Aristotle, *History of Animals* 3, 2: 511b. Aristotle's account of Syennesis is replicated and extended in [Hippocrates], *The Nature of Bones* 8: IX, 174 L. For a discussion of the problems raised by these accounts, see Duminil 1983: 67–73. C. R. S. Harris (1973: 20–1) discusses only Aristotle's account.

84 C. R. S. Harris 1973: 21–8; Duminil 1983: 92–101, with comments on the textual difficulties in Aristotle's account; Althoff 1999: 64–77.

85 Aristotle, *Enquiry into Animals* 3, 2: 511b = Diogenes, DK 31 B 6.

86 Windsor, Royal Library 19097v. Illustrated in Da Vinci 1977: pl. 16A.

87 Plutarch, *Table Talk* 6, 2: 687B; 8, 9; 731B–734D and p. 36 here.

88 Philostratus, *Lives of the Sophists* 536.

89 Heeg 1913; Sudhoff 1915–16.

90 [Hippocrates], *Letters* 10–17; Rütten 1992. Cf. the equally dubious tale of Anaxagoras' dissections, Plutarch, *Pericles* 6.

91 Jacobs and Rütten 1998: 124–5.

92 Democritus, DK 68 A 151; [Hippocrates], *Nature of the Child* 31: VII, 540 L. Cf. also [Hippocrates], *Regimen* 1, 30: VI, 504 L.; [Aristotle], *Problems* 10, 14: 892b.

93 Democritus, DK 68 A 158–9; Holmes 2010: 202–7, 216–27.

94 Leucippus, DK 67 B 2 from *On Mind*.

95 Wellmann 1929; Longrigg 1993a: 93–7; Craik 1998a: 163–7. The parallel may also be the result of a similar educational situation in which a master's teachings are encapsulated in a striking sentence that requires elucidation to be properly understood.

96 Jouanna 1988: 11–24.

97 [Hippocrates], *Ancient Medicine* 20, 2: I, 620–2 L.

98 R. Thomas 2000.

99 See pp. 22–4 here. Rechenauer 1991; Craik 2001b; Jouanna 2005.

100 For Aristophanes' medical jokes, see Gil and Rodriguez Alfageme 1972; Cordes 1994: 51–63; Rodriguez Alfageme 1995: 569–83. The earliest stage presentation entitled 'The Doctor' is perhaps to be credited to Dinolochus, a Sicilian, around 480 BC; far more are known from the fourth century, for example by Antiphanes and Aristophon (Sanchis Llopis 2000). Anaxandrides' *Pharmakomantis*, 'The Drug-seer', may have involved a similar satire.

101 Simon 1978; Padel 1995; Guardasole 2000; Craik 2001a; Kosak 2004; Ceschi 2009; Holmes 2010: 228–74.

102 Euripides, *Medea* 109 (some mss. read 'black-spleened'); Galen, 5, 317.

103 Clement of Alexandria, *Selections* 6, 749 = Euripides, fr. 909 Nauck.

104 Sophocles, *Philoctetes* 266–7, 632.

105 Ibid. 1326, 1328.

106 Ibid. 649–50.

107 Ibid. 1333, 1437. For the importance of the sequence of healers, see Jebb 1898: 205; Winnington-Ingram 1980: 302.

108 Edelstein and Edelstein 1945 (hereafter simply Edelstein 1945): T. 588–91; Radt 1999: 57–8; Garland 1992: 125; R. Parker 1996: 184–6; Connolly 1998.

109 Sophocles, *Oedipus* 1–150; Herodotus, *History* 1, 105; [Hippocrates], *Airs, Waters and Places* 21–2: 2, 74–82 L.; R. Thomas 2000: 33–6; Jouanna 2005.

110 Anonymus Londinensis, 12, 36–13, 20(?) (Phasidas); 8, 10–34 (Timotheus); 13, 21–47 (Aegimius); 11, 42–12, 8 (Thrasymachus); 14, 12–18, 8 (Plato). Phasidas, Timotheus and Thrasymachus are known only from this papyrus. The most recent editor, Daniela Manetti, reads Phasitas; earlier editors preferred Phasilas.

4 HIPPOCRATES, THE HIPPOCRATIC CORPUS AND THE DEFINING OF MEDICINE

1 Rütten 1993; Leven 1994; Nutton 1995e; D. C. Smith 1996; Lederer 2002; Schubert 2005; Rütten 2007.

2 The choral setting, *Serment*, by the composer Iannis Xenakis (1981), can be heard on the selection of his *Choral Music* (Hyperion: CDA 66980, 1998), or on *Messiaen and his Pupils* (Chandos: CHA 9663, 1999); the CD-Rom is Rütten 2007. It should also be noted that the ancient form of the *Oath*, in its original Greek, is rarely taken, and that what medical schools call the Hippocratic *Oath* may be any one of its later reworkings and revisions. Its provisions, however, are usually invoked only in debates about abortion and euthanasia (cf. Carrick 1985).

3 Edelstein 1967: 3–63; Flashar and Jouanna 1997; the strongest defence of authenticity was mounted by Lichtenthaeler (1984).

4 W. D. Smith 1979.

5 R. R. R. Smith 1990; Rubin Pinault 1992; Nelson 2005. The background is given by Speyer (1971) and Lefkowitz (1981).

6 Wenkebach 1932–3; Soranus, *Life*: *CMG* 4, 175–8: tr. Rubin Pinault 1992: 6–8; Rütten 1992.

7 Sherwin-White 1978: 260–1, 285; Jouanna 1999: 37–9; see pp. 261–2 here. Hippocrates did not live in the present town of Cos, which was built in 366/365 BC, but in the settlement now known as Astypalaia ('old town') several miles away across the island. Hippocrates may have discoursed under a plane tree, but the tree shown to tourists and photographed as the genuine tree (or, if any botanical objection is pressed hard, its descendant) is in the wrong location entirely.

8 Plato, *Protagoras* 311b–c; Aristotle, *Politics* 4, 4: 1326a. This does not, however, prove that Hippocrates ever resided or taught at Athens. For Asclepiads on Cos, see pp. 261–2 here.

9 Plato, *Phaedrus* 270c–d. 'Nature' here could be interpreted as 'what the soul really is'.

10 Joly (1961) summarises earlier discussions; W. D. Smith 1979: 31–9; Lloyd 1991: 194–223; Solbakk 1993: 170–203.

11 Phaedrus' words, and especially the use of the particle γέ (a cogent emendation for τέ in the manuscripts), are meant by Plato to suggest that not every doctor would agree with Hippocrates' formulation.

12 This is the interpretation of Solbakk (1993: 90–118), stressing Plato's general usage of 'the whole'.

13 Given Plato's ironic reference to meteorology (270a) and his dislike of earlier cosmological theories, he is unlikely to have taken 'the whole' in a cosmological sense (which it often bears in Presocratic discussions). The suggestion that 'the whole' may mean both body and soul together (Griswold 1986: 281, n. 38) is excluded by Plato's distinction between the two spheres of rhetoric and medicine (at 280a). Similarly, Plato's emphasis on understanding interactions suggests that he is thinking of more than a merely anatomical understanding of the body and its parts.

14 Jouanna 1999: 59. Many scholars have seen a link here with *Ancient Medicine* (20: I, 620–2 L.), which demands that the physician should know about 'nature', and the relationship between the body and food, drink and habit: but there the author derives his understanding of nature from medicine, whereas the *Phaedrus* passage implies the converse, that it is knowledge of nature that explains the body.

15 Soranus of Cos, according to the biography of Soranus of Ephesus, *Life* 3, found in the Coan archives that he was born in 460/459 BC, 'Olympiad 48, year 1, when Abriadas was "Monarchos"'; his death date is placed variously by Soranus between 375 and 351. The former date could well be right; the latter is far more dubious.

16 Galen, 18A, 731; W. D. Smith 1979: 127–8; Lloyd 1991: 205.

17 P. Potter 1993; Roselli 1999; Tuplin 2004. Since no strictly medical work by Ctesias is known to have survived, he may have made this comment in one of his historical works, but there is no sure proof that he mentioned Hippocrates there. Jouanna (1999: 61) rightly notes that the high medical quality of these two tracts is worthy of the traditional image of Hippocrates.

18 The Greek here can be interpreted to mean either that the reason that follows immediately is Hippocrates' own but is not expressed in his exact words, or that the reason itself is that of Aristotle/Meno.

19 Anonymus Londinensis 5, 35–6, 44.

20 Texts are set out in W. H. S. Jones' 1947 edition of Anonymus, pp. 5–6. Meno's work was in several books, and included discussion of diseases and therapies as well as of underlying theories. The author of the papyrus, however, always refers only to Aristotle as his source, and may also have modified his wording. Cf. Manetti (1999a), tentatively arguing that Meno's work and what is here ascribed to Aristotle may have been two different things.

21 This passage (6, 43–7, 40) must now be consulted in the re-edition by Manetti (1996). The writer twice declares that Aristotle's view of Hippocrates' beliefs differs from his own.

22 Manetti (1996: 302–5) stresses that Anonymus had no difficulty in reconciling in his own mind two tracts with a somewhat diverse approach to the humours, and finds a parallel in the contemporary medical papyrus P. Strasbourg, inv. 26.

23 Galen, 15, 25–6.

24 For *Aphorisms*, see Manetti 1996: 295, n. 2; for *Regimen*, see W. D. Smith 1979: 50–8; for *Breaths*, see Jouanna 1988: 39–49.

25 Manetti 1999a.

26 He bases his account of Hippo's theories on two separate treatises (11, 13). Thivel (1981: 357–69), seeing in this section a mixture of different Hippocratic tracts, claims that this shows that this section is a later addition to Meno's work, because the Hippocratic Corpus was not known as such before the early third century. That, of course, does not exclude the likelihood that certain blocks of material were already circulating together before then.

27 Aristotle, *Enquiry into Animals* 3: 511b–513a; Lloyd 1991: 404–8; cf. Anonymus Londinensis 19, 1–17, apparently quoting from *The Nature of Man*.

28 For the authors' use of Ionic, see p. 45 here.

29 See the lists of titles contained in the major manuscripts and the Aldine as set out by W. H. S. Jones (1923–31: II, lvii–lxvi). Note that the index in ms. V lists more texts than are contained in the Aldine or V itself.

30 Kudlien 1989; W. D. Smith 1979: 177–246; Irigoin 1997: 191–210; Jouanna 1999: 56–71.

31 For the *Testament*, see Deichgräber 1970: 88–107; *Sevens*, VIII, 634–73; IX, 433–66 L.; new edition of chapters 1–12 by West 1971; cf. Mansfeld 1971; for *On Wounds*, see Witt 2009.

32 Lonie 1981: 43–50; Deichgräber 1933.

33 H. Bruun 1997; Jouanna 2000: xxviii–xxxi, xxxix–xlv, suggesting that one author was responsible for the cases in *Epidemics* 5, 1–50, and another for those in 5, 51–106 and in 7. Those in 5, 51–106 are largely repeated verbatim in 7, but neither recension corresponds exactly to what the author had originally written. Both books are thus in a sense composite productions.

34 Grensemann 1982, 1987.

35 Unless stated otherwise, I follow the datings suggested by Jouanna (1999: 373–416) and Golder (2007).

36 Disagreement over the dating, purpose and even unity of some treatises can be wide: cf. the possibilities suggested for *Anatomy* by Craik (1998b: 166), plumping for a fourth-century date. *Sevens* has been located anywhere from the late sixth century BC to the early first century BC. Even *Airs, Waters and Places*, which at first sight can be situated in a familiar historical situation, has been dated anywhere from the 440s to the 390s BC.

37 Strabo, *Geography* 14, 19; Pliny, *Natural History* 29, 2, 4; Soranus, *Life* 4. Libraries are known from the imperial period at the Asclepieia at Pergamum and Cos (see L. Robert 1969: I, 179–81): did this legend arise to explain the absence of genuinely Hippocratic material from an earlier Coan library?

38 [Galen], *Commentary on the Hippocratic Oath*, p. 80 Rosenthal.

39 Byl 1995; Chang 2005.

40 W. D. Smith 1979: 199–215; Fraser 1972: 364–9; von Staden 1989: 453–6; Vallance 2000.

41 That anonymous blocks of diverse material could also circulate together before the creation of the Alexandrian Library is clear from a work such as *Diseases of Women*.

42 For the Greek, see Diels 1970; Jouanna 1996c, 1999; Golder 2007; for the Latin, see Kibre 1985; MacKinney 1952; Galvao-Sobrino 1996; for the Arabic, see Weisser 1989.

43 Whether in the fifth and fourth centuries these (or most) medical treatises originally circulated anonymously is a moot point. Aristotle certainly could name the authors of some medical treatises, but there is no trace within the Corpus of the sphragistic devices used by poets and prose writers to identify their authorship. Was this a sign of a sense of communal ownership of this learning?

44 F. Adams (1849) bears the title *The Genuine Writings of Hippocrates*. W. D. Smith 1979; for Galen's Hippocratism, see pp. 224–5 here. It is also clear that Galen's choice of *The Nature of Man* as the canonical text was shared by many earlier Hippocratics, even if their interpetations of it differed (Lloyd 1991: 408).

45 Edelstein 1967: 133–44; Lloyd 1991: 194–223.

46 Van der Eijk 1997b, 2005b: 1–8.

47 W. H. S. Jones 1923–31: IV, IX–XII; Manetti 1999b.

48 Cf. [Hippocrates], *Epidemics* 6, 8, 7: V, 344 L., incorporating 'data from the small writing tablet'.

49 The standard edition of the Corpus remains that of E. Littré (1839–61). Bibliographies of modern studies of Hippocrates are provided by Maloney and Savoie (1982), Bruni Celli (1984) and Fichtner (1984). Jouanna (1999) is a magisterial survey. E. D. Phillips (1973: 39–121) and Golder (2007) are more medically orientated; P. Potter (1988) offers a succinct introduction.

50 Berger (1970: pl. 162–3) shows both sculptures.

51 Cordes (1994) surveys the evidence from literary texts; Edelstein (1967) sets Hippocratic medicine in a broad context.

52 Berger 1970; Hillert 1990: 209–17; Krug 2008.

53 Heraclitus, DK 22 B 58; Aeschylus, *Agamemnon* 848–50; Plato, *Republic* 426b and *Laws* 933a; cf. also for incantations, Pindar, *Pythian* 3, 47–53; Sophocles, *Ajax* 582–3. In general, see Edelstein 1967: 238–9; Jouanna 1999: 154–6, 222–32.

54 Herodotus, *History* 3, 129–38; see p. 87 here.

55 [Hippocrates], *Art* 1: VI, 2 L., with Mann 2012. Edelstein (1967: 107) gives other examples. See Jouanna 1988; Jori 1996: 317–32.

56 [Hippocrates], *Ancient Medicine* 1–2: I, 570–4 L.; Schiefsky 2005.

57 [Hippocrates], *Breaths* 1, 4: VI, 92 L.; Jouanna 1999: sect. ii, 3. On Hippocratic causation, see Lloyd 1979: 49–58; 1987: 114–24; Hankinson 1998a: 51–69; Jouanna 2005.

58 [Hippocrates], *Prognostic* 1: II, 110–12 L.

59 A good example of this, from within the Corpus, is *Sevens*, whose explanations are difficult to align with those of, for example, *Breaths* or *The Art*.

60 [Hippocrates], *Ancient Medicine* 20, 1: I, 620 L. Cf. the attack on Melissus in *The Nature of Man* 1; cf. Longrigg 1993a: 87–9.

61 Contrast, for example, *Regimen* 1, 2–5: VI, 468–78 L., which opens with a discussion of the principles of fire and water that govern the universe, and *Fleshes* 1–2: VIII, 584 L., which begins with similar cosmological speculations.

62 [Hippocrates], *Ancient Medicine* 20, 2; 14, 1–6; 16, 1–17, 3; 23: I, 622; 600–4; 606–12; 634 L.; Hankinson 1992a.

63 [Hippocrates], *Ancient Medicine* 3, 1–6; 12, 1–2: I, 574–8; 596–8 L.

64 Ibid. 9, 1–2: I, 588 L. Cf. Edelstein 1967: 109; Lloyd 1987: 124–31.

65 [Hippocrates], *Ancient Medicine* 4, 2: I, 578–80 L. Cf. p. 97 here.

66 [Hippocrates], *The Nature of Man* 22 = *Regimen in Health* 7: VI, 84–6 L.; *Nutriment* 34: IX, 110 L.; *Aphorisms* 1, 3: IX, 110 L.

67 Galen, 1, 23–6 K.

68 Aristotle, *Rhetoric* 1, 12; [Hippocrates], *Regimen* VI, 594–606 L. Cf. Plutarch, *Consolation for Apollonius* 15: 110C, quoting Euripides, *Suppliant Women* 1109–14, denouncing those who 'by foods, drinks, and magical charms' seek to prolong their lives, albeit in physical discomfort.

69 For the general background, see Temkin 1971; Wohlers 1999. Two recent studies of the whole treatise have very different aims: Laskaris 2002; Lo Presti 2008. For another denunciation of temple medicine, see *The Diseases of Girls* 1, 8: VIII, 468 L., deriding the advice of priests to dedicate costly clothing to Artemis as a means of reducing the physical and mental suffering of girls before menarche.

70 [Hippocrates], *The Sacred Disease* 1, 1–23: VI, 352–8 L.

71 Ibid. 1, 32–8: VI, 360–2 L.

72 Ibid. 5, 1; 15, 1: VI, 368; 390 L.

73 Ibid. 1, 45–52, 3: VI, 364 L.

74 Ibid. 1, 24–45: VI, 358–64 L. Others were prepared to offer prayers to the gods if need be, but still placed the major responsibility for treatment with the physician ([Hippocrates], *Regimen* IV, 89: VI, 652 L.).

75 For causal necessity, see ibid. 5, 6 and 6, 2; 8, 5–6; 13, 11; 14, 6; 17, 8: VI, 370; 376; 386; 388; 392 L.

76 Edelstein 1967: 210–19; Kudlien 1977; Jouanna 1999: 258–75; but there is no trace, as yet, of the Stoic (and later Galenic) view of the beneficent purpose of the divine Creator.

77 [Hippocrates], *Regimen* 4, 87: VI, 640–2 L.

78 Ibid. 4, 89, 90: VI, 652; 656–8 L.

79 Conversely, Gorrini (2005) argues that the doctors' failure in the plague of Athens led directly to a burgeoning of healing cults.

80 Temkin 1991; Flashar and Jouanna 1997.

81 [Hippocrates], *Prognostic* 1 and 25: II, 112, 188 L.; Edelstein 1967: 72–5, 95–8.

82 [Hippocrates], *Fractures* 36: III, 540 L.; *Diseases of Women* 1, 71: VIII, 150 L.

83 [Hippocrates], *Joints* 33; 35; 78: IV, 154; 158; 312 L.

84 [Hippocrates], *Diseases* 1, 1: VI, 140–2 L.; *Joints* 147: IV, 212 L.; *The Nature of Man* 1: VI, 32 L.; Edelstein 1967: 99–101.

85 [Hippocrates], *Joints* 42: IV, 184 L.; *Law* 1: IV, 638 L.

86 Edelstein 1967: 3–63; Lichtenthaeler 1984; Jouanna 1999: 43–52; von Staden 2007; a new text of the *Oath* is given by Jouanna 1996c; and translated in Jouanna and Magdelaine 1999: 70–1.

87 [Hippocrates], *Epidemics* 1: II, 636 L.

88 [Hippocrates], *Physician* 1: IX, 206 L.; *Law* 5: IV, 642 L.; cf. Dean-Jones 2010.

89 Edelstein 1967: 26–30; Rütten (1997: 72–7) lists the variant interpretations of this passage.

90 Edelstein 1967: 9–15; Bellemare 1999. To relate this clause solely to abortion or euthanasia is unduly restrictive.

91 [Hippocrates], *Nature of the Child* 13: VII, 488–90 L.; *Diseases of Women* 68–9; 72; 78: VIII, 142–6; 152; 184 L.; cf. Plato, *Theaetetus* 149b. In general, Riddle 1992a; King 1998: 132–56. The *Oath* forbids only the giving of *phthoria*, a vaginal pessary which destroys the foetus, and some (e.g. Keller 1988) have seen this as allowing other methods of abortion, such as drugs which induce a miscarriage and are consequently of less danger to the mother. But in the overall ethical context of the *Oath* this interpretation is unlikely, and it is easiest to take the abortive pessary as representing all abortive methods.

92 The date of the *Oath* cannot be easily determined: Edelstein (1967: 55) put it in the second half of the fourth century; Jouanna (1999: 402), more cautiously, says fifth or fourth century; von Staden (2007) gives reasons for a somewhat later date.

93 Rightly emphasised by Temkin 2002: 21–8.

94 Von Staden 1996a: 404–37.

95 Rütten 1993: 51–4. The writer of Papyrus Oxyrhynchus 4970, around AD 100, thought all young doctors should take it at the beginning of their education, and he, or more probably another person, seems to have deliberately cut out this passage to preserve it in some way.

96 Cato, *To His Son*, fr. 1 = Pliny, *Natural History* 29, 7, 14; Plutarch, *Life of the Elder Cato* 23, 4.

97 Von Staden 1996a, 2007; Temkin 1991.

98 Libanius, *On the Doctor-Poisoner* 9; Nutton 1995a. W. H. S. Jones (1928) is still worth consulting. The plea by Scribonius Largus (see pp. 187–8 here) for the *Oath* to be sworn is self-evidently proof that it was not.

99 Deichgräber 1970; Nutton 1993a.

100 Edelstein (1967) famously thought it was a Pythagorean document. Few would now agree, although some Pythagorean influence remains a possibility (see Bellemare 1999; Temkin 2002: 4).

101 This 'law' (or, equally, 'custom') has no legal authority. We know of no such enactment by any city in Antiquity enforcing such an obligation, and much to refute such an interpretation. It refers simply to the 'lawful custom' or 'tradition' of this specific medical grouping.

102 For a contract to be a 'medical clysterer' (P. London 43), see Rémondon 1964.

103 Jouanna 1999: 43–6. For the phrase, see Renehan 1975: 156–7.

104 Plato, *Laws* 720a. Cf. [Hippocrates], *Law* 1: IV, 638 L., proclaiming that the best doctor is one trained from childhood.

105 Theopompus, *Histories*, *FGrH* 115 F 103; Andromachus, cited by Galen, 14, 42; for Galen, see W. D. Smith 1973; Aristides, *The Asclepiads* 11; *To the Rhodians, on Concord* 45.

106 Sherwin-White 1978: 75; W. D. Smith 1979: 214–19. Dr. Klaus Hallof, Berlin, reports an unpublished Coan inscription, of Roman date, in which a doctor traces his lineage back through generations to Hippocrates and Asclepius.

107 I stress 'was being', for not every writer in the Corpus would assent to the same degree to all these summary propositions.

108 Holmes (2010) develops some of these formulations. How much the Hippocratic Corpus itself contributed to the creation of an acknowledged technical language of medicine is a more difficult question. Certainly, by 340 BC a playwright such as Menander could expect his audience to enjoy the fake technicalities of the doctor in his *Shield* (433–64).

109 Roselli 1998: 15, pointing out the divergence from the normal picture of Hippocrates as the founder of human medicine, in a direct line from Apollo and Asclepius. Another tradition, found in Late Antiquity, sees Hippocrates as the rediscoverer of the true medicine established by Asclepius (or, in some versions, Noah); see Nutton 2012b.

110 I stress that it is *a* standard, and not the only one; other doctors adhered to different theories and approaches, and by no means all accepted the authority of the Corpus. But few rejected its information entirely, even if, in Galen's view, Hippocratics in his day were in a minority. Cf. *L'Année Epigraphique* 1997: 1527 for an inscription attesting Hippocrates' wide reputation.

5 HIPPOCRATIC THEORIES

1 In the headings of this and the next chapter, 'Hippocratic' is used in the chronological sense of 'contemporary with Hippocrates'.

2 The question of the authorship of the whole document has been effectively settled by Manetti (1994). Her re-examination of the papyrus shows that this was the work of the actual scribe and not a copy of something by an earlier writer. Identification with any known medical writer is thus highly improbable. Cf. also, for the authorship of the original doxography, Chapter 4, n. 20.

3 Anonymus Londinensis 4, 25–31. The terminology used here is Aristotelian, and need not reflect the original words of the earlier authors. 'Residues', for instance, does not occur in the Hippocratic Corpus. But that is no reason to reject the classification of Aristotle, who had far greater access to medical information from the fifth and fourth centuries than we have, in favour of a later Galenic one that privileged the theory of the four humours and whatever might seem to have led up to that theory.

4 Mansfeld 1994; Mansfeld and Runia 1996; Manetti 2009a.

5 Anonymus Londinensis 9, 38–44; 20, 30–42.

6 Ibid. 8, 9–35.

7 Or Abas – the second letter is not visible on the papyrus: 8, 35–44.

8 The first version of his name is given by Anonymus Londinensis 20, 1–21, and by Celsus, *On Medicine* 3, 9, 3, and the Homeric scholium to Δ 515, ed. Erbse 1974: 222; the second by Galen, 1, 144 and 15, 436. Celsus and Galen both note his treatment of fever by heating the patient, provoking vomiting and then giving large amounts of roast pork and wine, and then repeating the treatment if it seemed not to work, a somewhat rash therapy according to Celsus, although welcomed by those whom treatment by the followers of Herophilus and Erasistratus had not helped. The Homeric scholiast claims that he did this to remedy a deficiency.

9 Anonymus Londinensis 4, 31–40. Cf. Jouanna 1974: 508–10, for doubts on the validity of the evidence of Anonymus.

10 Anonymus Londinensis 4, 40–5, 34.

11 [Hippocrates], *Regimen in Acute Diseases* 1: II, 224 L.; Galen, 15, 418–20; 426–8.

12 [Hippocrates], *Internal Affections* 35–8; 52–4; 10–12: VII, 252–60; 298–302; 188–98 L. Cf. Jouanna 1974: 16–24, 493–500.

13 Lonie 1965. Modern political conflicts have also contributed to this division, with modern Greek medical historians tending to dismiss Cnidian medicine as inferior to Coan, and Turkish historians doing the reverse. For the historiographical background, see Lonie 1978.

14 See pp. 57–8 here.

15 W. D. Smith 1973; Thivel 1981; Di Benedetto 1986: 70–88. This is not to deny the existence of certain groupings, of both people and texts (cf. Jouanna 1974; Grensemann 1975).

16 [Hippocrates], *On Breaths* 10, 1 and 12, 1: VI, 104; 108 L.

17 Craik 1998b: 25–9.

18 Both men and women are subject to the same natural laws. Although the typical patient is usually male, female patients can also stand for men as well, and there is no suggestion, like that made later by Aristotle, that woman is in some way an incomplete and inferior

version of man. But many authors would share the view of the writer of *Diseases* 1 that women had often different diseases from men, and that their treatment (in part as a consequence) should often be carried out in different ways. See Dean-Jones 1994: 41–7, 110–21; King 1998: 21–74.

19 [Hippocrates], *Fractures* 1: III, 412–14 L.

20 [Hippocrates], *Ancient Medicine* 20, 2: I, 620–2 L.; *Regimen* 1, 2: VI, 468–72 L.

21 [Hippocrates], *Fleshes* 1, 1–3, 8: VIII, 584–8 L.

22 Ibid. 19, 1–7: VIII, 608–14 L.

23 [Hippocrates], *Sevens*: VIII, 634–72; IX, 433–66 L. West (1971), noting Near Eastern parallels, placed it very early; Mansfeld (1971) very late, arguing that navigational wind rose mentioned in Chapter 3 would not have been in use before the late Hellenistic period.

24 Cf. the much later comment of Pliny (*Natural History* 7, 1, 17) that 'nature has even imposed some of its laws on diseases'.

25 [Hippocrates], *Regimen* 1, 2, 2: VI, 470 L.

26 II, 1–92 L. For the date, see Jouanna 1996a: 79–82. General background is provided by R. Thomas 2000: 28–101.

27 [Hippocrates], *Airs, Waters and Places* 4: II, 18–22 L.

28 Ibid. 19, 5; 24, 1–10: II, 72; 86–92 L. On the question of the unity of authorship with *The Sacred Disease*, see H. Bruun 1997; Jouanna 2003.

29 [Hippocrates], *Airs, Waters and Places* 16, 23, 24: II, 62–6; 82–92 L. Note also the ingenious suggestion (ch. 14: II, 58–60 L.) that the long-headed Macrocephali became like this over time: a practice of binding the heads of children at first 'forced' them into an unnatural shape, but over time nature took over, and they no longer had need of such restraints, since this shape was transmitted in the semen of their fathers, which was drawn from all parts of the body.

30 Lieber 1996: 451–76, although not all her speculations are equally convincing.

31 The title (which may not be original) does not refer to epidemic disease in the modern sense but to 'visitations', either of disease or, somewhat less likely, of the physician.

32 [Hippocrates], *Epidemics* 1, 1: II, 598–604 L.

33 Ibid. 6, 7, 1: V, 330–6 L. Translation based on Grmek (1989: 305–6), who identifies the disease with diphtheria.

34 The author of *Epidemics* 7 and of the second part of *Epidemics* 5 tries to relate some cases to the season of the year and the rising or setting of the sun and stars. But where places are mentioned they serve more as addresses than explanations of disease.

35 Grmek 1979: 318. The point is not greatly affected if one agrees with Grmek that the author of *Epidemics* 1 and 3 was also responsible for two further sections, *Epidemics* 2, 3, 1 and 6, 7, 1.

36 [Hippocrates], *The Nature of Man* 9, 5: VI, 56 L.

37 Note, especially, *Humours* 12–19: V, 492–500 L. At *Humours* 7: V, 486 L. there is a clear allusion to the sufferers from the cough at Perinthus (*Epidemics* 6, 7, 7: V, 340 L.), and the final chapter (20: V, 500–2 L.), a parallel version of *Epidemics* 6, 3, 23–4, 3: V, 304–6 L. (unless this passage represents a late addition to the text while circulating in manuscript), has convinced some scholars that the two treatises (together with *Epidemics* 2 and 4) were written by the same person.

38 [Hippocrates], *Aphorisms* 3, 1–23: IV, 486 L.; the diseases of age constitute 3, 24–31: IV, 496–502 L.

39 [Hippocrates], *Diseases of Women* 2, 3: VIII, 238–40 L.

40 There were, of course, other presuppositions that led to the belief that the female body was in many ways different from that of the male (cf. Lloyd 1983: 58–86).

41 Di Benedetto 1986: 225–47; Edelstein 1967: 253–60. Metraux (1995) draws attention to contemporary developments in sculpture that show a concern for anatomy, but R. Osborne

(2011: 37–40) argues that they display little interest in muscles as such rather than in the articulation they represent. The dating of the tiny tract *Anatomy*: VIII, 536–40 L., which shows evidence at least of some observations on animals, is much disputed. Craik (1998b) suggests it is a fragment of a fourth-century redaction of material that may go back to the fifth: less plausibly, Jouanna (1999: 530) sees it as a pastiche of late Hellenistic or even Roman date, in part because it is unknown to lexicographers before Galen.

42 Duminil 1983; Skoda 1988.

43 [Hippocrates], *Joints* 41: IV, 180 L., with the comments of W. Pagel (a specialist in tuberculosis as well as a distinguished medical historian), cited by C. R. S. Harris 1973: 100–1. Cf. also Di Benedetto 1986: 239–41.

44 [Hippocrates], *The Sacred Disease* 11, 3–4: VI, 380 L.

45 Plutarch, *Roman Questions* 111: 290A; Aesop, Fables 16. 'Staggers' may be the result of infestation by the parasite *Taenia coenurus* or of eating rye grass affected by various fungi.

46 [Hippocrates], *The Sacred Disease* 13, 8: VI, 386 L.

47 [Hippocrates], *Epidemics* 6, 4, 6: V, 308 L.; *Internal Affections* 23: VII, 224 L. The author of *Glands* (VIII, 556–74 L.) shows a reasonable acquaintance with glands, even if he then classifies the brain as one of them.

48 [Hippocrates], *The Nature of the Child* 29: VII, 530 L.; King 1998: 34.

49 Anaxagoras, DK 59 B 21a: perhaps alluded to by [Hippocrates], *Regimen* 1, 11, 1 and 12, 1: VI, 486–8 L.; and *Ancient Medicine* 22, 3: I, 626 L.

50 [Hippocrates], *Regimen* 1, 13–24: VI, 488–96 L.

51 [Hippocrates], *Ancient Medicine* 22, 4: I, 628 L. Aristotle (*Generation of Animals* 2, 4: 737b) disputes the view that the womb acts like a cupping glass.

52 [Hippocrates], *Diseases* 4, 51–2: VII, 584–92 L.

53 King 1998: 33–5.

54 Ibid. 214–22. The notion of a 'wandering womb' may have originated in the fact that a prolapse of the uterus is extremely common in animals, especially cows, sheep and goats.

55 Lloyd 1971: 345–60; Lonie 1981: 77–86.

56 [Hippocrates], *Ancient Medicine* 1: I, 570–723 L.; *The Nature of Man* 1: VI, 32–4 L.

57 Cf., for the role of what we would term organs in the creation and transmission of fluids, *Ancient Medicine* 22: I, 626–34 L.

58 Thivel (1981: 279–383) gives a systematic study of the notion of humours, comparing it also with the theories in Anonymus Londinensis and in early philosophy.

59 Note the 'scientific soliloquy' of the author of *Epidemics* (6, 2, 5: V, 278–80 L.) as he muses on the relationship between various diseases and fluxes upwards or downwards, 'questions that require thought'.

60 [Hippocrates], *Ancient Medicine* 18, 1; I, 612 L., although his explanation of what these 'extremely clear' signs reveal is not that of other writers in the Corpus.

61 Brooks *et al.* (1962) offer interesting arguments for the theory of humours anticipating homoeostasis.

62 Menstruation, according to the author of *The Nature of the Child*, is simply 'a fact of her original construction' (see King 1998: 29–31).

63 [Hippocrates], *Coan Prognostics* 537, 541 L.: V, 706, 708 L.; Dean-Jones 1994: 136–44. By contrast with the generally favourable view of menstruation among the Hippocratics, Aristotle (*Enquiry into Animals* 7, 1: 582b) described it as a painful illness in itself.

64 Craik 1998a: 14–16.

65 [Hippocrates], *Affections* 1: VI, 608 L.; *Diseases* 1, 2: VI, 142 L.

66 [Hippocrates], *Airs, Waters and Places* 10: II, 42–50; *The Sacred Disease* 15: VI, 388 L.

67 [Hippocrates], *Haemorrhoids* 1: VI, 436 L.

68 Jouanna 1999: 317.

69 See pp. 21, 29 here.

70 [Hippocrates], *Ancient Medicine* 18–19, 24: I, 612–20, 634–6 L. For this author, it is the qualities, not the fluids themselves, that cause disease.

71 Anonymus Londinensis 11, 42–12, 2.

72 Anonymus Londinensis 18, 30–8. Blood becomes thicker or thinner as a result of changes in the flesh; bile is called an 'ichor' or 'serum' of flesh, which leaves it ambiguous whether this is a deformation, but the comment (at 20, 22) that he thought bile 'useless' suggests that he believed it could exist in the body in a harmless form; phlegm is said to be produced by 'rains', which implies that it too is not naturally present in the body.

73 [Hippocrates], *Airs, Waters and Places* 19; 24, 1–3: II, 70–2; 86–8 L.

74 Craik 2001b.

75 Not just among the body's constituents. The author of *Regimen* (3, 69: VI, 606 L.) propounded the novel theory that health depended also on a balance between food and exercise.

76 [Hippocrates], *The Sacred Disease* 8–10: VI, 376–80 L.; *Places in Man, passim.*

77 [Hippocrates], *Aphorisms* 1, 3–6: IV, 458–62 L.

78 [Hippocrates], *The Nature of Man* 4: VI, 40 L.

79 [Hippocrates], *Regimen* 1, 12–24: VI, 488–96 L.

80 Although the extent of the debt to Heraclitus is disputed: cf. Joly (1984: 27), 'no great influence', with Thivel (1981: 273), 'the author is a Heraclitean'.

81 Thivel 1981: 302–17, 369–84.

82 Jouanna 1961.

83 [Hippocrates], *Ancient Medicine* 20, 1: I, 620 L.

84 Those that emphasised the opposition between bile and phlegm could be easily assimilated to a four-element theory of disease on the assumption that in any one particular tract the author had chosen to concentrate only on this pair of opposites. Hence, for example, the easy acceptance of *Airs, Waters and Places* or *Epidemics* 1 and 3 within the canon of genuine Hippocratic works. For the use of opposites, see Lloyd 1971.

85 At what point the notion of humours became joined to that of elements, and they became seen as the four major constituents of the body, is not clear. Hippo of Croton, for instance (Anonymus Londinensis 11, 32–7), saw disease as resulting from the action of hotness and coldness on the body's natural moisture. Some doctors long continued to use humours to refer to any of the body's fluids (as in *Humours*: VI, 470–502 L. and p. 125 here).

86 [Hippocrates], *Diseases* 4, 3: VII, 544 L.

87 Anonymus Londinensis 20, 1–21; 25–37.

88 Ibid. 19, 15–48.

89 'Proportion' is a reminder of the Empedoclean and Pythagorean notions of a mathematical universe. 'Blending' here refers to the choice of ingredients, 'mixture' to their formation as a single substance.

90 [Hippocrates], *The Nature of Man* 42–3: VI, 38–40 L.: tr. Longrigg.

91 Ibid. 2, 4–5: VI, 36 L.

92 Ibid. 7, 8–9; 13: VI, 50; 64 L. Words involving 'necessity' are found eighteen times in this treatise.

93 Ibid. 9, 2: VI, 52 L.

94 Ibid. 15, 1; 7, 4–5; 16, 2–3: VI, 66; 48; 72–4 L.

95 Ibid. 9, 1–2: VI, 54 L. The exception is when many people fall ill with the same condition: in which case the cause is something in the air (ibid. 9, 3–4: VI, 54–6 L.). But if many individuals fall ill with different conditions, then the reason lies with the individual.

96 Ibid. 24: VI, 86 L.

97 Given the linkage via the Pythagoreans of mathematics, order and beauty, this is perhaps hardly surprising. Many texts in the Corpus, especially in the *Epidemics*, also

stress numbers and ratios with a precision that is foreign to the modern doctor, and that implies a search for a mathematical certainty or confirmation of diagnosis and treatment.

98 Schöner (1964) has a splendid map of the ramifications of this concept, but he is misleading when he implies that this scheme of four was in some way standard in the Corpus. Jouanna (2006, 2007) shows how the theory became further enlarged in Late Antiquity.

99 [Hippocrates], *Aphorisms* 3, 20; 22: IV, 494 L. (with the reading given by W. H. S. Jones 1923–31: IV, 128); IV 496 L.

100 [Hippocrates], *Airs, Waters and Places* 10, 12: II, 50 L.

101 Aristophanes, *Birds* 14; *Assemblywomen* 251; Sophocles, *Women of Trachis* 573. Langholf 1990: 46–50, 267–9. See also Müri 1953; Flashar 1966; Rütten 1992.

102 Kudlien 1967: 76–86.

103 Anonymus Londinensis 12, 30–5.

104 [Hippocrates], *The Nature of Man* 7, 9: VI, 50 L. A date between 410 and 400 BC is possible, on the grounds that black bile is not a familiar humour in *Epidemics* 1 and 3, but is so in *Epidemics* 2, 4 and 6, of c.399–5.

105 The author of *Affections* (36: VI, 246 L.) may represent a slightly different stage, talking of using specific types of drugs to expel bile, phlegm, black bile or water to reduce the imblance of those who are naturally inclined to be bilious, phlegmatic, melancholic or watery. The author of *Diseases* (1, 3: VI, 144 L.) similarly equivocates between black bile as a disease and as a fluid.

106 [Aristotle], *Problems* 30, 1: 953a–955a; Klibansky *et al.* 1964; Pigeaud 1988; van der Eijk 2005b: 279–98.

107 For the fragments of Rufus, *On Melancholy*, see Sideras 1994: 1181–2; Ullmann 1994: 1316–17; Pormann 2008. Galen, *On Black Bile*: 5, 104–48: tr. M. Grant 2000: 19–36. In general, see S. W. Jackson 1986; Arikha 2007.

108 Even if they were rejected by Galen as fantastic.

109 See pp. 58–60 here. In his *Enquiry into Animals* (3, 3: 512b) Aristotle quoted almost verbatim the description of the vascular system in Chapter 11: VI, 58–60 L., and attributed it to Polybus.

110 Sabinus ascribed everything from Chapter 16 onwards to Polybus, and Galen agreed, but rejecting also Chapter 11 (the passage quoted by Aristotle) as 'wholly bad and inconsistent with what was said in *Epidemics* 2': for their arguments, see Jouanna 1999: 62; W. D. Smith 1979: 166–72.

6 HIPPOCRATIC PRACTICES

1 The Greek word *technites*, from which we get 'technician', applies to all sorts of non-agricultural workers, from potters to dramatic performers. There was a considerable discussion in fifth- and fourth-century Greece, exemplified in Plato's dialogues and in *The Art*, as to just what constituted a *techne* (see Edelstein 1967: 87–110; Horstmanshoff 1976; Temkin 1977: 137–53; Jouanna 1988: 168–90; Jori 1996; Pleket 1995).

2 See p. 40 here. The Hippocratic treatise *The Surgery* (III, 272–337 L.) deals only in passing with the arrangements for the surgery itself; cf. *The Physician* 2: IX, 206–8 L. and *The Use of Liquids* 1: VI, 118 L. In later periods, the word *ergasterion*, 'workshop', is frequently found applied to a doctor's place of work, just as to any other craftsman's shop or industrial premises. Aeschines (*Oration* 1, 124) claims that the same building could be a doctor's surgery or a smithy, a laundry, a carpenter's shop or a brothel: it took its name from the trade carried on inside, not from any particular architectural feature.

3 The *Constitutions* incorporate material that is likely to come from a variety of physicians working in the same place. At Perinthus (*Epidemics* 2, 3, 1: V, 100 L.) a group of physicians arrive together. The author of *Prorrhetic* I cites (his own?) cases from Cos and

Odessus (34, 72: V, 518, 528 L.); the author of *Epidemics* 5, 1–50: V, 204–36 L. worked in Central Greece; the cases in *Epidemics* 7: V, 364–468 L., partly reworked in *Epidemics* 5, 51–106: V, 236–58 L., come from a doctor travelling in N. Greece and the central Aegean, often as part of a group (see F. Robert 1989). Chang (2005) points out that most of the cities named would have had wealthy patients.

4 Herodotus, *History* 3, 129–37; see p. 63 here.
5 Plato, *Gorgias* 455b; 456b; Xenophon, *Memoirs* 4, 2, 5; Cohn-Haft 1956; Nutton 1988: VI, 9–23; Jouanna 1999: 370–2.
6 Cohn-Haft 1956: 33–45.
7 Amundsen and Ferngren 1977.
8 Indeed, given the high failure rates recorded in *Epidemics* 1 and 3 (60 per cent fatalities), one might wonder why anyone should agree to, let alone pay for, such treatment. Even if allowance is made for the selective nature of such case records (perhaps chosen in order to avoid similar outcomes or to warn of likely failure in future) and for the possibility of payment only by results (cf. *Precepts* 4 and 6: IX, 254–8 L.), the question still remains.
9 [Hippocrates], *Precepts* 4: IX, 268 L.; Plato, *Gorgias* 456b; cf. [Hippocrates], *The Nature of Man* 1, 3: VI, 34 L. Similar claims for originality or effectiveness would have to be made if a doctor wished to earn money by attracting students who would pay him fees.
10 Edelstein 1967: 91–4; see pp. 96–7 here.
11 The playwright Alexis (fl. 350–300), fr. 146 Kassel-Austin (from his *The Woman Treated with Mandragora*). Cf. [Hippocrates], *Regimen in Acute Diseases* 2: II, 238 L.
12 [Hippocrates], *Prognostic* 1: II, 110 L.; *Epidemics* I, 1: II, 598 L.; cf. *Aphorisms* I, 1: IV, 458 L.
13 The author of *Art* (7: VI, 10–12 L.) comments on the difficulty of ensuring that patients understand and follow instructions. Cf. Jouanna 1999: 134–7.
14 [Hippocrates], *Prognostic* 1: II, 110 L.; Edelstein 1967: 65–85. Many of the authors in Horstmanshoff (2010) also emphasise that the didactic element in Hippocratic writings, including *Prognostic*, is aimed at patients as well as fellow practitioners.
15 Cf. [Hippocrates], *Affections* 13: VI, 220 L., arguing that if the doctor adds nothing bad by his treatment the death of a patient is not his fault.
16 Vegetti 1996; Fausti 2005.
17 [Hippocrates], *Prorrhetic* 2, 1: IX, 6 L. The use of present participles implies that this prediction is made in public, the marketplace, while the traders are selling their wares, and when they may be apparently well.
18 Among the inscriptions from the medico-religious building at Elea (see p. 258 here) is one of an *iatrom* [...]. Supplementation to *iatrom[antis]* (medical prophet) is tempting, but far from certain. Cf. Aeschylus, *Agamemnon* 1623; *Eumenides* 62; *Suppliant Women* 263; Aristophanes, *Plutus* 11, all but the first applying to gods.
19 [Hippocrates], *Prorrhetic* 2, 2–3: IX, 8–14 L.
20 Cf. [Hippocrates], *Joints* 42; 68; 78: IV, 184; 282; 312 L., where the author claims that his methods are more safe, if less flashy, than those of his competitors. Cf. also *Prorrhetic* II, 2: IX, 10 L., for 'competitions in forecasting'.
21 The author of *Prognostic* (1: II, 110–12 L.) wants to include both terms under the word *pronoia* ('forethought'), which is not otherwise found in the medical parts of the Corpus; elsewhere it usually means taking care, rather than understanding what is to come.
22 But this ideal of precision is often qualified in practice by the difficulty of understanding the individual: [Hippocrates], *Ancient Medicine* 9, 2–4; 12, 2; 20, 2: I, 588–90; 596; 622 L.; *Places in Man* 41, 1–2: VI, 330 L.; Holmes 2010: 150–62.
23 [Hippocrates], *Places in Man* 44: VI, 338 L.; *Aphorisms* I, 1: IV, 458 L.; *Affections* 13: VI, 220 L.
24 [Hippocrates], *Prognostic* 1: II, 112 L.; *Epidemics* 1, 1: II, 632–6 L.

25 E.g. 'Patients who suffer torpor after chills are not entirely in their senses'; [Hippocrates], *Prorrhetic* 1, 35: V, 518 L., repeated at *Coan Prognoses* 90: VI, 602 L.
26 P. Potter 1989; the whole of Baader and Winau (1989) is also relevant.
27 [Hippocrates], *Prorrhetic* 2, 2: IX, 8 L; Storer 2005. A desire to avoid similar outcomes in the future may also explain the presence of a large number of cases ending in death or involving medical failure of some sort. This attitude is openly admitted at *Joints* 47: IV, 212 L.; cf. also *Epidemics* 5, 27, 2: V, 226 L. See von Staden 1990.
28 [Hippocrates], *Epidemics* I, 23: I, 668–70 L., slightly adapted.
29 The formulation is that of Holmes (2010: 126). The Hippocratic writers show no real grasp of the significance of the pulse, although it was noted (e.g. *Places in Man* 3, 2: VI, 280 L.) and Aegimius of Elis (fl. 380 BC) wrote a book on the throbbing of blood vessels (Galen, 8, 498).
30 [Hippocrates], *Head Wounds* 11: III, 220 L.
31 [Hippocrates], *Head Wounds* 19: III, 252–4 L.
32 [Hippocrates], *Prognostic* 2: II, 114 L. The medical historian C. R. S. Harris claimed to have saved the life of his colleague A. L. Rowse by recognising in him the *facies Hippocratica* and demanding urgent intervention.
33 Jouanna 1999: 294–9.
34 The belief antedated such texts in the Corpus as *The Eight-month Child* and *The Seven-month Child* (VII, 432–60 L.) and survived the observations by Aristotle (*Enquiry into Animals* 7, 4: 584a–b) and others that some children born in the eighth month had survived.
35 Hanson 1997.
36 Cf. Craik 2001c. See pp. 22–4 here.
37 Rechenauer 1991; Jouanna 2005.
38 Solbakk 1993; Cordes 1994: 140–52; R. Brock 2000; Kosak 2000.
39 For the three different blocks of the *Epidemics*, see p. 60 here. In general, see Baader and Winau 1989; Langholf 1990: 222–54; Jouanna 2000: Introduction.
40 This method of diagnosis is certainly apparent in Galen (S. W. Jackson 1969).
41 In some treatises, notably *Internal Affections* and *Diseases* II, a variety of statements about illnesses, from the head downwards, are juxtaposed as if they offer different varieties of a single disease, a procedure said by Galen (15, 427–8) to be characteristic of the Cnidians. But this is a loose nosography at best, and one easily capable of being used alongside one that stressed individuality (e.g. *Places in Man* 34: VI, 326 L.). Cf. von Staden 2002b.
42 Cf. [Hippocrates], *Prorrhetic* 2, 2–4: IX, 10–14 L., advising the physician to repeat an examination at a similar time and place to reduce the possible variation. A major study in English along the lines of Koelbing (1977) would be valuable (cf. E. D. Phillips 1973: 62–72; Jouanna 1999: 141–76; Holmes 2010, offering many subtle insights).
43 [Hippocrates], *Diseases* II, 48: VII, 72–4 L.; *Diseases of Women* I, 71: VIII, 150 L.; *Sterile Women* 233: VIII, 416 L. For the same attitude in later authors, cf. Herophilus, frag. 51 von Staden.
44 [Hippocrates], *Prorrhetic* 2: IX, 34–6 L.
45 [Hippocrates], *Art* 3, 2; 8, 1–7: VI, 4–6; 12–14 L. Cf. *Epidemics* I, 11: II, 636 L.: 'help, or do not harm'.
46 Plato, *Republic* 360e–361a.
47 [Hippocrates], *Places in Man* 24: VI, 316 L.
48 [Hippocrates], *Fractures* 36: III, 540 L.
49 [Hippocrates], *Affections* 13: VI, 220 L.; *Fractures* 9: III, 452 L.
50 Berger 1970; pl. Figure 6.2 here.
51 [Hippocrates], *Oath*: IV, 630 L.; *Physician* 14: IX, 220 L.
52 [Hippocrates], *The Nature of Man* 11, 1–6: VI, 58–60 L. Only in the Appendix to *Regimen in Acute Diseases* is it accorded prominence in therapy (cf. 4: II, 402 L.).

53 [Hippocrates], *Epidemics* 5, 6, 3: V, 206 L.

54 Brain 1986: 158–72; cf. ibid. 112–20, concluding that venesection was not the principal method of therapy at this time.

55 Majno 1975: 186–8, 221–4.

56 [Hippocrates], *Diseases* 2, 12: VII, 22 L.; *Internal Affections* 18: VII, 212 L.; *Vision* 3–5: IX, 154–8 L.; *Joints* 11: IV, 106 L.

57 [Hippocrates], *Joints* 11: IV, 106 L.

58 [Hippocrates], *Epidemics* 5, 7, 1–4: V, 206–8 L.

59 [Hippocrates], *Joints* 2–8: IV, 80–98 L., with a sound understanding of the principles of the lever and of the difference between emaciated and well-muscled patients. The writer has treated both sports injuries (4; 11: IV, 86; 106 L.) and congenital dislocations, which have more serious consequences among the young (28: IV, 138 L.). He probably also wrote *Fractures*.

60 [Hippocrates], *Instruments of Reduction* 38: IV, 382–6 L., deriving in part from *Joints*. Despite the traditional title most of the book is taken up with manual treatment of dislocations. The best modern discussion of Hippocratic orthopaedics and surgery is Di Benedetto's (1986: 248–302); cf. also Craik 2010.

61 [Hippocrates], *Joints* 72: IV, 296 L., specifically recommended for someone practising in a populous city. The similar recommendation (47: IV, 202 L.) to obtain pressure by using a beam inserted into a hole in the wall also implies that this is to be done at a particular location. Contrast *Decorum* 8: IX, 236 L. The development of a rack for stretching the limb, shown in the illustrations to the Nicetas codex of Apollonius of Citium (ninth century, but dependent on drawings from the sixth century, if not much earlier), probably took place a generation or two after this. Cf. Di Benedetto 1986: 290–6; and here pl. 10.1.

62 [Hippocrates], *Joints* 42–3: IV, 182–8 L. The depictions of this and similar operations in the Nicetas codex suggest a high chance of serious injury to the patient, and even death from disarticulation of the neck.

63 [Hippocrates], *Head Wounds* 2, 5–7, 5: III, 190–210 L.

64 Ibid. 14, 5–8: III, 240–2 L.

65 The author assumes throughout that the doctor will already know about other aspects of medicine, but will involve himself with trephining only 'of necessity' (21, 1: III, 256 L.). The author of *Epidemics* 5, 1–50 shows himself to be a generalist with a reasonable command of surgery, although not all his operations succeed, and is perhaps even acquainted with *Head Wounds* (cf. *CMG* I, 4, 1, p. 53). For the fragments of *On Wounds*, see Witt 2009.

66 Craik 1995a, 1995b; Edelstein 1967: 303–17; Wilkins 2005; Wöhrle 1990.

67 [Hippocrates], *Ancient Medicine* 3, 4–6: I, 576–80 L.

68 Ibid. 5: I, 580–2 L. Cf. Lonie 1977.

69 Although some later authors thought that the Pythagoreans invented dietetics in the sixth century, this is likely to be an anachronism (Iamblichus, *Life of Pythagoras* 163).

70 Plato, *Republic* 406a–c; *Protagoras* 316d. Cf. [Hippocrates], *Epidemics* 6, 3, 18: V, 302 L.

71 Anonymus Londinensis 9, 20–36. Unless, of course, the doxographical author himself created the opinions of Herodicus out of mere hints in the original. Manetti (2005) warns that the papyrus is too fragmentary at this point to be sure that it refers to Herodicus of Selymbria; Jones' text, based on Diels' emendations, is misleading in its apparent completeness.

72 Plato, *Republic* 405d–406c; [Hippocrates], *Regimen* I, 1: VI, 466 L., talking of 'many' writers on the subject; Democritus, DK 58 A 33. Jori (1993) argued that Plato's context puts this change in the last quarter of the century, but this may be slightly too late.

73 Soranus, *Life of Hippocrates* 2; Porphyry, *Commentary on Iliad*, 11, 514. The situation is complicated by the orthographical confusion, already apparent by AD 50, between

Herodotus and Prodicus, alleged to have taught Hippocrates rhetoric. Pliny (*Natural History* 29, 2, 2) has Prodicus as the pupil of Hippocrates and the founder of the art of massage.

74 Craik (1995b), W. D. Smith (1999) and Thivel (1999) independently suggested that the historical Hippocrates might have contributed to the development of dietetics.

75 [Hippocrates], *Art* 6, 2: VI, 10 L. The author of the *Oath* also specifies the use of diets as the prime method of therapy.

76 The fourth book of *Regimen* (VI, 640–62 L.) deals specifically with dreams; those that foretell the future are left to specialist interpreters, but others can be understood by the doctor to indicate an excess or deficiency within the body (88, 7: VI, 640–2 L.).

77 Ibid. 1, 32, 2; III, 68: VI, 508; 594–604 L. For Diocles, who gave detailed advice on an appropriate diet throughout the day (fr. 182 van der Eijk), see p. 124 here.

78 Ibid. 1, 2: VI, 468–72 L. Note Plato's comment (*Republic* 406c–407e) that when craftsmen pay attention to a proper lifestyle they are viewed with amusement, but the wealthy are not. The universalist claim at *Regimen* 3, 69: VI, 604–6 L. is gainsaid by what follows.

79 [Hippocrates], *Regimen* 3, 67; 72–8: VI, 592–6; 610–24 L.

80 It should be emphasised that this is not entirely the same as removing the cause in modern medical practice: accurate diagnosis of the condition explains both what is wrong and how the imbalance can be rectified. There are occasional traces of homoeopathic treatment (e.g. *Places in Man* 42: VI, 334–6 L.).

81 [Hippocrates], *Regimen* 2, 39–56: VI, 534–70 L.; *Ancient Medicine* 3–4: I, 574–80 L.

82 Jouanna (1999: 129) cites the court speech of Antiphon, *On the Member of the Chorus*, for an instance of a drug intended to improve a condition that killed the recipient. Theophrastus (*Investigation into Plants* 9, 16, 8) cites Thrasyas of Mantinea for his invention of a drug based on hemlock and poppy juice that would bring about a peaceful death.

83 Studies on Hippocratic pharmacology are remarkably rare, e.g. Aliotta *et al.* 2003; Totelin 2009. A short survey in English is Stannard (1961).

84 As Lloyd (1983: 126–8) pointed out, the Hippocratic writers do not concern themselves with the questions of identification and differentiation found in, for example, Theophrastus.

85 Respectively, [Hippocrates], *Diseases of Women* 16: VIII, 854 L.; *Affections* 54: VI, 264 L. and *Diseases of Women* II, 110: VIII, 238 L.; *Affections* 43: VI, 252 L. Riddle (1992b: XIV, 37) argues that only 10 per cent of the drugs recorded in the Corpus have no place in modern guides of medical botany and pharmacognosy.

86 [Hippocrates], *Diseases of Women* 1, 78 and 91; VIII, 176 and 220 L. Cf. King 1998: 153.

87 [Hippocrates], *Diseases of Women* 129; 64 and 78; 198: VIII, 276; 132 and 190; 382 L.

88 Ibid. 110: VIII, 236 L.

89 In amenorrhoea sexual intercourse is often recommended as a way of opening the blocked female tubes (e.g. *Superfoetation* 4: VIII, 478 L.) and causing the blood to flow freely again (cf. Dean-Jones 1994: 126–35).

90 Von Staden 1992c; Andò 1999; Gourevitch 1999a.

91 King 1998: 153.

92 King 1998: 145–56. Contrast Riddle 1992b: XIV, XV.

93 Plato, *Republic* 426b, viewing drugs, cautery, cutting, chants and amulets as on the same level.

94 Contrast [Hippocrates], *Diseases* 2, 12: VII, 20 L. with *Places in Man* 40: VI, 330 L.

95 [Hippocrates], *Coan Prognoses* 2, 304: V, 650 L.

96 [Hippocrates], *Epidemics* 2, 3, 2: V, 104 L. The words obelised 'I pass over most things', although present in the Greek tradition by AD 800, are suspect, so Robert Leigh tells me.

97 Von Grot (1899) discusses the drugs under broad categories. In *Diseases* and *Affections* various treatments for the same condition are juxtaposed without further comment.

98 Stannard 1961: 508–9. In general, see Goltz 1974; von Staden 2002b; Scarborough 2010.

99 [Hippocrates], *Diseases of Women* 136 and 78: VIII, 308 and 184 L.

100 Celsus, *On Medicine* 3, 9; Galen, 1, 214; 15, 436 = Erasistratus, fr. 213–14 Garofalo.

101 Girard 1990.

102 Only in the very much later *Decorum* (9: IX, 238 L.) do we find the statement that knowing drugs, how they work, and what, how much and when to prescribe is the beginning, middle and end of medicine.

103 Plato, *Laws* 470a–d. By saying that slave doctors would 'ordinarily' treat slaves he also leaves open the possibility that they would treat non-slaves. Where there was a choice, social pressures would probably mean that the wealthiest citizens would not seek to be treated by slaves, but for those lower down the social scale this must have been an option.

104 [Hippocrates], *Epidemics* 4, 2; 38: V, 144; 180 L.

105 Xenophon, *Memoirs* 2, 10, 2.

106 Jouanna 1999: 117.

107 [Hippocrates], *Precepts* 4 and 6: IX, 254–8 L. Cf. also the joke about the poor patient in Crates, fr. 14.

108 Lonie 1981: 43–54.

109 [Hippocrates], *Diseases of Women* 1, 62: VIII, 126 L.

110 Euripides, *Hippolytus* 293–6. The notion of 'women's networks of information', not necessarily available to males, should be used with caution; cf. Dean-Jones 1995.

111 Hyginus, *Fables* 274. The Latin has Agnodike; I give the form in which it would have been recognised in Greek.

112 King 1998: 181–5.

113 Plato, *Theaetetus* 149b–e: the text of the final (abortion) clause is clearly corrupt, but no cogent solution has so far been produced. The words are put into the mouth of Socrates, himself the son of the midwife Phaenarete. (Hanson (1996) notes that in the gynaecological treatises the attendants are generally assumed to be female. See also King 1998: 178–81.)

114 Hanson 1994. The suggestion that the Corpus reflects non-Athenian behaviour might save Plato's credit, but his comment is intended to have a wider relevance, as this is a custom enjoined by the goddess Artemis.

115 *IG* 2/32, 6873: Hillert 1990: 77–9. The word read as *maia* in the relief itself has been reread as a proper name (see *SEG* 33, 1983, 214).

116 Xenophon, *Household Management* 7, 37.

117 Flemming 2000: 383–91; Dasen 2004 (with wider reflections on birth and childcare); Laes 2011; H. Parker 2012.

118 Discussions of the literacy rate among Athenian women suggest that less than 5 per cent of them could read, but a wealthy professional like Phanostrate or the wife of a rich Athenian might well have been among that number. Cf. Demand 1994: 66.

119 Good 1994: 101–7.

7 RELIGION AND MEDICINE IN FIFTH- AND FOURTH-CENTURY GREECE

1 Pausanias, *Description of Greece* 8, 42, 7–9; Jost 1985: 90–7, for the setting and the adjacent mountain shrines. Both the date and the architect have been challenged: for a survey of the question, defending Pausanias, see Winter 1980. Cf. also Beard and Henderson (1995) for meditations on this temple.

2 Pausanias (*Description of Greece* 1, 3, 4) claims that Apollo the Warder-off of Evil had been unrecognised before being invoked at Athens to cure the plague. Cf. also 10, 11, 5, for a dedication at Delphi from the citizens of Cleonae, freed from the plague after a sacrifice ordered by the Delphic oracle.

3 This cult of Apollo is attested much earlier there, around 700 BC; see Jost (1985: 485–9), who argues strongly that Pausanias is wrong to link this dedication with the Thucydidean plague and is applying a feature of the cult in his own day to a remoter period when the god was 'Protector of Warriors'. If Pausanias is right, this region will have been among the (relatively few) parts of the Peloponnese affected, according to Thucydides (*History* 2, 54). It is, of course, impossible to tell whether Apollo is being thanked for ending the plague at the town or for protecting it when others nearby fell victim.

4 Thucydides, *History* 2, 47; 2, 51; 2, 53. For Delos, see ibid. 3, 104; Diodorus, *History* 12, 58. For parallels in other epidemics, see pp. 162, 288–9 here.

5 Garland 1992: 131; R. Parker 1996: 175; Verbanck-Piérard 2000; Gorrini and Melfi 2002; Gorrini (2005) stresses the paucity of evidence for such cults before 430 BC. Cf. also, for healing gods in Attica, nn. 42–3 below.

6 Edelstein 1945: the first volume lists only literary and epigraphic testimony (= T.); Semeria (1986: 931–58) adds the archaeological and numismatic evidence, but only for one area. Riethmüller (2005) provides plans and detailed discussion of the shrines in Greece, and, in vol. 2, a comprehensive listing and bibliography of shrines of Asclepius throughout the ancient world. Melfi (2007) concentrates on Greece. Iconography is covered at length by Holzmann (1984).

7 Edelstein 1945: II, 1–64.

8 Homer, *Iliad* 2, 729.

9 Hesiod, fr. 122 = T. 21; Homeric Hymn 16, 1–3 = T. 31; cf. Isyllus, *Hymn*, line 30 = T. 516.

10 The Asclepiads of Cos and Cnidus do not enter directly into this controversy for they traced their ancestry back to Asclepius' son Podalirius, returning from the Trojan War (T. 212–13). For the difficulties with this story, see W. D. Smith 1973. For the (disputed) stories about the births of Asclepius and Machaon, see T. 36–40.

11 Pausanias, *Description of Greece* 3, 26, 9 = T. 186; 4, 3, 2 = T. 190; 4, 30, 3 = T. 191. Strabo (*Geography* 8, 4, 4 = T. 715) calls it a temple of Asclepius.

12 Graf 1996. For another example of a cult with two apparently different geographical foci, see L. G. Mitchell 2001. The Messenian association of the cult of Machaon with Nestor appears to be post-Homeric (information from Maria Elena Gorrini).

13 Edelstein 1945: T. 7; Jost 1985: 495–9.

14 Eusebius, *Preparation for the Gospel* 3, 14, 6 = T. 13; Pausanias, *Description of Greece* 2, 26, 7 = T. 36. Apollophanes the Arcadian wished to know whether Hesiod had been right to say that Asclepius was the child of a Messenian.

15 The 'recall' of Asclepius and his sons to their central sanctuary at Messene may have been a deliberate attempt to create a local Pantheon for the new city (Pausanias, *Description of Greece* 4, 31, 10–12). The absence, before c.300 BC, of a shrine of Asclepius at Naupactus, home to many Messenian exiles in the 450s (ibid. 10, 38, 9–13 = T. 444), suggests that Asclepius was not strongly linked with Messene in the fifth century.

16 Pausanias, *Description of Greece* 2, 26, 4 = T. 19; 8, 25, 11 = T. 17. This story was already being propagated in the late fourth century BC (see *IG* 4, 2, 128, iv, 40–50 = T. 32).

17 Strabo, *Geography* 9, 5, 17 = T. 714; 8, 6, 15 = T. 735.

18 Strabo, *Geography* 8, 4, 4 = T. 715 (later, and perhaps more accurately, assigned to Machaon by Pausanias); Herondas, *Mime* 2, 97 = T. 714a; cf. 4, 2 = T. 482. This evidence is doubted by the Edelsteins (1945: II, 239–40), but see now Aston 2004; Riethmüller 2005: 1, 91–208, 279–324.

19 Pausanias, *Description of Greece* 2, 27, 1–7 = T. 739; Burford 1969; Tomlinson (1983) argues that this was not the famous sculptor and inventor of the Canon, as Pausanias thinks; Riethmüller 2005: 1, 230–40.

20 Plato (*Ion* 530e = T. 560) provides the earliest unequivocal evidence for these contests, the Asclepieia: earlier games are known at Epidaurus in the late sixth century (Pindar,

Nemean 5, 95–7 = T. 556), with boxing and the pancration, but, despite the ancient commentries on this passage (T. 557–9), it is not entirely certain that these games were then held in honour of Asclepius.

21 Aristophanes, *Wasps* 122–3 = T. 733; Garland 1987: 115–17, 208–9. Garland (1992: 120) suggests that Telemachus was the founder of this shrine as well as of that in Athens itself; certainly the scenes on his monument link the two together, although the inscription itself does not mention any role for him in its foundation.

22 Garland 1992: 116–35, 201–5; Aleshire 1989, 1991; Connolly 1998; King 1998: 99–113; R. Parker 1996: 175–85, commenting also on a newly discovered plate painted with the baby Asclepius and the word 'Epidaurus'; Riethmüller 2005: 1, 241–75; Wickkiser 2008.

23 See p. 52 here; T. 587–90. Connolly (1998) argues strongly that the tradition that he was host to the god is a late invention based on knowledge of the Paean.

24 Plato, *Phaedo* 118A = T. 524; for later discussion of the reasons, see T. 526–30, with Most 1993. For a payment of a cock to Asclepius, cf. the story in Artemidorus, *Dream Book* 5, 9 = T. 523.

25 The inscription on Telemachus' monument was in part published as *IG* 2², 4960 (T. 720); important new fragments, partially translated by Garland (1992: 118), are most accessible in *SEG* 25, nos. 226, 3. R. Parker (1996: 101) suggests that Telemachus may have been an Epidaurian resident in Athens; Garland (1992: 122, cf. 203) that Telemachus or a family member had been healed at Epidaurus, but, if so, Telemachus never tells us. The monument itself was set up some time, and perhaps over twenty years, after Asclepius' arrival. It is highly likely that Telemachus' name is also to be restored at *IG* 2², 4355 as 'the first to sacrifice'. Wickkiser (2008) stresses the political element in this decision and in the subsequent spread of the cult, but her argument that it also reflects dissatisfaction at the failures of the new 'Hippocratic' medicine seems forced.

26 R. Parker 1996: 181; Aleshire 1989: 15 (not in Edelstein 1945).

27 T. 716–99. For Arcadia, see Jost 1985: 493. Graf (1996: 188) suggests an early arrival of Asclepius also in Central Italy (cf. pp. 161–4 here).

28 Pugliese Carratelli 1939–40: 178, 188, 195; Aleshire 1989: 68; Graf 1985: 62–3. Note also the (apparently unique) instance of a village with a healing spring on the island of Icaros changing its name to reflect that of the god (L. Robert 1969: 549–68).

29 Aleshire 1989: 8; R. Parker 1996: 345; Clinton 1994: 17–34. The first clear evidence for the Epidauria does not, however, appear until later (cf. T. 564–5; Aleshire 1989: 82, 90–2).

30 Connolly 1998.

31 R. Parker 1996: 175. Pausanias (*Description of Greece* 1, 31, 6) records an altar to Athena Hygieia in the countryside at Acharnae but the cult in his day, around AD 170, was now that of Athene of Horses. He also notes a statue of Athena Paionia in a shrine of Dionysus in Athens (1, 2, 5) and an altar of Athena Paionia at the Amphiaraon, near Oropus (1, 34, 3).

32 Stilwell 1976: 493, 466.

33 Jost 1985: 500–4, 208.

34 Pausanias, *Description of Greece* 2, 27, 7 = T. 739; Burford 1969: 41–51. The meaning of the cult title Maleatas is very obscure. Isyllus (*Hymn*, lines 29–30 = T. 516, with Kolde 2003) implies a link with Apollo Maleatas also for Tricca (but by reverse influence from Epidaurus?).

35 Graf 1985: 260.

36 Plutarch, *Roman Questions* 94: 286D = T. 708. One modern response to Plutarch (Graf 1992) stresses the liminality of the cult in the functional opposition between city and countryside; not all have concurred. Cf. Riethmüller 2005: 1, 360–81.

37 Habicht 1985: 37–63; Zunino 1997: 139–89, 281–4.

38 This is in part why Jost (1985: 489) prefers to explain Apollo's title as referring to his role as a military protector.

39 N. Ehrhardt 1989; cf. for Erythrae, Graf 1985: 250, n. 251. Apollo also heads the names in the Hippocratic *Oath* (IV, 628 L.).

40 Livy, *History* 4, 25 (following a plague); cf. 29, 7 and 40, 51.

41 Strabo (*Geography* 14, 4, 6–7), referring to the cult at Miletus and on Delos, claims the word means 'Healer', but his etymology could be learned speculation: an alternative is a link with 'oulios', 'deadly', with the adjective used apotropaically. For Elea, see Ebner 1966; Fabbri and Trotta 1989. As 'pholarchs', the doctors headed the cult organisation.

42 Demosthenes, *Oration* 21, 52. Votive offerings depicting parts of the body have also been found in shrines of Aphrodite and Artemis Kalliste, and, from the Roman period, of Artemis Kolainis, Hercules and Zeus the Most High (see van Straten 1981: 105–22). Whether the votive plaque to Demeter at Eleusis (*IG* 22, 4639) was given in gratitude for healing or for enlightenment is disputed (cf. van Straten 1981: 122 and pl. 56; and, for healing dedications to Demeter at Mesembria, in Thrace, 106, pl. 59–60).

43 Kutsche 1913: 48–52; Kearns 1989: 171; Gorrini and Melfi 2002. The author of *The Diseases of Young Women* (1, 8: 468 L.) appears to be attacking some of the cult practices at Brauron on the grounds that they are unlikely to be of any benefit to young women.

44 For a list of votive offerings at this shrine like those of the Athens Asclepieion, see *IG* 7, 303. See also Karidas 1968; Krug (1985: 153) gives a small clear plan.

45 [Hippocrates], *Regimen* 4, 89; cf. also 90: VI, 652, 658–60 L. Significantly, Asclepius is missing from this list.

46 For wealth, see Aleshire 1989: 46–8, 96–100, 163 (on property given by Demo, a priest). R. Parker (1996: 179) notes that the recorded Asclepio- names from Athens first appear at the end of the fifth century. For details of the sanctuaries in Greece, see Riethmüller 2005: 2, 1–315.

47 The state of war between the Athenians and the Peloponnesians perhaps prevented any formal religious embassy until the truce of 421. The memory of the plague would still have been strong among Athenian religious authorities when they were called upon to approve the new cult (Gorrini 2005).

48 How far formal adoption by Athens helped to propagate the cult among Athenian allies and beyond is an open question; cf. Kolde 2003; Wickkiser 2008.

49 The texts of tablets 1 and 2, *IG* 4, 2, 121–2 are most accessible in Edelstein 1945: T. 423; the badly damaged tablets 3 and 4, *IG* 4, 2, 123–4 are translated (along with the others) in LiDonnici 1995. Cf. Dillon 1994, 1997: 73–80; Pecere and Stramaglia 1996. The older discussions by Weinreich (1909), Herzog (1931) and Edelstein (1945: II, 139–80) are still valuable. Guarducci (1978: 143–66) surveys healing inscriptions in general.

50 Edelstein 1945: T. 423, nos. 3, 4, 9.

51 Valerius Maximus, *Wonderful Stories* 1, 1, 19 = T. 797; for a cure, see also T. 423, 11; 21; 36. But the Epidaurian tablets are remarkably free of stories alleging some form of guilt or religious offence as the cause of falling ill.

52 Respectively, Edelstein 1945: T. 423, 3; 5; 15; 16; 37; 38 and T. 431; T. 423, 6 and 7; T. 423, 4; 9; 11; 18; 20; 22; 32 and the later T. 438 (Rome) and T. 442 (Lebena); T. 423, 28; T. 423, 26 and T. 424; T. 423, 21; 31; 34; 39; 42; for the goblet, see T. 423, 10; for the lost boy, see T. 423, 24.

53 Ibid. T. 423, 1–2.

54 For Rome, see ibid. T. 438; for Lebena, see T. 439–42; for Pergamum, see H. Müller 1987. The minor inscriptions of Asclepian cures from Athens, Epidaurus, Lebena, Pergamum and Rome are conveniently republished by Girone (1998). No cure inscription survives from Cos, although that shrine was said to be adorned with such records.

55 Aleshire 1989: 113–369 (seven inventories from Athens, from *c*.350–100 BC); van Straten 1981, 1992.

56 King 1998: 102–13, although not all of her ideas fit the Greek context. Cf., for discussions of Asclepius cures in the context of modern psychiatric healing and of folk medicine, Castrén 1989; Tick 2001. Prêtre and Charlier (2009) offer modern medical interpretations.

57 For the importance of 'holiness' and 'purity', note the inscription at the entrance to the shrine at Epidaurus (T. 318, 336), and for its resonances with the words of the Hippocratic *Oath*, see von Staden 1996a, 2007.

58 Edelstein 1945: T. 423, 11.

59 Aleshire 1989: 28–30. Similar buildings have also been found at many other healing shrines, e.g. the Amphiaraon at Oropus (cf. Krug 1985: 131–61 for plans).

60 Edelstein 1945: II, 138–73.

61 At the later shrine of Pergamum, the 'Rufinian grove', if within the precinct itself, can hardly have consisted of more than a few trees. Riethmüller 2005: 1, 378–80.

62 For parallels with later Christian healing shrines, cf. Sheils 1982: 9–54, 153–64, 385–414.

63 Edelstein 1945: T. 423, 25; 33. Pausanias, *Description of Greece* 10, 38, 13 = T. 444.

64 Respectively, Edelstein 1945: T. 423, 22; 15; 19; 32; 31. The effort involved in making the pilgrimage may have also served to validate the expectations of a cure.

65 Pausanias, *Description of Greece* 9, 39, 2; for the Amphiareion, see n. 44 above. One may suspect also some borrowings between the cults.

66 The repair of the goblet and the recovery of the child (p. 110 here) are exceptions, but both could, in context, be seen as restoring wholeness.

67 Peek 1969a: 112, no. 242, suspecting a link with the priest in *IG* 4, 2, 534, 535 and 540.

68 It was forbidden either to die or to give birth within the sacred precinct itself; around AD 150 the Colonnade of Cotys was refurbished to cater for the parturient and the dying.

69 *Sylloge Inscriptionum Graecarum* 3, 596: *I. Olympia* 62.

70 Aleshire (1989: 99) succinctly disposes of the theory that the 'drachma for Asclepius' was a tax on all citizens that created a fund out of which the public physicians were paid. An entrance fee to suppliants at the shrine is more likely, but her estimate of fifteen to twenty suppliants per day raises problems of its own. If she is right, visitors to the shrine on the occasion of any festival would not pay this tax, which would be levied only on those actually consulting the god.

71 For the public physicians, see *IG* 2², 772 = T. 552; for the relief, see *IG* 2², 4359, with Aleshire 1989: 94–5; there is a good picture in Bertier (1972: frontispiece).

72 The two lists of names were originally the same, but the relationship with the figures is far from clear (cf. Cohn-Haft 1956: 57, n. 13).

73 For these men, see pp. 124–5 here.

74 Erasistratus (fr. 29 Garofalo) reported that in the sanctuary of the temple of Apollo at Delphi around 280 BC hung a leaden 'tooth-puller', proof, he thought, that one ought to extract teeth when they could be removed easily and safely.

75 Aleshire 1989: 65–6. It cannot entirely be ruled out that the dedication of instruments was meant to represent the treatment previously given the patient, and that the writing tablets were the equivalent of prescriptions. If these were given by medical men, then another seven doctors or surgeons can be added to her list of medical donors.

76 *IG* 2², 483.

77 Sherwin-White (1978: 275) advises caution as the shrine was merely one of several places where such public documents were set up, and the doctors had their main centres of activity elsewhere. But the participation of doctors in the cult is known from the later Hellenistic and Roman periods. Cf. also a fragment of an honorary decree for a doctor erected at the Amphiaraon at Oropus (Petrakis 1997: no. 240).

78 [Hippocrates], *The Sacred Disease* 1: VI, 354–64 L. Cf. Edelstein 1967: 205–46; R. Parker 1983: 211–34; Jouanna 1999: 260–79.

79 The author of *Regimen* (4, 87: VI, 642 L.) accepts the validity of prayer, while at the same time counselling medical intervention, and claims to have discovered all there is to know about diet with the god's help (4, 93: VI, 602 L.). But that is not the same as offering to cure solely through prayer and incantation, for that implies a greater degree of control over divine action.

80 See also p. 65 here.

81 H. W. Miller 1953; Nörenberg 1968; Schölkopf 1968; Kudlien 1977; Jouanna 1999: 278–9.

82 Euripides, fr. 294 Nauck = 292 Nauck: the first group are treated 'traditionally' (see Guardasole 2000: 84–6). Cf. the opening attempt by the Hippocratic author to define 'divine' (*The Sacred Disease* 1: VI, 352 L.). Some diseases, notably mental afflictions and epidemics, continued to be viewed as in some way caused by the gods, as well as having a physical explanation, and belief in one explanation in one case did not preclude the other in another.

83 [Hippocrates], *Regimen* 4, 87: VI, 642 L.

84 Ibid. 87; 89; 90: VI, 642; 652; 656–8 L. The Athenian doctor Euenor (fl. 322 BC) commended the medicinal virtues of the spring at the Amphiaraon (Athenaeus, *Sophists at Dinner* 2, 46d).

85 Lanata 1969; R. Parker 1983: 208–13.

86 And, of course, many so-called 'irrational' prejudices remained and were often justified by 'rational' argument (see Lloyd 1979). Other healers, such as the pharmacologists and rootcutters, occupy an intermediate place on the spectrum between medicine and magic.

87 See R. Parker 1983: 215, citing Plato, *Cratylus* 405a–b, for an assertion that purification serves the same ends in both medicine and mantic of making man 'pure in both body and soul'; Hoessly 2001.

88 Cf. Graf 1997: 30–5. The relationship of religion, magic and healing in the ancient world is notoriously difficult, both conceptually and textually, since the great bulk of our information comes from the Roman Imperial period, and there is a temptation to elide chronological differences. For a range of interpretations, see also Edelstein 1967: 205–46; Lanata 1969; Luck 1985; Faraone and Obbink 1991; Lanternari 1994; Dickie 2001.

89 [Hippocrates], *Prorrhetic* II, 1: IX, 8 L.

90 Graf 1997: 25–6, 35 (from the city of Teos c.470 BC, cursing those who harm it or its citizens through deadly '*pharmaka*' [spells]); but Meiggs and Lewis (1969: no. 30, p. 65) translate '*pharmaka*' simply as poisonings. Note the (much later) defence of Apollonius of Tyana against a charge of magic when curing a plague at Ephesus (Philostratus, *Life of Apollonius* 8, 7, 9–10): his forecasting of the plague was the result of his own perceptions, but the cure itself was wrought by Hercules, a healing god.

91 [Galen], *Commentary on the Hippocratic Oath*, fr. 2a–e Rosenthal.

92 Cf. R. Parker 1996: 184: 'The truest explanation for the rise of Asclepius may be that he was, as it were, in partnership with Hippocrates.'

8 FROM PLATO TO PRAXAGORAS

1 Celsus, *On Medicine*, pref. 8.

2 What he did mean is far from clear, especially as he goes on (pref. 9) to praise some eminent physicians for using their 'knowledge of nature' to improve dietetics. However, a belief in the Hippocratic authorship of *Ancient Medicine* could have led Celsus to conclude that Hippocrates rejected speculative hypotheses in medicine.

3 Plato, *Second Letter* 314d.
4 Athenaeus, *Sophists at Dinner* 2, 59C, a fragment of the comic poet Epicrates, has often been interpreted to show that he came to Athens.
5 Anonymus Londinensis 20, 25–50.
6 Plato, *Timaeus* 84a, 84d–e, perhaps also alluding to the theories of the author of *The Sacred Disease?* See also Lloyd 1968; Craik 2001b.
7 Plato, *Timaeus* 82a–e.
8 Ibid. 82e–83a.
9 Ibid. 84a–c.
10 H. W. Miller 1962. Longrigg (1993a: 242) notes that Thrasymachus of Sardis, according to Anonymus Londinensis (11), believed that blood changed into the harmful bile and phlegm with changes of temperature. But (ibid. 112) this is still some way from Plato's idea of the degeneration of tissues, and then of the individual parts back down into their constituents.
11 Plato, *Timaeus* 81b–e.
12 Ibid. 75a–76d. Some protection is given by hair, 'sufficient to provide shade in summer and shelter in winter, but not to impede perception', which then raises questions about baldness.
13 Ibid. 69e.
14 Plato, *Laws* 4, 720d–e; 9, 857d; Williams 1973; R. Brock 2000.
15 Plato, *Timaeus* 44d–45b, 69e–72d.
16 Ibid. 86b–89d; Plato's views on madness are discussed in Simon (1978) and W. V. Harris (forthcoming).
17 Anonymus Londinensis devotes more space, four columns (XIV–XVIII), to Plato's ideas in the *Timaeus* than to those of any other author.
18 See pp. 228–9, 236–7 here.
19 Todd 1976.
20 Chalcidius (*c.* AD 400), *Commentary on Plato's Timaeus* 246; pp. 256–7 Waszink, discussed on pp. 48–9 here; Lloyd 1991: 164–93.
21 One might compare their different uses of medical information in their ethical discussions (see Jaeger 1954).
22 Aristotle, *On Sensation* 436a; *On Breathing* 480b; van der Eijk 1999c, 2005b.
23 This hypothesis was not as strange as it might seem to us, since the discovery that the nerves originated in the brain was not made for another generation.
24 For the Aristotelian sections of Anonymus Londinensis, see pp. 58–9, 72; Galen, *Avoiding Distress* 15–17: tr. Nutton 2012a takes as paradigmatic the loss of the Aristotelian and Peripatetic material in the fire of 192 from his own library and, more importantly, from the imperial libraries, which meant that the rarities were gone for ever.
25 Theophrastus, *Enquiry into Plants* 4, 3; Amigues 2010; see also *The Oxford Classical Dictionary*, ed. 3: 238, s.v. bematists.
26 Ross 1971: 112–14; for the ostrich, see Aristotle, *The Parts of Animals* 4, 13: 697b.
27 Aristotle, *The Parts of Animals* 1, 5: 644b–645a.
28 Longrigg 1993a: 161; cf. Gotthelf 1985; Gotthelf and Lennox 1987.
29 Aristotle, *Enquiry into Animals* 1, 16: 494b.
30 Kollesch 1997; Oser-Gröte 2004.
31 C. R. S. Harris 1973: 121–56. One should remember that this is also the first Greek description of the heart to refer to chambers.
32 Aristotle, *Parts of Animals* 3, 4: 666b.
33 Aristotle, *Enquiry into Animals* 3, 3: 514a.
34 Lloyd 1983: 94–104; Dean-Jones 1994: 81; Föllinger 1996.
35 He wrote a work, now lost, on 'Health and Disease', and possibly others. Cf. van der Eijk 1999e.

36 Moraux 1984: 729–72.

37 Scarborough 1978; Fortenbaugh and Gutas 2002; Fortenbaugh *et al.* 2003; Debru 2005; van der Eijk 2005; Amigues 2010; Galen, *Avoiding Distress* 17: tr. Nutton 2012a records the loss of rare Theophrastan treatises in 192; by comparison, his work on plants was easily available. A major project co-ordinated by Professor van der Eijk will examine the place of medicine in the Peripatetic tradition, and vice versa.

38 Kollesch 1997: 370.

39 Galen, 2, 281–2 = Diocles, fr. 17; cf. also fr. 24. The fragments of Diocles are cited from van der Eijk 2000–1, which supersedes Wellmann 1901.

40 Quotations from Pliny, *Natural History* 26, 6, 10–11 = fr. 3; and Anonymus Bruxellensis, *On the Seed* = fr. 2 van der Eijk.

41 Van der Eijk 2000–1: II, xxxi–xxxviii. The older theory of Jaeger that he was much younger than Aristotle is based on very doubtful evidence (see von Staden 1992b).

42 Diocles, fr. 23c–d van der Eijk, with the commentary at II: 39–41, pointing also to the divergences from the theory attacked by Aristotle (*Generation of Animals* 746a).

43 Wellmann 1901: 234; against the attribution, see C. R. S. Harris 1973: 105–6; van der Eijk 2000–1: I, xi, who does not include this passage among the fragments of Diocles.

44 Diocles, fr. 40, 6 van der Eijk.

45 His notions of embryology included a belief in both male and female seed, and in an embryo that was formed in forty days and then developed faster in the womb for boys than girls (see fr. 40–8 van der Eijk).

46 For bandages, see fr. 162, 166 van der Eijk; for the spoon, see fr. 167 van der Eijk, with the drawing in Krug (1985: 101). The so-called Dioclean spoon, now in the Meyer-Steineg collection at Jena, is a modern forgery (or a copy of a lost original) (Salazar 2000: 49, 102).

47 For poisons, see fr. 215 van der Eijk; for vegetables, see fr. 200; cf. fr. 193–211; for *Rhizotomikon*, see fr. 204; for pharmacology, see fr. 145–8; for a prescription, see fr. 221 = P. Antinoopolis 123.

48 Fr. 65–71 van der Eijk. Caelius Aurelianus complained that he regulated the patient's diet according to the number of days of illness (fr. 92 van der Eijk).

49 Fr. 97, 143 van der Eijk; W. D. Smith 1979: 181–9. Hippocratic texts possibly known to him are *Aphorisms*, fr. 55b; *Epidemics* 3, fr. 57; *Prognostic*, fr. 64; and *Joints*, fr. 162–3, but the linkage is made clear only by later authors. For the apparent citation of *The Eight-month Child* and *Nutriment* (fr. 40, 5), see van der Eijk's commentary *ad loc.*

50 Diocles, fr. 27, 51 van der Eijk.

51 Diocles, fr. 27, 40 van der Eijk; the different version given in fr. 183a, 6 does not come from a genuine work by Diocles.

52 Diocles, fr. 95, 98, 102 van der Eijk. But note that Diocles speaks only of the thick artery and offshoots coming from it and the heart. His vascular anatomy is still sketchy.

53 Diocles, fr. 74, 80; cf. fr. 101, 107 van der Eijk. The words 'psychic *pneuma*', however, may not be those of Diocles himself.

54 Jaeger 1913; Verbeke 1945.

55 Diocles, fr. 51, 53, 89, 92, 182 van der Eijk.

56 Diocles, fr. 183: 40, 5; 41 van der Eijk.

57 Diocles, fr. 168, although the conditions mentioned are all directly related to the womb and to childbirth (fr. 168–75 van der Eijk).

58 Diocles, fr. 180–1 van der Eijk.

59 Diocles, fr. 185 van der Eijk.

60 Diocles, fr. 176–7, 188, 191, 195, 200, 222–3, 225, 228–9, 233 van der Eijk. Several other unassigned fragments are likely to come from this work.

61 Diocles, fr. 176 van der Eijk 1996, noting also the modification of Galen's position with regard to this passage from Diocles in *On Medical Experience* 13, 4–5: tr. Walzer and Frede 1985: 109 = Diocles, fr. 16, cf. fr. 49.

62 Galen, *On Examining the Physician* 5, 2: *CMG* Suppl. Or. 4, 69; *On Medical Experience* 13, 4. Pleistonicus was a pupil of Praxagoras but his home town is not recorded. They were presumably included among 'all the ancient doctors', whose works Galen claims to have had copied extremely accurately before they were lost in the fire of 192; *Avoiding Distress* 15: tr. Nutton 2012a.

63 The most recent edition is by Garofalo (1997).

64 Anonymous Parisinus 8, 1, 1–4 = Erasistratus, fr. 180 Garofalo; Diocles, fr. 87 van der Eijk; Praxagoras, fr. 67 Steckerl; [Hippocrates], *Places in Man* 14: VI, 303 L.

65 Van der Eijk 1999b.

66 Galen, *On Medical Experience* 13, 4: tr. Walzer and Frede 1985: 70 (not in van der Eijk: should one read Dieuches for Diogenes?).

67 Fragments in Bertier (1972). Mnesitheus, fr. 10, 11 B.: for the Hippocratic method of division, see p. 57 here.

68 Diocles, fr. 40, 2; 27, 5 van der Eijk.

69 Mnesitheus, fr. 12–14 B.

70 Fragments in Steckerl (1958). Praxagoras, fr. 50–2, 54–60 St.; Phylotimus, fr. 12 St.

71 Galen, 2, 141 = Praxagoras fr. 21 St.; Rufus, *The Names of Parts* pp. 165–6 Dbg = fr. 22 St., linking with older ideas about fluids.

72 Galen, 10, 260 = Praxagoras, fr. 97 St.; venesection, Galen, 11, 163 = Mnesitheus, fr. 5 B. = Dieuches, fr. 3 B. = Praxagoras, fr. 98 St.; prognosis, Galen, 9, 728 = Praxagoras, fr. 93 St.; Galen, 9, 775 = Pleistonicus, fr. 24 St.

73 Galen, 9, 728 = Praxagoras, fr. 93 St.; Plutarch, *Questions about Nature* 26: 918D = Mnesitheus, fr. 16 B.

74 Dieuches, fr. 15 B.; Praxagoras, fr. 105–8, 113 St.; Phylotimus, fr. 21 St.; Pleistonicus, fr. 6 St.; Herophilus, T. 255 von Staden.

75 Mnesitheus may have written a whole tract on hellebore (fr. 48 B.). Cf. Pliny, *Natural History* 25, 21, 47–25, 61; J. André 1955; Girard 1988. Both black and white hellebore were still noted in *The British Pharmaceutical Codex* for 1907 (although by then the rhizome of the white variety was recommended only in a powder to keep moths away). From the 1950s, extracts have been used against hypertension (see Trease and Evans 1978: 619–20).

76 Caelius Aurelianus, *Acute Diseases* 3, 17, 164 = Praxagoras, fr. 109 St. Early editors read 'magnificam', 'magnificent', but 'manificam' is more likely. Details of other surgical treatments advocated by this group of doctors are scanty; Celsus and Galen report that both Diocles (fr. 165 van der Eijk) and Phylotimus (fr. 23 St.) devised a successful way of resetting a dislocated femur.

77 Porphyry, *Homeric Questions* 165 Schrader = Praxagoras, fr. 36 St. With the possible exception of fr. 120, none of his fragments deals specifically with the properties of foods, although diets are recommended as part of the healing process.

78 Cf. the slightly later discussions about dietetics as the third part of medicine by the Alexandrian commentators on Homer (Erbse 1974: III, 222).

79 Mnesitheus, fr. 18–20 B.; Dieuches, fr. 13–18 B.

80 Dieuches, fr. 19 B.

81 Scarborough 1970.

82 Phylotimus, fr. 4–21 St. I take the numbers in fr. 11 to refer only to one book, 13, *pace* Steckerl (112–13), who prefers two separate books, 3 and 10. For another (late) Hellenistic writer on dietetics, the Erasistratean Hicesius, see Gourevitch 2000.

83 Phylotimus, fr. 11, 12 St.

84 Galen, 15, 136 = Dieuches, fr. 4 B.

85 The one surviving fragment of Mnesitheus' treatise on the *Constitution of the Body* (fr. 17 B.), although revealing little about his own dissections, seems to depend heavily on Aristotle.

86 Although his authorship of a treatise on *Foreign Diseases* (fr. 63 St.) suggests that he spent some time away from Cos, either as a student or, later, as a travelling physician. His dates are disputed. If he is the father of Praxagoras, son of Praxagoras, named on a Coan contribution list of *c.*260 BC (Sherwin-White 1978: 102), he was active in the last quarter of the fourth century and the first decades of the third, which would agree with the evidence for influence from Aristotle and Diocles.

87 Sherwin-White 1978: 216; for Phylotimus and his family, see ibid. 105, 195.

88 Although it is highly likely that he was acquainted with the writings of Hippocrates and traditions about him, proof is singularly elusive (see Nickel 2005).

89 Praxagoras, fr. 15 St.; Phylotimus, fr. 1–2 St.

90 Praxagoras, fr. 10–11 St. The word that later is used for 'nerves', *neura*, can also mean ligaments and sinews, but the association with sensation suggests that Praxagoras thought of them as our 'nerves'.

91 Praxagoras, fr. 7, 8, 9, 11 St.; cf. Solmsen 1961.

92 Praxagoras, fr. 85 St.; for Diocles, see p. 123–4 here. Longrigg (1993a: 174–5) argues for a substantial influence of Diocles and Sicilian medicine on Praxagoras, although he allows for some independence. An alternative view is that both Diocles and Praxagoras were working out the consequences of Aristotle's ideas, for example that *pneuma* and the source of sensation were located in the heart.

93 Pleistonicus, fr. 3 St.; Phylotimus, fr. 2 St.; Herophilus, see pp. 134–5 here.

94 C. R. S. Harris 1973: 110–13.

95 Praxagoras, fr. 26–8 St.

96 See p. 155 here.

97 *Planudean Anthology* 273 = Crinagoras, poem 52, ed. Gow and Page 1968. It is tempting, but unnecessary, to see a link between this epigram and poem 22, referring to a recent incident on Cos, and to conclude that Crinagoras had seen this statue during a visit to Cos.

98 This is not to deny that many texts still lack a known author, either by accident or because their authors wished to associate their ideas with a famous name, as with the so-called *Letter* of Diocles to King Antigonus (fr. 183 van der Eijk), with its unusual seasonal medicine.

99 See Chapter 3, n. 97 here.

9 ALEXANDRIA, ANATOMY AND EXPERIMENTATION

1 Edelstein 1967: 247–302; Kudlien 1969; Fraser 1972: I, 335–56; Longrigg 1981, 1988, 1993a: 177–219; von Staden 1989, 1992a; Flemming 2003; Lang, forthcoming.

2 The fragments of Herophilus are collected by von Staden (1989); those of Erasistratus by Garofalo (1988).

3 Although Erasistratus, through his father, was connected with the court at Antioch in Syria, no ancient source associates his anatomical investigations with that city, referring to dissections taking place only in Alexandria. For the dubious story that links his medical activity with the Seleucids, his alleged discovery of the love of Antiochus I for his stepmother Stratonice, see p. 365, n. 57 here.

4 See pp. 217–18 here.

5 See p. 127 here.

6 For Galen, 2, 890, as emended at *CMG* 5, 2, 1, 38, see p. 367, n. 101 here; for his gynaecological experience, see Soranus, *Gynaecology* 1, 35; 4, 14 and 36.

7 This is the formulation of Viano (1984).

8 Von Staden 1989: 43, with T. 9–11; Garofalo 1988: 20, 60–1. The weakness of the tradition as historical evidence is pointed out by Scarborough (1985b).

9 Kudlien (1969) stresses the new importance of careful observation of a wide range of phenomena.

10 R. Parker 1983: 33–41; Teles, *On Exile* 31, 9 Hense.

11 Edelstein 1967: 274–81.

12 Carlino 1999; French 1999.

13 Herodotus, *History* 2, 86–9; Diodorus, *History* 1, 91–2.

14 Fraser 1972: I, 70–4.

15 Although no source specifies the origin of the corpses, save that they were criminals, the continuation elsewhere of Greek taboos about violating a corpse and the ways in which Greek justice systems worked suggest that the bodies were far more likely to be of non-citizen Egyptians or foreigners than of Alexandrian Greeks; Flemming 2003: 452. For the apartheid or 'frontier' mentality, cf. von Staden 1989: 29.

16 Weeks 1970; von Staden 1989: 1–22; Nunn 1996: 42–53.

17 Longrigg (1993a: 187) rightly points out that the brain and often other organs were removed crudely or by being first liquefied inside the body.

18 The accounts in Herodotus and Diodorus (see n. 13 here) certainly show a good general knowledge of embalming procedures, and must have been obtained at least through an interpreter, but they say next to nothing about the precise information that an anatomist would need to know.

19 Cf. Nunn 1996: 43–4.

20 Fraser 1972: part II and 305–35 for patronage; von Staden 1989: 26–31.

21 Poets and litterateurs were, directly or indirectly, useful for propaganda, while many of the discoveries of Hellenistic scientists had a practical, military value.

22 Menecles of Barca, *FGrH* 270 F 9: his list of exiles comprises 'grammarians, philosophers, geometers, musicians, painters, teachers, doctors and many other craftsmen'.

23 But, as far as I know, there is no evidence that any of the medical scholars who visited Alexandria ever consulted these manuscripts there. For the story of the Library, see Fraser 1972: 320–34; Canfora 1987; el-Abbadi 1992; Vallance 2000. Galen's references (in his commentaries on *Epidemics* III: 17A, 606–7 and *The Nature of Man* 1, 44: 15, 105, 109) are critically reviewed by W. D. Smith (1979: 199–204).

24 For the founding of the Museum, see Fraser 1972: 312–20.

25 Naphtali Lewis 1963.

26 Most 1981; Langholf 1986; Lang 2009.

27 Pfeiffer 1968: 98. Fraser (1972: 318) thinks it likely that provision was made for lecturing on the premises of the Museum, although he rightly notes that 'much would be effected by means of informal discussion and conversation'. Vallance (2000) is very sceptical.

28 Von Staden 1989: 458, 478, 486.

29 Longrigg 1993a: 179.

30 Celsus, *On Medicine*, pref. 23–6 = Herophilus, T. 63a von Staden 1989.

31 For the (lost) treatise on vivisection, see Galen, 19, 55: tr. P. N. Singer 1997: 25. There may be traces of it still in Arabic. But note that at 12, 252 Galen distinguishes between those kings who experimented on condemned criminals and pharmacologists who reported potentially dangerous drugs of which they had no experience. The former, he argues, did nothing wrong. His allusion may extend beyond the pharmacological experiments of Attalus III and Mithridates.

32 John of Alexandria, *Commentary on Galen, On Sects*, p. 57 Pritchet; Agnellus, *Commentary on Galen, On Sects* 23; p. 92 Westerink = Herophilus, T 63b–c von Staden 1989. Agnellus and John depend on the same material, which, at the very least, shows that the story was known in Late Antique Alexandria, although a direct dependence on Celsus is unlikely. Galen is their most favoured source.

33 Tertullian, *On the Soul* 10, 4 = Herophilus, T. 66 von Staden 1989.

34 Lloyd 1991: 356–7; Grmek 1996. The author of the (implausible) story in the Jewish Talmud (*Tosefta Niddah* 4: 17; Babylonian Talmud, *Niddah* 30b) that Cleopatra carried out anatomical experiments on pregnant female slaves to see the various stages of the formation of the foetus also insists that these unfortunates were condemned criminals. There may be a link with the story that, when preparing for a possible suicide, she tested poisons on slaves. Cf. Scarborough 2012: 7–8.

35 Dates for both Herophilus and Erasistratus are imprecise (see von Staden 1989: 43–50; Garofalo 1988: 18–21, placing both men in the period 330/320–260/250 BC, and noting that some of Erasistratus' experiments presuppose some of Herophilus' discoveries).

36 Galen, 10, 28; 8, 723 = Herophilus, T. 10–11 von Staden 1989. Although the belief in a link with Praxagoras is not as strongly based as one might like, it certainly predates Galen.

37 Von Staden 1989: 427–42.

38 Respectively, Herophilus, T. 79; 122–3; 124; 90–2, 98–9 von Staden 1989; for the pineal gland, cf. Galen, *Anatomical Procedures* IX 3: 2, 723 = p. 569 Garofalo: tr. C. Singer 1956: 233. Cf. P. Potter 1976.

39 Respectively, Herophilus, T. 86–9; 60a–b; 95; 61, 101–14 von Staden 1989.

40 Herophilus, T. 115–18, with von Staden's (1989) discussion, p. 240.

41 Ibid. T. 60, 95–6, 115; 119–20; cf. 54 von Staden 1989, although Galen and others thought his descriptions somewhat careless. See also C. R. S. Harris 1973: 178–81.

42 Von Staden 1989: 260–7; but note Longrigg (1993a: 200–2) argues for *pneuma* alone.

43 Herophilus, T. 80–5, 121–5 von Staden 1989.

44 Herophilus, womb T. 61, 114; *rete mirabile* T. 121; liver T. 60 von Staden 1989.

45 Ibid. T. 193–202 von Staden 1989.

46 Ibid. T. 80, 212–13 von Staden 1989.

47 C. R. S. Harris 1973: 186–95; von Staden 1989: 262–88.

48 For water-clock, see Marcellinus, *On Pulses* 11 = Herophilus, T. 182; for definitions, see T. 163, 177, 187–8 von Staden 1989. A direct influence from Aristoxenus of Tarentum, the pupil of Aristotle, although often suggested by modern scholars, is not attested in the ancient sources; the 'musicians' are perhaps more likely to have included scholars in Alexandria.

49 Herophilus, T. 237–8; 234; 58–9 von Staden 1989, with Hankinson 1990, 1998a: 297–302.

50 Herophilus, T. 232; cf. 233 von Staden 1989, for Galen's complaint that he limited treatment to remedies indicated by the 'instrumental' parts of the body and not by its 'homoeomerous' tissues as well.

51 Ibid. T. 248–9 von Staden 1989.

52 Ibid. T. 255 von Staden 1989. By being quickly excreted it could thus be taken in large amounts (Girard 1988). For identification, see Raven 2000: 79–81.

53 Ibid. T. 230, 229 von Staden 1989.

54 Ibid. T. 42–8. T. 42 and 44 von Staden 1989 interpret these 'neutral things' as therapies, but Galen (T. 45 and 48) extends this to cover causes, signs and symptoms, as well as states that are neither fully healthy nor ill, such as convalescence or old age.

55 Strabo, *Geography* 10, 5, 6 = fr. 4A G.; Galen, *On the Opinions of Hippocrates and Plato* 8, 3, 7 = fr. 289 G. But the latter passage could be simply Galen's way of reconciling divergent notices about what Erasistratus had discovered, based on no sound information.

56 The report that he promised an ointment to one of the Ptolemies (fr. 12 G.) is far from conclusive proof that he worked in Alexandria, even if it is interpreted to mean that he dedicated his book *On Gout* to a Ptolemy.

57 *Pace* Fraser 1969; contrast Lloyd 1975. For the variant names in the story of the cure of the lovesick Stratonice, see Galen, *On Prognosis* 6: 14, 630–4, with Nutton 1979: 195; Mesk 1913; Hillgruber 2010.

58 Erasistratus, fr. 5–8 G.; Scarborough 1985b.
59 Galen, *On Habits* 1: *CMG* Suppl. Or. 3, 12–14 = fr. 247 G., from *On Paralysis*, Book 2. Erasistratus is here associated with Hippocrates as 'most glorious'.
60 Galen, 5, 548 = Erasistratus, fr. 201 G.; Lonie 1975: 136–42.
61 Galen, 11, 153 = fr. 198 G. That he could see the join with the naked eye is unlikely, but it was a logical inference.
62 Erasistratus, fr. 42, 289 G. Garofalo (1988: 26) notes that a belief, shared with Aristotle and his school, that the brain was cold and bloodless may well have influenced his first thoughts.
63 For Greek experimentation, see von Staden 1975; Lloyd 1991: 70–99.
64 Galen, 2, 646 = fr. 52 G., with C. R. S. Harris 1973: 379–88.
65 Anonymus Londinensis 33, 43 = fr. 76 G.
66 For Erasistratus' views on humours, see W. D. Smith 1982; for his teleology, see von Staden 1997c.
67 With the possible exception of fr. 158 G. = Oribasius, *Synopsis, for Eustathius* 2, 32, none of the quotations of him by the Byzantine encyclopedists is taken directly from his writings; see Garofalo's (1988) index of sources.
68 Cf. Garofalo 1988: 47 for evidence of his familiarity with some Hippocratic treatises.
69 Vegetti 1993, 1998b: 92–9.
70 Von Staden 1997c: 199–208.
71 Erasistratus, fr. 140–2 G.
72 Ibid. fr. 119–33, 144, 284 G.
73 Ibid. fr. 86–8; 76 G.
74 Ibid. fr. 74, 93, 96, 109, 150, 198 G. By acting as a pump the heart also sends out nutriment and *pneuma*, so that the processes of nutrition and respiration are not entirely governed by a vacuum.
75 W. D. Smith 1982. Galen (8, 191 = Erasistratus, fr. 192 G.) complained that Erasistratus made no mention of 'black bile'.
76 Erasistratus, fr. 195, 240, 248–50, 162; cf. 229 G.
77 Ibid. fr. 248 G.
78 Garofalo (1988: 27; fr. 176–7 G.) argues that he continued to attribute mental disorders, such as phrenitis and lethargy, to problems affecting the meninges; he located the cause of apoplexy (fr. 174 G.) in the brain.
79 Ibid. fr. 195–6 G.
80 Ibid. fr. 109 G. Each side of the heart, according to Erasistratus, belonged to a different vascular system and did not communicate with the other. For *pneuma* drawn in by a vacuum process, see fr. 103–8 G.
81 Ibid. fr. 47–9 G. The reconstruction of his views has to be made largely on the objections to them by Galen (cf. C. R. S. Harris 1973: 195–233; Furley and Wilkie 1984: 26–37; Garofalo 1988: 33–43).
82 For possible links with other Peripatetics, see Scarborough 1985b.
83 Erasistratus, fr. 195 G.
84 Ibid. fr. 195; 169; cf. 162, 185 G., for plethora, an excess of blood, as the cause of disease. But fr. 168 G. suggests that Erasistratus also accepted other general causes of disease. The new Cologne Papyrus 327 explains 'burning fever', *kausos*, as caused by the entrance of 'fluid' (i.e. probably blood) from veins into the arteries, thereby blocking the flow and distribution of *pneuma*. This long fragment on fever, copied in the early second century BC, is likely to come from an Erasistratean source, and possibly even from Erasistratus himself, although it contains none of the specific technical terms associated with Erasistratus.
85 That Galen's own conclusion was wrong also points up the difficulty of this experiment, as modern replications of it have shown (see C. R. S. Harris 1973: 379–88).

86 Erasistratus, fr. 63 G.; Brain 1986.

87 Erasistratus, fr. 156–67, 231 G.; to which add Galen, 11, 176; W. D. Smith 1982. Galen has great fun with Erasistratus' preference for fasting as a way of drawing excess blood back into the veins.

88 Erasistratus, fr. 63–4, 66, 161–2, 267–8 G.

89 Ibid. fr. 253 G.

90 Ibid. fr. 184b G.

91 Ibid. fr. 117–18, 162, 247 G.

92 Brain 1986; Vallance (1990: 22–30) suggests that Asclepiades (see pp. 171–3 here) derived some of his theories from Erasistratus. For the new Cologne fragment, see n. 84 here.

93 Especially in *On Venesection, against the Roman Erasistrateans* (11, 187–249: tr. Brain 1986: 38–66), where Galen claims that they have now gone over to wholesale bleeding.

94 [Hippocrates], *The Heart*: IX, 80–92 L.; the quotation comes from Chapter 10. The most accessible English translation is that of I. M. Lonie in Lloyd 1978: 347–51. Important discussions are by C. R. S. Harris 1973: 83–94; Lonie 1975; Manuli and Vegetti (1977: 101–13) argue for a date around 350 BC; Duminil 1983: 299–302.

95 Lonie 1975: 10–15.

96 Ibid. 2–4; Manuli and Vegetti (1977) emphasise its Platonic teleology and language.

97 [Hippocrates], *The Heart* 2: IX, 78 L. The problem, already noted by Plato (*Timaeus* 91a), was familiar even to non-medics (cf. Plutarch, *Table Talk* 7, 1: 697F–700B).

98 The author's decision to place the 'ruling part' of the soul in the left ventricle might suggest a date as late as the first century BC (cf. Lonie 1975: 149–53).

99 Galen (18A, 7) makes him a contemporary of Herophilus. For his general standing as an anatomist, see Galen, 5, 651; 8, 212; 15, 134.

100 Rufus, *The Names of Bodily Parts* p. 142 Dbg; Galen, 3, 203; 4, 646; Soranus, *Gynaecology* 1, 57.

101 The attribution to Eudemus is found only in a mediaeval Latin version of Galen's *On the Anatomy of the Womb* (3, 2), not in any Greek manuscript (see Nickel 1971: 38, 72). For Euenor, see p. 130 here.

102 Marganne 1981: 55–60.

103 Galen, 5, 651; 15, 134; 18A, 7; cf. 8, 212.

104 Rufus, *The Names of Bodily Parts* p. 134 Dbg.

105 Celsus, *On Medicine*, pref., 12–53.

106 Apollonius, *On Joints*: CMG 11, 1, 1, p. 80. But von Staden (1989: 445–6) can show no anatomical discovery or investigation by the later Herophileans. The comment of Andreas (ibid. An. 5 = Cassius the Iatrosophist, *Problems* 58 Ideler) seems to have been made in passing, and not to come from a work on anatomy or necessarily to be based on his own dissections.

107 P. Potter 1993.

108 For the development of pulse doctrine by the Herophileans, see von Staden 1989: 446–8.

109 Celsus, *On Medicine*, pref., 26. This defence of experimentation on criminals stands in opposition to what 'plerique proponunt'.

110 Cicero, *Academics* 2, 122; Celsus, *On Medicine*, pref., 40–4, 74–5. Deuse (1993: 835–7), noting that Celsus is likely to have been repeating an Empiricist account of the debate, suggests that these standard epistemological objections were at some point countered by the supporters of anatomy. But, if they were, neither Celsus nor Galen refers to them, and they did not lead to any consistent anatomical dissections of human subjects.

111 Cf. Lennox 1994.

112 Edelstein (1967: 286) notes the weakness of the argument that only by anatomy could one learn about the body: other methods had been, and would be, found (cf. Celsus, *On Medicine*, pref., 43), and only after the introduction of dissection would anyone have thought to claim it as 'essential'.

113 Celsus, *On Medicine*, pref., 43.
114 Galen, 6, 480; 13, 605.

10 HELLENISTIC MEDICINE

1 Pfeiffer 1968: 97–8, 283; Fraser 1972: 317–19.
2 Algra *et al.* 1999; a good selection of translated texts is given by Long and Sedley (1987).
3 There exists no large-scale study of medicine in this period: Flemming (2003) and Rihll (2010) offer brief surveys in English; Kudlien (1979) and Massar (2005) are well-documented accounts of the social history of medicine in this period. Cf. Holmes 2009.
4 Schmidt 1924; Raschke 1978: 650–76, 904–1055.
5 Lloyd 1983: 119–26; Scarborough 1978; Amigues 2010.
6 Diocles, fr. 177 van der Eijk.
7 Erasistratus, fr. 35 G. (Garofalo (1988: 72) casts doubt on the existence of a specific tract called *On Causes*.) For his poison tract, see frs. 270–84 G.
8 Erasistratus, fr. 280 G.; for an autopsy on a dropsical patient, see fr. 251 G.
9 For Herophilus himself, see p. 155 here.
10 Dioscorides, *Materia medica*, pref. 1. For surviving fragments of his pharmacology, see von Staden 1989: 473 and fr. An. 18–42. For Heraclides' view, see p. 152 here.
11 Ibid. 516 and fr. Ma. 1–16.
12 Effe 1974.
13 Nicander, ed. Gow and Scholfield 1953; Jacques (2002, 2007) are fundamental, not least because of their commentaries.
14 Kudlien 1970b; cf. also the *Hedypatheia* of Archestratus of Gela, 'the Hesiod of foods' (fl. 350 BC): tr. Wilkins and Hill 1994; Olson and Sens 2000; and the (much later) Heraclitus of Rhodiapolis, 'the Homer of medical poetry', *TAM* 2, 2, 910.
15 Jacques 1979, 2002, 2007. Not everyone could understand his language easily, and his poems were later often accompanied by interpretative commentaries or by simpler summaries.
16 Most 1981: 109; Langholf 1986; Lang 2009; for Posidippus' *Iamatika*, 95–101, see Bing 2004.
17 Galen, 14, 214, 237.
18 Pliny, *Natural History* 25, 3, 6–7; Galen, 14, 283–5. Cf. also Galen, 14, 150, an alleged letter of Zopyrus to Mithridates, offering him a condemned criminal on whom to try out an antidote for snakebite; Watson 1966; Totelin 2004. Cf. also n. 23, below.
19 Pliny, *Natural History* 25, 3, 5–7.
20 Ibid. 25, 26, 62, which does not prove that Crateuas was in his service, *pace* Wellmann 1897. Collins (2000) is a beautifully illustrated survey of illuminated manuscripts of ancient pharmacology, with a good bibliography.
21 Heraclides, fr. 1–5 Gu.; Antiochis, *TAM* 2, 2, 595; H. Parker 2012: 373–4.
22 Ibid. fr. 7 Gu., although if the title alludes to Herophilus' description of hellebore as 'the general', it could be simply dealing with other herbs. He wrote at least two other large works on pharmacology (fr. 6–7, 37–8 Gu.).
23 Heraclides, fr. 25 Gu.; Ullmann 1972b. Cleopatra's *Cosmetics* was cited by Galen through Statilius Crito and perhaps directly. Plutarch, *Ant.* 71, 6–8; Dio, *Hist.* 51, 11, 12; and Galen, 14, 237 also claim that she tested the poison that killed her on maids (or condemned criminals) – see Marasco 1995b. H. Parker (2012) suggests that the cosmeticist was not the same as the queen.
24 Michler 1968, 1969; Marganne 1998.
25 The last two books of Celsus, *On Medicine*, are the major literary source for Alexandrian surgery (see Mazzini 1999; Sabbah and Mudry 1994: 103–210).

26 Dasen 1993; Garland 1995.
27 R. Jackson 1994. Oribasius (*Medical Collections* 49, 4–6) gives a very detailed description of an instrument devised by Andreas of Carystus to reduce dislocated limbs, which neatly demonstrates the links between Alexandrian medicine and technology (see Drachmann 1963: 171–3; and, for later developments, 173–85).
28 Apollonius of Citium, ed. Kollesch and Kudlien 1965.
29 W. D. Smith 1979: 212–22; P. Potter 1993.
30 Cf. Stückelberger 1994. A good selection of the illustrations in colour is given by Waugh *et al.* (1984). Schöne (1896) gives the complete set of illustrations in black and white.
31 Herophilus, fr. 261–6 von Staden.
32 Von Staden 1989: 453–5. The glossary of Bacchius (fl. 230 BC), covering at least eighteen Hippocratic texts, was particularly influential (ibid. fr. Ba 12–76); for Zeno and the sign controversy, see ibid. fr. Zn 5–6; W. D. Smith 1979: 199–201.
33 The earliest compiler of a Hippocratic glossary, according to Erotian (Hippocratic *Glossary*, pref.), was Xenocritus of Cos, whose dates are unknown, but who was possibly a younger contemporary of Herophilus.
34 Marganne 2001.
35 Heraclides, fr. 73–97 Gu. For Empiricist use of Hippocrates, see Deichgräber 1965: 220–52.
36 Nelson (2005) ingeniously suggests that two of the earliest of these writings, the *Speech from the Altar* and *The Embassy*, originally formed part of the *Coan History* of Macareus (fl. 250 BC).
37 [Hippocrates], *Speech at the Altar*; *Decree*; *Letters* 1–9; IX, 404; 400; 312–20 L. Pellicer (2000) discusses the later artistic representations of this refusal to attend the sick, universally endorsed by later Greek authors, despite its obvious clash with the sentiments of the Hippocratic *Oath*. For an artist's linkage of the *Epidemics* with the Athenian plague, see Figure 4.1 here.
38 Texts most accessible in W. D. Smith (1990); Rubin Pinault (1992) offers texts and translations of the later *Lives* and a discussion of their relationship with the *Letters*. Fundamental is Rütten (1992).
39 Flashar 1962: 338–40. The major quotations from *Airs, Waters and Places* (1, 8–12; 19–20: 859b–860b; 861b–862a) come in sections that seem later than the rest. Humours play a relatively restricted role outside the 'Hippocratic passages', and most attention is given to bile, phlegm and black bile.
40 The range of possibilities is wide: Forster (1928) thought that the work could not be earlier than the first century BC and possibly a good deal later. Marenghi (1964) argued that sections 1, 6–9, 14, 27, 31–5, 37 and 38 were genuinely Aristotelian. Jouanna (1996b: 286) assigns it to the middle of the fourth century without further argument, referring merely to Louis (1991). But Louis, although (pp. XVIII, XXIV) claiming authorship by Aristotle, elsewhere is more nuanced: at pp. XXIX–XXX, he gives sections 1, 2, 7, 10, 14, 18, 21, 26, 28, 30, 32–3 and 35–6 to the young Aristotle, and parts of 4, 13 and 15 to him at a later date; while other sections he places in the middle and late third century BC. The contrast with Marenghi is eloquent: only five or six passages are considered by both scholars to go back to Aristotle.
41 Flashar (1962: 338–40) summarises the links he sees between the two corpora.
42 I follow in general Flashar (1962: 303–58), who argued that Aristotle's own collection of *Problems* is now lost and cannot be identified for certain with any section of this book; and, on grounds of language, style, Peripatetic influences and doctrine, that much of this book goes back to around 250 BC (largely excluding the long treatise-like expository answers, but retaining the short 'question–question' group). He pointed to the absence of any reference in the medical sections to any of the discoveries of Herophilus and

Erasistratus, but warned against placing any weight on this omission in order to determine the date of composition.
43 [Aristotle], *Problems* 1, 1: 859a.
44 For cabbage, see ibid. 3, 17: 873a; for diseases, see 7, 8: 887a. This appears to be a longer reworking of the question at 1, 7: 859b.
45 [Aristotle], *Problems* 30, 1: 953a. Klibansky *et al.* 1964; Pigeaud 1988; Rütten 1992: 188–213.
46 Flashar 1962: 316–20, 327–31.
47 [Aristotle], *Problems* 1, 1 and 30, 8: 859a, 956a.
48 Ibid. 1, 46: 865a. Section 5, 1–41: 880b–885b deals specifically with questions about fatigue, both after exercise and during one's normal life.
49 Ibid. 14, 1–15: 909a–10b. For the direct borrowings from *Airs, Waters and Places*, see Jouanna 1996a: 152–4, 1996b, noting the Aristotelian reworking of certain words and phrases. For other borrowings, see Bertier 1989.
50 [Aristotle], *Problems* 1, 7: 859b.
51 Ibid. 1, 32–3: 863a.
52 Ibid. 1, 55–6: 866a–b.
53 Ibid. 9, 9–10 and 12: 890a–b.
54 Ibid. 1, 31: 863a.
55 Ibid. 1, 45: 864b.
56 Ibid. 4, 1–32; 31, 1–29; 11, 1–62; 35, 1–10; 6, 1–7: 876a–880b, 957a–960a, 898b–906a, 964b–965a, 885b–886a.
57 Ibid. 13, 6: 908a; 1, 12 and 30, 14: 860b and 957a.
58 But the Hippocratic four-humour theory as expounded by Galen can be found here only with difficulty, for there are no discussions of the consequences of an excess or deficiency of blood, or of venesection.
59 Von Staden 2000; Nutton 2000a: 139–46; van der Eijk 2005b.
60 Lucretius, *On the Nature of Things* 6, 665–6, 769–830, 1090–286. Parallels with earlier Greek authors are most easily found in C. Bailey 1947: 1723–44.
61 Demetrius (P. Herculaneum 831) recommended improving one's physical state as a way of combating the passions and errors of the soul. Lucretius' description of the plague has, of course, an artistic and a philosophical function in his poem that goes far beyond the merely medical.
62 Nutton 1975; von Staden 1982.
63 Von Staden 1989: fr. Ba. 78, with his discussion on pp. 478–9, 482; a Herophilean school at the temple of Men Karou near Laodicea (Strabo, *Geography* 12, 8, 20) lasted for several decades at least, beginning in the late first century BC.
64 There are also very many writers on medicine and surgery whose names are known but who cannot be forced into the straitjacket of association with a particular sect (cf. von Staden 1999: 88–90).
65 It remains a moot point how far the ancients' historiography of Hellenistic philosophy in terms of schools and sects influenced medical historiography.
66 Deichgräber 1965 (fundamental); Frede 1987: 243–60; Hankinson 1995.
67 Deichgräber 1965: fr. 5–8. For Philinus, see ibid. fr. 134–42.
68 For Serapion, see ibid. fr. 143–53; for Ptolemy of Cyrene, see ibid. fr. 166–7; for Glaucias of Tarentum (fl. 175 BC), see ibid. fr. 154–62; and Heraclides; for Lycus of Naples (fl. AD 60), see ibid. fr. 256–65.
69 Ibid. fr. 279–81. For the Sceptic Sextus Empiricus (fl. AD 200), see ibid. fr. 298–306; A. Bailey 2002; Floridi 2002.
70 Ibid. fr. 10b, 1 = Galen, *Outline of Empiricism* 1: tr. Walzer and Frede 1985: 23–4.
71 The Greek word 'dogma' can mean both 'decision' and 'belief', and in the epistemological debates of the time was often contrasted with true knowledge. Hence their opponents

could be lumped together as 'Dogmatics' or 'Logicians', even though they differed equally strongly among themselves as to just what constituted a true cause or how it might be identified.

72 The contemporary historian Polybius (*Histories* 12, 25d) sourly commented that, for all their pretensions to superior knowledge, the Logical physicians faced with a patient were just as helpless as someone who had never read a case history.

73 Galen, *Outline of Empiricism* 2 = Deichgräber 1965: fr. 10b: tr. Walzer and Frede 1985: 24–5.

74 Deichgräber 1965: 291–9.

75 Ibid. 298–305.

76 See p. 135 here.

77 The arguments and counterarguments are most easily found in Galen's *Outline of Empiricism* and *On Medical Experience* (tr. Walzer and Frede 1985).

78 Glaucias wrote a treatise called *The Tripod*, about 'The three things', but Empiricists themselves debated the extent to which Serapion had recognised the doctrine of similarities as one of the constituent parts of medicine (Deichgräber 1965: 83, 165).

79 Ibid. 301–5.

80 There is some slight evidence from the Roman period for the participation of doctors in inquests and police investigations, but these would appear to be in cases of assault, where wounds could be viewed externally, and did not involve an internal, pathological autopsy.

81 Celsus, *On Medicine*, pref. 40–4; Deichgräber 1965: fr. 66–70.

82 For their Hippocratic exegesis, see ibid. fr. 309–65, esp. fr. 310 for their characterisation of Hippocrates.

83 Galen, 12, 534, 989; 13, 462; 17A, 735 = T. 9, 6, 11–12 Gu.

84 Fragments are cited according to Guardasole (1997 = Gu. T. 14–25, fr. 1–18a Gu.), hence his portrayal among the greats of pharmacology in the introductory pages of the Vienna Dioscorides. Galen (12, 989; 13, 502 = T. 14; 17 Gu.) names Mantias as his teacher.

85 Celsus, *On Medicine* 7, 7, 6 = fr. 46 Gu.; cf. fr. 43–5, 47 Gu. for other surgical recommendations.

86 Von Staden 1999: 100–4. Guardasole (1997) and Deichgräber (1965: fr. 169–248) offer a more positive impression of Caelius' opinions.

87 Heraclides T. 29–32 and fr. 73–97 Gu.

88 Galen, 11, 796 = T. 23 Gu. Cf. Galen, *Outline of Empiricism* 8: tr. Walzer and Frede 1985: 34–6. Others had a much higher regard for Andreas and his books (see p. 143 here).

89 Wellmann 1916; Wendel 1943. Given his grammatical and lexicographical interests, Pamphilus may have collected synonyms for plants from a variety of native languages, including Egyptian.

90 Erasistratus, fr. 279 Garofalo.

91 Deichgräber 1965: fr. 146; cf. fr. 153. In his attack on Pamphilus, Galen (12, 251) denounces ostensibly medical books that gave instructions for making love philtres or poisons, bringing about an abortion or sterility, inducing favourable or unfavourable dreams, or merely causing something nasty to happen, such as binding an opponent in a law suit so that he could not speak properly. But there is no reason to conclude from this that Andreas or Serapion, in recommending un-Galenic remedies, would have also accepted the rest of this medical magic.

92 The basic study remains Wellmann (1889).

93 Wellmann 1921; Röhr (1923: 35–76) emphasises that notions of sympathy and antipathy were accepted by many who would have rejected magic.

94 Edelstein (1967: 232–5) warns that a belief in sympathetic remedies, widespread among Greek writers on medicine and philosophy from the late fourth century BC on, should

not be interpreted as a descent from rational medicine, since the theories on which it was based were very different from those of the magicians and depended on the conceptions of the workings of the universe adopted by Stoics, Peripatetics and others.

95 Pliny, *Natural History* 30, 1, 1–6, 18. A major study of magic in Pliny is still a desideratum, despite much good recent work on the *Natural History*; cf. also Gaillard-Seux 2003: 15–44. The magical papyri are most accessible in the English translation by H. D. Betz (1992). Cf. Graf 1997; Karenberg and Leitz 2002.

96 Van der Toorn 1985: 70–2; Ferngren 2000; see p. 292 here.

97 Hull 1974; Kee 1986: 24–6, 75–83.

98 Josephus, *Antiquities* 8, 44–9, expanding on 1 *Kings* 4, 29–34. A Latin history of medicine depending on both Jewish and Greek sources is published in Nutton (2012b).

99 Kudlien 1979: 65–72. Cf. Figure 6.3 here.

100 See Chapter 3, n. 27–32. For later Greek medical books in Egyptian temples, see Hanson 2005.

101 Galen, 13, 776–8, copying from the much earlier Greek pharmacologist Heras. The recipes were variously headed 'By Hermon, the sacred scribe' or 'From the inner sanctuary'.

102 Respectively, Galen, 13, 287; 13, 1038; 13, 204; 12, 879; 14, 178; 13, 338, cf. 133–4; 14, 182, cf. 180.

103 Kudlien 1979: 46, 68.

104 Ibid. 20–2.

105 Diodorus, *History* 1, 82, 3, based on a report of *c*.300 BC.

106 Kudlien 1979: 32–4.

107 Nutton 1977: 194.

108 Nutton 1996.

109 Pliny, *Natural History* 20, 100, 264; Galen, 14, 183, although the readings are suspect.

110 *I. Delos* 1573.

111 *I. Delos* 1547.

112 Mastrocinque 1995; Marasco 1996; Massar 2005: 51–64; Hillgruber 2010.

113 The inscriptional evidence for medical families in one place becomes more abundant in the Hellenistic period, but this may not indicate a new development, particularly given the older tradition of Asclepiad clans of healers.

114 The Egyptian evidence is most easily found in Harrauer (1987: 89–90); the inscription was published by A. Martin (1984).

115 *SEG* 23, 1873: no. 305.

116 Kudlien 1979: 7.

117 Sherwin-White 1978: 270–1. Later on, in the Roman period, Xenophon and his family ranked among the 'first citizens' on Cos; see below, p. 260–1.

118 Cicero, *On Duties* 1, 72. Comments like this go back in the Greek world at least to Aristotle (*Nicomachean Ethics* 1, 13, 7: 1102a).

119 Pleket 1995.

120 Römer 1990.

121 Nutton 1995d: 14.

122 Around AD 210, Origen imagined that a typical town would have a substantial variety of different healers (*Homily 13 on Luke*, p. 208 Fournier). For parallels, cf. Cipolla 1976: 67–124; Wear 2000: 22–5.

123 The list in Cohn-Haft (1956) is supplemented by Nutton 1977: 218–26; Nutton 1981b; Roesch 1984; Massar 2001; Samama 2003: 38–42, and by the general account in Massar 2005: 30–50, 65–103.

124 Massar 2001: 184.

125 Jouanna 1999: 370–1.

126 Sherwin-White 1978: 265–71; Massar 2001: 182.

127 *I. Creticae* IV, 168 and I, 7, around 217 BC. His wife erected a statue to him at Gortyn (*SEG* 43, 2000: no. 50).

128 Massar 2001: 183, citing *I. Histriae* 26; *IG* 5, 1, 1145 (letters sent from the Laconian town of Gytheion to a doctor in Sparta).

129 Pliny, *Natural History* 29, 6, 12; see p. 164 here.

130 *IG* 12, 1, 1032. Teles (*On Exile*, p. 26 Hense) asked rhetorically whether if a doctor was voted out of his post in favour of a drug seller it was a disgrace and a misfortune to him or to the public who failed to elect him.

131 Kudlien 1979: 55–8; Massar 2001: 187–91.

132 Massar 2001.

133 The only figure recorded for a salary in an inscription, 1,000 drachmas a year (Cohn-Haft 1956: 38; Massar 2001: 185), is about four or five times the annual wages of a mason. This sum was assured before any patients had to be seen.

134 Nutton 1981b: 14–16; Massar 2001: 191–7.

135 [Hippocrates], *Precepts* 12: IX, 266 L. *Physician* 2: IX, 208 L. warns against ostentatious, gleaming bronze furniture in the surgery; cf. Nutton 1985a: 36–7.

136 Jouanna 1999: 371.

137 Ibid. 404–6, 380; Dean-Jones 2010.

138 [Hippocrates], *Physician* 1: IX, 204 L.; *Precepts* 14: IX, 270 L.

139 [Hippocrates], *Precepts* 6 and 4: IX, 258, 254–6 L.

140 Edelstein (1967: 321) argued strongly that it was the *patient* who loved the art, since the next sentence, which talks of patients recovering simply through a belief in the goodness of the physician, explains the rare word. But the sentence could equally well explain why the doctor by being kind is a friend to his art: *because* the patient recovers thereby and the reputation of medicine is therefore boosted (Temkin 1991: 27–33).

141 [Hippocrates], *Precepts* 8: IX, 262–4 L.

142 [Hippocrates], *Decorum* 5 and 1: IX, 232, 226 L.

143 [Hippocrates], *Decorum* 2: IX, 226–8 L.; *Precepts* 10: IX, 266 L.

144 [Hippocrates], *Decorum* 3, 5–6: IX, 228; 232–6 L.

145 Ibid. 7–18; 236–44 L.

146 Deichgräber (1970: 88–107) is fundamental. For the date, see Jouanna 1999: 415. An English version of the *Testament* is given by W. H. S. Jones (1928: 59–60) and by MacKinney (1952: 16–19, Document K.), but the latter's arrangement is confusing and shows no knowledge of the non-Latin variants. On the *Testament* in Arabic, see Deichgräber (1970: 108–13), who discusses a reworking of this treatise by Rhazes (d. 925). Kibre (1985) has no entry for this work, although (92) she includes one ms. of it as coming from *De Arte*, and lists another (198) under *Praecepta*. Her third entry under this heading is a ms. of *De Visitando Infirmum*.

11 ROME AND THE TRANSPLANTATION OF GREEK MEDICINE

1 Nutton 1993e, 1995c. J. M. André (2006) gives a full but very traditional account based on the literary sources; Hanson (2006) is a fine short account.

2 J. N. Adams 1982, 1995; Sabbah 1991; Boscherini 1993b; Mazzini 1997: I, 123–71; Migliorini 1997; Debru 1998; Langslow 2000.

3 For Celsus, see Langslow 1994; for Caelius Aurelianus, see Urso 1997; Mudry 1999.

4 For recipes by Scribonius Largus preserved in Greek, see p. 174 here.

5 Orth 1925; Migliorini 1997: 21–94.

6 Langslow 1999. The linguistic point still stands whether or not one believes that here Plautus is taking over material from Greek comedy, not commenting directly on the Roman scene.

7 Boscherini 1993b: 31–44. For the possibility that some of these words came into Latin via Etruscan, see Boscherini 1970: 19–120.

8 See pp. 46–7, 150–2 here. Cf. the bilingual inscription published by A. Martin (1984).

9 Ebner 1966; D'Arms 1970.

10 *CIL* 11, 1979–80 = *CIE* 3731–2. The presumed archaeologically determined date, the second half of the seventh century BC, would appear to rule out any connection of Rutile Hipucrates (*CIE* 10017), from Tarquinii, with the historical Coan Hippocrates.

11 Krug (1985: 31–6) has useful remarks about Etruscan medicine; Sterpellone 2002; van der Meer (1987) dates the liver to 150–19 BC.

12 Cicero, *In Defence of Cluentius* 40, 178; cf., for the Greek equivalent, the *periodeutes*, Modestinus, *Digest* 27, 1, 6, 1; Galen, 12, 844; Ramsay 1941: 191, an inscription from Lystra set up by a Quintilla Ancharena to Ancharenus Petronius and Anenius 'called *periodeutes*'.

13 Although, as the epitaph of L. Sabinus L. l. Primigenius shows (*CIL* 11, 5836 (*ILS* 7794)), the travelling doctor, '*medicus fora multa secutus*', was still in existence. For a doctor with a civic salary, cf. *CIL* 11, 3007 (*ILS* 2542), an ex-military doctor 'with a salary' of the 'most splendid city of the Ferentans'. For a *sevir*, note the plutocratic and somewhat absurd P. Decimius P. l. Merula of Assisi (*CIL* 11, 5399–400 (*ILS* 5369, 7812)).

14 Dench 1995: 159–66.

15 They had a fearsome reputation: according to Plutarch (*Table Talk* 5, 7: 680D–E), a mere glance from an angry Thibian could kill.

16 See Nutton 1985b: 138–9; Dench 1995; for the modern Marsi, see Norman Lewis 1989.

17 See p. 108 here.

18 Valerius Maximus, *Remarkable Facts and Stories*, is the major account = Edelstein 1945, T. 848. Ovid (*Metamorphoses* 15, 622–744 = T. 850) and the anonymous author of *Famous Men* (= T. 849) add minor details. Valerius depends heavily upon Livy (see Bloomer 1992), whose account survives only in an abridgment of Book 11 = T. 846, but he may also have drawn on Varro's *Religious Antiquities*.

19 For Telemachus, see pp. 106–7 here; for Archias, see Pausanias, *Description of Greece* 2, 26, 8 = Edelstein 1945: T. 801.

20 But Ovid (*Metamorphoses* 15, 722) calls the temple one of Apollo. Livy knew of a temple of Asclepius at Antium in 170 BC (*History* 43, 4, 7 = Edelstein 1945: T. 844), but the summary of his account is too brief to show whether he was Valerius' source for calling it a temple of Asclepius. Ovid's version implies an earlier temple of Apollo, later taken over by Asclepius, and is perhaps preferable. However, the Latin form of the name, Aesculapius, seems to represent an early form of the Greek, and possibly much earlier contacts with the cult.

21 Degrassi 1986. The votive offerings are of a type of pottery common in the late fourth to early third century BC; an alternative explanation is that this was at this period a healing shrine of a local deity, taken over and massively remodelled in honour of Asclepius in the first half of the second century BC.

22 When the Roman ambassadors reached Epidaurus they were instructed in the precise rites that must be followed at their shrine. For the rites, see also Festus, *On the Significance of Words* 268 Lindsay = Edelstein 1945: T. 509. On liminality, see Graf 1992: 160–7.

23 Ovid, *Fasti* 1, 290–4 = Edelstein 1945: T. 855. The text of Pliny, *Natural History* (29, 1, 16), implies that there was a second temple to Asclepius built at the same time outside the city, but this may be simply his misremembering of the story of the temple at Antium. Cf. Edelstein 1945: II, 252, n. 8, accepting a knowledge of Asclepius in Rome well before 292 BC.

24 Suetonius, *Claudius* 25, 2 = Edelstein 1945: T. 858. Besnier (1902) requires considerable updating.

25 T. W. Potter 1985; Comella 1981; Beard *et al.* 1998: 12–13, 69–70.

26 Pliny, *Natural History* 29, 6, 12–14.

27 The alternative is to say that the Romans were inviting a member of a new occupational group to come and establish that craft within Rome, rather in the way that mediaeval monarchs invited particular types of craftsmen to settle in their domains. On either interpretation, Archagathus' arrival is unique in its official backing.

28 For a variety of interpretations, see Nutton 1986: 47; von Staden 1996b: 369–75.

29 Little weight should be placed on Dionysius of Halicarnassus, *Roman Antiquities* 1, 10; cf. 10, 53.

30 Celsus, *On Medicine* 5, 19, 27; Caelius Aurelianus, *Chronic Diseases* 4, 1, 7; P. Merton 115 = Marganne 1981: no. 206.

31 Astin 1969; Gruen 1992: 52–83; von Staden 1996b: 375–94.

32 Pliny, *Natural History* 29, 6, 14; for the *Oath* as conspiracy, see Plutarch, *Cato the Elder* 23, 3–4.

33 Pliny, *Natural History* 29, 6, 15; the additional details in Plutarch, *Cato* 23, 5, 6 may be correct.

34 W. H. S. Jones 1957; Boscherini 1993a.

35 Cato, *On Agriculture* 127, 1–3.

36 Von Staden 1996b: 387–94.

37 Nutton 1993c.

38 Pliny, *Natural History* 25, 5, 9–10; 26, 33, 51; 26, 6, 11; Galen, 14, 30.

39 For the moralising in Pliny, see Nutton 1986; Hahn 1991; Beagon 1992.

40 Rawson (1985) and Gruen (1992) describe the cultural context of Hellenisation. MacMullen (1991) is typically trenchant.

41 Horace, *Epistle* 2, 1, 156; cf. Ovid, *Fasti* 3, 101f.

42 Brunt 1988.

43 Pliny, *Natural History* 29, 8, 16. His statement lacks corroboration, and may misrepresent the ban of 161 BC on Greek philosophers and rhetoricians. But if doctors were expelled from Italy they were soon back.

44 Marasco 1995a.

45 Hallof *et al.* 1998: 105–9, with a good discussion of the political background.

46 *IG* 22, 3780, with the comment at *SEG* 37, 1987: n. 151. Marasco (1995a: 38–9) argues that the medical allusions and references in the poet Lucilius (fl. 135 BC) are to be connected with his membership of the Hellenophile circle of the Scipios.

47 Cicero, *2nd Proceedings against Verres* 3, 28.

48 Cicero, *Letters to His Friends* 13, 20; cf., for his own experience of him, ibid. 16, 4 and 9 (although Asclapo does not appear to have been greatly successful).

49 *CIL* 10, 388.

50 Suetonius, *Julius* 42; *I. Ephesos* 4101, with Knibbe 1981–2; Brugmann 1983. For Hellenistic precedents, see p. 156 here.

51 Suetonius, *Augustus* 59; Cassius Dio, *History* 53, 30.

52 Nutton 1971b; 1981b: 14–22.

53 Nutton 1986.

54 Nutton 1985a: 39–40.

55 Nutton 1992: 38–9. That some of these Greek names may hide non-Greeks, and that slaves trained in medicine were regularly given Greek names, only confirms the strength of the identification of medicine as something Greek. A more favourable view is held by Kudlien (1986a) and Korpela (1987).

56 Eusebius, *Ecclesiastical History* 5, 1, 49; Galen, 14, 621–3: tr. Nutton 1979: 91–3; *Lives of the Fathers of Merida* 6, 11 Garvin. For the city of Rome itself, Korpela (1987) provides a detailed list of names and putative statuses from literary as well as epigraphic texts.

57 The date of this very fragmentary rescript is either 93–4 or 108–9. On the stone it follows an imperial decision of 75 granting certain privileges to doctors, masseurs and teachers, but, as Fischer (1979) pointed out, there is no clear proof that the 'slaves most disgracefully dispatched' were students of medicine or that the 'teachers' were medical teachers.

58 Justinian, *Code* 6, 43, 3, 1; 7, 7, 1, 5a. These rulings, of 530–1, are best interpreted as offering a definitive solution to long-standing legal problems of joint ownership rather than a response to an immediately pressing social problem.

59 Justinian, *Digest* 38, 1, 27: nor to spend his days watching theatrical performances put on for him by his ex-slaves.

60 Nutton 1986.

61 Pliny, *Natural History* 25, 5, 9–10; 26, 33, 51; 26, 6, 11.

62 Pliny, *Natural History*, Books 7 and 20–32. His authorities for each book are listed in Book 1.

63 Sabbah and Mudry 1994; Celsus' date is hard to determine precisely. Columella, Quintilian and the Elder Pliny, writing at the latest in the 70s, know his work, and he cites recipes from Heras of Cappadocia and Antonius Musa, both writing in the last quarter of the first century BC. In his references to the Methodists he says nothing about Thessalus, which suggests that he was writing before AD 50. A comment that Cassius, 'the most ingenious doctor of our age', had recently died (*On Medicine*, pref. 69) gives a little more precision, if he is the same as Cassius of Centuripae, who was known to Scribonius Largus, writing in the 40s. A date for Celsus in the reign of Tiberius (AD 14–37) is thus probable.

64 Celsus, *On Medicine*, pref. 8–11.

65 Ibid. 7, pref. 3. Celsus is not troubled by the Greek names of these modern surgeons.

66 Langslow 1994; von Staden 1996b: 394–408.

67 C. F. Schultze (1999), arguing that he was a doctor, notes Celsus' expertise in understanding and criticising medical texts, as well as evidence for him at times putting theory into practice. (The first-person singular is used 240 times.) But while this might entitle him to be called a *medicus* by moderns, Celsus' own silence and the flexible boundary between healer and layman argue against him being so called by his contemporaries.

68 Celsus, *On Medicine* 3, 4, 10, but not, of course, ruling out appropriate rewards.

69 Celsus, *On Medicine*, pref. 65; those who are in charge of *valetudinaria* (sc. for slaves, see p. 264 here) cannot pay full attention to individuals and must resort to common characteristics, as if they were treating dumb animals or foreigners ignorant of the subtle reasoning of medicine. A similar complaint is made at 3, 4, 8–16.

70 Celsus' rationality should not be confused with that of the Rationalists: his claim is that all doctors require the ability to reason and form an independent judgment.

71 Although these benefits are not much greater than non-Greek versions of medicine that rely on herbs and other practical aids to the treatment of wounds and diseases (*On Medicine*, pref. 1; cf. 4, 13, 3; 5, 28, 7; 6, 9, 7 for country remedies superior to those of *medici*).

72 Celsus, *On Medicine*, pref. 4–5; von Staden 1996b: 403–5, 2009a, b, 2010.

73 The granting of citizenship to doctors in Rome (see p. 167 here) may also have been a means of controlling the flow of doctors, by ensuring some form of registration.

74 Pliny, *Natural History* 7, 37, 124. While a switch of career is not impossible, Pliny's hostility to Asclepiades as a Greek doctor advises caution.

75 Apuleius, *Anthology* 4, 19.

76 Cicero, *On the Orator* 1, 14, 62. An alternative translation applies Crassus' 'we' to members of his circle and not necessarily to himself alone.

77 Pliny (*Natural History* 7, 37, 124) has him dying in extreme old age from falling downstairs. Rawson 1982; Gourevitch 1987; Pigeaud 1991: 42–7. I am not convinced by the chronological and genealogical speculations of Polito (1999).

78 Celsus (*On Medicine*, pref. 11) says that Themison in his old age departed somewhat from Asclepiades' views, and that this was 'recent' (*nuper*); the notorious chronological vagueness of this term, whose meaning might range from days to decades, does not help in deciding between dates, except to cast doubt on a career for Themison ending much before the 50s BC. But the text of Pliny, *Natural History* (29, 5, 6), is defective at the crucial point, and the evidence that Themison was a direct pupil of Asclepiades is far from clear. Little can be drawn from the cognomen of a doctor honoured at Alexandria in AD 7 (Römer 1990), even if one could be sure that it was given him at birth out of homage to Themison.

79 Pliny, *Natural History* 26, 7, 12, the prime source for the datings by earlier scholars (e.g. Wellmann 1908b; R. M. Green 1955). Polito's argument (1999: 55) that Pliny derived his dating from a confusion with that of Asclepiades of Myrlea (cf. Suda, s.v. Asclepiades) is possible, but far from proven, given the uncertainties in the career of that grammarian.

80 Pliny, *Natural History* 29, 5, 6.

81 As well as Themison of Laodicea in Syria, his pupils included the Sicilian T. Aufidius, Philonides of Dyrrachium and Nicon of Acragas (Stephanus, *Geography* s.v. Dyrrhachium).

82 See p. 194 here. Cf. also L. Manneius of Tralles (p. xxx here), whose epithet 'wine-giver' recalls a favoured therapy of Asclepiades.

83 A translation of some fragments is given by R. M. Green (1955); a more up-to-date listing is provided by Vallance (1993: 711–27), to which add reference in the following note.

84 Galen, *On My Own Opinions* 6, 6: tr. Nutton 2001: 77; Boudon-Millot and Pietrobelli 2005: 178.

85 He rejected in particular the doctrine of 'critical days', although probably not the notion of crises.

86 Leith 2012. Vallance (1990: 122–30) prefers a link with the mechanism of Erasistratus, with whose work he was extremely familiar, although he did not agree with some of his ideas, particularly on therapy.

87 Benedum 1967.

88 Galen, 11, 163.

89 For wine, see Pliny, *Natural History* 23, 19, 31–2; Sextus Empiricus, *Against the Mathematicians* 7, 91; Caelius Aurelianus, *Acute Diseases* 2, 58; cf. as 'wine-givers', L. Manneius, p. 194 here, and Argaios Argaiou Pambotades, *Epigrammata Graeca* 853, from Athens.

90 Scribonius Largus, *Drug Recipes*, pref. 3–4; Celsus, *On Medicine* 3, 4, 2.

91 Celsus, *On Medicine* 3, 4, 3.

92 Caelius Aurelianus, *Acute Diseases* 1, 116–54; 3, 34; *Chronic Diseases* 3, 127; 149.

93 Cassius the Iatrosophist, *Problems* 40.

94 König and Whitmarsh (2007: 3–39) offer a sophisticated discussion of the multiple identities of the Greeks in the Roman Empire.

12 THE CONSEQUENCES OF EMPIRE: PHARMACOLOGY, SURGERY AND THE ROMAN ARMY

1 Juvenal, *Satires* 3, 62: the doctor and the masseur figure in the list of occupations given at lines 75–6, along with the grammarian, the tightrope-walker and the magician. For their geographical origins, see Nutton 1986: 37–8; Korpela 1987; Noy 2000; Figure 17.6 here.

2 Cf. the Greek doctors Hermogenes (*RIB* 461) and Antiochus at Chester (p. 186 here). The findspots of the inscriptions indicate a link with the army (see Figure 18.2 here).

3 Scribonius Largus, *Drug Recipes* 97, against gout and pains in the side; originally devised by Philo(nides) of Catania, it was used also by Largus against epilepsy and madness.

4 Galen, 10, 7–8: tr. Hankinson 1991: 5–6. The tradition of publishing one's advice to a monarch goes back at least to Hellenistic times, and is represented today by a whole series of almost certainly pseudonymous tracts directed to such figures as King Antigonus of Macedon, Ptolemy and Maecenas.

5 Scribonius Largus, *Drug Recipes*, pref. 1; 13.

6 Ibid. 59, 60; 31, 177; 97, 177; 70, 175, 268, 271. Another doctor on the expedition was C. Stertinius Xenophon (see pp. 260–1 here).

7 Ibid. 163. Whether he was there as an army doctor on a short service contract or was brought along as the private physician of a general or leading courtier is unclear; cf., for a private doctor to a governor, *CIL* 3, 12116.

8 Largus, *Drug Recipes* 163, 171. Baldwin (1992) prefers an African origin.

9 Sconocchia 1983: viii; 1993: 856–9, 890–908. The Greek recipes do not entirely correspond to the Latin. For his possible bilingualism, see Langslow 2000: 51–2.

10 Sconocchia (1983) is the best edition; there is no English translation.

11 Rinne 1896; Schonack 1913.

12 For the torpedo, see Largus, *Drug Recipes* 11; 162.

13 Ibid. 70 (quinsy); 59–60 (dentifrices, all with a cachet of use by the imperial family).

14 Evershed *et al.* 2004; Künzl 2002.

15 Galen, 12, 753; Bartels *et al.* 2006.

16 Touwaide 2012.

17 Largus, *Drug Recipes* 91, 94 (Valens); 202, 213, 239 (Meges).

18 Ibid. 122, 172.

19 Ibid. 12.

20 Ibid. 12.

21 Ibid. 13, 17. Recipes for epilepsy involving gladiator's blood and the like continued to be recommended long after the ending of gladiatorial displays (Temkin 1971: 12–14, 22–4; Moog 2002).

22 The *Preface* is translated into English by Hamilton (1986) and Pellegrino and Pellegrino (1988). Neither is entirely reliable. The essential study remains Deichgräber (1950). See also n. 28 here.

23 Largus, *Drug Recipes*, pref. 1–3.

24 Cf. Celsus, *On Medicine*, pref. 10, 64 and 66.

25 Largus, *Drug Recipes*, pref. 5; 199. Celsus, a near-contemporary, uses the word '*professio*' in a similar way, referring (*On Medicine*, pref. 11) to the development of 'this healthgiving profession of ours'.

26 Korpela 1995.

27 Largus, *Drug Recipes* 199; pref. 1–3.

28 Mudry 1997. Nowhere does Largus assert that the *Oath* was actually taken, and his own argument suggests that it was not, or at least irregularly.

29 The first printed edition of his book appeared only in 1529, made from a manuscript that immediately vanished; the first commentary was published in 1655. Not until 1974 did a Latin manuscript of his work come again to light, in the Chapter Library of Toledo, and not until 1983 did a good modern edition appear in print.

30 The standard edition, incorporating some pseudonymous material, is Wellmann (1906–14). The best English translation is that of Beck (2005). Some older editions and handbooks call the author Pedacius, the reading of some manuscripts, but Pedanius is far better attested and suggests that he or his family had gained Roman citizenship by associating with Pedanius Secundus, consul in 43 and later governor of Asia, or his brother, consul in 60.

31 For Lucius, 'the Teacher' of Tarsus (fl. 60), who taught Asclepiades Pharmacion and Statilius Crito, see Fabricius 1972: 190–2.

32 Dioscorides, *Materia medica*, pref. 4. See Scarborough and Nutton 1982: 213–17; Riddle 1985.

33 Dioscorides, *Materia medica*, pref. 1–2. For Crateuas, fragments of whose writings were later copied on to some of the pages of the Vienna Dioscorides, see p. 143 here. Sextius Niger, active in the first half of the first century AD, was a Roman who wrote in Greek (Wellmann 1889; Stannard 1965). Galen (11, 797) considered both Crateuas and Niger essential reading for the would-be pharmacologist.

34 Dioscorides, *Materia medica*, pref. 8–9.

35 Raven 2000. For botanical names, see Aufmesser 2000; Beck 2005.

36 Dioscorides, *Materia medica* 2, 129. For problems of identification, see Raven 2000.

37 Dioscorides, *Materia medica*, pref. 5; Riddle 1985: 24–131. Ancient book-rolls, it should be remembered, did not have page marks or indexes; some authors, like Largus and Pliny in his *Natural History*, tried to help the reader by providing a preliminary table of contents.

38 Riddle 1980, 1985: 168–217; Reeds 1991; Collins 2000; Cronier 2009.

39 Reeds 1991.

40 For the wider Roman encyclopaedic tradition, see Stahl 1962; French 1994: 196–295.

41 For Pliny as an author on pharmacology, see J. André 1956; Stannard 1965; Morton 1986; Scarborough 1986. Beagon (2005) comments on his ideas on the human body.

42 Müntzer 1897; Scarborough 1986.

43 Pliny, *Natural History* 27, 1, 2.

44 Pliny, *Natural History* 25, 1, 1–3, 7; and p. 145 here.

45 Galen, 14, 2. His poem was re-edited by Heitsch (1964: 7–15; cf. Heitsch 1963: 26–39). Whether he or his son is the royal doctor to whom Erotian dedicated his Hippocratic glossary is unclear.

46 Galen, 14, 31–42; 13, 988. A new edition of the poems of Damocrates is being prepared by Sabine Vogt.

47 Galen, 13, 441. Fragments of Asclepiades are listed by Fabricius 1972: 192–8, 247–53.

48 Fabricius 1972: 185–9.

49 For Crito's career, see p. 262 here. Fragments in Fabricius 1972: 190–2.

50 [Galen] *The Properties of the Centaury*; Nutton 2010b. The closest parallel is another text from this period, also written in Greek but surviving mainly in Latin, the *Letter on the Vulture*, ed. Möhler 1990, but this contains much more magical material.

51 One surviving tract is [Galen], *Substitute Drugs* 19, 721–47, whose author mentions several other writers of the late Hellenistic period.

52 Crito took part in Trajan's campaigns on the Danube (see p. 262 here).

53 For the use of friendly towns, see Caesar, *Civil Wars* 3, 78; 87; 101.

54 R. Jackson 1988: 130–2. Vegetius (*Epitome* 1, 6; 1, 22), evidently based on much earlier doctrine, advised close attention to the healthiness of the prospective site and the adequacy of the water supply.

55 R. Schultze 1934; Watermann 1974: 113–27; Dolmans 1993; Wilmanns 1995: 103–7 and pl. 7; Breitwieser 1998: 42–59; Baker 2004. The scepticism of Baker (2002) is unjustified in the light of the excavations at the Danubian fortress of Novae.

56 Pitts and St Joseph 1985.

57 R. W. Davies 1970b; Wilmanns 1995: 108–16. A new inscription records the building of a new hospital near Aleppo (Syria) for an auxiliary cohort in 108/9 (Jarry 1985: 114).

58 Knörzer 1970; Watermann 1974: 167–72.

59 R. W. Davies 1970a. *An. Ep.* 1995, 1259a–e comes from a similar barrel destined for the hospital of the auxiliary fort at Arrabona.

60 R. Jackson 1988: 134.

61 Richmond 1968: 86, but not all agree with his interpretation.

62 Accepted, however, by A. Johnson 1983: 157–64.

63 Cassius Dio (*History* 68, 14, 2) implies major treatment in tents immediately to the rear of the battlefield; cf. also *Life of Alexander Severus* 47, 2: 'he visited the sick in their own tents'. The famous relief on Trajan's column shows a soldier being treated on or near the field. For medicine while on campaign, see Velleius Paterculus, *History* 2, 114, 2; Tiberius as general allowed his sick troops to use his own doctors, his kitchens, his bath and his own carriage or litter. A similar story, ostensibly of a much earlier period, is told by Livy (*History* 8, 36, 6–8).

64 Bowman and Thomas 1991.

65 Youtie and Winter 1951: no. 468.

66 R. Jackson 1988: 131.

67 Wilmanns 1995: 108, 115. Hospitals, *valetudinaria*, are otherwise known only for the large slave households and landed estates of the Later Republican and Early Imperial periods.

68 For the numbers, see Wilmanns 1995: 68–70; a legion had 5,600 men, an auxiliary unit between 500 and 1,000. The Rome fire brigade had four doctors per cohort of 1,000 men (*CIL* 6, 1058, 1059); the ratio of doctors to men in the other urban units is not known.

69 *CIL* 9, 1617. Ammianus, *History* 16, 6, 2 records the career of a doctor who was promoted to be the centurion guarding the public buildings of Rome.

70 Respectively, *CIL* 6, 31172; 13, 1833. Cf. Galen, 12, 557, 580 for Antiochus, 'a splendid camp doctor' and author of a recipe.

71 R. W. Davies 1969, 1972; Wilmanns 1995: 117–24, 233. At Aquincum Marcius Marcellus, a doctor, describes himself as being 'under the bandager and veteran Valerius Praesens', *An. Ep.* 2008: 1123.

72 Nutton 1970.

73 R. W. Davies 1969: 88–94; Wilmanns 1995: 75–102.

74 *CIL* 3, 14216, 9. At the other extreme of age, Caius Papirius Aelianus, *medicus ordinarius* in the Third Legion at Lambaesis, N. Africa, was buried, aged 85, in an elegant grave (*CIL* 8, 18314).

75 Justinian, *Code* 10, 53, 1; Numisius almost certainly joined up on a short-term contract. For a doctor who had a later civil career, see *CIL* 9, 3007; M. Ulpius Telesporus served auxiliary cavalry units in Africa and Germany before becoming town physician at Ferentium (Italy).

76 Nutton 1968; Wilmanns 1995: 176; Clackson and Meissner 2000.

77 Lucian, *How to Write History* 16, 24, if he is not a figment of Lucian's satirical imagination.

78 For Antiochus and Hermogenes, see n. 76 here; [Habr]ocomas, *RIB* 1028; Hymnus, *CIL* 13, 5208; Onesiphorus, *CIL* 8, 2874; Zosimus, *CIL* 13, 6621.

79 Galen, 13, 604.

80 Künzl 1982: 80–5; 1996. Note *IG* 14, 1717, a Greek inscription to an '*organopoios*', possibly an instrument-maker. For earlier developments in medical and surgical instruments, see p. 144 here.

81 Celsus, *On Medicine* 7, 5, 1–3; R. Jackson 1988: 128.

82 Plutarch, *Precepts of Health* 16: 131A–B; Renehan 2000.

83 Paul, 6, 88; Schöne 1909; Salazar 2000: 10–53. In the Ephesus medical 'contests' of the second century one of the categories was called 'Instruments', probably for the invention of new instruments (*I. Ephesos* 1161).

84 Plutarch, *Life of Cato the Younger* 70, 6.

85 The headline, 'Knowledge from learning [...] from the days of Galen, Father of Catgut Sutures', comes from an advert for Curity Sutures in *Surgery, Gynecology and Obstetrics* (91, 2: 1950), and is wrongly based on his preference for thin silk sutures at 10, 942–3. For his operations, see 10, 409–23.

86 Galen, *On Examining the Physician* 14: *CMG* Suppl. Or. 4, 134–7. Archaeological evidence also reveals successful (and some unsuccessful) setting of fractured limbs.

87 Galen, 2, 631–3: tr. C. Singer 1956: 192–3; *On the Opinions of Hippocrates and Plato* 1, 5, 1–5: *CMG* 5, 4, 1, 2, 73–7.

88 Toledo-Pereyra 1973: 371–5, under the misapprehension that the treatise described was by Galen. Cf. also the divisions of surgery as described around AD 180 in P. Oxy. 4972.

89 R. Jackson 2002a: 91–2.

90 R. Jackson 2002a; De Carolis 2009.

91 Galen, *On Examining the Physician* 9, 7: *CMG* Suppl. Or. 4, 104–5. This is more plausible than his much later claim to have had no fatalities at all (13, 600). For others' successful treatment of gladiators' wounds, see 10, 378. Cf., for similar doctors, *CIL* 6, 10172–3; *IG* 14, 1330. Had the doctor commemorated by a club of gladiatorial fans at Ephesos (*I. Ephesos* 3055) also served in this way?

92 R. Jackson 1988: 123–5; Majno 1975: 186–8, 367, 399–400. Honey, also recommended, would have had bactericidal effects and promoted healing (Majno 1975: 115–20, 370). For early dentistry, see Hoffmann-Axthelm 1981, 1985.

93 Celsus, *On Medicine* 7, 26; MacKinney 1965: 80 and pl. 82.

94 Justinian, *Digest* 50, 13, 1, 3 (from Ulpian, *c.*AD 200).

95 Celsus, *On Medicine* 7, 16. Majno (1975: 362–5) points out that these procedures presuppose effective ligaturing of the blood vessels with tourniquets and with various types of forceps.

96 Pliny, *Natural History* 6, 28, 105; Bliquez 1996.

97 Krug 1985: 103; Finch (2011) presents new evidence from Pharaonic Egypt of a prosthetic toe.

98 Marganne 1998: 96–119; R. L. Grant 1960; Sachs and Varelis 2001a, 2001b. Galen had planned a major treatise on surgery, but no trace of it remains, unless it became the final two books of the *Method of Healing*.

99 Eunapius, *Lives of the Philosophers* 499; Augustine, *City of God* 22, 8; John of Ephesus, *Lives of the Eastern Saints* 38, with S. A. Harvey 1984: 88.

100 Harig (1971) pointed out that the provision of hospitals for estate slaves or for the great slave households in Rome itself in the last century of the Republic and the Early Empire similarly reflected the growing importance of these slaves, and the increasing costs of supplying replacements.

101 Vegetius, *Epitome* 1, 88. The hospital in the fortress at Luxor, Egypt (el-Saghir 1986: 115) may have been used well into the fourth century, but I know of no clear evidence for the use of legionary hospitals in the fifth century.

13 THE RISE OF METHODISM

1 See pp. 165–6 here.

2 Pliny, *Natural History* 29, 5, 6–11.

3 Pliny, *Natural History* 29, 5, 9; 29, 8, 26–7. For analyses of Pliny's rhetoric, see p. 379, n. 41 here.

4 Vettius Valens also founded his own sect (Pliny, *Natural History* 29, 5, 8). Menecrates, *IG* 14, 1759; Leonides or Leonidas, [Galen], *Introduction* 4: 14, 684, famous as a surgeon and pharmacologist. An alternative explanation for the epithet is that he was taught by another 'episynthetic', Agathinus. For the history of the Empiricists in the Roman period, including prolific authors such as Menodotus of Nicomedia and Theodas, see Deichgräber 1965: 203–19, 407–18.

5 The Greek word for 'sect', '*hairesis*', simply means 'choice' (von Staden 1982).

6 Celsus, *On Medicine*, pref. 53, emphasising it as a 'way' of classifying observations; Galen, 2, 343.

7 Galen, 10, 53–4: tr. Hankinson 1991: 27–8; 18A, 25. He also wrote at least one *Introduction to Medicine* and another tract on *Disorders of Body and Soul*. For Methodism in Egyptian papyri, see Leith's commentary on Papyrus Oxyrhynchus 4971.

8 Galen, 10, 909–16, with Benedum 1971. For Crito, see p. 262 here. For the possibility that he is the Methodist author of *The Properties of the Centaury*, above p. 181, see Nutton 2010b.

9 For Soranus, see p. 199 here. That he taught Attalus is revealed by Galen, 10, 911.

10 *CIG* 3283. Petzl (1983: 537) dates it to the second century, but a late first-century date cannot be excluded. There are good photos in Benedum 1978; Conrad *et al.* 1995: 43.

11 Rubinstein 1985.

12 Tecusan 2004. The promised second volume of commentary has not appeared.

13 [Galen], *Introduction* 4: 14, 684; Galen, 10, 52–5: tr. Hankinson 1991: 27–8; Agnellus, *Commentary on Galen's On Sects* 4 = John of Alexandria, *Commentary on Galen's On Sects*, pref.: p. 16 Pritchet. The first citation shows that this genealogy was already formed by the late second century, and is implied also by Celsus' opposition to it (n. 16 here).

14 Van der Eijk 1999d.

15 See p. 170 here. If the Alexandrian honorand in AD 7 (Römer 1990) is this Themison, the neat master–pupil–pupil triad is impossible.

16 Celsus, *On Medicine*, pref. 54; cf. 11 and 62. For Celsus' date, see p. 376, n. 63 here. The earlier Celsus is placed – a date under Tiberius, 14–37, is often favoured, although without firm grounds – the harder it becomes to see Thessalus as the first real Methodist.

17 Pliny, *Natural History* 29, 5, 8–9.

18 Galen, 10, 35; 51–2: tr. Hankinson 1991: 19, 26–7; 18A, 271.

19 [Galen], *Introduction* 4: 14, 684; cf. Diller 1936b. The question is largely one of semantics: how to decide at what point doctrines become truly Methodist.

20 *CIL* 12, 1804; Tarsus, see n. 22 here.

21 Bean and Mitford 1970: no. 38.

22 For Artorius, see Caelius Aurelianus, *Acute Diseases* 3, 14; for Arius, see Galen, 12, 776, 829; 13, 857; Dioscorides, *Materia medica*, pref., suggesting doctrinal differences with the other pharmacologists named in the next sentence.

23 Dioscorides, *Materia medica*, pref. 2.

24 Plutarch, *Table Talk* 6, 2: 687B; and 8, 9: 731B, 733B.

25 Lucretius, *On the Nature of Things* 6, 1090–286; for his possible sources, see C. Bailey 1947: 1718–44.

26 Celsus, *On Medicine*, pref. 11; Pliny, *Natural History* 29, 5, 6. Pigeaud (1993: 571) notes that, according to Caelius Aurelianus (*Chronic Diseases* 2, 215; 3, 65; 5, 51), the break came around the time of the composition of *Chronic Diseases*, Book 2, although it was far from complete.

27 Moog 1995. There is, however, no clear proof that Themison himself ever gave it the name of the 'Method'.

28 Celsus, *On Medicine*, pref. 64; at 54, Celsus implies that his followers were wrong to appeal to Themison's authority for denying that the knowledge of any cause whatever has a bearing on treatment.

29 Soranus (*Gynaecology* 1, 1 and 3) modified this slightly, allowing that a knowledge of the natural workings of the body and of anatomy might be valuable, but only as evidence of erudition. Of itself, it was useless in practice.

30 Caelius Aurelianus, *Acute Diseases* 3, 188; cf. 2, 44 and 52.

31 Caelius Aurelianus, *Chronic Diseases*, pref. 3, who also notes that this was not a new distinction, and that others had described the treatment of chronic diseases such as gout and epilepsy, but not as part of a systematic study of chronic diseases.

32 Celsus, *On Medicine*, pref. 55; later descriptions of Methodist doctrine give four stages (Galen, 1, 195: [Galen], *Introduction* 3: 14, 680), beginning with 'onset'. Whether Celsus

was in error, considered 'onset' irrelevant to his discussion or did not know of this slightly later division is a moot point.

33 Cf. Caelius Aurelianus' comments at *Acute Diseases* 1, 16, 155; Leith (2008: 582–4) distinguishes between observing a three-day period, possibly involving alternate fasting and feeding (cf. Galen, 10, 536, where such a procedure could be accepted by an Erasistratean doctor), and basing a system of therapy on it. The latter is likely to have been an innovation of Thessalus.

34 Celsus, *On Medicine*, pref. 65–6; 3, 4, 9–10.

35 Celsus, *On Medicine*, pref. 73, a nice example of Celsus' strategy of setting his own brand of 'rational' medicine as a mean between two extremes.

36 Pigeaud 1991: 26–8.

37 Galen, 10, 52; 67–74: tr. Hankinson 1991: 27, 34–8; for Galen's insistence on the distinction, see 10, 85–93: tr. Hankinson 1991: 43–7.

38 Pliny, *Natural History* 29, 5, 9, perhaps dependent on the opening words of the letter to Nero; see Galen's citation of it, 10, 8: tr. Hankinson 1991: 6. Cf. also Galen's parody, 10, 11–12: tr. Hankinson 1991: 7–8.

39 Galen, 10, 4–5 (some revealing snobbery), 11–12, 22: tr. Hankinson 1991: 4–5, 7–8, 13.

40 Galen, 1, 83: tr. Walzer and Frede 1985: 11–12; 10, 5: tr. Hankinson 1991: 4–5; 10, 781, 927.

41 Galen, 18A, 271; 10, 35: tr. Hankinson 1991: 19.

42 Galen, 1, 82: tr. Walzer and Frede 1985: 11; 1, 192–3; 10, 35: tr. Hankinson 1991: 19; [Galen], *Introduction* 3: 14, 681–2; Caelius Aurelianus, *Chronic Diseases* 2, 145.

43 Galen, 10, 250–2 (from Thessalus' *Surgery*).

44 [Galen], *Introduction* 3: 14, 680.

45 Galen, 1, 71; 96–102: tr. Walzer and Frede 1985: 6, 17–19. But this to a Methodist is not the same as saying that one must take the season or age of the patient into account; they see merely the intensity of the disease, and its appearance might vary (cf. Galen, 1, 80: tr. Walzer and Frede 1985: 10).

46 Edelstein 1967: 183–4; Nutton 1990c.

47 Pigeaud 1991: 43–6; 1993: 594–7.

48 Note the emphasis on the immediate and visible appearance of any commonality even when the things themselves may not be thought similar (P. Oxyrhynchus 3658; [Galen], *Medical Definitions* 17: 19, 353; Galen, 1, 81–2: tr. Walzer and Frede 1985: 10–11).

49 Galen, 10, 263–5; 535–43; Leith (2008) argues that this pattern need not be slavishly followed and allowed for variation.

50 At 6, 839–43, Galen allows, for the sake of argument, the validity of an atomic universe and of an explanation of disease in terms of fluidity or stricture, but (6, 872) rejects entirely the notion of 'mixed' conditions.

51 E.g. Caelius Aurelianus, *Chronic Diseases* 2, 145; *Acute Diseases* 2, 147. Cf. Galen, 10, 53: tr. Hankinson 1991: 27; 18A, 269.

52 Caelius Aurelianus, *Acute Diseases* 2, 147.

53 Galen, 10, 52–8: tr. Hankinson 1991: 27–30; Gourevitch 1991: 66–70, noting also that Caelius showed no embarrassment at putting forward both Methodist and non-Methodist definitions of various diseases. In the absence of modern tests that identify diseases by their causal agent, ancient disease classifications were groupings of symptoms and syndromes; some were relatively stable, others more debatable, like modern discussions on the status and reality of various forms of mental illness or of ME.

54 Gourevitch 1991: 64–6, citing [Galen], *Medical Definitions* 16–17: 19, 353, and the use of '*intelligentia*' by Caelius. Galen ([Galen], *Introduction* 5: 14, 684) reports that the Methodists believed medicine to be entirely a 'science', but only, he goes on immediately to say, because they had, in his view, a totally false view of what a science was. Their science was not something that was certain and infallible by the rules of reason.

55 Frede 1982; Lloyd 1983: 182–200; Hankinson 1998a: 318–20.
56 Sextus, *Outlines of Pyrrhonism* 1, 240. This does not mean, as Edelstein (1967: 186–9) argued, that Methodism derived its philosophical basis from Scepticism.
57 Galen, 1, 98 (without naming those converted to the truth): tr. Walzer and Frede 1985: 18; 10, 53: tr. Hankinson 1991: 27–8; cf. [Galen], *Introduction* 4: 14, 684.
58 Galen, 10, 53: tr. Hankinson 1991: 27; he took over a variety of therapies from Soranus (12, 414; 493–5; 956; 987; 13, 42), but not necessarily directly. The standard edition of Soranus' writings is that of Ilberg (1927), but this does not include the citations in later authors.
59 The best account of Soranus is that of Hanson and Green (1996).
60 Suda, s.v. Soranos; Caelius Aurelianus, *Acute Diseases* 2, 130; Soranus, *Gynaecology* 2, 44, which implies that this book was written away from Rome, perhaps back in Ephesus. Soranus rejects the view of others that Roman women overindulge in sex and drink.
61 Caelius Aurelianus, *Acute Diseases* 3, 124; *Chronic Diseases* 5, 30; Soranus, *Gynaecology* 2, 6, and, for anatomy, which he regarded as largely useless for practice but gave a good impression of one's learning, ibid. 1, 3. For parallels, see p. 263 here.
62 Marcellus, *On Drugs* 19, 1; Tzetzes, *Chiliads* 6, 300–2, linking him also to Rufus.
63 Detailed lists, obtained mainly from quotes in the writings of others and from bibliographies compiled by Arabic authors (but often deriving from good sources), can be found in Michler (1975) and Ullmann (1978a: 76). The *Life* (ed. Ilberg 1927: 175–8, and translated by Rubin Pinault 1992: 7–8) is attributed to a Soranus, but this may be a redaction of a *Life* by Soranus of Cos, whose discoveries are cited in sections 3 and 4. For philosophy, see Podolak 2010.
64 Bendz (1990–3) is the most recent edition, not entirely replacing Drabkin (1950), which has an English translation.
65 Contrast the approaches of Urso (1997) and the various authors in Mudry (1999).
66 The standard edition remains that of Ilberg (1927). There is an excellent English translation by Temkin (1956). The more recent edition and translation in the French Budé series (Burguière *et al.* 1988–2000) is useful for its notes.
67 Metrodora, tr. Del Guerra 1994; her date and sex are disputed; cf. Congourdeau 1994; H. Parker 1997.
68 For the *Gynaecology* of Caelius, see Drabkin 1951. The *Gynaecia* of Mustio/Moschion (ed. Rose 1882) was widespread in the Middle Ages in both East and West. It is a compendium based on a fuller text of Soranus than we possess, but was first composed in Latin (Mustio) and later (ninth or tenth century?) translated into Greek (Moschion). Dasen (2004) has an excellent bibliography.
69 For specula, see Longfield-Jones 1986; for abortion, cf. Tertullian, *On the Soul*, 25, in part deriving from Soranus' lost *On the Soul* (see Polito 1994; Podolak 2010); for child-rearing, cf. the patristic material assembled by Buell (1999); for satirists' jokes, see *Greek Anthology* 15, 19; Martial, *Epigrams* 6, 36.
70 Soranus, *Gynaecology* 1, 3–4, although the presence of lanolin, one might think, would keep the hands smooth.
71 Flemming (2000: 385–91) lists women called '*medica*' and '*iatrina*' on inscriptions; supplemented by Laes (2011). For literary sources, see Flemming 2007b; H. Parker 2012.
72 Antiochis, *TAM* 2, 2, 595, with Heraclides, fr. 1–5 Gu.; Hygia, *CIL* 6, 4458 (note also 4473, a female slave assigned to the palazzo's hospital); Restituta, *IG* 14, 1751.
73 *CIL* 6, 9477; Figure 17.7 here; another '*iatromea*' is *CIL* 6, 9478.
74 Galen, 14, 641–7: *CMG* V 8, 1, 110–17; Eunapius, *Lives of the Philosophers* 465.
75 It may be significant that in the many meditations on, and reformulations of, the birth stories in the Gospels the absence of medical attention at the birth of Jesus is hardly, if ever, noted.

76 Censorinus, *On Birthdays*; Tertullian, *On the Soul* 37–8. Riddle (1992a) places excessive weight on the secret networks of women. Contrast Dean-Jones (1995). There is much to ponder in M. H. Green (2008).

77 Soranus, *Gynaecology* 4, 7–8.

78 For this debate, see Soranus, *Gynaecology* 3, 1, 1–5.

79 For general surveys of gynaecology in Rome, see Gourevitch 1984a; Flemming 2000; Dasen 2004.

80 *IG* 12, 5, 199, cf. Samama 2003: 7; a 'women's doctor' is not one of the subspecies of doctor, like the 'clinical' or the 'ocular' doctor, recorded on inscriptions or papyri. And was Soranus writing for women, or, more plausibly, for the male head of the household seeking appropriate advice and assistance for his wife and other female members?

81 The list in Flemming (2000: 385–91) excludes both Zosime and Panthea. See also Laes 2011; H. Parker 2012.

82 *IGRR* 3, 376, on the base of a statue erected to her in the main square by her husband Asclepiades. For Panthea, see ibid. 4, 507. For Antiochis, see n. 72 here.

83 *CIG* 3736, from Bithynia. Was Vettianus himself a doctor? Her name suggests that she had been his freedwoman and pupil.

84 *CIL* 14, 2019.

85 Künzl 1995, 2002: 21–4.

86 Flemming 2000.

87 Soranus, *Gynaecology* 1, 4, 17 (an error shared with other doctors, perhaps because of a confusion with the pathological state of atresia); 1, 4, 12 (the result of a superficial dissection that suggested a continuity between the utero-ovarian ligament and the rear of the ureter).

88 Respectively, ibid. 1, 15, 48–16, 56; 1, index (missing in the text as we have it); 1, 18, 59 and index; 2, 5, 76; 2, 22, 118; 2, 12, 88 and 14, 95.

89 Lloyd 1983: 182–200.

90 Soranus, *Gynaecology* 3, 2, 17–19.

91 Ibid. 1, 6, 29.

92 Ibid. 1, 6, 29; 1, 8, 33. The last view goes against a general belief that saw menstruation as essential for female health.

93 Ibid. 1, 8, 33. As one learns from 3, 13, 47, any lack of tone in the uterus handicaps conception.

94 Ibid. 3, 14, 49; 3, 11, 43–12, 46; 4, 15, 84–8.

95 Ibid. 3, 3, 25. This condition, our 'nymphomania', is found more often in men; see the discussion in Caelius Aurelianus, *Acute Diseases* 3, 18. Cf. also Rufus of Ephesus, pp. 64–84, 119–21 Dbg.

96 Soranus, *Gynaecology* 4, 5, 26–9. See also King 1998: 213–38.

97 Soranus, *Gynaecology* 4, 2, 60–3, 62.

98 Ibid. 4, 3, 62–70. Caesarean section was not practised in Antiquity; see Gourevitch 2004.

99 Respectively, Caelius Aurelianus, *Acute Diseases* 1, 111 and 3, 35; 3, 165; 3, 137, cf. p. 126 here; *Chronic Diseases* 1, 118 and 130, cf. p. 177 here; Soranus, *Gynaecology* 4, 12; cf. Pliny, *Natural History* 28, 6, 33. Lloyd 1983: 168–82.

100 Soranus, *Gynaecology* 3, 10, 42; Caelius Aurelianus, *Chronic Diseases* 2, 151; 3, 78.

101 Caelius Aurelianus, *Chronic Diseases* 2, 44–8; Drabkin 1951.

102 Caelius Aurelianus, *Chronic Diseases* 1, 155; 162–5; Lloyd 1983: 177, n. 222.

103 Caelius Aurelianus, *Chronic Diseases* 1, 162–5 (although Soranus is not explicitly mentioned as his Greek source); 4, 13, with Nutton 1998.

104 Nutton 1990c.

105 Galen, 14, 599–605: *CMG* 5, 8, 1, 148–56.

14 HUMORAL ALTERNATIVES

1 The fragmentary remains of Pneumatism were collected first by Matthaei (1808) and later by Wellmann (1895). Neither included the writings of Aretaeus or Anonymus Londinensis (on whom see p. 211 here).

2 Galen, *On Cohesive Causes* 1, 2: *CMG* Suppl. Or. 2, 54–5 (Arabic and English); 134 (Latin).

3 Kudlien 1962, 1968b.

4 W. D. Smith 1979: 231–4.

5 Galen, 1, 486; [Galen], *Introduction* 2 and 9: 14, 676, 698.

6 C. R. S. Harris 1973: 238–41.

7 Oribasius, *Medical Collections* 9, 5 and 12: *CMG* 6, 1, 2, 6; 12–14.

8 Galen notes his embryology at 4, 612; his views on pulse at 8, 646; 750–7.

9 Galen, 1, 457.

10 [Galen], *Definitions*: 19, 347; cf. Caelius Aurelianus, *Acute Diseases* 2, 53.

11 Athenaeus, cited by Oribasius, *Medical Collections*, Libr. inc. 39: *CMG* 6, 4, 139; 141, from *On the Healthy Diet*.

12 For pulses, see Galen, 7, 749, 754, 786, 935–6; for fevers, see 7, 367.

13 For medical aspects of bathing and for new archaeological material, see R. Jackson 1990b, 1992; Künzl 1986.

14 Agathinus, reported by Oribasius, *Medical Collections* 10, 7: *CMG* 6, 1, 2, 49–53.

15 Suda, s.v. Archigenes. Mavroudis (2000) is an exhaustive study.

16 C. R. S. Harris 1973: 251–7; Mavroudis 2000: 55–68.

17 Fabricius 1972: 198–9.

18 For amulets, see Galen, 12, 874; 13, 256.

19 Kudlien 1963, 1970a; Oberhelman 1994, but omitting the Galenic material discussed below. Since the Pneumatists may have continued well into Late Antiquity (the Roman doctor Alexander styles himself 'Christian and Pneumatist' (*CIG* 9792), unless the epithet means 'man of the Spirit'; cf. *CIG* 9578), an early date for Athenaeus does not necessarily entail one for Aretaeus.

20 [Alexander], *On Fevers* 1; 92; 97; 105 Ideler. For the date, see Tassinari 1994. If the description of the ascetic seeker after wisdom, Aretaeus, *Chronic Diseases* 2, 29, alludes to Christians, this would prove a later date, but this is far from certain, for there were pagan ascetics also.

21 Aretaeus, *Chronic Diseases* 4, 13, 20.

22 Galen, *A Sketch of Empiricism* 10: tr. Walzer and Frede 1985: 39–40 = Deichgräber 1965: 75–9.

23 Galen, 12, 312.

24 The most recent edition is that by C. Hude (ed. 2, *CMG* 2, 1958). The older edition (Leipzig: C. Cnobloch, 1828), by K. G. Kühn (assisted by the young Wilhelm Dindorf), is still valuable for its notes and indexes. The only English translation remains F. Adams (1856).

25 Deichgräber 1971; Roselli 2005.

26 Respectively, Aretaeus, *Acute Diseases* 1, 5; 2, 3; and *Chronic Diseases* 2, 2.

27 Idem, *Chronic Diseases* 1, 11.

28 Garofalo 1997.

29 Anonymus Londinensis (esp. cols. 23–4 and 32–4), but his emphasis on 'emanations', a term familiar in Epicurean philosophy, warns against a simple identification.

30 'Pneumatism' could, on this argument, be merely an ahistorical, classificatory term.

31 The ps. Galenic tract *Medical Definitions* (19, 346–462), written between 70 and 150, has often been considered a Pneumatist work, but although some of its definitions may go back to a Pneumatist source it cannot be properly described as such (see Kollesch 1973).

32 Strabo, *Geography* 14, 19; Pliny, *Natural History* 29, 2, 2; Soranus, *Life of Hippocrates* 4, from Andreas' *The Descent of Medicine*. The mss. of the *Life* have him burning the archive at Cnidus, which may be another variant of the story.

33 Largus, *Drug Recipes*, pref. 5; see p. 177 here.

34 Marganne (2001) lists twenty-two Hippocratic papyri, mostly from Late Antiquity.

35 Roselli 1988; Glycon, *IGRR* 4, 507 ('Hippocrates died well; but he is dead no longer; nor I, no less famous than old Hippocrates'); Clement of Alexandria, *Miscellany* 2, 20. In general, see Kudlien 1989; Temkin 1991: 126–45.

36 For the Coan coins (from the first two centuries) and mosaic, see Hillert 1990: 24–9 and pl. 1, 2 and 5; for Ostia, see Meiggs 1973: 233–4, 562–4, arguing for a date around 120; Hommel (1957, 1970) ingeniously suggests a link with a physician to the Emperor Marcus Aurelius in the 160s.

37 *Griechische Versinschriften* 1632, probably from this period.

38 *IG* 9, 1, 881 (before AD 200). I am not entirely convinced of the authenticity of the inscriptions referring to Hippocrates and reported by Peek (1969b: 33–4) to have been found in the stoa of the ancient baths on the island of Nisyros.

39 L. Robert 1962: 220, n. 374.

40 The obscurity of much of *Nutriment* (IX, 94–121 L.) and its late vocabulary raise extremely difficult problems of interpretation. Cf. Galen's belief in the methods of Hippocratic forgers, *Commentary on Epidemics I*: *CMG* 5, 10, 1, 213; *Commentary on Epidemics VI*: *CMG* 5, 10, 2, 2, 355; and his story of the spoof passage invented by Lucian for explication by an Alexandrian teacher, *Commentary on Epidemics I*: *CMG* 5, 10, 1, 402.

41 Erotian, *Hippocratic Glossary*, pref.: the work as we have it has undergone later redaction (see Ilberg 1893; Nachmanson 1917, 1918). For the Andromachi, see p. 181 here.

42 Aulus Gellius, *Attic Nights* 3, 16, 8, quoting *Nutriment* 42. His learned circle in Athens expected its members to be acquainted with medical themes as part of general culture (see the condemnation of the unfortunate disputant who confused 'veins' and 'arteries', ibid. 18, 10, 8, and Marcus Aurelius, *Meditations* 2, 2).

43 Galen, *Commentary on Epidemics II*: *CMG* 5, 10, 2, 1, 11; 16; 167.

44 Anonymus Londinensis 6, 6–7, 7; cf. p. 59 here.

45 W. D. Smith 1979: 234.

46 Galen, 15, 21.

47 Ilberg 1890; Pfaff 1932a; W. D. Smith 1979: 235–40; Manetti and Roselli 1994: 1617–35; Manetti 2009b; von Staden 2009b.

48 Galen, *Commentary on Epidemics VI*: *CMG* 5, 10, 2, 2, 212; 293; Pfaff 1932b.

49 Galen, 18A, 248. For Julian's bias against Sabinus, see 18A, 255.

50 For Galen's comments about prognosis, see, for example, 7, 487; 14, 600–5: *CMG* 5, 8, 1, 72–5; *On Examining the Physician* 3, 17–4, 5; 5, 18–19: *CMG* Suppl. Or. 4: 60–2; 78–9; *On Medical Terminology* 29; Meyerhof and Schacht 1930–1.

51 Lloyd 1991: 398–416.

52 Suda, s.v. Rufus; Damocrates, cited by Galen, 14, 119, calling him 'an excellent man, skilled in his art'. His dates are assured from Pliny, *Natural History* 24, 28, 43; 25, 49, 87.

53 The identification is strongly urged by Kudlien (1975), not least because Rufus himself wrote a poem on plants (Galen, 11, 796 K.). For Me(n)nius or M(a)enius Rufus, see the recipe copied by Asclepiades Pharmacion, *apud* Galen, 13, 1010 K. Neither *nomen* is as yet found among Ephesian names. The mention of Rufus of Ephesus by Galen (5, 105: tr. M. Grant 2000: 19) among the 'recent' doctors is too vague to bear any weight. Swain (2008: 114) suggests that Rufus was mentioned in Crito's *Getica*, and, more speculatively, that he may have had links with the court. In general, see Nutton 2008b.

54 Rufus, *Medical Questions* 65–72: tr. A. J. Brock 1929: 123–4; *On the Names of Bodily Parts*, p. 151 Dbg. For Asia Minor, see *Medical Questions* 29–33: tr. A. J. Brock 1929: 117–18.

55 The old discussion of his writings (Ilberg 1930) is not entirely superseded by the studies listed in n. 60 here.

56 Quotation from *On the Names of Bodily Parts*, pref. The standard edition is that of Daremberg and Ruelle (1879 = Dbg), which also contains many of the fragments preserved by later authors. More recent editions of the treatises named are: *On Gout*, ed. Mørland 1933; *On the Names of Bodily Parts*, ed. Kowalski 1960; *On Diseases of the Kidneys and Bladder*, ed. Sideras 1977.

57 Gärtner 1962 (with an excellent commentary), 1970. A partial English translation is A. J. Brock (1929: 113–24).

58 For botany, see Rufus, p. 292 Dbg = Galen, 11, 796; 12, 425; for plague, see Oribasius, *Medical Collections* 44, 17 (for buboes); *Synopsis* 6, 25. His prophylactic potion ('I've never seen anyone who's drunk it not survive') is recorded by Paul of Aegina (*Seven Books* 2, 35 = p. 439 Dbg). But not everyone will believe his claim that the way to distinguish between plague caused by bad air and that by foul exhalations from the underground is to see whether birds or animals die first (p. 352 Dbg).

59 Respectively, Mørland 1933; Ullmann 1983, 1978c (but not all the cases are necessarily those of Rufus, despite Ullmann's title). For a discussion of other material from Arabic sources, see Ullmann 1994.

60 For general studies of Rufus' medicine, see Abou Aly 1992; Sideras 1994; Thomassen and Probst 1994.

61 Rufus, *Medical Questions* 3, 16: tr. A. J. Brock 1929: 115.

62 Galen, 16, 636; 19, 57–8: tr. P. N. Singer 1997: 27; *Commentary on Epidemics VI*: *CMG* 5, 10, 2, 2, 174, 411. He accepted *Aphorisms* as a genuine work of Hippocrates, Stephanus, *Commentary on Aphorisms* 1, pref.; but fr. 6 (p. 295 Dbg) is a Renaissance pastiche.

63 Ibid. 13: tr. A. J. Brock 1929: 123–4.

64 Galen, 5, 105: tr. M. Grant 2000: 19; Rufus, 354–60, 454–9, 519 Dbg; Ullmann 1978b: 72–7; Pormann (2008) offers a comprehensive discussion of this tract, its sources and influence, as well as a text and translation of the surviving fragments.

65 Rufus, *Medical Questions* 13: tr. A. J. Brock 1929: 123–4. Cf., for another example of interrogation, *On Gout* 2. Rufus, fr. 311: p. 511 Dbg, may come from a treatise on *Hippocratic Medicine*, but other sources are possible.

66 Rufus, *On the Names of Bodily Parts* 8–10. This method was followed by some of Galen's teachers. Cf., for Rufus' anatomical terminology, Lloyd 1983: 149–67.

67 Many of the shorter titles preserved in Rhazes may in fact be merely section headings from this big work (see the discussion in Ilberg (1930) and Ullmann (1994)).

68 Rufus, pp. 463; 464–8; 500; 504; 524–9 Dbg, with Ullmann 1974.

69 In general, on his treatise *On Bringing Up Children*, see Ullmann 1975; Pormann 1999.

70 Rosenthal 1975: 204; cf. Apuleius, *Apology* 45 and Pliny, *Natural History* 32, 47, 135.

71 The particular problems of homosexuals are discussed in a fragment quoted by Qusta ibn Luqa (ed. P. Sbath, *Bulletin de l'Institut d'Egypte* 23, 1941, p. 134).

72 *I. Ephesos* 1161–9, 4101b. The four classes, *suntagma*, *cheirourgia*, *problema* and *organa*, appear to deal, respectively, with medical recipes, surgery, an impromptu topic for debate and (new?) instruments, but other translations are possible.

73 For the Museum, see *I. Ephesos* 3239, with Nutton 1995d: 7–9.

74 See the surveys on aspects of culture in Bowman *et al.* (2000: 875–1008). The cultural context, although without direct reference to Rufus, is discussed in König 2005; Gill *et al.* 2009.

75 *TAM* 2, 2, 910 = *IGRR* 3, 733; cf. 732.

76 *CIG* 3311 = Petzl 1983: 536.

77 *Griechische Versinschriften* 2020 (cf. 445 for another medical poet); *Bulletin épigraphique* 1983, 426.

78 [Galen], *Medical Definitions*: 19, 346–462, with Kollesch 1973; [Galen], *Introduction*: 14, 674–797 (for its surgery, see p. 188 here); Galen, 4, 489–93; cf. for his own summary of the *Method of Healing*, Garofalo 1999, and for another surviving tract on fevers, Tassinari 1994.

79 *Greek Anthology* 7, 158, probably to be identified with his verse *Iatrica*, *Medical Matters*, in forty books; Heitsch 1964: 16–22; von Wilamowitz-Moellendorff 1928; Wellmann 1934. Marcellus was later patronised by the famous orator and consul Herodes Atticus.

80 [Galen], *Whether What Is in the Womb Is a Living Being*: 19, 158–81 (the peroration, 179–81, is full of literary and historical allusions; last edition, by H. Wagner, diss. Marburg, 1914); [Galen], *How the Foetus is Ensouled* (ed. Kalbfleisch 1895: tr. Wilberding 2011) is possibly by the Neoplatonist Porphyry; for Asclepiades, see p. 181 here.

81 Galen, 19, 8: tr. P. N. Singer 1997: 3, with the emendation of Cornarius, Γαληνοῦ for-νὸς, to bring it into line with the subtitle of the *Introduction*. The ms. reading gives the heading simply as 'By Dr. Galen'. Cf. the story at *On My Own Opinions* 1: *CMG* 5, 3, 2, 54–6; Boudon-Millot and Pietrobelli 2005: 172.

82 Galen, 10, 457: 4, 22: tr. May 1968: 559.

83 W. D. Smith 1979.

84 Galen, 18B, 926–7; *Anatomical Procedures* 14, 1: p. 184 Dkw.

85 For Lycus, see Galen, 18B, 927; for Quintus, see Galen, *Anatomical Procedures* 14, 1: p. 184 Dkw. Hunain ibn Ishaq in the mid-ninth century believed that a commentary on *The Nature of the Child*, preserved in Syriac, had been originally written by Pelops; Bergsträsser 1925: 36, no. 108.

86 Galen, 15, 136; W. D. Smith 1979: 68.

87 Rosenthal 1956; Nutton 2012c. The case for Galenic authorship is argued by Strohmaier (1970, 2004) and Jouanna (1991), but Galen's failure to mention any such commentary, or, indeed, to make use of the *Oath* in any of his writings on medical deontology is a major objection. This commentary is oddly neglected by modern students of Asclepius.

88 Oribasius, *Medical Collections* 9, 15–20: *CMG* 6, 1, 2, 15–20.

89 Ibid. 9, 10: *CMG* 6, 1, 2, 11. The Galenic passage comes in the commentary of *Airs, Waters and Places* (information from Prof. G. Strohmaier).

90 Antyllus, ibid. 9, 9 and 11: *CMG* 6, 1, 2, 11–12; Galen, ibid. 9, 10: *CMG* 6, 1, 2, 11–12. Cf. Borca 2000; Nutton 2000b.

91 For this treatise, which survives in Arabic, and in partial translations in Hebrew and Latin, see Ullmann 1977; Wasserstein 1982: 157–64; Jouanna 1996a: 133–48. An edition by G. Strohmaier is forthcoming in the *CMG* series.

92 Galen, *Commentary on Epidemics II*: *CMG* 5, 10, 1, 321.

93 Galen, 2, 280–2: tr. C. Singer 1956: 30–1, distinguishing between a (fanciful) earlier age when anatomical knowledge was passed from father to son and the modern task of restoring that tradition; Grmek and Gourevitch 1994.

94 Galen, 18A, 113, 123; *Commentary on Epidemics II*: *CMG* 5, 10, 1, 312.

95 Galen, 19, 29–30: Boudon-Millot *et al.* 2007: 151–3: tr. P. N. Singer 1997: 12–13.

96 Galen, 19, 25–31: Boudon-Millot *et al.* 2007: 147–53: tr. P. N. Singer 1997: 11–13; 2, 1–2: tr. C. Singer 1956: 31–2.

97 I follow the reading of the Arabic at *Anatomical Procedures* 1, 1: 2, 218 = 5, 7 Garofalo. See Nutton 1987; Grmek and Gourevitch 1988, 1994.

98 Galen, *Commentary on Epidemics II*: *CMG* 5, 10, 1, 312.

99 Galen, 14, 614–19: *CMG* 5, 8, 1, 84–7; 19, 13–15: Boudon-Millot *et al.* 2007: 138–9: tr. P. N. Singer 1997: 5–6 (although the list of Galen's works prepared by the Arabic translator Hunain gives the number as five). The man's name is spelled variously in the manuscripts.

100 Boudon 2001, 2002; Boudon-Millot 2007: 153–4 (a new Greek text), with her commentary.

101 Galen, 19, 16: Boudon-Millot *et al.* 2007: 153: tr. P. N. Singer 1997: 7. The treatise *On the Anatomy of the Womb* (2, 887–908) was given a modern edition and commentary by Nickel 1971: *CMG* 5, 2, 1.

102 Galen, *On My Own Books* 4, 34–8: Boudon-Millot *et al.* 2007: 153.

103 Ibid. 4, 37: Boudon-Millot *et al.* 2007: 153: tr. P. N. Singer 1997: 9–10, with Debru 1995a; König 2005: 254–300; Gleason 2009.

15 THE LIFE AND CAREER OF GALEN

1 A good biography of Galen in English is still lacking: Sarton (1954) is full of error. Better are Temkin (1973: 10–63), W. D. Smith (1979) and P. N. Singer (1997: vii–xliii). The most detailed accounts are by Schlange-Schöningen (2001), Hankinson (2008: 1–148) and the introductions to Boudon-Millot *et al.* (2007); P. N. Singer (2012). Nutton (2010a) attempts some contextualisation.

2 The time of year is clear from 15, 599–600, 'just entering my 29th year' at the autumn equinox, but the year itself is disputed. His first Roman stay is firmly dated to 162–6 by the external evidence for the Parthian campaign of Lucius Verus of 162–6: Verus was away during the first winter of Galen's stay in Rome, and had not returned when Galen left hurriedly three years later (14, 613; 647; 649: *CMG* 5, 8, 1, 83; 116–19). At the end of his life (19, 15–16: tr. P. N. Singer 1997: 6) Galen stated that his refutation of his Roman opponents during his first months took place when he was in his 34th year and that he had returned home 'when 37 years had been completed since my birth' – that is, he was born in 129, confirmed now by *Avoiding Distress* 34: tr. Nutton 2012a, where he puts his arrival in Rome 'in my thirty-third year', i.e. aged 32. However, in the earlier commentary on *Joints* (18A, 347) he remarked that he had stayed in Rome since his 32nd year – that is, he was born in 130 – but this then requires an extremely long return journey to Pergamum of over a year. For a more detailed exposition of this chronology, without the evidence of *Avoiding Distress*, see Nutton 1973.

3 Habicht 1969; Koester 1998.

4 The occupations of his grandfather and great-grandfather are given at *Avoiding Distress* 59: tr. Nutton 2012a. How wealthy Galen was is hard to determine. His comments at 5, 37–52 (tr. P. N. Singer 1997: 117–25) indicate substantial wealth, although only half that of his friend, who was among the wealthiest of the 40,000 male inhabitants of Pergamum (cf. 5, 49–50: tr. P. N. Singer 1997: 123–5). For the possibility that his retainer as an imperial doctor was HS 200,000, and that he had equestrian status, see Christol and Drew-Bear 2004: 111. For his father's farms, see 6, 546, 552: tr. Powell 2003: 66, 69; 6, 755, 783; 11, 336; 14, 17–21; 18A, 49; and for meteorology, see Jouanna 2007: 314–15.

5 Galen, 5, 40–50; cf. also 5, 17: tr. P. N. Singer 1997: 119–21, 107–8; 6, 755. He mentions no brothers or sisters, or a wife: given the example of his parents and his belief that people needed to be on the same intellectual highway for affection to develop between them (cited by al-Mas'udi, *Muruj al-dhahab*: tr. Meisami 1989: 275–6), it is likely that Galen never married.

6 Galen, 6, 552: tr. Powell 2003: 52; 6, 755, 783; 8, 587; 14, 17; 19, 40 and 59: tr. P. N. Singer 1997: 18, 27. His name is known only from Byzantine sources (Suda, s.v. Galenos; Tzetzes, *Chiliads* 12, 8), but there is no strong reason for doubt.

7 For the two men, see Diller 1936a. The poem to the sun (*CIG* 3546) also contains Euripidean allusions, and would bear out Galen's comments on his father's learning. If his father was an Aelius, it is tempting to associate his citizenship with his architectural achievements during Hadrian's reign. The origin of the name Claudius found in the printed Greek editions is obscure. A very late scribe of one tract in Vlatadon 14 does give that *nomen*, but it is not found in any other MS of the treatise concerned, and no author,

Byzantine, Arabic or Latin, appears to know of it. Two contemporary architects called Nicon is a coincidence, three is even more unlikely.

8   For his moral example, *Avoiding Distress* 58–64: tr. Nutton 2012a. For other fathers coming with their sons to school, cf. Horace, *Satires* 1, 6, 81; Epictetus, *Discourses* 2, 14, 1.

9   Galen, 5, 41: tr. P. N. Singer 1997: 119; 6, 755; 783; 8, 587; 19, 43: tr. P. N. Singer 1997: 19–20; *Avoiding Distress* 58–62: tr. Nutton 2012a. For toys, see 3, 262: tr. May 1968: 193. For the Arabic story, see Rosenthal 1975: 34, with which cf. 6, 756; 19, 59: tr. P. N. Singer 1997: 32.

10   Galen, 10, 609; 14, 608: *CMG* 5, 8, 1, 78 (pl.); 16, 223; 19, 59: tr. P. N. Singer 1997: 27. By Late Antiquity the story had changed, and some thought Galen's move to medicine had been ordained by an oracle (Lenz 1959: 115). For Galen's belief in Asclepius, see p. 218 here and von Staden 2003.

11   For Nicon's death, see Galen, 6, 756. For Galen's wealth, see Galen, 5, 44–7, 59: tr. P. N. Singer 1997: 20–1, 28; 10, 609; note also the feeble denial that Galen's personal wealth had not helped his career (10, 561).

12   See pp. 217–19 here. Lopez Ferez 2010: 371–9; W. D. Smith 1979: 62–77. Galen's stay at Corinth was brief, since he found his intended teacher, Numisianus, was no longer there.

13   Nutton 1993b, to which add the reference at Galen, 13, 631; for a (later) non-medical awareness of the cachet of a stay at Alexandria, see Nutton 1972.

14   Nutton 1993b. For astronomy, see pp. 272–3 here. I am grateful to Gotthard Strohmaier for information from the unpublished commentary on *Airs, Waters and Places*.

15   P. Giessen 43; *L'Année Epigraphique* 1968: 159; 1992: 341. [Soranus], *Introduction* pp. 244–5 Rose recommends beginning medical education at the age of 15.

16   See p. 263 here.

17   Galen, 14, 608: *CMG* 5, 8, 1, 77, should not be pressed to mean that Galen was intended for a career as a professional philosopher; Bowersock (1969, 2010a) puts Galen into the right context, although Galen usually contrasts the errors of 'sophists' with the appropriate methods of the philosopher–doctor. See also Kollesch 1981; Swain 1996: 357–79. Doctors figure in Plutarch's *Table Talk*, and medical themes are discussed in Aulus Gellius' *Attic Nights* and Athenaeus' *Sophists at Dinner*. The conceit goes back, of course, to Plato's *Symposium*, in which Dr Eryximachus participates.

18   Nutton 1971b, 1995d. Note also a new inscription of a doctor member of the Ephesus Museum (*I. Ephesos* 3239).

19   For his writings on grammar, see Galen, 19, 48: tr. P. N. Singer 1997: 22. They included a work on *Clarity and Unclarity* and another on *Attic Shibboleths* (Herbst 1911).

20   Nutton 2011: 254.

21   For the library, see Wilkins 2007; Nutton 2009; and above p. 4 here. His writings in Greek amount to approximately 10 per cent of all surviving Greek literature before AD 350. Precise details are impossible, because his own catalogue of his books (19, 8–48: tr. P. N. Singer 1997: 3–22; important additions in Boudon-Millot *et al.* 2007) omits several works that he believed had been totally lost, especially after the fire of 192. The Arabic scholar–translator Hunain ibn Ishaq (809–77) listed fifty Galenic works not included by Galen in his own catalogue (Bergsträsser 1932). Fichtner (1990) gives 434 separate titles, not all of them genuine. Taking an ancient book-roll as the equivalent of thirty printed pages, I estimate that he wrote/dictated two or three pages a day over a working life of some sixty years, on top of his other activities. The standard edition, by Kühn (1821–33), contains a Greek text with subjoined Latin translation; discoveries since then, especially of versions in Latin or Arabic, have added another 20 or 30 per cent to its approximately 16,000 pages, and others are still in prospect. The introduction to Boudon-Millot *et al.* (2007) provides the best summary of the textual history of his

writings, including information on Vlatadon 14, and is supplemented for Arabic sources by Boudon-Millot (2011).

22 Galen, *On Examining the Physician*, *CMG* Suppl. Or. 4, *passim*. The prospective patient should not be acutely ill, since the process of investigation takes time.

23 Galen, 9, 804; 10, 19: tr. Hankinson 1991: 11; 10, 406; similar abuse, using the same occupational categories, was levelled against the Christians (Origen, *Against Celsus* 3, 55).

24 Lloyd 1991: 398–416; Jouanna 2010.

25 See p. 54 here; Deichgräber 1970: 31–51; Jouanna 1997.

26 Lloyd 1991: 398–417.

27 W. D. Smith 1979; Manetti and Roselli 1994; Flemming 2008. They occupy five fat volumes in Kühn's edition of the Greek (1821–33), and the rediscovery of several genuine commentaries in Arabic, such as that on *Epidemics* 2 and much of that on *Epidemics* 6, more than makes up for the presence in Kühn of spurious commentaries on *Humours* and *Nutriment*.

28 Galen, 18B, 318–22.

29 Galen, 17B, 345–56, an excellent example of Galen's mixture of genius and perversity.

30 Galen, *Avoiding Distress* 23–8: tr. Nutton 2012a; Deichgräber 1956.

31 Manetti and Roselli 1994.

32 The importance of the Galenic search for authenticity is emphasised by W. D. Smith 1979.

33 Galen, 19, 62–157. An edition of this text is being prepared by Lorenzo Perilli; see Perilli 2007.

34 For *Prorrhetic*, see *CMG* 5, 9, 2, 32–3; and for Galen's comments on this work and *Coan Prognoses* in his commentary on *Epidemics* 3, see *CMG* 5, 10, 2, 1, 62–4. The discussion of Manetti and Roselli (1994: 1550–2) is more accurate than W. D. Smith's (1979: 155–60). For Galen's view of *Ancient Medicine*, see *CMG* 5, 10, 1, 220.

35 For earlier attempts to distinguish between authentic and non-authentic works by Hippocrates, see W. D. Smith 1979; Kudlien 1989: 364–5. In view of the importance given to *The Sacred Disease* in modern scholarship, it is interesting to note that Galen did not count it a genuine work of Hippocrates (cf. Grensemann 1968: 48).

36 Barnes 1990; for Heraclitus, see p. 215 here; was the moralising poetaster Sarapion (Oliver 1936) also a doctor?

37 Galen, *On Medical Experience*, ed. Walzer 1944; translation repr. in Walzer and Frede 1985: 49–106; *On My Own Opinions*, ed. Nutton 1999, *CMG* 5, 3, 2; full Greek text in Boudon-Millot and Pietrobelli 2005.

38 The first treatise is lost in Greek; the second, *Avoiding Distress*, came to light in Greek in 2005 – see Boudon-Millot *et al.* 2010: tr. Nutton 2012a. For logic, see Stakelum 1940; Bobzien 2002; Barnes 2007.

39 Galen, *That the Best Physician is Also a Philosopher*: 1, 53–63: tr. P.N. Singer 1997: 30–4. This is the general message of Temkin (1973).

40 Galen, 5, 41–5; cf. 68; 19, 59: tr. P. N. Singer 1997: 119–21, 132, 27.

41 Galen, *On My Own Opinions* 2, 1–3, 1: *CMG* 5, 3, 2, 56–62; 131–45; Boudon-Millot and Pietrobelli 2005: 172–3.

42 Von Müller 1895; Strohmaier 1998; Galen, *Introduction to Logic*, ed. Kalbfleisch 1896: tr. Kieffer 1964; *On Fallacies*, 14, 582–98: tr. Edlow 1977; ed. and tr. Ebbesen 1981, 1, 79–87; 2, *passim*.

43 Rescher 1965, 1966; Moraux 1984: 706, n. 99.

44 Walzer 1949; Gero 1990. For his philosophy in general, see Barnes and Jouanna 2003; Hankinson 2008: 49–241. For his eclecticism, contrast Hankinson (1992b) with Donini (1992: 3502–4), who calls it simply fudge.

45 Lloyd 1996; for definitions, see Hood 2010.

46 Moraux 1984: 735–85.

47 DeLacy 1988; Galen, *On My Own Opinions* 3, 1; 7, 1–5; 13, 1–15, 9: *CMG* 5, 3, 2, 58–61; 76–81; 102–25; Boudon-Millot and Pietrobelli 2005: 173, 178–9, 185–9.

48 Galen, *On My Own Opinions* 2, 1–3: *CMG* 5, 3, 2, 56–9: Boudon-Millot and Pietrobelli 2005: 172–3; Hankinson 1989; Flemming 2009.

49 Barnes 1991; Hankinson 1991.

50 Hankinson 1991: 373–403.

51 See Frede's *Introduction* to Walzer and Frede 1985.

52 Galen, *CMG* 5, 10, 2, 2, 483–7. For children, see Walzer 1962: 154–61. In general see Gill 2010; and the introductions in P. N. Singer (2012), which also contains new information taken from Galen's observations of animals.

53 For Arria, see Galen, 14, 208; for demonstrations, see 14, 627: *CMG* 5, 8, 1, 96–7.

54 Galen, *On Examining the Physician* 9, 4–6: *CMG* Suppl. Or. 4, 103–5, where Galen claims to have challenged his competitors for the post to replace the intestines of a monkey as effectively as he had just done (13, 599; 18B, 567). 13, 599 also shows another way in which Galen established his reputation quickly.

55 Galen's formulation at 13, 599 and 18B, 567 suggests that this was a local 'High Priest' of the imperial cult at Pergamum rather than the high priest of the province of Asia (Schlange-Schöningen 2001: 84–94).

56 Galen, 13, 599. L. Robert (1940a) remains fundamental. Note also L. Robert's discussion (*Bulletin épigraphique* 1962, no. 294) of the high priest's right to give a gladiatorial show. Cf., for other doctors involved with the games and shows, *IG* 4, 365; *CIG* 6, 10085; 10171–3. *CIL* 3, 12925 = *ILS* 5119 is the epitaph of a gladiator who died 'under treatment'. On Cos around AD 50 twenty-four gladiators were killed in the games given by a local worthy; Bosnakis and Hallof 2008: 224. For the rising costs of gladiators, see the decree of the senate on this subject (*ILS* 5163).

57 Galen, 2, 345: tr. C. Singer 1956: 62; 3, 287: tr. May 1968: 215; 5, 160: tr. Furley and Wilkie 1984: 205; 8, 304; 10, 378; 11, 227; 13, 599; 18B, 567, although not all of these may be references to his time at Pergamum. Cf. Scarborough 1971; Schlange-Schöningen 2001: 97–102. New palaeopathological evidence of gladiators from Ephesus throws much light on Galen's activities (see *Sunday Times Magazine*, 15 December 2002), suggesting that their diet aimed to add bulk.

58 This version (Galen, *On Examining the Physician* 9, 4–7: *CMG* Suppl. Or. 4, 102–5 = Meyerhof 1929: 77, with a more accurate translation) is preferable to that in 13, 600, which claims that no gladiator died in his first term. Cf. also 8, 304: tr. Siegel 1976: 139, for his personal observation of a gladiator who died a day after being wounded in the left ventricle of the heart. Galen's figure may refer solely to deaths in training.

59 Galen, 10, 455; 18A, 347. For his possible travels, see Nutton 1973: 165–70.

60 Galen, 14, 622: *CMG* 5, 8, 1, 92–3. It remains, of course, possible that this *stasis* broke out when he was already in Rome. The word is never applied to an external war (and hence speculation about a Parthian invasion, let alone a civil war between the Pergamenians and the Galatians, is foolish); for local rivalries, cf. Dio Chrysostom, *Orations* 38–51; Pliny, *Letters* 10, 48; 81–2; Suda, s.v. Cephalion = *FGrH* 93 T 1; *Epigrammata graeca* 877b. Galen himself wrote a short tract *On Concord*, very much a political term (19, 46: tr. P. N. Singer 1997: 21). But the word can also indicate any sort of local commotion (*Acts* 24, 5).

61 Galen, 14, 605–19: *CMG* 5, 8, 1, 74–89.

62 Ibid. 14, 612–13; 625–6; 629: *CMG* 5, 8, 1, 80–3; 94–9; Debru 1995a.

63 For Victorinus, see Galen, *CMG* 5, 9, 1, 265: *CMG* Suppl. Or. 2, 77; for Martius, see 16, 457.

64 Galen, 14, 599–605; 625; 648: *CMG* 5, 8, 1, 69–75; 94–5; 116–19. One would love to know when he wrote *On Slander* 19, 46 (tr. P. N. Singer 1997: 21), in which he included some details of his own life.

65 Galen, 19, 15: tr. P. N. Singer 1997: 6, with Nutton 1973: 159. For reactions to the plague in Asia Minor, see Lucian, *Alexander* 36; Lane Fox 1986: 231–5.

66 Galen, 19, 17: tr. P. N. Singer 1997: 7, with Nutton 1973: 169.

67 Galen, 14, 649–50: *CMG* 5, 8, 1, 118–21; 19, 17–18: tr. P. N. Singer 1997: 7–8. For Lucius' death, cf. Historia Augusta, *Verus* 9, 10; *Marcus Aurelius* 14, 7. The account in Aelian (fr. 206 Hercher) implies a sudden death, perhaps from a stroke akin to what he had had in 166 (Fronto, *Letters* 2, 6).

68 Schlange-Schöningen (2001: 138–42) notes that there is no clear proof that Galen returned to Rome before late 169, when he would have been sent back by Marcus from Aquileia. But the implication of the wording at Galen, 14, 650: *CMG* 5, 8, 1, 118–19 is that Galen was 'left behind' in Rome when Marcus departed.

69 Galen, 19, 18: tr. P. N. Singer 1997: 7–8; 14, 4: tr. A. J. Brock 1929: 197; 14, 650: *CMG* 5, 8, 1, 118–21.

70 Galen, 14, 650; 661–5: *CMG* 5, 8, 1, 118–21; 130–5.

71 Horstmanshoff 1995; Gourevitch 2001a. For the frightened politicians, see *CMG* 5, 10, 2, 2, 494; for athletes, see 2, 632: tr. C. Singer 1956: 192 with *CMG* 5, 4, 1, 2, 74–6; 3, 890: tr. May 1968: 526; 6, 446: tr. R. M. Green 1951: 274; 8, 254; 10, 407; 490; 608; 671; 11, 227; 18A, 348. In what language did he address his patients? Although his style has very few Latinisms in it, and although, with one dubious exception (Galen, 14, 183), he never cites a Latin book, one can hardly believe that he was not fluent enough in Latin to communicate with those who had no Greek, even if most of the higher circles in which he moved in Rome consisted of fellow Greeks and those fluent in Greek. Cf. Adams 2008.

72 Meyerhof 1929: 85, from *How to Profit from One's Enemies*. For a gift of 400 gold pieces for curing the wife of Boethus, see Galen, 14, 647: *CMG* 5, 8, 1, 116–17. For New Year gifts to one's doctor not counting as payment, see Justinian, *Digest* 19, 5, 26, 1.

73 E.g. 'friends and pupils', Galen, 19, 10: tr. P. N. Singer 1997: 3; 'friends and colleagues' (or 'pupils'), 17A, 576. Andorlini (2000) neatly aligns Galen's methods of exposition with the evidence of papyri and tomb reliefs. For the charlatan, see Meyerhof 1929: 83, from *On Diseases Hard to Cure*.

74 Nutton 1973: 167; Harig 1987–8.

75 Galen, *On Morals*: tr. Walzer 1949: 67. For the importance of this passage for dating other psychological texts, see P. N. Singer 2012.

76 *Avoiding Distress* 54: tr. Nutton 2012a; for the move to Campania, ibid. 10–11: tr. Nutton 2012a.

77 Galen, 19, 46: tr. P.N. Singer 1997: 21, included by him among his moral treatises. For his attitude to Severus, 14, see 216–17.

78 Galen, 14, 212–14. *On Theriac, for Pamphilianus*, which probably dates from the Severan period, is unlikely to be genuine (see Nutton 1997a).

79 See pp. 210, 245 here; note his variations in the story of his diagnosis of lovesickness. At *On Prognosis* 6: 14, 630–5 (*CMG* 5, 8, 1, 100–5), it is a woman in love with an actor; later, in his commentary on *Prognostic* (*CMG* 5, 9, 2, 218), it is a man in love with a woman. The former account is more likely to be true because of its circumstantial detail.

80 Galen, *On My Own Opinions*, 11, 1–4: CMG 5, 3, 2, 90–3; Boudon-Millot and Pietrobelli 2005: 182–3, with Debru 1995b.

81 Nutton 1991b.

82 For the legends of Galen's death, see Nutton 2001; Strohmaier 2007.

83 For the Alexander quotation and its relationship to *On My Own Opinions* 1, 4–2, 3: CMG 5, 3, 2, 56–9; Boudon-Millot and Pietrobelli 2005: 172–3, with the discussion at *CMG* 5, 3, 2, 37–9. That this tract was, as Arabic authors claimed, Galen's last work seems established from the cross-references within it, including one to *On My Own Books*.

84 The accident described in 14, 212–14 took place at the Secular Games, which were held only in 204. The reference to Aelius Antipater (14, 218) must predate his fall from grace following his governorship of Bithynia, datable to between 205 and 211. For the authenticity of *On Theriac*, see Swain 1996: 430–2, and, at greater length and with different arguments, Nutton 1995b, 1997a; against, Strohmaier 2007: 395–6. If the author was not Galen, he was also a doctor with links to Alexandria who had served at court for twenty-five years or more.

85 Galen, 14, 660: *CMG* 5, 8, 1, 128–9. But most of the *Meditations* were written long before Galen came on the scene.

86 Galen, *On Examining the Physician* 9, 19: *CMG* Suppl. Or. 4, 112–13. But Aulus Gellius, who shows greater familiarity with Latin than with Greek literature, made his visit to Attica before Galen visited Athens.

87 Galen, 10, 909–16; König 2005: 254–300; Mattern 2008; Rosen 2010.

88 See p. 263 here.

89 Cf. Wilkins 2011. His quotations from Scribonius Largus are taken at second hand (see p. 175 here) and may derive from Greek works by Largus. More complicated is a reference to Pliny in a lemma at 14, 183.

90 *Avoiding Distress* takes the form of a letter to a school-friend from Pergamum who had also spent time in Rome and who had remained in touch with him throughout his life.

91 The sole exception is at 6, 424: tr. R. M. Green 1951: 261, referring to springs N.E. of Rome as 'near us'.

92 Galen, 14, 23; 6, 665, 697: tr. Powell 2003: 116, 130; 6, 802; cf. 10, 832, 14, 28, and, for Galen's first taste of Falernian, see 8, 774.

93 For Severus and Caracalla, see Galen, 14, 217; for aqueducts, see 17B, 159; for roads, see 10, 632–3.

94 Galen, *On Examining the Physician*: *CMG* Suppl. Or. 4, *passim*; Meyerhof 1929: 84 (from *How to Profit from One's Enemies*).

95 Galen, 14, 641–7: *CMG* 5, 8, 1, 110–17; 11, 242, perhaps to be identified with Valerius Diodorus, author of a lexicon to the Attic orators.

96 Horstmanshoff 1995; Mattern 2008.

97 Galen, 8, 224–5: tr. Siegel 1976: 107. For the drug, see 6, 429: tr. R. M. Green 1951: 264; 13, 129. The *Advice to an Epileptic Boy* (11, 357–78: tr. Temkin 1934) is avowedly a letter to a patient he has never seen.

98 Athenaeus, *Sophists at Dinner* 1, 1e; 26c–27d; 3, 115c–116a; Wilkins 2007. In general, see Braund and Wilkins 2000: 476–502.

99 Sharples 1982; Todd 1976; Nutton 1984b: 319–23; Tieleman 1997; Fazzo (2002) is cautious.

100 Eusebius, *Ecclesiastical History* 5, 28, 13–14; Gero 1990.

101 Origen, *Philokalia* fr. 2, 2; R. M. Grant 1983. For the possibility that Clement of Alexandria knew some of Galen's philosophical writings, see Havrda 2011.

102 For Gargilius, see the introduction to Maire (2002); for the Berlin papyrus, see Hanson (1985: 39–47). Cf. Riddle 1984.

16 GALENIC MEDICINE

1 Frede 1981.

2 Von Staden 2002a. Galen's discussions of the unity of medicine are found in this tract (*CMG* Suppl. Or. 2, 22–9; 115–29) and in *On the Constitution of the Art of Medicine* 1, 224–303.

3 Galen, 2, 225, 343, 643–6: tr. C. Singer 1956: 5, 61, 197–9; 8, 213; *On Examining the Physician* 9, 23; 14, 1–4: *CMG* Suppl. Or. 4, 114–15, 134–7.

4 *The Anatomy of Bones* 2, 732–88: tr. C. Singer 1952; Garofalo and Debru 2005; *The Anatomy of Nerves* 2, 831–56: tr. Goss 1966; Garofalo and Debru 2008; *The Anatomy of Veins and Arteries* 2, 779–830: tr. Goss 1961; Garofalo and Debru 2008; *The Anatomy of Muscles* 18B, 926–1026: tr. Goss 1963; Garofalo and Debru 2005; *Anatomical Procedures*, Books 1–9: 2, 215–731: tr. C. Singer 1956; Books 9–15: tr. Duckworth 1962. In general, see Rocca 2008.

5 Galen, 3, 1–4, 366: tr. May 1968; 5, 181–805: *CMG* 5, 4, 1, 2.

6 Galen, *Compendium of the Timaeus*, ed. Kraus and Walzer 1951; *Commentary on Medicine in the Timaeus*: *CMG* Suppl. 1, 1934.

7 Galen, 3, 98–9: tr. May 1968: 118–19.

8 Galen, 13, 605–8; for the phrase, cf. 6, 480: tr. Powell 2003: 39.

9 Galen, 19, 55: tr. P. N. Singer 1997: 25; Ormos 1993.

10 Galen, 2, 218, 220: tr. C. Singer 1956: 2–3. Cf. Rufus, *On the Names of Parts*, p. 134 D–R.

11 Galen, 2, 220–2, 385: tr. C. Singer 1956: 3, 77; 13, 604; 609.

12 Galen, 2, 220–6; 323; 383–6: tr. C. Singer 1956: 3–5, 51, 76–7; *Anatomical Procedures* 11, 4: p. 86 Dkw.

13 Galen, 2, 905, with Nickel's (1971) commentary, *CMG* 5, 2, 1, 93–4, 103–6; cf. 4, 228; 3, 551; 3, 363: tr. May 1968: 662–3, 352, 256.

14 Galen, 14, 627: *CMG* 5, 8, 1, 96–7; 2, 222–3: tr. C. Singer 1956: 3–4. For the usefulness of different animals for showing different structures, see *On Problematical Movements* 11, 21–2, with Nutton 2011: 360–2.

15 Galen, 2, 690: tr. C. Singer 1956: 218.

16 Information from the late Hugh Cott, FRZS, who referred me to Sikes (1971: 217–18). A slightly different conclusion was reached independently by Scarborough (1985c) and Gourevitch (2001a: 159–60). See also Hankinson 1988. For his other animal subjects, see Rocca 2002: 89.

17 Debru 1994; Grmek 1996: 101–22.

18 Galen, 18B, 953–4; 2, 234–5: tr. C. Singer 1956: 2–3; see 3, 96 and 225: tr. May 1968: 117–18, 182, for the change of mind.

19 Rocca 2002, 2003, 2008; Manzoni 2001.

20 May (1968: 42, 771–2) lists what she believes to be Galen's anatomical discoveries. As well as those mentioned in the text, they are, among the muscles, platysma myoides, panniculus carnosus, levator palpebrae superioris and popliteus, and possibly the anastomoses of the superior and inferior gastric vessels.

21 Good examples in *On Problematical Movements* (Debru 2002; Nutton 2011).

22 Galen, 2, 36–8: tr. A. J. Brock 1916: 59–61; Temkin 1977: 162–6.

23 His work on Hippocratic anatomy (19, 55: tr. P. N. Singer 1997: 25) is now lost.

24 Galen, 2, 646–8: tr. C. Singer 1956: 199–200; 4, 734–5: tr. Furley and Wilkie 1984: 181–3.

25 Galen, 2, 634–41: tr. C. Singer 1956: 193–7; he saw the beating of the living heart in the slave of Marullus (2, 631–3: tr. C. Singer 1956: 192–3).

26 Galen, 4, 733–4: tr. Furley and Wilkie 1984: 179–81, with C. R. S. Harris 1973: 380–9, for modern repetitions of the experiment.

27 For his final view, see *On the Formation of the Foetus* 3: 4, 662–72; *On My Own Opinions* 11: *CMG* 5, 3, 2, 90–3; Boudon-Millot and Pietrobelli 2005: 182–3 (both implying that the brain was formed last). But in the former passage Galen's (unusual) change of view is from one that considered that the three organs were formed simultaneously (expressed in *On Seed* 1, 8–9: *CMG* 5, 3, 1, 92–4); in the latter from one that accepted the priority of the heart. On this problem, see Debru 1995b; Nutton 1999: 177–9.

28 This was the message of *On the Opinions of Hippocrates and Plato*, 5, 211–805: *CMG* 5, 4, 1, 2. Plato had not specified the liver as the seat of the appetitive soul.

29 Mani 1959: I, 61–104, 12.

30 Galen, 2, 9–24: tr. A. J. Brock 1916: 17–39.

31 The first book of *On the Natural Faculties* (2, 1–73: tr. A. J. Brock 1916: 2–113) is Galen's most vigorous defence of vitalism.

32 Galen, 5, 521, 534–5: *CMG* 5, 4, 1, 2, 385; 393–5.

33 C. R. S. Harris 1973: 333–8.

34 Galen, 2, 828; 3, 509; 4, 243–6: tr. May 1968: 331, 670–2. Galen claims no credit for this discovery, and there were others, like Lycus (see p. 220 here), who had investigated the foetus before him.

35 Galen, 2, 207: tr. A. J. Brock 1916: 321; 3, 455; 521; 539: tr. May 1968: 300–3; 337–8; 346.

36 C. R. S. Harris 1973: 2–3, 268; Debru 2008.

37 Both the stomach and the hot heart were perceived by Galen as cooking organs, changing the qualities of the material originally presented to them.

38 Galen, 4, 703–36: tr. Furley and Wilkie 1984: 144–83.

39 Although the *rete mirabile* is not found in humans, it appears in ungulates, on which Galen certainly experimented (Rocca 2002, 2003), and was named by Herophilus or his followers (T. 121 von Staden). Galen was thus following a long tradition in seeking a role for this organ. I am not convinced by Prioreschi (1996b) that Galen was not thinking of the *rete mirabile*.

40 Temkin 1977: 154–63, pointing out that Galen referred only rarely to a 'zotic *pneuma*' and only on one occasion – and very tentatively at that – to 'nutritive *pneuma*'.

41 Galen, *On My Own Opinions* 5, 1–7: *CMG* 5, 3, 2, 66–73; 175–6; *On Temperaments* 1, 509–694: tr. P. N. Singer 1997: 202–89.

42 Manuli and Vegetti 1988.

43 Schöner 1964; I. W. Müller 1993; Klibansky *et al.* 1964.

44 Debru 2002; Nutton 2011.

45 Kovačič 2001; Flemming 2007a.

46 Hankinson 1988, 1989.

47 Galen, 3, 904–7: tr. May 1968: 532–4; Walzer 1949: 23–37.

48 Galen, 4, 365–6: tr. May 1968: 733.

49 Ibid. 3, 606; 4, 153–8: tr. May 1968: 382, 625–8. In general, see Flemming 2000: 255–358.

50 Galen, 3, 899–901: tr. May 1968: 530–1.

51 Flemming 2000: 314–21. This belief in the general physiological unity of mankind may explain why Galen devotes little space to gynaecology as such in his writings.

52 Galen, 11, 137; 10, 181–4, 342; 13, 467–8.

53 Galen, 14, 641–4: *CMG* 5, 8, 1, 110–15.

54 Galen, 14, 218; 12, 440; 14, 662–4: *CMG* 5, 8, 1, 130–3.

55 Galen, 2, 343: tr. C. Singer 1956: 61; 8, 56; 8, 213; *On Examining the Physician* 9, 9–13: *CMG* Suppl. Or. 4, 106–9.

56 Galen, 16, 566–8.

57 Galen, *The Soul's Dependence on the Body* 1, 767–817: tr. P. N. Singer 1997: 150–76; P. N. Singer (2012) argues that the apparent physicalist position on the soul adopted in this tract is merely a repetition of others' views.

58 Sappho, fr. 31, ed. Page; Catullus, *Poems* 51, is a Latin version.

59 Philemon, fr. 106, cf. 204 K–A.

60 Galen, *Commentary on Epidemics VI*: *CMG* 5, 10, 2, 2, 483–7.

61 Galen, 14, 635–40: *CMG* 5, 8, 1, 104–11.

62 Galen, 14, 630–5: *CMG* 5, 8, 1, 100–5. For the variant versions of the story of Antiochus and Stratonice, see p. 157, n. 57 here.

63 Galen, 5, 30; 34: tr. P. N. Singer 1997: 114–15.

64 Manuli and Vegetti 1988: 65–214; Barras *et al*. 1995; Gill 2010; and the discussions in P. N. Singer 2012.

65 Galen, *Commentary 4 on Epidemics VI*, 8–10: *CMG* 5, 10, 2, 2, 197–207. Cf. the advice in [Hippocrates], *Decorum*, on p. 158 here.

66 See pp. 157–8 here.

67 Jouanna 1997; Mattern 2008.

68 Galen, *On Prognosis* 14, 599–673: *CMG* 5, 8, 1; *On Examining the Physician* 4, 4–5, 19: *CMG* Suppl. Or. 4: 64–79. For a fragment of a pre-Galenic treatise on prognosis, but in the same Hippocratic tradition, see Andorlini 2009: 15–35.

69 Galen, 14, 602, 620: *CMG* 5, 8, 1, 70–1; 90–1.

70 Nutton 1993c.

71 Galen, 9, 587–607.

72 Galen, 8, 394–6 (only two cases); 9, 597.

73 Galen's treatises on the pulse occupy over 1,000 pages (8, 453–9, 549); the *Synopsis* (8, 453–92) is translated in P. N. Singer 1997: 325–44. Marcellinus, Schöne 1907: a *CMG* edition by H. von Staden is in press.

74 For these pulses, see Galen, 8, 553–66 and 9, 488; 9, 509–11; 8, 553 and 827–35; 9, 78; 303–7; 546.

75 Galen, 14, 661: *CMG* 5, 8, 1, 130–1.

76 Galen, 8, 511–14; 900–16.

77 Barnes 1991; emphasised from the point of view of a modern clinician by Johnston 2006.

78 Hankinson 1998a: 374–9; 1998b.

79 Galen, 18B, 1–42.

80 Cf. the case history of the sufferer from fever, in Galen, *On Examining the Physician* 8, 5–8: *CMG* Suppl. Or. 4, 94–9.

81 Galen, 17B, 355–6; *On Examining the Physician* 5, 10; 5, 18; 14, 4: *CMG* Suppl. Or. 4, 72–3, 78–9, 136–7. For examples of disobedience, see 9, 218–20; 14, 635–41: *CMG* 5, 8, 1, 104–11.

82 Galen, 10, 909–16; cf. 9, 218.

83 This is particularly evident in the late *Art of Medicine* (1, 407–12), *On My Own Books* (19, 8–48) and *On the Order of My Own Books* (19, 49–61: tr. P. N. Singer 1997: 394–6, 8–48, 49–61) and in *On My Own Opinions* (*CMG* 5, 3, 2; Boudon-Millot and Pietrobelli 2005).

84 Meyerhof 1929: 83.

85 For the law, see Below 1953: 122–34. For Galen's friendships, see 14, 612: *CMG* 5, 8, 1, 80–1 (Sergius Paullus); *On Regimen in Acute Diseases According to Hippocrates* 1: *CMG* Suppl. Or. 2, 76–7; *Commentary on Regimen in Acute Diseases* 3, 59: *CMG* 5, 9, 1, 265 (Aufidius Victorinus).

86 Galen (7, 836–80) classified all diseases into five general categories: disorders of conformation, of the number of parts, of the size of parts, of relative position and of dissolution of continuity.

87 Galen, 10, 390.

88 Galen, 7, 766–804: tr. Theoharides 1971, although Galen thought of it more as a terminal state than a disease. Contrast the title of his major nosographical work (*On Affected Parts*, 8, 1–452).

89 Above all, see Galen, 9, 550–941. Cf. Lloyd 2009.

90 Galen, 8, 194–5; his master Pelops compared this to the result of scorpion bite or the sting of a deadly spider (8, 196).

91 Galen, 1, 582; 5, 696: *CMG* 5, 4, 1, 2, 519; 8, 230–2; 17B, 541–3; 648–50 (following a Hippocratic aphorism); 18A, 96; *CMG* 5, 10, 2, 2, 462–4.

92 Galen, 12, 365 and p. 174 here; cf., for the fisherman, 4, 497; 8, 72; 421.

93 Galen, 10, 943, 986, 990; Mani 1991.

94 Galen, *On Examining the Physician* 14; *CMG* Suppl. Or. 4, 134–7.

95 Galen, 2, 631–3: tr. C. Singer 1956: 192–3; 5, 181–2, with the improved text at *CMG* 5, 4, 1, 2, 72–6; 5, 910: tr. P. N. Singer 1997: 304; Ostia, 18A, 348.

96 Galen, 18B, 318–628; 18A, 300–767.

97 Galen, *On Venesection, against Erasistratus* 11, 148–86; *On Venesection, against the Erasistrateans in Rome* 11, 187–249. The Erasistrateans now argued that Erasistratus had simply failed to mention bleeding alongside his customary method of fasting (11, 195). A third treatise, *On Venesection* (11, 250–316), was written in the 190s or even later. All are translated in Brain (1986).

98 Galen, *On Examining the Physician* 10, 1: *CMG* Suppl. Or. 4, 116–17. For the general principles of Galen's therapeutics, see Johnston 2006; van der Eijk 2008.

99 Galen, 6, 664: tr. Powell 2003: 116; *The Thinning Diet* 66: tr. P. N. Singer 1997; 315; cf. also 1, 624.

100 Galen, 12, 948; 12, 443–5.

101 Galen, 6, 486, 664: tr. Powell 2003: 41, 116; and *The Thinning Diet* 66: tr. P. N. Singer 1997: 315. Note Galen's own experience, when young, of being compelled to chop wood to keep warm (6, 134: tr. R. M. Green 1951: 79).

102 Galen, 6, 499; cf. 523: tr. Powell 2003: 46, 56; *On the Thinning Diet* 40–1: tr. P. N. Singer 1997: 310–11.

103 Galen, 6, 486, 539–40, 669: tr. Powell 2003: 41, 63–4, 119; 11, 142.

104 Athenaeus, *Sophists at Dinner* 1, 1e; 26c–27d; 3, 115c–116a; Nutton 1984b; Braund and Wilkins 2000; Wilkins 2007.

105 Respectively, Galen, 6, 602: tr. Powell 2003: 90; 11, 390, 17B, 155, 161, 163, 182; 6, 738–40: tr. Powell 2003: 148.

106 Galen, 14, 21–3: partially tr. A. J. Brock 1929: 200.

107 For cereals, see, for example, Galen, 6, 514: tr. Powell 2003: 53; 6, 811; 10, 468; *On the Thinning Diet* 40–1: tr. P. N. Singer 1997: 310–11; for wine, see 6, 334–9: tr. R. M. Green 1951: 204–6; 6, 800–6; 10, 833–7, with L. Robert 1980: 319–37.

108 Galen, 14, 18; 11, 663.

109 Powell (2003) is more informative and accurate than M. Grant (2000), although Grant translates more texts. *The Thinning Diet* is translated in P. N. Singer (1997: 305–24). For Galenic dietetics in general, see Grimaudo 2008.

110 Galen, 6, 663: tr. Powell 2003: 115.

111 Galen, *On Barley Soup*, 6, 816–31: tr. M. Grant 2000: 62–7.

112 Galen, 6, 596–602: tr. Powell 2003: 88–9; 11, 367–8.

113 Galen, 6, 332–4: tr. R. M. Green 1951: 201–3; *CMG* 5, 10, 2, 2, 465; the milky diet of the centenarian peasant (6, 343: tr. R. M. Green 1951: 210) was not recommended.

114 Galen, 1, 23–7: tr. P. N. Singer 1997: 45–7; 5, 820, 874–5, 894, 909: tr. P. N. Singer 1997: 59, 86–7, 96–7, 304; 17B, 361.

115 Galen, *CMG* 5, 10, 2, 2, 494.

116 Galen, 5, 899–909: tr. P. N. Singer 1997: 299–304. Cf. also 5, 806–98: tr. P. N. Singer 1997: 52–99.

117 *ILS* 8157.

118 Yegül 1992, 2010; R. Jackson 1990b; DeLaine and Johnston 1992; Fagan 1999, 2006.

119 Galen, 10, 536; 11, 393.

120 Galen, 6, 182–9: tr. R. M. Green 1951: 110–14; 10, 702–16; cf. p. 209 here.

121 Barnes 1997; Jacques 1997; van der Eijk 1997a; von Staden 1997b.

122 Riddle 1985; Debru 1997. Cf. pp. 174–9 here.

123 Galen, *On My Own Opinions* 9, 1–3: *CMG* 5, 3, 2, 84–9; Boudon-Millot and Pietrobelli 2005: 181–2; Harig 1974; Jacques 1997; Vogt 2008.

124 Röhr 1923: 96–133; Touwaide 1994.

125 Galen, *On My Own Opinions* 9, 1–3; 12, 10: *CMG* 5, 3, 2, 84–6; 102; Boudon-Millot and Pietrobelli 2005: 180–1.

126 Galen, 11, 379–12, 377; 12, 378–13, 361; 13, 362–1058.

127 Galen, 13, 362–3. *On Antidotes* 14, 1–209, and *On Theriac, for Piso* 14, 210–94, both date from the early third century.

128 Debru 1997.

129 Fabricius 1972; H. Parker 2012.

130 Goltz 1976: 29–30, 129; cf. Galen, 13, 126–36.

131 Jacques 1997; Touwaide 1997.

132 Harig 1974.

133 Ibid. 195–212.

134 Galen, 10, 209–17.

135 Galen, 1, 383: tr. P. N. Singer 1997: 382.

136 Galen, 11, 336.

137 *Avoiding Distress* 6 and 31–7: tr. Nutton 2012a.

138 Galen, 12, 172; 216; 227; 14, 6: tr. A. J. Brock 1929: 199. For the date, see Nutton 1973: 169–70. By contrast, N. Europe contributed little to his pharmacopoeia, apart from the *radix britannicus* (probably dock), mead and *melka*, a kind of yoghurt from N. Lombardy.

139 Galen, 12, 169–75: tr. A. J. Brock 1929: 192–5; cf. Hasluck 1929: 671–88, and, for the text, see Harig 1987–8.

140 Galen, 10, 143, 942.

141 Galen, 14, 9–10; 59; 61; 211.

142 Galen, 14, 3–4; 216. The curious notion that Marcus was a drug addict derives from a misunderstanding of Galen's Greek at 14, 3–4: tr. A. J. Brock 1929: 197; see Hadot 1984.

143 Galen, 14, 66; 82–105; Meyerhof 1929: 85; *Avoiding Distress* 6 and 31–7: tr. Nutton 2012a.

144 Galen, 14, 217. For the authenticity of this tract, see Nutton 1995b, 1997a.

145 Galen, *On Examining the Physician* 12, 2–8: *CMG* Suppl. Or. 4, 124–9.

146 Galen, 14, 26; 10, 791; 13, 570–2; 703; 14, 6.

147 Galen, 12, 918; 14, 30.

148 Galen, 14, 30.

149 Galen, 12, 909; 13, 636–40.

150 See above, p. 218.

151 *Miracles of St. Artemius* 21; Timarion 28; Temkin 1973: 67–8.

17 ALL SORTS AND CONDITIONS OF (MAINLY) MEN

1 Kudlien 1979, 1986a; Nutton 1985a; Pleket 1995. There is much valuable information in Gourevitch (1984b). For the Egyptian evidence, see Hirt 1996. Gummerus (1932) is the best repertory of the epigraphic evidence for the Western half of the Empire, but he never published a second collection dealing with the East, on which see Samama (2003).

2 See p. 177 here. Cf. Lindemann 1999: 11.

3 Phaedrus, *Fables* 1, 14; cf. Martial, *Epigrams* 1, 47; 8, 74.

4 As a whole series of jokes never failed to point out; for example *Palatine Anthology* 11, 115–17; 119; 121–6; Martial, *Epigrams* 10, 77; 11, 71; Menander, *Monostichs* 379 Jäkel; *The Lover of Laughter* 175–89; 221–2.

5 Philo, *On the Flight* 13.

6 Justinian, *Digest* 48, 19, 38, 5; 48, 8, 3, 2; 48, 8, 4, 2. In the Greek world, and arguably later, there were other local jurisdictions.

7 Ulpian, cited in Justinian, *Digest* 50, 13, 1, 3, from around 210.

8 See pp. 156–8 here. Cf. Lucian, *The Disowned Son* 180.

9 Suetonius, *Julius* 42; *Augustus* 59.

10 The Emperor Hadrian, following earlier enactments by Vespasian and possibly Trajan, confirmed the universal freedom of all doctors from local taxation and personal liturgies (Justinian, *Digest* 27, 1, 6, 8; cf. 50, 4, 18, 30).

11 P. Oxyrhynchus 40. Cf. the legal decision in Justinian's *Code* 10, 53 (52), 1, of *c*.215, restoring an army doctor to his civilian privileges on his return from (short-term) service 'if you are included in the number of those given the concessions for doctors'. Parallels from Egypt suggest that the applicant had to bring some form of proof of his assertion.

12 Justinian, *Digest* 27, 1, 6, 2–4. This section on immunities is based on Nutton 1971b, 1973.

13 For this college, and for a possible college at Constantinople, see *Theodosian Code* 13, 3, 8–9; Nutton 1973: 207–12.

14 Justinian, *Digest* 27, 1, 6, 4; 27, 1, 6, 6; 50, 9, 1; 50, 13, 1.

15 For example, in 362 the Emperor Julian (*Letter* 75b), in order to propagate 'the saving art of medicine', freed all doctors from civic liturgies, but the case of the doctor Philo, forced to act as a councillor at Rhosus (Syria), shows how easily the law could be evaded, despite the claim of Libanius (*Letter* 723) that 'even if the Rhosians knew Philo was a doctor, though he himself might be weak, the law is strong'.

16 For Rome, see *ILS* 5481; the scribe Telesphorus is recorded on both a Greek and a Latin inscription (*IGUR* 1673 and *CIL* 6, 9566). For Ephesus, see *I. Ephesos* 719; Engelmann 1990.

17 *CIL* 5, 6970 (Turin); *I. Ephesos* 719; cf. L. Robert 1960: chs 9 and 18; *I. Ephesos* 719; for tombs, see *I. Ephesos* 2304.

18 *Palatine Anthology* 9, 675.

19 *I. Ephesos* 1161–9, 4101b (contests). It is possible that a similar contest was held at Smyrna. Another inscription (*I. Ephesos* 1386) records a decision about fees, but it is unfortunately so badly damaged that no secure conclusion can be drawn about its contents.

20 Engelmann (1990) traces the career of a doctor who became *Grammateus* and *Prytaneus* of the city before ending as Asiarch. He or his son presided over the medical games of 153/4. Another doctor, Publius Aelius Menander, who won sections at several of the contests, was a member of the religious college of the Kouretes (*I. Ephesos* 1980). For a tax-immune doctor Cleandros Bretennios as a holder of various religious offices and a councillor, see *I. Ephesos* 946, with 941 and 964; and for a wife and a daughter of a doctor as priestess of Artemis, see *I. Ephesos* 3233, 3239.

21 Römer 1990; cf. *Bulletin épigraphique* 1992, n. 622. For the variety of other practitioners at Alexandria, cf. Fulgentius of Ruspe, p. 9 Helm; Historia Augusta, *Forty Tyrants* 7, 4; 8, 1, with Syme 1971: 18–29.

22 Ovid, *Fasti* 3, 809–21.

23 See pp. 245, 155, 162 here.

24 L. Robert 1940b: 135; 1969: 934–8; Kudlien 1983.

25 P. Thmouis 1, 123 and 128; *IGLS* 788, with Hirt 1996: 88–92; for the Jewish evidence, see Preuss 1978: 35–6.

26 Fabbri and Trotta 1989.

27 Cicero, *In Defence of Cluentius* 14, 40; *CIL* 11, 5836 = *ILS* 7794; Boon 1983; Feugère *et al.* 1985; R. Jackson 1990a, 1996; Voinot 1999, 1999–2000.

28 Respectively, Galen, 13, 90; 13, 281; 13, 281; 12, 786; 13, 1031, cf. 11, 681; 12, 104; 13, 287; 13, 294; 13, 1038; 13, 204; 13, 1036; 14, 180, 182.

29 Galen, 13, 1031.

30 Plutarch, *Table Talk* 7, 1 and 8, 9. Other medical themes are discussed at length (ibid. 3, 4; 3, 6; 5, 7; 6, 1–3; 6, 8). He also wrote a treatise *On Keeping Well* 122B–137E. Cf. Boulogne 1996.

31 Cf. also Plutarch, *On Keeping Well* 15: 129D, warning his readers not to display their knowledge of medical terminology ostentatiously in the sickroom.

32 Galen, 14, 612; 626–7; 651–2: *CMG* 5, 8, 1, 80–3; 94–7; 120–1; Debru 1995a. Cf. p. 208 here for Athenaeus' recommendation of medicine and medical history to his learned readers.

33 Apuleius, *Apology* 48–52.

34 Marx 1877; cf. Migliorini 1997: 21–94.

35 Seneca, *On Benefits* 6, 15, 4; *Letters* 15, 2; 15, 4.

36 Galen, *On Examining the Physician*: *CMG* Suppl. Or. 4; Nutton 1985a, 1990b.

37 Seneca, *On Benefits* 6, 15, 4; Cicero, *On Duties* 1, 150–1; cf. Brunt 1973.

38 Cassius Dio, *History* 81, 7, 1: Gellius was a legionary commander in Syria; cf., for his father, Nutton 1971a; Christol and Drew-Bear 2004.

39 Galen, 14, 660: *CMG* 5, 8, 2, 128–9; Ovid, *Fasti* 3, 809–21. Kühn (1827–8: 2, 373, citing Eustathius, *Commentary on Odyssey* T. 135) noted that doctors would be then on the same level as pastry cooks and cake-makers.

40 Galen, 1, 38–9: tr. P. N. Singer 1997: 52.

41 Hirt 1996: 99–116, 159–98.

42 Vettius Valens, 1, 37–9; cf. the later lists printed in Pingree's 1986 edition (Appendix I, 387–8). A similar list is given in Hermes Trismegistus (71, 18; 74, 20; 97, 8 Gundel). For the Quinquatrus, see Ovid, *Fasti* 3, 809–21.

43 Vettius Valens, 1, 20; 1, 17. Cf. also Hermes, 65, 19 Gundel; Ptolemy, *Almagest* 4, 4, 3–12; Hephaestion, *Apotelesmatica* 2, 19; 15–16.

44 Firmicus Maternus, *Handbook of Astrology* 8, 29, 5; 8, 24, 14; 4, 10, 3.

45 Ibid. 8, 26, 12; 5, 2, 17; 8, 28, 3; 8, 25, 10. According to Hermes Trismegistus, 74, 20 Gundel, the (rare) conjunction of Mercury, the sun and Jupiter may produce a 'medicosophist or medicogeometrician in a royal palace'.

46 Nutton 1992: 45–7; Kudlien 1986a: 57–64.

47 Suetonius, *Augustus* 81; Cassius Dio, *Histories* 53, 30; Pliny, *Natural History* 29, 6. For the Samian inscription, see Hermann 1960: 141. His name is found on a Pompeian graffito (Della Corte 1959: 91) and he is also the alleged author of a Late Antique Latin tract, *De herba vettonica, On Betony*. See also Michler 1993.

48 Pliny, *Natural History* 29, 5, 8; 29, 8, 20.

49 Martial, *Epigrams* 6, 31; 11, 71; *Palatine Anthology* 15, 19. In general, see Brecht 1931: 45–9; P. Ehrhardt 1974.

50 Tacitus, *Annals* 12, 66–7; cf. 2, 69, 5 with Griffin 1997: 251.

51 The qualification for the status of a knight was property worth 400,000 sesterces; of a senator 1 million. Both were way beyond the dreams of the average citizen. That Pliny (*Natural History* 29, 5, 7) here refers to Xenophon and not to an otherwise unknown brother Quintus is argued by Kaplan (1978). For family members among the 'first citizens', see Bosnakis and Hallof 2008.

52 Sherwin-White 1978: 283–5, 85; Kaplan 1978; a new inscription from Cos (Bosnakis and Hallof 2008) contains a letter of Claudius praising him for 'saving my life' and 'never falling short in his reverence for me or his concern for you'.

53 *FGrH* II B 200, with Russu 1972; Fabricius 1972: 190–2; Scarborough 1985a.

54 *I. Ephesos* 719. Cf. *Journal of Roman Studies* 93, 2003: 251.

55 Robert and Robert 1954: 167. He was known to Galen, and commemorated on coins of Heraclea (Benedum 1971; Figure 17.3 here).

56 Nutton 1971a; Christol and Drew-Bear 2004, who suggest also that his rank of *ducenarius*, equal to that of a minor imperial governor, indicates that he was paid 200,000 sesterces a year as an imperial doctor. His benefactions were not confined to his native city.

57 Other imperial doctors and benefactors include Servilius Damocrates at Blaundus in Lydia (Cichorius 1922: 432–3), and Ser. Sulpicius Hecataeus at Cnidus (*I. Knidos* 90). For Titus' doctor staying at Herculaneum, see Catalano 1966: 270–3.

58 *CIL* 11, 3943. Since he was born in 87, he must have obtained his citizenship in his twenties, as Trajan died in 117.

59 Pliny, *Letters* 10, 5–7; 10. 'Clarissimus' ('very distinguished') frequently indicates senatorial rank.

60 Pliny, *Letters* 10, 11. Had Marinus felt upstaged by the grant of citizenship to a mere masseur? His name, Postumius Marinus, shows that he himself had already obtained citizenship.

61 Pleket (1995: 31) points out the high percentage of civic doctors coming from the upper reaches of local society. This is perhaps not entirely surprising, given that these posts were voted on by the councils, to which many family members and friends would have belonged.

62 For embassies, see *IG* 14, 1934; *IGRR* 3, 534; Justinian, *Digest* 27, 1, 6, 8.

63 *Athenische Mitteilungen* 17, 1892: 198, with the comments of L. Robert 1969: 5, 692–4.

64 Respectively, Pleket 1958: no. 10; Galen, *CMG* 5, 10, 1, 401; *CIG* 4379c, with L. Robert 1932: 103–7. Many of Galen's teachers had studied at Alexandria, as had Rufus and Soranus (see pp. 214, 199 here) and the young man with diet problems (Galen, 7, 635).

65 Meyerhof 1929: 84.

66 *ILS* 7796; Kudlien (1986a: 35) doubts whether all these *seviri* were freedmen.

67 One must also allow for the fact that one might adopt or be given a Greek name because it was expected that doctors would be Greek, just as owners of pizza parlours pretend to Italian names.

68 One example can stand for them all: a recently published inscription from Spain (*Hispania Epigraphica* 4, 1994: p. 65, no. 146) records a doctor C. Argentarius Heraclides, son of Erasistratus. The combination of two famous medical names cannot be accidental.

69 Voinot 1999.

70 For decuries, see *CIL* 6, 3984; 8904; *IGUR* 30 (from the 180s); cf. also *CIL* 6, 8504; Korpela 1987: 70–81, although his statistics are to be treated with care; Kudlien 1986a: 92–117.

71 Juvenal, *Satires* 3, 77. Martial's doctors likewise bear Greek names. Cf. Figures 17.5–6 here.

72 *IG* 14, 1934; Hillert 1990: pl. 15.

73 For Rimini, see p. 188 here; there are good pictures in R. Jackson 2002a; cf. Michaelides 1984, 1988. For Pompeii, see Eschebach 1984.

74 *ILS* 5369; 7812.

75 *CIL* 9, 1655; 1971. Cf. *Journal of Roman Studies* 93, 2003: 247, n. 217.

76 Whether it was only the rich who employed a variety of doctors from different sects is an intriguing question.

77 Respectively, *IG* 9, 2, 1276; *IG* 5, 1, 1245; *CIL* 9, 3895 (even if 'Chirurgus' is a *cognomen* and not an occupational title, it should indicate at least his father's ambitions for him); *CIL* 9, 3895.

78 Galen, 8, 197; Dio, *Orations* 8, 7; 9, 4. The relationship of St Paul with St Luke, the doctor, may not be entirely explained by their shared Christian belief. Cf. also *IG* 14, 2019, set up by Tertianus to Archelaus of Nicomedia, who 'laboured often with me on my journeys', possibly as his doctor or as his partner.

79 *TAM* 5, 1, 671; *Griechische Versinschriften* 655, with Pausanias, *Description of Greece* 10, 32, 9.

80 For Pompeii, see Eschebach 1984; Bliquez 1994; for Stabiae, see Galen, 10, 363–72; for Sorrento, see *L'Année Epigraphique* 1951: no. 201.

81 Hirt 1996: 159–208; Kudlien 1986a; Pleket 1995.

82 Gauckler 1895: pl. III, no. 2 = *CIL* 8, 2109; Hillert 1990: pl. 30; for Modius Asiaticus, see Hillert 1990: pl. 22; cf. also, for another high-quality portrait from Rome, ibid. pl. 16; for Agathemerus, see Figure 17.1 here.

83 Forrest 1972: 314. Later, St John Chrysostom (*Homily on Acts* 52; *Patrologia Graeca* 60, 365) assumes it normal for a local physician to take pupils.

84 Seneca, *Letters* 40, 5; 104, 19. Dio of Prusa thought these itinerants should be accepted *faute de mieux* (*Orations* 8, 7; 9, 4).

85 Galen, 11, 300; Plautus, *Menaechmi* 946–56 (perhaps reflecting a Greek original); cf. P. Oxy. 4001; P. Ross. Georg. III 2. Plutarch (*On Progress in Virtue* 11: 81F) implies that the most seriously ill were treated at home. The rooms in the House of the Surgeon at Pompeii fronting on to the street and with restricted access to the domestic rooms and garden at the rear would appear to have been where he worked, and are reminiscent of the typical layout of a doctor's house in 1940s England. The patients entered the larger surgeon's house at Rimini (De Carolis 2009) from the street and were seen in a more private room: there was also a toilet and separate washing facilities. The doctor and his family lived on the well-appointed upper floor.

86 *IG* 2², 2237; 2243; 2245; *IG* 5, 1, 159 (Sparta); 5, 2, 50 (Tegea).

87 Macridy 1912: 54, no. 27; for festivals, see Hiller von Gärtringen 1906: no. 100.

88 Paribeni and Romanelli 1914: 60, n. 49; Dio Chrysostom, *Orations* 33, 6.

89 *Hispania Epigraphica* 4, 1994, no. 286.

90 Plato, *Laws* 916 A–B; doctors might be called upon to examine also for the stone and strangury. Cf. the fragments of Rufus of Ephesus, *On the Sale of Slaves*: tr. Rosenthal 1975: 204.

91 P. Oxyrhynchus 896. *BGU* 647, AD 130, is a medical report signed by the owner of an *iatreion* at Karanis, Minicius Valerianus. Cf. also Worp 1982: 227–8.

92 P. Oxyrhynchus 39, with Hirt 1996: 146–8; Cohn-Haft 1956: 68–72; Nutton 1981b: 213–15; Roesch 1984.

93 *Acts* 3, 2; 8, 6; 9, 39; 14, 8; cf. also, for healers who were opposed to the apostles, 8, 9; 19, 13.

94 Cf. Jerome, *Letters* 50, 5, 1, on the surgery as a place for general gossip.

95 Cf. Galen's quack dentist, Meyerhof 1929: 83; p. 245 here.

96 Plutarch, *How to Detect a Flatterer* 32: 71A; Augustine, *City of God* 1, 18; John Chrysostom, *Homilies: Patrologia Graeca* 51, 55; 61, 506; 62, 132; 63, 212; 655–6.

97 Galen, 18B, 685–7.

98 Hence the very detailed instructions in the Hippocratic *Surgery* and, still more, in Galen's commentary, on the exact details of bandaging.

99 Hillert 1990: pl. 23; 187–93 (instruments). A tomb relief from fourth-century BC Athens, Figure 17.8 here, was later, *c.*AD 100, reworked to represent a doctor by the insertion of panels showing book-rolls and instruments; Krug 2008: 36. Do the military insignia on the tomb of the *archiatros* Asclepiades (Hillert 1990: pl. 26) mean that he served in the army at some point?

100 Ibid. pl. 32.

101 Galen, *On Examining the Physician*, passim: *CMG* Suppl. Or. 4.

102 Like the pseudo-Galenic *Definitions* 19, 346–462; Kollesch 1973.

103 Andorlini 1999; Fischer 2000c; Hanson 1997.

104 W. D. Smith 1979. Cf. Augustine, *Against Faustus* 33, 6; Temkin 1991: 42–3.

105 Diocles, fr. 183a van der Eijk, rightly labelled dubious. For the variants, see Opsomer and Halleux 1985.

106 Galen, *On Examining the Physician* 10: *CMG* Suppl. Or. 4, 116–19.

107 [Galen], 14, 674–797; p. 188 here.

108 Galen, 11, 151, who derided the argument as ignorant and foolish. Strato was the pupil and close associate of Erasistratus, to be distinguished from his contemporary the natural scientist Strato of Lampsacus.

109 Galen, 14, 613–20: *CMG* 5, 8, 1, 82–91.

110 Galen, 15, 441–6. See also Barb 1950; Deichgräber 1976. Galen's discussion of divination in his *On the Opinions of Asclepiades* (2, 29: tr. A. J. Brock 1916: 47) has unfortunately not survived.

111 Galen, 12, 357.

112 Ptolemy, *Tetrabiblos* 1, 3, 15–16; cf. Manuli 1980. Ptolemy is praised by Galen in the commentary on *Airs, Waters and Places* (see Toomer 1985: 199, although he considers this an interpolation). But note the references to Galen's use of Ptolemy preserved in al-Mas'udi, *Kitab al-tanbih* (tr. Carra de Vaux, Paris: Imprimerie nationale, 1896: 181). A later Greek summary of Ptolemy associated the two men chronologically; Boudreaux 1912: 95.

113 Galen, 9, 911–16; cf. also *CMG* 5, 10, 2, 2, 244. For Galen's considerable knowledge of astronomy, see 5, 654; Cooper 2011a, 2011b: 61–76; and the treatises *On the Seven-month Child*, ed. Walzer 1935; and the (as yet unpublished) *Commentary on Airs, Waters and Places* discussed by Toomer 1985; Wasserstein 1982: 88–9.

114 Galen, 11, 792; 797–8; 12, 207; 249–51; cf. his comments on Roman astrologers in Toomer (1985: 198–9), where Galen refers to his (lost) work on Hippocratic astronomy.

115 Galen, 9, 913. Cf. Barton 1994b; Nutton 2008a.

116 Juvenal, *Satires* 6, 581: cf. *Greek Anthology* 11, 164.

117 Barton 1994a: 186–91.

118 Andorlini 2003.

119 Ptolemy, *Tetrabiblos* 3, 12, 147–8; Barton 1994a: 189–94. This arrangement became a standard part of mediaeval medical knowledge, and is frequently depicted visually in medical mss. throughout Europe: for example London, Wellcome 40 (Latin); Wellcome 349, fol. 22 r. (German); Aberystwyth, Mostyn 88 (Welsh); London, British Library, Arundel 251, fol. 46 (German); Jurina 1985: pl. 197 (German printed calendars).

120 *CIL* 10, 1497; Pliny, *Natural History* 29, 5, 9.

121 [Galen] 19, 529–73, quotation from 545. On this tract, see Weinstock 1948. The so-called *Astrologia Ypocratis*, a Latin version of this text, may be a Latin translation of a recension of this text (Thorndike 1960).

122 Galen, 19, 530 = Diocles, fr. 64 van der Eijk.

123 [Galen], 19, 530. The headings at *Epidemics* 2, 5 and 2, 6 refer to physiognomy, and appropriately describe these sections, which link physical appearance with types of illness – those suffering from dropsy have grey eyes – but this quotation is not found there. *The Nature of Women* 1 talks about the medical significance of skin colour. But 'physiognomy' may well be used here in an older sense to mean simply 'knowledge of nature' (cf. Clement, *Miscellany* 1, 121, 135; Fulgentius, *Virgilian Summaries* 84, 10–11 Helm), and is thus creatively misinterpreted by the author (cf. Schöne 1910).

124 On Galen and physiognomics, see 2, 622–45: tr. P. N. Singer 1997: 254–66; 5, 464–5, with DeLacy's commentary at *CMG* 5, 4, 1, 2, 654; Barton 1994b; Popović 2007; Swain 2007.

125 *Prognostica Galieni*, Montpellier, Faculté de Médecine Ms. 185, fol. 1r.; Vatican, Ms. Reginensis Latinus 1324, fol. 66r.

126 Galen, 9, 900–41. The notion that some of the numbers recorded in the calculations of significant events in the *Epidemics* might rest on as flimsy a foundation as the climacterics of the astrologers was, of course, anathema to him.

127 Especially Galen, 9, 911, where Galen allows that the Egyptian discoveries of the influence of the moon on sickness and health are 'most true'.

128 Galen, 9, 934.

129 Galen, 12, 291.

130 Galen, 12, 249.

131 Galen, 11, 792–8.

132 Keyser 1997; although as Jouanna (2011) points out, Galen was prepared to modify his dislike when faced with their apparent success.

133 For the astrological medical handbook of Nechepso, see Firmicus Maternus, *Astrological Handbook* 4, 16; Aetius, *Tetrabiblos* 1, 19; Thessalus, *On Plants* 1; P. Bingen 13. A recipe for a plaster of Nechepso is given at Aetius, *Tetrabiblos* 15, 2 (see Wellmann 1907: 536).

134 Galen, 12, 207 K. For examples of gems of this sort, carved with the snake-god Chnoubis, sometimes with the inscription 'for the stomach', see Festugière 1975: 155–7. Cf. Julius Africanus, *Cestoi* 1, 4–5 Viellefond, for an amulet to stop bleeding.

135 See p. 175 here.

136 Friedrich 1968; Leith 2006. Although the tract is dedicated to an Emperor Claudius, there are very strong grounds for doubting the Methodist's authorship (see Diller 1936b: 181; *contra*, Sconocchia 2000, but somewhat implausibly). When it was written is disputed; Gundel and Gundel (1966: 153) assign it in the late first century; Pingree (1976: 83) to the third or fourth century. Whether true or false, the career of the author is meant to indicate that he came from a respectable level of society. Cf. Festugière 1939.

137 Galen, 12, 251; Wellmann 1934.

138 Wellmann 1908a: 772–7.

139 Africanus, *Cestoi* 1, 4–5 Viellefond. Pliny (*Natural History* 34, 50, 166) knows of the use of such plaques. A similar combination of types of remedy is found in Africanus' fragments of veterinary medicine (*Cestoi* 3, 1–36).

140 Ullmann 1972a, 1973.

141 Kaimakis 1976. For Marcellus, see p. 217 here.

142 Galen, 12, 874; 13, 256; Alexander of Tralles, *Handbook* 1, 12: I, 567 Puschmann. According to the biography in the Suda, Archigenes also wrote much on '*Physika*' – that is, sympathetic remedies and the like. Röhr (1923: 97–133) points to the overlap between medical and magical explanations of drugs, especially in the notion of sympathy/antipathy.

143 Historia Augusta, *Caracalla* 5, 7. In the Middle Ages there circulated at least three different Latin versions of a tract on such medical herbs and precious stones attributed to Galen, which was composed originally in Greek at some point before the ninth century, when it was translated into Arabic (Thorndike 1963).

144 Merkelbach 1994. On magic and medicine in general, see pp. 113–14, 175 here; Moreau and Turpin 2000; Dickie 2001; Janowitz 2001; Karenberg and Leitz 2002.

145 *Acts* 13, 6–12, with Nock 1972: 308–30; *Acts* 8, 9–11; cf. 18, 13, with M. Edwards 1997.

146 Ammianus, *History* 16, 8, 1; 19, 12, 14; cf. 26, 31, 1–4; 28, 1, 26–9.

147 These three therapies are chosen deliberately to exemplify different levels of acceptability to the modern medical profession. The astral Galenist I met when giving a seminar at the Exeter University Centre for Complementary Medicine.

148 Scribonius Largus, *Drug Recipes* 17; Galen, 12, 342 (a variant remedy); Celsus, *On Medicine* 3, 23, 7; Alexander, *Seven Books* 1, 15: I, 571–3 Puschmann, ascribed to Marsinus the Thracian; Moog 2002.

149 Justinian, *Digest* 50, 1, 13, 1, 3.

150 For Cythera, see pp. 268–9 here; Tarragona, *CIL* 2, 4313–14 = Alföldi 1975: 442 and pl. 95, 1; 444 and pl. 102, 2, the memorial of a twelve-year-old charioteer whose 'inmost viscera were consumed by fiery diseases the hands of doctors could not overcome'.

18 MEDICINE AND THE RELIGIONS OF THE ROMAN EMPIRE

1 There is no comprehensive study on the interaction between religion and medicine in the Roman world. There are valuable insights in Edelstein 1967: 205–46; Temkin 1991. Krug (1985: 120–79) and R. Jackson (1988: 138–59) are good on the archaeological and epigraphic evidence, particularly from the N.W. provinces of the Empire.

2 See p. 260 here; cf. also the Oulioi (from Apollo Oulios) at Velia. The high percentage of doctors called Apollonius and Asclepiades is also striking.

3 Theophrastus, *Characters* 16.

4 See pp. 112–14 here.

5 Galen, Kudlien 1981; Plutarch, *On Superstition* 12: 171A–B; cf. 7: 168C, deriding the superstitious man who sends his doctor away when he is ill.

6 P. Oxyrhynchus 3078; C. Nissen 2001. Note the cynical comment at Tacitus, *Histories* 4, 81: if the man who claimed to have been advised by Sarapis to seek a cure from the emperor was healed, that would redound to the emperor's credit; if not, he could be mocked as a credulous fool.

7 Nock 1972: 720–35; Lane Fox 1986: 102–67.

8 Coventina, *RIB* 1522–34; Pausanias, *Description of Greece* 4, 34, 7, hinting at the transformation of the mainly military cult of Apollo Korythos into a healing cult in the Roman period.

9 [Galen], *Commentary on the Hippocratic Oath* (fr. 2a–e Rosenthal) gives a detailed description of the image of Asclepius and explains his attributes. For iconography, see p. 355, n. 6 here. Nock 1972: 414–45 (quotation, from A. B. Cook, on p. 425); S. Mitchell 1999.

10 The festival of the Robigalia took place on 25 April, with, as its central element, a sacrifice to Robigo (Blight or Mildew) to protect the crops from blight. Ovid, *Fasti* 4, 905–42, with Latte 1960: 67–8. For Fever, see *Dea Febris*, Valerius Maximus 2, 5, 6; Wissowa 1909.

11 Judeich 1898: 7; Deichgräber 1956: 35–8.

12 *Mark* 5, 13; cf. *Luke* 13, 11; *Matthew* 9, 32–3; 12, 22; 17, 14–20; Tatian, *Against the Greeks* 16. For Jewish beliefs, see Eitrem 1950; Brown 1972: 131–2; Kee 1986: 21–6; van der Toorn *et al.* 1995; Ferngren 2000, 2009. For Babylonia, see Kinneir Wilson and Reynolds 1990: 187. For demons in Egyptian medicine, see Nunn 1996: 103–5. The Greek Plutarch (*On Superstition* 7: 168C) claimed that a belief that demons caused disease was characteristic of the superstitious.

13 Kotansky 1994: 58–71.

14 For the introduction of a foreign god, cf. the bilingual (Latin and Greek) dedication to Asclepius by a military tribune at Lanchester (*RIB* 1072).

15 *RIB* 141, 146, 150 (Bath); 305 (Lydney), cf. 616–17 (near Lancaster). Does the small altar to Minerva found in Coventina's well at Carrawburgh (*RIB* 1543) imply that Venico, the donor, identified the local goddess with Minerva, or is this a chance collocation, the result of the way in which the whole site was destroyed?

16 Manetho, *Egyptian History* fr. 11 (not included in Edelstein 1945; cf. P. Oxyrhynchus 1381 = Edelstein 1945: T. 331, with updated bibliography in Girone 1998: 171–93); Damascius, *Life of Isidore* 302 = Edelstein 1945: T. 826.

17 Beard *et al.* 1998: 344; cf. 317–18, on syncretism, which is no new feature, but endemic in earlier Greek religion.

18 Croon 1967; Ginouvès 1994. An inscription from the Aquae Albulae near Rome, *CIL* XIV, 3911 + *L'Année Epigraphique* 2000: 380, records the cure of a wounded horse at the spring.

19 Servius, *Commentary on Aeneid* 7, 84; cf. Seneca, *Letters to Lucilius* 41, 3.

20 *RIB* 149; 139, 146, 147; Thévenot 1968: 97–116, 200–21. In general, see Kötting 1950.

21 Dio, *History* 77, 15, 6; *I. Ephesos* 802. Halfmann 1986: 226–9; Riethmüller 2005: 2, 690.

22 A survey of the evidence, literary, archaeological and numismatic, for healing shrines, of all types, is a desideratum. Riethmüller (2005: vol. 2) gives an exhaustive listing of shrines of Asclepius.

23 These divinities might be called upon in any combination, e.g. *CIL* 5, 6414–15, invoking Asclepius, Bona Valetudo (Good Health) and Mars; *I. Cret.* 1, 27 (Lebena), a dedication to Zeus, Sarapis and Asclepius, the healer of Titane and Lebena. Cf. *Journal of Roman Studies* 93, 2003: 271–2.

24 For healing deities in one region, see Breitwieser 1998: 77–104; C. Nissen 2009.
25 For Asclepian cure inscriptions from Epidaurus, Pergamum, Lebena and Rome, see Girone 1998.
26 Herzog and Schatzmann 1932.
27 *I. Cret.* 1, XVII, 21 = Edelstein 1945: T. 791.
28 Philostratus, *Life of Apollonius* 1, 7 = Edelstein 1945: T. 816; L. Robert 1973; Ziegler 1994.
29 Pausanias, *Description of Greece* 2, 27, 6; cf. 2, 27, 1 for the continuing prohibition; Burford 1969: 80 and Figure 3.
30 Marcus Aurelius, in Fronto, *Correspondence* 3, 10.
31 Habicht 1969: 6–18; A. Hoffmann 1998. When the complex was finished is less clear, but certainly by 150. Habicht's commentary on no. 101 lists the evidence for Hadrian as Asclepius: a century earlier, the Emperor Claudius had likewise been associated on Cos with Asclepius as a result of his benefactions to the island (*IGRR* 4, 1053). The evidence of the Arabic version at Galen, 2, 224 (= pp. 11–12 Garofalo) shows that the vulgate reading of the benefactor's name as Costunius is the result of a (relatively simple) copyist's error.
32 Lucian, *Icaromenippus* 24 = Edelstein 1945: T. 569; Galen, 13, 272.
33 Ziegenaus and De Luca 1968–84. The reputation of the 'grove of Rufinus' lasted well into the sixth century (see Feissel 1999: 265–7).
34 Habicht 1969: 102 is a dedication to Asclepius by a doctor to a troupe of actors. An earlier theatre, erected under Trajan, was soon demolished to make way for the new monumental gateway (see A. Hoffmann 1998: 43).
35 Philostratus, *Life of Apollonius* 4, 34 = Edelstein 1945: T. 792; Meier 2009.
36 For incubation, see pp. 109–10 here. Incubation was a common feature of many other cults around the Empire, and many gods are recorded in votive inscriptions as having acted by sending orders or dreams (see Nock 1972: 45–8).
37 H. Müller 1987; Weinreich 1909: 77–81; C. P. Jones 1998.
38 Galen, *Commentary on Medical Statements in the Timaeus*, CMG Suppl. 1, 33.
39 Aristides, *Orations* 48, 21.
40 Aristides, *Orations* 47–52, although only a fragment of the last is extant: tr. Behr 1968. Note also Festugière 1975: 89–125.
41 Aristides, *Orations* 48, 3 and 8. C. P. Jones 1998; Lane Fox 1986: 159–63; Holmes 2006; Petsalis-Diomidis 2010; Israelowich 2012.
42 Aristides, *Orations* 48, 37–45.
43 Ibid. 48, 47–8.
44 Galen, 17B, 137.
45 Aristides, *Orations* 48, 38; 51, 19; 48, 20.
46 Ibid. 49, 18.
47 Ibid. 49, 8–10.
48 Ibid. 49, 14–15.
49 Ibid. 47, 73. For Satyrus, see p. 217 here.
50 Ibid. 47, 75; cf. 47, 27.
51 Ibid. 47, 63; 48, 73.
52 Ibid. 47, 73; 48, 34.
53 *Mark* 5, 24–34; *Luke* 8, 43–8; *Matthew* 9, 20–2.
54 *ILS* 3411; *ILS* 3513.
55 Varinoglu 1989: 42–3.
56 See p. 231 here; Kudlien 1981.
57 Galen, 3, 812: tr. May 1968: 491.
58 Galen, *CMG* 5, 10, 1, 108. For treatments, see 10, 971–2; 11, 314–15: tr. Brain 1986: 98. For his acceptance of others' cures by Asclepius, see 6, 869; *Sketch of Empiricism* 10: tr. Walzer and Frede 1985: 40–1.

59 [Galen], *Commentary on the Hippocratic Oath* fr. 1 c: p. 60 Rosenthal.

60 Artemidorus, *Dream Book* 4, 22: 255, 12–13 Pack.

61 *ILS* 2194; L. Robert 1937: 386–8.

62 Rufus, cited by Oribasius, *Medical Collections* 45, 30, 11–14: *CMG* 6, 2, 1, 192 = Edelstein 1945: T. 425.

63 Aelian, fr. 100 = Edelstein 1945: T. 405; Diogenes of Oenoanda, fr. 15 Smith.

64 A statue of Asclepius, from Hierocaesaraea in Lydia (*TAM* 5, 2, 1254), bore on its base the famous Homeric line that one doctor was worth many other men. At the fortress of Novae on the Danube a shrine to Asclepius was erected within the hospital, *L'Année Epigraphique* 1998: 1130–5; 1999: 1331–8.

65 See p. 216 here.

66 *TAM* 2, 3, 910 (*IGRR* 3, 733, cf. 732); for his writings, see p. 216 here.

67 *Bulletin de correspondence hellénique* 1886, 215; L. Robert 1937: 256. For the healing shrine at Nysa, see Strabo, *Geography* 1, 1, 44.

68 *IGRR* 4, 520.

69 *IGRR* 4, 1278; Merkelbach 1972.

70 A selection of examples: at Euromus, in Caria, Menecrates gave five columns to the temple of Zeus (*CIG* 2714); at Didyma, C. Pomponius Pollio was chosen as official interpreter of the oracle of Apollo (Nutton 1969); Leontidas, *archiatros* at Hermione in S. Greece, was guide to the shrine (*IG* 4, 723); while on Lesbos, Bresos, son of Bresos, *archiatros*, continued family tradition by holding a multitude of priestly and civic offices (*IG* 12, 2, 484); at Iulia Gordos (Lydia), a doctor was hierophant in a Dionysiac college (*TAM* 5, 1, 744; cf. *IGRR* 4, 1383, for another hierophant); at Ephesus, Attalus Priscus, scion of a long line of *archiatri*, was a councillor and a high temple official (*I. Ephesos* 622). It goes almost without saying that the holding of a priesthood of Asclepius was not confined to doctors.

71 For the civic doctors, see p. 256 here; Pleket 1995: 31. C. Nissen (2009: 155) rightly warns that what may have been a civic title could easily be attributed to any local doctor of note.

72 This characterisation of the second century was made by Dodds 1965; Bowersock 1969: 74; *contra*, MacMullen 1981.

73 Van Straten 1981; MacMullen (1981: 32–3) emphasises the ubiquity of the (mainly lost) written and inscribed records of such cures.

74 The cynical Diagoras (in Cicero, *On the Nature of Gods* 3, 89) remarked that the universally joyous tone of votive inscriptions was only possible because those who thought differently were now dead. MacMullen (1981: 48–52) warns against over-interpretation of this data.

75 Lactantius, *Divine Institutions* 1, 3.

76 See pp. 109, 162 here.

77 *IGRR* 1, 767; 4, 360; 4, 1498; *IG* 22, 4533; Wiseman 1973: 143–83. The novelist Xenophon (*Ephesian Stories* 1, 6) has the parents of his lovers consult the oracle at Claros to discover the reason for their apparent illness. For these oracles in general, see Lane Fox 1986: 171–82, 231–41; L. Robert 1969: 393–430.

78 Gordon *et al.* 1993: 150; cf. also 149 for a statue of Mercury, set up to aid the harvest and as 'a health-giving remedy', that had driven away a plague of locusts.

79 *Epigrammata Graeca* 1034 Kaibel; Lane Fox 1986: 232–3.

80 Lucian, *Alexander* 36; L. Robert 1980: 404, drawing attention to similar apotropaic messages found elsewhere, such as 'Let no evil enter: Hercules dwells within'.

81 Lucian, *Alexander* 9. Petsalis-Diomidis (2010: 12–66) and Bendlin (2011) are extremely sceptical about the historicity of the details in Lucian's account, noting the mixture of fact and fantasy in Lucian's similar account of the Syrian Goddess.

82 Ibid. 6; 15–17; 19; 29. For Apollonius as a healer, see Philostratus, *Life of Apollonius* 3, 44; 4, 1; 4, 10; 4, 45 (a story also told of Asclepiades of Bithynia).

83 Lucian, *Alexander* 46.
84 L. Robert 1980: 393–421.
85 Lucian, *Alexander* 5; 22; 24.
86 L. Robert 1980: 393–421; Lane Fox 1986: 241–50.
87 Aristides, *Orations* 47, 70–3.
88 Ibid. 47, 75–7; 49, 37.
89 Chaniotis 1995. The inscriptions are conveniently collected by Petzl (1994).
90 *TAM* 5, 1, 331.
91 See pp. 59, 110 here.
92 MacMullen (1981: 32) cites contemporary examples from Syria and the countryside around Pergamum.
93 Cf. Kudlien 1978.
94 Kee 1986: 9–26; Lieber 2000.
95 Kahn 1975.
96 *Job*, chs 4, 5, 8 and 20.
97 2 *Chronicles*, 16, 12.
98 Jesus b. Sirach, *Ecclesiasticus* 38, 1–15. Allan (2001: 390–1) discusses textual variants in the Hebrew.
99 Vermes 1973.
100 For plants, see *Enoch* 8, 3.
101 Josephus, *Jewish Antiquities* 8, 42–9; cf. 1 *Kings* 4, 33. Moses the magician seems to be a later development in the sources (Gager 1972).
102 General surveys include: Moule 1965; Vermes 1973; M. Smith 1978; Kee 1983, 1986; Helm 2000; John 2001. Pilch (2000), while stressing that the aim of the Gospel narratives is to provide convincing proof of the Christian message, also suggests ways in which 'healing' could have taken place.
103 *Mark* 10, 46–52; *Matthew* 9, 1–8; *Mark* 5, 25–34 = *Luke* 8, 43–8; *Matthew* 8, 28–34; *Luke* 17, 14–50. On demonology in the Gospels, see Böcher 1972; Ferngren 2000.
104 *Matthew* 8, 1–4; *Luke* 17, 11–19.
105 *Mark* 5, 22–43 = *Luke* 8, 41–56; *Matthew* 9, 18–26; *Luke* 7, 11–17; 11, 1–44. For the notion of a healing power going out from Jesus, see *Mark* 5, 30; *Luke* 6, 19; 8, 46.
106 *Matthew* 8, 5–13; *Luke* 7, 1–10.
107 *Mark* 6, 7 and 13; *Luke* 9, 2 and 6; *Matthew* 10, 1 and 8.
108 See pp. 294–5 here. For a pagan example of a miracle serving to legitimate the healer, cf. Tacitus, *Histories* 4, 81, a blind man sent by Sarapis to be cured by Vespasian in AD 69.
109 Temkin 1991: 103.
110 The comment of *Mark* (5, 26) that the woman with the issue of blood had spent all her money on doctors is found only in some younger mss. at *Luke* 8, 26, and is now usually omitted as a later interpolation to harmonise the two versions.
111 Paul, *Colossians* 4, 14. On the vexed question of the relationship of Luke's medical knowledge to his theologico-historical writing, I agree with Cadbury (1919) that there is nothing that would mark Luke out from any educated man of the time as particularly skilled or interested in medicine for its own sake. The focus and intent of his Gospel and *Acts* are theological, not medical.
112 Paul, 1 *Timothy* 5, 23; James, *Epistle* 5, 14–15.
113 Helm 2000.
114 *John* 9, 3; cf. 5, 14.
115 Amundsen (1996: 158–75) points out that Tatian does not exclude dietetics or surgery, and explains Tatian's understanding of the links between pharmacology and magic.
116 Cyprian, *On Death* 9; cf. Tertullian, *On the Soul* 30.
117 For Simon Magus, see p. 277 here; Hippolytus, *Apostolic Constitutions* 16. The strong prohibition may reflect the closeness (some pagans might even say the identity) of the

miraculous healing promised in the Gospels. Cf. also Apollonius of Tyana's desire to separate his activities as a wonder-worker from the magician's, and Apuleius' attempt in the *Apology* to distinguish between what he was doing (medicine and investigative research) and what his opponents alleged (magic).

118 For example *Matthew* 4, 24; 8, 1–17; 9, 18–36.

119 *Acts* 3, 1–11; 5, 14–16.

120 *Acts* 8, 7–8 (note the belief of Simon Magus in the 'power' of the Apostles, *Acts* 8, 9–24).

121 *Acts* 9, 34–42.

122 *Acts* 14, 8–18; 19, 12.

123 For repetition of the Gospel stories, see, for example, *Gospel of the Nazareans*; Hennecke *et al.* 1963: I, 148–52; *Letter of the Apostles* 5: I, 193–4; and the early papyrus Gospel, I, 96. By 400 the ps. Clementine (*Recognitions* 6: II, 537) boasted that news of Jesus' miracles, confirmed by many travellers, had reached the ears of the Emperor Tiberius.

124 *Acts of John* 30–3: Hennecke *et al.* 1963: II, 222–3; *Acts of Andrew*: II, 400–2. The dubious historicity of these events does not diminish the evangelical function of these stories.

125 *Acts of Peter*: Hennecke *et al.* 1963: II, 276–7. The combination of motives in this story is illuminating.

126 Although the writers themselves use the miracles to demonstrate the power and authority of Jesus as an incentive towards conversion, and are not emphasising the ability of Christianity to offer physical healing (John 2001; Ferngren 2009), their readers or hearers may well have gained that impression. Cf. Frend 2005.

127 Eusebius, *Ecclesiastical History* 1, 13; cf. the story of the conversion of Iberia in the Caucasus by a healing miracle performed on its queen, Theodoret (*Ecclesiastical History* 1, 24).

128 Eusebius, *Ecclesiastical History* 7, 18. The comments of Eusebius, an eyewitness, imply that the word 'Saviour' was engraved on the base. For the identification of the statue with Asclepius and Hygieia, see Dinkler 1980: 32–4. Or would this have been a statue of a less familiar personage (an emperor?). For a statue erected to ward off plague, see *SEG* 57, 2007, 2064.

129 First emphasised by Harnack 1892: 37–152; Nock 1972: 308–30; MacMullen 1981: 50, 168–9; 1985: 25–31. The point is not affected by Ferngren's (1992, 2009) demonstration that New Testament writers and most subsequent preachers laid stress far more on the eternal salvation offered to the believer than on physical healing, and that to posit Christian healing as an antagonistic alternative to secular healing is exaggerated. But without earlier reports of healing miracles (whether true or invented) the growth (resurgence?) of interest in miracles and miracle stories in the fourth and fifth centuries requires considerable explanation (van Uytfanghe 1981). Nor until the consolidation of doctrine in the fourth century should one make a strict distinction between orthodox and heretical belief; and, even today, popular Christianity may differ substantially from what theologians prescribe.

130 For the theological background, see Greer 1986: 118–28; Holman 2001.

131 See Schürer 1987: II, 525–8, for the charity chest and its distributors.

132 *Genesis* 21, 33. For the later traditions, see Preuss 1978: 444.

133 Baron 1948: 91. MacMullen (1981: 155) gives references to similar hostels at pagan sites.

134 *Luke* 10, 30–7; *Matthew* 25, 35–45, perhaps deriving from a Midrashic interpretation of *Psalm* 119, 19; *Matthew* 10, 8, almost certainly Matthew's own expansion of his source material.

135 *Acts* 4, 34–5; 6, 1–6.

136 Eusebius, *Ecclesiastical History* 4, 23; 6, 43.

137 Ibid. 7, 22. The Greek is more precisely translated as 'fearing the transmission and the sharing in death'.

138 T. S. Miller 1997: 51.

139 Bowersock 2010b.

140 Cyprian, *Letters* 62, 4; Lane Fox 1986: 530–42.

141 Julian, *Letter* 22 = Sozomen, *Ecclesiastical History* 5, 16; Kislinger 1984. The office of high priest was filled by a wealthy and influential local magnate, who presided over the main festivals and games: it was not, like the Christian and Jewish priesthoods, held by men who devoted themselves entirely to religious cults.

142 Theodore Lector, *Ecclesiastical History* 59.

143 In the apocryphal *Acts of Pilate* 1 (Hennecke *et al.* 1963: I, 451; probably written in the late second century), Pilate is made to say, after hearing of Jesus' miracles, that the Jews were wrong to think of him as a sorcerer operating through demons, for he was acting through the god Asclepius. (Not in Edelstein 1945.)

19 MEDICINE IN THE LATER ROMAN EMPIRE

1 For the disappearance of alternative views, see pp. 302–3 here.

2 Maire 2002 and p. 235 here; Kalbfleisch 1895; Kudlien 1968c. For the medical poem of Q. Serenus, often placed around 220, see p. 5 here.

3 Viellefond 1970.

4 Björck 1944: 7–12; Doyen-Higuet 1984.

5 Lane Fox 1986: 516–42. For hagiography in general, see Howard-Johnston and Hayward 1999.

6 Prudentius, *The Garland* 10, 498; cf. Fulgentius, p. 9 Helm; Augustine, *City of God* 22, 24. Evidence put forward to show the continuation of anatomy in the Byzantine world (Bliquez and Kazhdan 1984; Browning 1985 (to which add Anastasius of Sinai, *Questions* 92: *Patrologia graeca* 89, 930)) is unconvincing. Most of it repeats passages from Galen, and only Bliquez and Kazhdan's (1984) reference 2 (Theophanes, *Chronography* 11, 16–20) seems historical. Even here, the peculiar circumstances of the incident advise caution about applying it more generally.

7 Temkin 1991. Note the church elder from Tyre (Eusebius, *Ecclesiastical History* 10, 4, 11) who quoted the definition of the true doctor from *Breaths* 1: 'he sees terrible things, touches things that are unpleasant, and grieves personally at the misfortunes of others'. This became a favourite quotation among Christians (Jouanna 1988: 102).

8 Brown 1978; Cameron 1993; Bowersock *et al.* 1999.

9 Nash Williams 1950: no. 92 and Figure 75.

10 Sharpe 1964; Jacquart and Thomasset 1985: 8–22. Nonetheless, medicine may be the largest exception to the equation of literacy with ecclesiastical needs, and one should not assume that most owners of medical books were clerics.

11 For the college and its problems, see Nutton 1977: 208–10; 1981b: 19–21.

12 Justinian, *Code* 6, 43, 3, 1; 7, 7, 1, 5a.

13 Nutton 1991a.

14 Fischer 1980; J. N. Adams 1995.

15 Philostorgius, *Ecclesiastical History* 8, 10; Aetius (*Tetrads* 6, 12) reports Posidonius' opinions on the 'Ephialtes', a feeling of suffocation that some believed was occasioned by being throttled by a demon.

16 Temkin 1977: 202. His division between tradition and empiricism seems to me less helpful.

17 Editions: Oribasius, ed. J. Raeder, *CMG* 6, 1–3; Aetius, *Tetrads* 1–8, ed. A. Olivieri, *CMG* 8, 1, 2; 9–16, ed. A. Garzya, *CMG*, forthcoming; Paul, *Seven Books*, ed. J. L. Heiberg, *CMG* 9, 1, 2. Their methods of compilation are discussed by van der Eijk (2010).

18 Baldwin 1975.

19 Respectively, Paul, *Seven Books* 6, 65–6; 77–8; 120; 82; 88; 45. Arabic authors also later gave Paul the soubriquet 'the Obstetrician'.

20 Ibid. 6, 96, from Soranus, 6, 33.

21 F. Adams 1844–7. Two decades later this recourse to the past for insights into practical therapy for the present had fallen out of fashion. Ancient medicine had become ancient history (Gourevitch 1999b).

22 Palladius, *Commentary on Epidemics VI*: II, 157 Dietz. The essays in Garofalo and Roselli (2003) show a variety of ways in which Galenism developed in this period.

23 See p. 194 here.

24 Temkin 1991: 231–5; Duffy 1984. The best edition is Puschmann (1878–9).

25 Cunningham 1986.

26 Wolska-Conus 1989; Westerink 1964; Duffy 1984; Dickson 1998. Rouché (1999) offers important caveats.

27 Temkin 1932; Beccaria 1971; Iskandar 1976; Lieber 1981; Marasco 2010; Pormann 2010. A substantial bibliography of Late Antique Alexandrian medicine is given by Palmieri (2002), to which should be added Garofalo and Roselli (2003).

28 The tracts were: *On Sects*; *Art of Medicine*; *Synopsis on the Pulse*; *Method of Healing, for Glaucon*; *Collection 1* (*Anatomy for Beginners, sc. On Bones*; *On Muscles*; *On Nerves*; *On Veins and Arteries*); *On Elements*; *On Temperaments*; *On the Natural Faculties*; *Collection 2* (*On Causes and Symptoms*); *On Affected Places*; *Collection 3* (*The 16 Books on the Pulse*); *On the Differences between Fevers*; *On Crises*; *On Critical Days*; *Method of Healing*; *On the Preservation of Health*. Three texts, *On Sects*, *Synopsis on the Pulse* and *On the Preservation of Health*, may not have been translated into Syriac, and the last may not have formed part of the syllabus until the Muslim period.

29 For Greeks in Ravenna, cf. the sale document, dated 578, witnessed by the son of Leontius, 'doctor at the Greek *schola*'. For the Ravenna commentaries, see Palmieri 2001, 2002.

30 Gundert 1998; Garofalo 1994; Boudon 2001; Savage-Smith 2002; Jouanna 2006, 2007, 2010.

31 Garcia-Ballester 1993.

32 Anonymus, *Exposition of the Whole World* 37; Nutton 1972.

33 Eunapius, *Lives of the Philosophers* 497–8. For other *iatrosophists*, see Bowersock 2010a.

34 Palladas, *Greek Anthology* 11, 281.

35 Eunapius, *Lives* 497–8.

36 Libanius, *Letters* 1208, 1358; cf. 843.

37 It is preserved in Greek in a variety of recensions and compilations, such as Galen, 19, 574–601, 602–8; Ideler 1841: 1, 307–16 and in an Arabic translation. Theophilus (*On Urines*, pref.) criticised it as incomplete, but not too much should be made of this. Arabic authors preserve fragments of other works by Magnus on prognosis and on fever. For his literary productions, see *Greek Anthology* 16, 270; West 1982.

38 Pithis 1983; Masullo 1999.

39 Cassius Felix, *On Medicine*, ed. Fraisse 2002.

40 See p. 199 here; Bendz 1964; Pigeaud 1982; Roselli 1991; Urso 1997; Mudry 1999. A similar debate rages over the extent to which his *Gynaecology* reproduces sections from Soranus.

41 The fact that *On Acute Diseases* 1 covers a single disease, 'phrenitis', whereas the other books deal with six or seven, suggests that Caelius may have at least modified his original source. Whether the overall structure – definition, semiotics, diagnosis (including differentiation from similar conditions), area affected, treatment, comments on alternative therapies by distinguished doctors of the past – is that of Caelius or Soranus is hard to determine, although the latter seems more likely.

42 Cf. J. N. Adams 1995 for similar developments in Latin veterinary medicine.

43 Marcellus, *On Drugs*, ed. Niedermann; Rousselle 1990.

44 Alexander, *Handbook* 2, 475 Puschmann.

45 Ausonius, *Obituary of My Father; Family Poems* 1, 13.

46 Opsomer and Halleux 1991.

47 Cassiodorus, *Institutes* 1, 31, 2.

48 Baader 1989: 410.

49 Fischer 2000a, 2003. One of Oribasius' *Synopses* was also available in Latin, in two different recensions, as were a few works by Galen.

50 Riddle 1981.

51 Hugonnard-Roche 1989, 1997.

52 Bergsträsser 1925, 1932.

53 Ennodius, *Letters* 384, 437, 445; Procopius, *Wars* 5, 1, 38. Cf. the curious story that he believed he was being attacked by stone-throwing demons (Anon., *Life of S. Caesarius of Arles* 1, 41).

54 Anthimus, *On the Observance of Foods*, CML 8, 1: tr. M. Grant 1996.

55 [Zachary of Mytilene], *History* 7, 10f. A more flattering account of him can be found in Severus of Antioch, *Letters* 31, 85, 86.

56 Procopius, *Wars* 2, 26, 31; 2, 28, 8; cf. 8, 10, 11 for Tribunus' role in later negotiations.

57 *Chronicle of Siirt*, pp. 498, 537; Barhebraeus, *Ecclesiastical Chronicle* I, 117 Abbeloos and Lamy; Chabot 1902: 580–98.

58 *Life of St Nicholas of Sion* I, 40; II, 243 Anrich.

59 Markus 1990.

60 Alexander of Tralles, 2, 585 Puschmann; Honigmann 1944; Temkin 1991: 234–6.

61 Augustine, *Letter* 138. This confusion of magic and medicine was not confined to Christians; cf. pp. 258–9 here for the earlier trial of Apuleius.

62 Methodius, *On the Resurrection*. His model was Plato's *Symposium*.

63 Theodoret, *On Providence* 3; *Patrologia Graeca* 83: 593–5; *Letters* 1114.

64 Nemesius, *On the Nature of Man* 6, 14; Telfer 1955; Sharples and van der Eijk 2008.

65 Nutton 2001: 22–30.

66 Iṣidore of Pelusium, *Letters* 4, 125.

67 Hippolytus, *Apostolic Tradition* 16.

68 Eusebius, *Ecclesiastical History* 7, 3, 23.

69 *Inscriptiones Latinae Christianae Veteres* 1233.

70 Sozomen, *Ecclesiastical History* 8, 6; cf. 4, 24, an orthodox bishop deposed for failing to excommunicate a murderous quack.

71 Eusebius, *Ecclesiastical History* 8, 13, the model for other medical martyrdoms (see Peeters 1939).

72 Peeters 1929: 70; Anon., *Life of S. Pantaleon: Patrologia Graeca* 115, 449C; 'Vita SS. Cosmae et Damiani', *Analecta Bollandiana*, 1: 1882, 589. One redaction of their lives locates them at Aegeae, site of a famous temple of Asclepius (van Esbroeck 1981). In general, see Fitzgerald 1948; Magoulias 1954.

73 For the miracles of SS. Cyrus and John, who also took no fees, see Sophronius, *Miracles of SS. Cyrus and John*, *Patrologia Graeca* 77, 3; T. Nissen 1939; Marcos 1975.

74 Epiphanius, *A Cure-all for Heresy* 67.

75 Gregory, *Against Eunomius* 1, 42, 45; Philostorgius, *Ecclesiastical History* 15. Cf. Sozomen, *Ecclesiastical History* 3, 15.

76 Casey and Hoffmann (1999) cast doubt on the earlier view that posited considerable activity even in the fifth century.

77 Eusebius, *Life of Constantine* 3, 56; Sozomen, *Ecclesiastical History* 2, 5; Libanius, *Oration* 30, 39; Zonaras, *Epitome* 13, 12 = Edelstein 1945: T. 817–20. *IG* 4, 2, 438, of AD 355, is an inscription from Epidaurus protesting against the destruction of the temple of Aegeae. Cf. Chapter 18, n. 140 here.

78 Rufinus, *Ecclesiastical History* 2, 23–30; Socrates, *Ecclesiastical History* 5, 16; Eunapius, *Lives of the Philosophers* 472. For the *parabalani*, see p. 289 here.

79 Herzog 1939.

80 Habicht 1969: 20; Feissel 1999.

81 L. Robert 1980; for the significance of statues of Asclepius to Christians, see *Passion of the Four Crowned Saints*: *Acta Sanctorum*, 3 November. For another type of takeover, see Rohland 1977: 74–104.

82 Theodoret, *The Cure for the Ailments of the Greeks* 8, 22 = Edelstein 1945: T. 5.

83 Marinus, *Life of Proclus* 29 = Edelstein 1945: T. 562.

84 Caesarius, *Sermons* 52; 53.

85 Temkin 1991: 181.

86 Arnobius, *Against the Gentiles* 2, 5, implying that many still remained committed pagans.

87 Gregory of Nazianzus, *Oration* 7, 6–7. Gregory's evidence implies that the *Oath* was being sworn, but also that it was not compulsory, since he makes little of any direct refusal on the part of Caesarius. Some Greek manuscripts of the *Oath* from the ninth century onwards replace the pagan preamble with a Christian invocation.

88 Asmus 1911. Note also the Neoplatonic doctor Asclepiades, who wrote on the immortality of the soul (*IG* 14, 1424; Figure 17.5 here), and C. Calpurnius Macedo, 'a follower of Socrates and Plato', who 'knew well the tenets of Hippocrates' (of *c.*360) (Ramsay 1919). Doctors were still being denounced as pagans and heretics at Constantinople in the 550s (John of Ephesus, *Ecclesiastical History* p. 481 Brooks).

89 Suda, s.v. Jacobus; Malalas, *Chronicle* p. 370 Dindorf; *Paschal Chronicle*: *Patrologia Graeca* 92, 824A; Marcellus, *Chronicle* p. 88; Photius, *Library* 344A.

90 Asmus 1913; L. Robert 1948: 119–26; R. R. R. Smith 1990: 153–5.

91 Damascius, cited by Photius, *Library* 348B. Cf. the Jewish doctor in the reign of Justin II (565–78) who was alleged by the author of the *Life of S. Symeon the Younger* (p. 208 van der Ven) to have used sorcery, invoked demons and even employed a female ventriloquist as an oracle to foretell the course of a disease.

92 Sophronius, *Miracles of SS. Cyrus and John* 30; Photius, *Library* 352B; Suda, s.v. Gesios; Zachary of Mytilene, *On the Creation of the World*: *Patrologia Graeca* 75, 1060–106. Lectures on Galen's *On Sects* are ascribed to Gesius in Vatican, Pal. Lat. 1090, fols. 1–42v. For a possible reference on a papyrus from Petra, see Bowersock 2010a. In one recension of the *Life and Miracles of Cosmas and Damian* (mir. 20 Rupprecht), a learned doctor and sophist called Menas is healed by the saints when the learning of Galen and Hippocrates has failed.

93 Ibid.

94 Procopius of Gaza, *Commentary on Kings III*: *Patrologia Graeca* 87, 1165; *Letter* 102; Aeneas of Gaza, *Letter* 20. For the story of Asa, see p. 292 here.

95 Horden 1982 (repr. in 2008, XI); S. Mitchell 1993: II, 134–50.

96 Vikan 1984.

97 Victricius of Rouen, *In Praise of the Saints*; Herval 1968: 112–13, 139–40.

98 Augustine, *Letters* 98, 5; 227; *City of God* 22, 8; *Against Julian* 52; 162; Flint 1991: 301–6; MacMullen (1997) stresses the continuity of pagan and Christian practices.

99 *Miracles of St. Artemius*, pp. 3, 4, 22, 24, 26, ed. Papodopoulos-Kerameus: tr. Crisafulli and Nesbitt 1997: 79–85, 130–3, 140–5, 147–53; Kazhdan and Sherry 1998. The collection and circulation of specific blocks of healing-miracle stories end with those of Artemius, and may have been deliberately created as a counterweight to stories of pagan healing. Nonetheless, individual stories of miraculous healing continued to form part of most saints' lives.

100 John of Ephesus, *Lives of the Eastern Saints* p. 643 Brooks; S. A. Harvey 1984: 88.

101 Procopius of Gaza, *Commentary on Kings III*: *Patrologia Graeca* 87, 1165; Temkin 1991; Chirban 2010.

102 Nicetas, *Sermon*: *Patrologia Latina* 52, 866A; Caesarius, *Sermon* 52, although this does not exclude the possibility of seeking medical help from a 'proper' doctor (see Flint 1991: 149).

103 Brown 1988.

104 Diadochus of Photike, *On Spiritual Knowledge* 53–5: p. 115 Des Places.

105 E.g. Arbesmann 1954; Ambrose, *On Virginity* 42; *Letters* 80; Asterius, *Homily* 10, 4, 3: p. 137 Datema; Basil, *Letters* 8; Nilus of Ancyra, *Letters* 3, 33; Origen, *Homily on Leviticus* 8; Romanos, *Hymns* 8 and 60.

106 Asterius, *Homilies* 9, 1 and 13: pp. 115, 127 Datema; Basil, *Letters* 260, 263; John Chrysostom, *On Ananias* 2–3; Nilus of Ancyra, *Letters* 3, 327; Origen, *Homily 1 on Psalm 38*; *Homily 18 on Jeremiah*; *Homily 18 on Numbers*; *Homily 2 on Kings*; *Homily 13 on Luke 2*; by the mid-seventh century, George of Pisidia (*Hexaemeron* 1544, cf. 1388–9) could regard Christ as 'the Galen of the soul'. In general, see Frings 1959; Molland 1970.

107 See pp. 294–5.

108 T. S. Miller (1997: 77–85) suggests an Orthodox response to Arian proselytisation. Alternatively, the numbers requiring assistance may have overwhelmed the relatively domestic arrangements found in the third century (see p. 296 here). Crislip (2005) prefers a link with Pachomian monasticism in Egypt in the early fourth century.

109 *Paschal Chronicle*, under the year 350; cf. also under 360.

110 Epiphanius, *A Cure-all for Heresy* 75.

111 Gregory of Nazianzus, *In Praise of Basil* 63, 82; Holman 2001.

112 Basil, *Letters* 94; cf. 50.

113 Gregory, *In Praise of Basil* 63.

114 Palladius, *Dialogues*: *Patrologia Graeca* 47, 200, with Chrysostom, *Against Stagirius* 3, 13; *Homily on Matthew* 56; and *Paschal Chronicle*, under the year 360; the Sampson hospital, T. S. Miller 1990. For the metaphor, see Nilus of Ancyra, *Letters* 3, 33.

115 Jerome, *Letters* 77, 66.

116 Augustine, *Sermons* 356, 10.

117 Sternberg 1991.

118 Kelly 1995: 255–62.

119 Chabot 1902: 265; Vööbus 1970: 129, 159; 1982: 70.

120 In general, see Mentzou-Meimari 1982. For a doctor attending a hospital in a small town in N.E. Asia Minor, see *CIG* 9256. For new archaeological discoveries in the Near East, see *Bulletin épigraphique* 1989: 102, no. 971; Koenen 1996: 181; Hirschfeld 1992: 196–9; Fowden 1999: 94–5.

121 Sozomen, *Ecclesiastical History* 3, 16; Joshua the Stylite, *Chronicle* 26; 28; 41–3.

122 Schwartz 1922–74: II, 1, 405; Cyril of Scythopolis, *Life of S. Sabas* 73, with De Vaux 1964; T. S. Miller 1990.

123 Dols 1987: 372; Procopius, *Buildings* 2, 10.

124 *Life of St. Artemius* 25–6.

125 P. Cairo Maspéro 67151. In some, doctors brought along students, just as they did to a private house.

126 John of Ephesus, *Lives*, p. 669 Brooks; Sozomen, *Ecclesiastical History* 4, 27.

127 Vööbus 1970: 129, Canon 22; 1982: 76, Canon 47 (cf. Canon 36); J. P. Thomas (1987), for the Byzantine legislation. Horden (2008: ch. I) offers a judicious overview of the debate on the medicalisation of the ancient hospital.

128 Papathomas 2000; Papyrus Sorbonne 69.

129 Vööbus 1970: 80.

130 Dols 1987: 372; Vööbus 1965: 145–6.

131 On one occasion the *xenodokeion* itself served as a prison; John of Tella was imprisoned in a *xenodokeion* at Nisibis while he was being brought in captivity to Antioch (*Life of John of Tella*, p. 45 Brooks).

132 Vööbus 1967: 100–1; 1970: 93.

133 *Pace* Dols 1987: 375, misled by Vööbus' (1967) English translation of the Syriac 'malpana', '(theological) teacher', as 'doctor'.

134 [Athanasius], *Questions, for Antiochus* 103–4: *Patrologia Graeca* 28, 662 (probably to be dated around 500); summarised in Anastasius of Sinai, *Moral Questions*, 114: *Patrologia Graeca* 89, 765. For Aristotle, see pp. 147–8 here.

20 CONCLUSION

1 Galen, of course, claimed to be largely drawing on what Hippocrates had done but had only adumbrated in his writings.

2 Cantor 2002. Lectures on the *Aphorisms*, however, were still given in the nineteenth century. A change from a practical to a historical view of ancient medicine can be neatly seen in the differences between F. Adams (1844–7, 1849 and 1856).

3 Nutton 2002b.

4 Gourevitch 1999b; Weisz 2002.

5 Wolstenholme 1982: 95–6; Cantor 2002: 281–4; Weisz 2002: 267–9.

6 Lloyd 2001; Attewell 2007.

7 Lloyd 2003.

8 Helman 1978; Rippere 1981. For the six non-naturals, cf. p. 306 here.

9 Powell 2003; Manzoni 2001; Rocca 2003.

10 Kagan 1994.

11 *Times*, 6 May 2003: 8.

12 Nutton 1995e; D. C. Smith 1996; Lederer 2002; Schubert 2005; Rütten 2007.

13 Lloyd 2003.

14 Aulus Gellius, *Attic Nights* 18, 10, 1.

15 Cf. the Parable of the Good Samaritan, *Luke* 10, 30–6; *CIL* 6, 5197, Agathopus, a slave doctor, accompanied his master on his journey back from Lyons to Rome *c*.AD 25, only for the latter to die soon after his arrival.

16 Xenophon, *Household Management* 7, 37; Columella, *On Agriculture* 12, 1, 5.

17 Hanson 1996: 159–82; King 1998: 180–7, both severely critical of earlier hagiography. Other ways to uncover women's role in ancient healing are outlined by M. H. Green 1989; Flemming 2000; Dasen 2004; H. Parker 2012.

18 Ullmann 1978a, 1978b: 7–40; Garcia-Ballester 1982, 1994: 13–29; Siraisi 1981; Nutton 1997b; Reeds 1991; Bylebyl 1979: 335–70.

19 French 1999: 163–85. His criticism was toned down in the second (1555) edition and in his later notes.

20 Harvey 1628; Wear 1983; French 1997.

21 For Scantia, see *CIL* 10, 3980 (*ILS* 7805).

22 For Demetrius, see Galen, 14, 4: tr. A. J. Brock 1929: 197–8; for Thyrsus, see *CIL* 6, 6320, from the burial place of the slaves of the Statilii family, *c*.AD 40.

BIBLIOGRAPHY

Abou Aly, A. (1992) *The Medical Writings of Rufus of Ephesus*, PhD thesis, University of London.

Adams, F. (1844–7) *The Seven Books of Paul of Aegina*, 3 vols, London: The Sydenham Society.

—— (1849) *The Genuine Writings of Hippocrates*, London: The Sydenham Society.

—— (1856) *The Extant Works of Aretaeus, the Cappadocian*, London: The Sydenham Society.

Adams, J. N. (1982) *The Latin Sexual Vocabulary*, London: Duckworth.

—— (1995) *Pelagonius and Latin Veterinary Terminology in the Roman Empire*, Leiden: Brill.

—— (2008) *Bilingualism and the Latin Language*, Cambridge: Cambridge University Press.

Aleshire, S. B. (1989) *The Athenian Asklepieon, the People, their Dedications and the Inventories*, Amsterdam: J. C. Gieben.

—— (1991) *Asklepios at Athens: Epigraphic and Prosopographic Essays on the Athenian Healing Cults*, Amsterdam: J. C. Gieben.

Alföldi, A. (1975) *Die römischen Inschriften von Tarraco*, Berlin: De Gruyter.

Algra, K., Barnes, J. and Mansfeld, J. (1999) *The Cambridge History of Hellenistic Philosophy*, Cambridge: Cambridge University Press.

Aliotta, G., Piomelli, D., Pollio, A. and Touwaide, A. (2003) *Le Piante medicinali nel Corpus Hippocraticum*, Milan: Guerini e Associati.

Allan, N. (2001) 'The physician in Ancient Israel', *Medical History*, 45: 377–94.

Althoff, J. (1999) 'Aristoteles als Medizindoxograph', in van der Eijk 1999a: 57–94.

Amigues, S. (2010) *Théophraste, Recherches sur les Plantes: A l'Origine de la Botanique*, Paris: Belin.

Amundsen, D. W. (1996) *Medicine, Society and Faith in the Ancient and Medieval Worlds*, Baltimore: Johns Hopkins University Press.

Amundsen, D. W. and Ferngren, G. B. (1977) 'The physician as expert witness in Athenian law', *Bulletin of the History of Medicine*, 51: 202–13.

Andò, V. (1999) 'Terapie ginecologiche, saperi femminili e specificità di genere', in Garofalo *et al.* 1999: 255–70.

Andorlini, I. (1995) *Trattato di Medicina su Papiro*, Florence: Istituto Papirologico.

—— (1997) '*Specimina*' per il Corpus dei Papiri Greci di Medicina', Florence: Istituto Papirologico.

—— (1999) 'Testi medici per la scuola: raccolte di definizioni e questionari nei papiri', in Garzya and Jouanna 1999: 1–15.

—— (2000) 'Codici papiracei di *medicina* con scoli e commento', in M. Goulet-Cazé (ed.) *Le Commentaire entre Tradition et Innovation*, Paris: Vrin: 41–52.

—— (2001) *Greek Medical Papyri*, vol. 1, Florence: Istituto Papirologico.

—— (2003) 'Il papiro inedito PSI inv. 1702 (cod. pap. I d. C.): un anonimo del genere degli Iatromathematikà', in A. Garzya and J. Jouanna (eds) *Trasmissione e Ecdotica dei Testi medici greci*, Naples: D'Auria: 7–23.

—— (ed.) (2004) *Testi medici su papiro*, Florence: Istituto Papirologico.

—— (2009) *Greek Medical Papyri*, vol. 2, Florence: Istituto Papirologico.

Andorlini, I. and Marcone, A. (2004) *Medicina, Medico e Società nel Mondo antico*, Florence: Le Monnier Università/Storia.

André, J. (1955) 'Les Noms latins de l'hellébore', *Revue des Études latines*, 32: 174–87.

—— (1956) 'Pline l'ancien botaniste', *Revue des Études latines*, 33: 297–318.

André, J. M. (2006) *La Médecine grecque à Rome*, Paris: Tallandier.

Arbesmann, A. (1954) 'The concept of "Christus medicus" in St. Augustine', *Traditio*, 10: 1–28.

Arikha, N. (2007) *Passions and Tempers: A History of the Humours*, New York: Ecco.

Arnott, R. (1996) 'Healing and medicine in the Aegean Bronze Age', *Journal of the Royal Society of Medicine*, 89: 265–70.

—— (1997) 'Surgical practice in the prehistoric Aegean', *Medizinhistorisches Journal*, 32: 249–77.

Arnott, R., Finger, S., Smith, C. U. M., Lichterman, B. and Breitwieser, R. (eds) (2003) *Trepanation: History, Discovery, Theory*, Lisse: Swets and Zeitlinger.

Asmus, R. (1911) *Das Leben des Philosophen Isidoros von Damaskios aus Damaskos*, Leipzig: Teubner.

—— (1913) 'Der neuplatoniker Asklepiodotos der Grosse', *Sudhoffs Archiv*, 7: 36–42.

Astin, A. E. (1969) *Cato the Censor*, Oxford: Clarendon Press.

Aston, E. (2004) 'Asclepius and the legacy of Thessaly', *Classical Quarterly*, 54: 18–32.

Attewell, G. N. A. (2007) *Refiguring Unani Tibb: Plural Healing in Late Colonial India*, New Delhi: Longman Orient.

Attia, A. and Buisson, G. (eds) (2009) *Advances in Mesopotamian Medicine from Hammurabi to Hippocrates*, Leiden and Boston: Brill.

Aufderheide, A. C. and Rodriguez-Martin, C. (1998) *The Cambridge Encyclopedia of Human Paleopathology*, Cambridge: Cambridge University Press.

Aufmesser, M. (2000) *Etymologische und wortgeschichtliche Erläuterungen zu De materia medica des Dioscurides*, Hildesheim, Zurich and New York: Olms-Weidmann.

Baader, G. (1989) 'Die Tradition des Corpus Hippocraticum im europäischen Mittelalter', in Baader and Winau 1989: 409–19.

Baader, G. and Winau, R. (eds) (1989) *Die Hippokratischen Epidemien*, Stuttgart: Franz Steiner.

Bagnall, R. S. and Frier, B. W. (1994) *The Demography of Roman Egypt*, Cambridge: Cambridge University Press.

Bailey, A. (2002) *Sextus Empiricus and Pyrrhonean Scepticism*, Oxford: Clarendon Press.

Bailey, C. (1947) *Lucretius, De Rerum Natura*, Oxford: Clarendon Press.

Baker, P. (2002) 'The Roman military *Valetudinaria*: fact or fiction?', in R. Arnott (ed.) *The Archaeology of Medicine Proceedings of the Theoretical Archaeology Group 1998*, Oxford: Archaeopress: 69–80.

—— (2004) *Medical Care for the Roman Army on the Rhine, Danube and British Frontiers from the First through Third Centuries AD*, Oxford: Hadrian Books.

Baldwin, B. (1975) 'The career of Oribasius', *Acta Classica*, 18: 85–97.

—— (1992) 'The career and works of Scribonius Largus', *Rheinisches Museum*, 135: 74–82.

Barb, A. A. (1950) 'Birds and medical magic', *Journal of the Warburg and Courtauld Institutes*, 13: 318–22.

Bardinet, T. (1995) *Les Papyrus médicaux de l'Egypte pharaonique*, Paris: Fayard.

Barnes, J. (1990) *The Toils of Scepticism*, Cambridge: Cambridge University Press.

—— (1991) 'Galen on logic and therapy', in Kudlien and Durling 1991: 50–102.

—— (1997) 'Logique et pharmacologie: à propos de quelques remarques d'ordre linguistique dans le *De simplicium medicamentorum temperamentis ac facultatibus* de Galien', in Debru 1997: 3–34.

—— (2007) *Truth, etc. Six Lectures on Ancient Logic*, Oxford: Oxford University Press.

Barnes, J. and Jouanna, J. (eds) (2003) *Galien et la Philosophie*, Vandoeuvres: Fondation Hardt.

Baron, S. W. (1948) *The Jewish Community*, Philadelphia: Jewish Publication Society of America.

Barras, V., Birchler, T. and Morand, A.-F. (1995) *Galien: L'Âme et ses Passions*, Paris: Les Belles Lettres.

Bartels, E. M., Swaddling, J. and Harrison, A. P. (2006) 'An ancient Greek pain remedy for athletes', *Pain Practice*, 6(3): 212–18.

Barton, T. S. (1994a) *Ancient Astrology*, London: Routledge.

—— (1994b) *Power and Knowledge: Astrology, Medicine and Physiognomics Under the Roman Empire*, Ann Arbor: University of Michigan Press.

Bates, D. (ed.) (1995) *Knowledge and the Scholarly Medical Traditions*, Cambridge: Cambridge University Press.

Beagon, M. (1992) *Roman Nature: The Thought of Pliny the Elder*, Oxford: Clarendon Press.

—— (2005) *The Elder Pliny on the Human Animal: Natural History, Book 7*, Oxford: Clarendon Press.

Bean, G. E. and Mitford, T. B. (1970) 'Journeys in rough Cilicia', *Denkschriften der Akademie der Wissenschaften in Wien*, 102: 3.

Beard, M. and Henderson, J. (1995) *A Short Guide to the Classics*, Oxford: Oxford University Press.

Beard, M., North, J. and Price, S. (1998) *Religions of Rome, Vol. 1: A History*, Cambridge: Cambridge University Press.

Beccaria, A. (1971) 'Sulle tracce di un antico canone latino di Ippocrate e Galeno', *Italia medioevale e umanistica*, 14: 1–24.

Beck, L. Y. (2005) *Dioscorides of Anazarbus, De materia medica*, Hildesheim and New York: Olms-Weidmann.

Behr, C. A. (1968) *Aelius Aristides and the Sacred Tales*, Amsterdam: Hakkert; repr. in *P. Aelius Aristides, The Complete Works*, vol. II, Leiden: Brill, 1981.

Bellemare, P. M. (1999) 'The Hippocratic Oath: Edelstein revisited', in J. K. Coyle and S. C. Muir (eds) *Healing in Religion and Society from Hippocrates to the Puritans: Selected Studies*, Lewiston, Queenston and Lampeter: The Edwin Mellon Press: 1–64.

Below, K. H. (1953) *Der Arzt im römischen Recht*, Munich: C. H. Beck.

Bendlin, A. (2011) 'On the uses and disasdvantages of divination in oracles: oracles and their literary representation in the time of the Second Sophistic', in J. A. North and S. R. F. Price (eds) *The Religious History of the Roman Empire*, Oxford: Oxford University Press: 175–250.

Bendz, G. (1964) *Studien zu Caelius Aurelianus und Cassius Felix*, Lund: C. W. K. Glerup.

—— (1990–3) *Caelius Aurelianus, Celeres Passiones, Acutae Passiones*, Berlin: Akademie Verlag.

Benedum, J. (1967) 'Die balnea pensilia des Asklepiades von Prusa', *Gesnerus*, 24: 93–107.

—— (1971) 'Statilios Attalos', *Medizinhistorisches Journal*, 6: 264–77.

—— (1978) 'Markos Modios Asiatikos', *Medizinhistorisches Journal*, 13: 307–9.

Berger, E. (1970) *Das Basler Arztrelief*, Basle: Karger.

Bergsträsser, G. (1925) 'Hunain ibn Ishaq, über die syrischen und arabischen Galen-Übersetzungen', *Abhandlungen für die Kunde des Morgenlandes*, 17: 2.

—— (1932) 'Neue Materialien zu Hunain Ibn Ishaq's Galen-bibliographie', *Abhandlungen für die Kunde des Morgenlandes*, 19: 2.

Bertier, J. (1972) *Mnésithée et Dieuchès*, Leiden: Brill.

—— (1989) 'A propos de quelques résurgences des epidémies dans les problemata du corpus aristotelicien', in Baader and Winau 1989: 261–9.

Besnier, M. (1902) *L'Île Tibérine dans l'Antiquité*, Paris: A. Fontemoing.

Betz, H. D. (ed.) (1992) *The Greek Magical Papyri in Translation, Including the Demotic Spells*, ed. 2, Chicago: University of Chicago Press.

Betz, O. (1986) 'Der Aussatz in der Bibel', in Wolf 1986: 45–62.

Biggs, R. D. (1969) 'Medicine in Ancient Mesopotamia', *History of Science*, 8: 94–105.

Bing, P. (2004) 'Posidippus' *Iamatika*, in B. Acosta-Hughes, E. Kosmetatou and M. Baumbach (eds) *Labored in Papyrus Leaves: Perspectives on an Epigram Collection Attributed to Posidippus (P. Mil. Vogl. VIII 309)*, Cambridge, MA: Harvard University Press: 276–91.

Björck, G. (1944) *Apsyrtus, Julius Africanus et l'Hippiatrique grecque*, Leipzig: Harrassowitz.

Bliquez, L. J. (1994) *Roman Surgical Instruments and Other Minor Objects in the Archaeological Museum of Naples*, Mainz: Philipp von Zabern.

—— (1996) 'Prosthetics in Classical Antiquity', *ANRW*, II, 37(3): 2640–76.

Bliquez, L. J. and Kazhdan, A. (1984) 'Four testimonia to human dissection in Byzantine times', *Bulletin of the History of Medicine*, 58: 554–7.

Bloomer, W. M. (1992) *Valerius Maximus and the Rhetoric of the New Nobility*, Chapel Hill and London: University of North Carolina Press.

Bobzien, S. (2002) 'Pre-stoic hypothetical syllogistic in Galen's *Institutio Logica*', in Nutton 2002a: 57–72.

Böcher, O. (1972) *Christus Exorcista: Dämonismus und Taufe im Neuen Testament*, Stuttgart: W. Kohlhammer.

Bodel, J. (2000) 'Dealing with the dead: undertakers, executioners and potter's fields in ancient Rome', in Hope and Marshall 2000: 128–51.

Bodson, L. (1991) 'Le vocabulaire latin des maladies pestilentielles et épizootiques', in Sabbah 1991: 215–42.

Boon, G. C. (1983) 'Potters, oculists, and eye-troubles', *Britannia*, 14: 1–12.

Borca, F. (2000) 'Towns and marshes in the ancient world', in Hope and Marshall 2000: 74–84.

Born, G. V. R. (2002) 'The wide-ranging family history of Max Born', *Notes and Records of the Royal Society of London*, 56: 219–26.

Boscherini, S. (1970) *Lingua e scienza nel 'De agri cultura' di Catone*, Rome: Ateneo.

—— (1993a) 'La medicina in Catone e Varrone', *ANRW*, II, 37(1): 729–52.

—— (ed.) (1993b) *Studi di Lessicologia medica antica*, Bologna: Patron.

Bosnakis, D. and Hallof, K. (2008) 'Alte und neue Inschriften aus Kos, III', *Chiron*, 38: 205–42.

Bosworth, A. W. (2002) 'Vespasian and the slave trade', *Classical Quarterly*, 52: 350–7.

Boudon, V. (2001) 'Deux manuscrits médicaux arabes de Meshed (Rida tibb 5223 et 80): nouvelles découvertes sur le texte de Galien', *Comptes rendus de l'Académie des Inscriptions et belles Lettres*: 197–220.

—— (2002) 'Galen's On My Own Books: new material from Meshed, Rida, tibb. 5223', in Nutton 2002a: 9–18.

Boudon-Millot, V. (2007) *Galien, Tome I, Introduction générale. Sur l'Ordre des ses propres Livres. Sur ses propres Livres. Que l'excellent Médecin est aussi Philosophe*, Paris: Les Belles Lettres.

—— (2011) 'L'ecdotique des textes médicaux grecs et l'apport des traditions orientales', in R. Goulet and U. Rudolph (eds) *Entre Orient et Occident: La Philosophie et la Science gréco-romaines dans le Monde arabe*, Vandoeuvres: Fondation Hardt: 322–88.

Boudon-Millot, V. and Pietrobelli, A. (2005) 'Galien ressuscité: édition *princeps* du texte grec du *De propriis placitis*', *Revue des Études grecques*, 118: 168–213.

Boudon-Millot, V., Guardasole, A. and Magdelaine, C. (eds) (2007) *La Science médicale antique. Nouveaux Regards. Études réunies en l'Honneur de Jacques Jouanna*, Paris: Beauchesne.

Boudon-Millot, V., Jouanna, J. and Pietrobelli, A. (2010) *Galien. Tome IV. Ne pas se chagriner*, Paris: Les Belles Lettres.

Boudreaux, P. (1912) *Catalogus codicum astrologorum graecorum. Codicus Parisinorum pars tertia, Tome VIII.*, 3, Brussels: H. Lamertin.

Boulogne, J. (1996) 'Plutarque et la médecine', *ANRW*, 37(2): 2762–92.

Bowersock, G. W. (1965) *Augustus and the Greek World*, Oxford: Clarendon Press.

—— (1969) *Greek Sophists in the Roman Empire*, Oxford: Clarendon Press.

—— (2010a) 'Iatrosophists', in L. Galli Milič and N. Hecket-Noti (eds) *Historiae Augustae Colloquium genevense in honorem F. Paschoud septuagenarii*, Bari: Edipuglia: 83–91.

—— (2010b) 'Parabalani: a terrorist charity in late antiquity', *Anabases*, 12: 45–54.

Bowersock, G. W., Brown, P. and Grabar, O. (eds) (1999) *Late Antiquity*, Cambridge, MA: Harvard University Press.

Bowman, A. K. and Thomas, J. D. (1991) 'A military strength report from Vindolanda', *Journal of Roman Studies*, 81: 62–73.

Bowman, A. K., Garnsey, P. and Rathbone, D. (eds) (2000) *The Cambridge Ancient History, Vol. XI. The High Empire, A.D. 70–192*, Cambridge: Cambridge University Press.

Brain, P. (1986) *Galen on Bloodletting*, Cambridge: Cambridge University Press.

Bratton, T. L. (1981) 'The identity of the plague of Justinian', *Transactions and Studies of the College of Physicians of Philadelphia*, 5(3): 113–24, 174–80.

Braund, D. C. and Wilkins, J. (eds) (2000) *Athenaeus and his World: Reading Greek Culture in the Roman Empire*, Exeter: University of Exeter Press.

Brecht, F. J. (1931) *Motiv- und Typengeschichte des griechischen Spottepigramme, Philologus, Suppl.*, 22: 1.

Breitwieser, R. (1998) *Medizin im römischen Österreich*, Linz: Museum des Stadt Linz.

Brock, A. J. (1916) *Galen on the Natural Faculties*, London: Heinemann.

—— (1929) *Greek Medicine*, London: J. M. Dent.

Brock, R. (2000) 'Sickness in the body politic: medical imagery in the Greek polis', in Hope and Marshall 2000: 24–34.

Brooks, C. M., Gilbert, J. L., Levey, H. A. and Curtis, D. R. (1962) *Humors, Hormones and Neurosecretions*, Albany: State University of New York Press.

Brown, P. (1972) *Religion and Society in the Age of St. Augustine*, London: Faber and Faber.

—— (1978) *The Making of Late Antiquity*, Cambridge, MA: Harvard University Press.

—— (1988) *The Body and Society*, New York: Knopf.

Browning, R. (1985) 'A further testimony to human dissection in the Byzantine world', *Bulletin of the History of Medicine*, 59: 518–20.

Bruce-Chwatt, L. J. and de Zulueta, J. (1980) *The Rise and Fall of Malaria in Europe: A Historico-epidemiological Survey*, Oxford: Oxford University Press.

Brugmann, K. (1983) 'Edikt der Triumviri oder Senatsbeschluss?', *Epigraphica Anatolica*, 2: 47–73.

Bruni Celli, B. (1984) *Bibliografía Hipocrática*, Caracas: Ediciones del Rectorado Universidad Central de Venezuela.

Brunner, F. G. (1977) *Pathologie und Therapie der Geschwülste in der antiken Medizin bei Celsus und Galen*, Zurich: Juris Druck.

Brunt, P. A. (1971) *Roman Manpower, 225 B.C.–A.D.14*, Oxford: Clarendon Press.

—— (1973) 'Aspects of the social thought of Dio Chrysostom and the Stoics', *Proceedings of the Cambridge Philological Society*, n.s. 19: 26–34.

—— (1988) *The Fall of the Roman Republic*, Oxford: Clarendon Press.

Bruun, C. (2007) 'The Antonine plague and the third-century crisis', in O. Hekster, G. de Kleijn and D. Slootjes (eds) *Crisis in the Roman Empire: Proceedings of the Seventh Workshop of the International Network Impact of Empire (Nijmegen, June 20–24, 2006)*, Leiden and Boston: Brill.

Bruun, H. (1997) '*De morbo sacro* and *De aere aquis locis*', *Classica et Mediaevalia*, 48: 15–48.

Buell, D. K. (1999) *Making Christians: Clement of Alexandria and the Rhetoric of Legitimacy*, Princeton: Princeton University Press.

Burford, A. (1969) *The Greek Temple Builders at Epidauros*, Liverpool: Liverpool University Press.

Burguière, P., Gourevitch, D. and Malinas, J. (1988–2000) *Soranas d'Ephèse, Maladies des Femmes*, 4 vols, Paris: Les Belles Lettres.

Burke, P. F. (1996) 'Malaria in the Greco-Roman world', *ANRW*, II, 37(2): 2252–81.

Burkert, W. (1992) *The Orientalizing Revolution*, Cambridge, MA: Harvard University Press.

Byl, S. (1995) 'L'aire géographique des médecins hippocratiques', in van der Eijk *et al.* 1995: 225–35.

Bylebyl, J. J. (1979) 'Padua and humanistic medicine', in C. Webster (ed.) *Health, Medicine and Mortality in the Sixteenth Century*, Cambridge: Cambridge University Press.

Cadbury, H. J. (1919) *The Style and Literary Method of Luke*, Cambridge: Cambridge University Press.

Cameron, A. (1993) *The Mediterranean World of Late Antiquity*, London: Routledge.

Canfora, L. (1987) *La Biblioteca scomparsa*, Bari: Laterza.

Cantor, D. (ed.) (2002) *Reinventing Hippocrates*, Aldershot: Ashgate.

Caracci, P. (1964) 'Medici e medicina in Aquileia Romana', *Aquileia Nostra*, 35: 87–102.

Carlino, A. (1999) *Books of the Body: Anatomical Ritual and Renaissance Learning*, Chicago: Chicago University Press.

Carmichael, A. G. (1993) 'Plague of Athens', in Kiple 1993: 934–7.

Carrick, P. (1985) *Medical Ethics in Antiquity: Philosophical Perspectives on Abortion and Euthanasia*, Dordrecht: Reidel.

Carter, J. C. (ed.) (1998) *The Chora of Metapontum: The Necropoleis*, Austin: University of Texas Press.

Casey, P. J. and Hoffmann, B. (1999) 'Excavations at the Roman temple in Lydney Park, Gloucestershire, in 1980 and 1981', *Antiquaries Journal*, 79: 81–144.

Casson, L. (2001) *Libraries in the Ancient World*, New Haven: Yale University Press.

Castrén, P. (ed.) (1989) *Ancient and Popular Healing*, Athens: Finnish Institute in Athens.

Catalano, V. (1966) *Case, abitanti e culti ad Ercolano*, Rome: Bardi.

Cavenale, R. (2001) 'L'anesthésie chirurgicale dans l'antiquité gréco-romaine', *Medicina nei Secoli*, n.s. 13: 25–46.

Celli, A. (1933) *The History of Malaria in the Roman Campagna*, London: J. Bale.

Ceschi, G. (2009) *Il vocabolario medico di Sofocle: Analisi dei contatti con il Corpus Hippocraticum nel lessico anatomico-fisiologico, patologico e terapeutico*, Venice: Istituto veneto di scienze, lettere ed arti.

Chabot, J. B. (1902) *Synodicon Orientale*, Paris: Imprimerie nationale.

Chang, H.-H. (2005) 'The cities of the Hippocratic doctors', in van der Eijk 2005a: 17–72.

Chaniotis, A. (1995) 'Illness and cures in the Greek propitiatory inscriptions and dedications of Lydia and Phrygia', in van der Eijk *et al.* 1995: 323–44.

Chirban, J. T. (ed.) (2010) *Holistic Healing in Byzantium*, Brookline, MA: Holy Cross Orthodox Press.

Christol, M. and Drew-Bear, T. (2004) 'Caracalla et son médecin L. Gellius Maximus à Antioche de Pisidie', in S. Colvin (ed.) *The Greco-Roman East: Politics, Culture, Society*, New Haven: Yale University Press: 85–118.

Cichorius, C. (1922) *Römische Studien*, Leipzig: Teubner.

Cipolla, C. M. (1976) *Public Health and the Medical Profession in the Renaissance*, Cambridge: Cambridge University Press.

Clackson, J. and Meissner, T. (2000) 'The poet of Chester', *Proceedings of the Cambridge Philological Society*, 46: 1–6.

Clanchy, M. T. (1993) *From Memory to Written Record*, Oxford: Oxford University Press.

Clinton, K. (1994) 'The Epidauria and the arrival of Asclepius in Athens', in T. Hägg (ed.) *Ancient Greek Cult Practice from the Epigraphic Evidence*, Stockholm: Almqvist: 17–34.

Cohn-Haft, L. (1956) *The Public Physicians of Ancient Greece*, Northampton, MA: Smith College.

Collins, M. (2000) *Medieval Herbals: The Illustrative Tradition*, London: The British Library.

Comella, A. (1981) 'Tipologia e diffusione dei complessi votivi in Italia in epoca medio- e tardo-repubblicana', *Mélanges de l'École française de Rome*, 93: 717–803.

Congourdeau, M. H. (1994) 'Metrodora et son oeuvre', in E. Patlagean (ed.) *Maladie et Société à Byzance*, Paris: Les Belles Lettres: 57–96.

Connolly, A. (1998) 'Was Sophocles heroized as Dexion?', *Journal of Hellenic Studies*, 118: 1–21.

Conrad, L. I. (1981) *The Plague in the Early Middle East*, PhD thesis, Princeton University.

Conrad, L. I., Neve, M., Nutton, V., Porter, R. and Wear, A. (1995) *The Western Medical Tradition*, Cambridge: Cambridge University Press.

Cooper, G. M. (2011a) Galen and astrology: a marriage made in heaven', *Early Science and Medicine*, 16: 10–46.

—— (2011b) *Galen, De diebus decretoriis, from Greek into Arabic*, Farnham and Burlington: Ashgate.

Cordes, P. (1994) *Iatros: das Bild des Arztes in der griechischen Literatur von Homer bis Aristoteles*, Stuttgart: Steiner.

Corvisier, J. N., Didier, C. and Valdher, M. (eds) (2001) *Thérapies, Médecine et Démographie antiques*, Arras: Artois Presses Université.

Craik, E. M. (1995a) 'Diet, *diaeta*, and dietetics', in C. A. Powell (ed.) *The Greek World*, London: Routledge: 387–402.

—— (1995b) 'Hippocratic diaita', in Wilkins *et al.* 1995: 343–50.

—— (1998a) *Hippocrates, Places in Man*, Oxford: Clarendon Press.

—— (1998b) 'The Hippocratic treatise *On Anatomy*', *Classical Quarterly*, 48: 135–67.

—— (2001a) 'Medical reference in Euripides', *Bulletin of the Institute of Classical Studies*, 45: 81–95.

—— (2001b) 'Plato and medical texts; *Symposium* 185c–193d', *Classical Quarterly*, 51: 109–14.

—— (2001c) 'Thucydides on the plague: physiology of flux and fixation', *Classical Quarterly*, 51: 102–8.

—— (2010) 'The teaching of surgery', in Horstmanshoff 2010: 223–34.

Crisafulli, V. S. and Nesbitt, J. L. (1997) *The Miracles of St. Artemios*, Leiden: Brill.

Crislip, A. (2005) *From Monastery to Hospital: Christian Monasticism and the Transformation of Health Care in Late Antiquity*, Ann Arbor: University of Michigan Press.

Cronier, M. (2009) 'L'herbier alphabétique grec de Dioscoride: quelques remarques sur sa genèse et ses sources textuelles', in Ferraces Rodríguez 2009: 33–60.

424

Croon, J. H. (1967) 'Hot springs and healing Gods', *Mnemosyne*, 40: 225–46.

Cule, J. (1975) 'Pestis flava: y Fad Felen', in J. Cule (ed.) *Wales and Medicine*, Llandysul: Gomer Press.

Cunningham, A. (1986) 'The theory/practice division of medicine: two late-Alexandrian legacies', in T. Ogawa (ed.) *History of Traditional Medicine*, Osaka: Taniguchi Foundation: 303–24.

D'Arms, J. H. (1970) *Romans on the Bay of Naples: A Social and Cultural Study of the Villas and their Owners from 150 B.C. to A.D. 400*, Cambridge, MA: Harvard University Press.

Da Vinci, L. (1977) *Leonardo da Vinci: Anatomical Drawings from the Royal Collection*, Exhibition Catalogue, London: Royal Academy of Arts.

Daremberg, C. and Ruelle, E. (1879) *Oeuvres de Rufus d'Ephèse*, Paris: Imprimerie nationale.

Dasen, V. (1993) *Dwarfs in Ancient Egypt and Greece*, Oxford: Clarendon Press.

—— (ed.) (2004) *Naissance et petite Enfance dans l'Antiquité*, Fribourg: Academic Press.

David, A. R. (2010) 'Atherosclerosis and diet in Ancient Egypt', *The Lancet*, 375: 718–19.

Davies, M. (1988) *Epicorum graecorum Fragmenta*, Göttingen: Vandenhoeck & Ruprecht.

Davies, R. W. (1969) 'The medici of the Roman armed forces', *Epigraphische Studien*, 8: 83–9.

—— (1970a) 'Some Roman medicine', *Medical History*, 14: 101–6.

—— (1970b) 'The Roman military medical service', *Saalburg Jahrbuch*, 27: 84–104.

—— (1972) 'Some more military medici', *Epigraphische Studien*, 9: 1–11.

De Carolis, S. (ed.) (2009) *Ars medica. I ferri del mestiere. La* domus *'del Chirurgo' di Rimini e la chirurgia nell'antica Roma*, Rimini: Guaraldi.

De Vaux, R. (1964) 'Les Hôpitaux de Justinian à Jérusalem d'après les dernières fouilles', *Comptes rendus de l'Académie des Inscriptions et belles Lettres*: 202–7.

Dean-Jones, L. A. (1994) *Women's Bodies in Classical Greek Science*, Oxford: Clarendon Press.

—— (1995) '*Autopsia, historia* and what women know: the authority of women in Hippocratic gynaecology', in Bates 1995: 41–59.

—— (2010) '*Physician*: a metapaedogogical text', in Horstmanshoff 2010: 53–72.

Debru, A. (1994) 'L'expérimentation chez Galien', *ANRW*, II, 37(2): 1718–56.

—— (1995a) 'Les démonstrations médicales à Rome au temps de Galien', in van der Eijk *et al.* 1995: 69–82.

—— (1995b) 'L'ordre de formation des organes embryonnaires: la retractio de Galien', *Bulletin d'Histoire et d'Epistémologie des Sciences de la Vie*, 2: 156–63.

—— (ed.) (1997) *Galen on Pharmacology: Philosophy, History and Medicine*, Leiden: Brill.

—— (ed.) (1998) *Nommer la Maladie: Recherches sur le Léxique grécolatin de la Pathologie, Mémoires du Centre Jean Palerne*, 17.

—— (2002) 'Galen, *On the Unclear Movements*', in Nutton 2002a: 79–85.

—— (2005) 'Theophrastus' biological opuscula and the Hippocratic Corpus: a critical dialogue', in van der Eijk 2005a: 325–42.

—— (2008) 'Physiology', in Hankinson 2008: 263–82.

Debru, A. and Palmieri, N. (eds) (2001) *Docente Natura: Mélanges de Médecine ancienne et médiévale offerts à Jean Sabbah*, St Etienne: Université de St Etienne.

Degrassi, D. (1986) 'Il culto di Esculapio in Italia centrale durante il periodo reppublicano', in F. Coarelli (ed.) *Fregellae 2: Il santuario di Esculapio*, Rome: Qasar.

Deichgräber, K. (1933) *Die Epidemien und das Corpus Hippocraticum*, Berlin: Akademie Verlag.

—— (1950) *Professio medici: Zum Vorwort des Scribonius Largus*, Mainz: Steiner.

—— (1956) 'Parabasenverse aus Thesmophoriazusen II des Aristophanes bei Galen', *Sitzungsberichte der Akademie der Wissenschaften zu Berlin*.

—— (1965) *Die griechische Empirikerschule*, ed. 2, Berlin, Zurich: Weidmann.

—— (1970) 'Medicus gratiosus', *Abhandlungen der Akademie der Wissenschaften in Mainz, geistes- und sozialwissenschaftliche Klasse*: 195–309.

—— (1971) 'Aretaeus von Kappadokien als medizinischer Schriftsteller', *Abhandlungen der sächsichen Akademie der Wissenschaften*, 63: 3.

—— (1976) 'Ausgewähltes aus der medizinischen Literatur der Antike, I', *Philologus*, 101: 135–47.

Del Guerra, G. (1994) *Medicina e Cosmesi ad Uso delle Donne*, Milan: Mimesis.

DeLacy, P. (1988) 'The third part of the soul', in Manuli and Vegetti 1988: 43–63.

DeLaine, J. and Johnston, D. E. (1992) *Roman Baths and Bathing: Journal of Roman Archaeology, Suppl. series*, 37.

Della Corte, M. (1959) 'La scuola di Epicuro in alcune pitture Pompeiane', *Studi Romani*, 7: 126–45.

Demand, N. (1994) *Birth, Death and Motherhood in Classical Greece*, Baltimore and London: Johns Hopkins University Press.

Dench, E. (1995) *From Barbarians to New Men: Greek, Roman and Modern Perceptions of the Peoples of the Central Apennines*, Oxford: Clarendon Press.

Deuse, W. (1993) 'Celsus im Prooemium von "De medicina": Römische Aneignung griechischer Wissenschaft', *ANRW*, II, 37(1): 819–41.

Di Benedetto, V. (1986) *Il Medico e la Malattia*, Turin: Einaudi.

Dickie, M. (2001) *Magic and Magicians in the Greco-Roman World*, London: Routledge.

Dickson, K. (1998) *Stephanus the Philosopher and Physician: Commentary on Galen's Therapeutics to Glaucon*, Leiden: Brill.

Diels, H. (1970) *Die Handschriften der griechischen Ärzte*, repr., Leipzig: Teubner.

Diller, H. (1936a) 'Nikon', *RE*, 17(1): 507–8.

—— (1936b) 'Thessalos', *RE*, 2e Reihe, 6: 167–82.

Dillon, M. P. J. (1994) 'The didactic nature of the Epidaurian *iamata*', *Zeitschrift für Papyrologie und Epigraphik*, 101: 239–60.

—— (1997) *Pilgrims and Pilgrimage in Ancient Greece*, London: Routledge.

Dinkler, E. (1980) 'Christus und Asklepios: zum Christus-typus der polychromen Platten im Museo Nazionale Romano', *Sitzungsberichte der Heidelberger Akademie der Wissenschaften, philosophisch-historische Klasse*.

Dobson, M. J. (1997) *Contours of Death and Disease in Early Modern England*, Cambridge: Cambridge University Press.

Dodds, E. R. (1965) *Pagan and Christian in an Age of Anxiety*, Cambridge: Cambridge University Press.

Dolmans, M. T. R. M. (1993) *Valetudinaria Exercitus*, PhD thesis, University of Leiden.

Dols, M. (1987) 'The origin of the Islamic hospital: myth and reality', *Bulletin of the History of Medicine*, 61: 367–90.

—— (1992) *Majnun: The Madman in Medieval Islamic Society*, Oxford: Clarendon Press.

Donini, P. L. (1992) 'Galeno e la filosofia', *ANRW*, II, 36(5): 3484–504.

Doyen-Higuet, A. M. (1984) 'The Hippiatrica and Byzantine veterinary medicine', *Dumbarton Oaks Papers*, 38: 111–20.

Drabkin, I. E. (1950) *Caelius Aurelianus: On Acute and Chronic Diseases*, Chicago: University of Chicago Press.

—— (1951) 'Soranus and his system of medicine', *Bulletin of the History of Medicine*, 25: 503–18.

Drachmann, A. G. (1963) *The Mechanical Technology of Greek and Roman Antiquity*, Copenhagen: Munksgaard.

Duckworth, W. H. L. (1962) *Galen on Anatomical Procedures: The Later Books*, Cambridge: Cambridge University Press.

Duffy, J. M. (1984) 'Byzantine medicine in the sixth and seventh centuries: aspects of teaching and practice', *Dumbarton Oaks Papers*, 38: 21–7.

Duminil, M. P. (1983) *Le Sang, les Vaisseaux, le Coeur dans la Collection hippocratique*, Paris: Les Belles Lettres.

Duncan-Jones, R. P. (1996) 'The impact of the Antonine plague', *Journal of Roman Archaeology*, 9: 108–36.

Durand, J. M. (1988) *Maladies et Médecins: Archives royales de Mari 26*, Paris: Editions Recherche sur les Civilisations.

Dzierzykray-Rogalski, T. (1980) 'Palaeopathology of the Ptolemaic inhabitants of Dakleh oasis (Egypt)', *Journal of Human Evolution*, 9: 71–4.

Ebbell, B. (1967) 'Beiträge zur ältesten Geschichte einiger Infektionskrankheiten', *Skrifter utgitt av det Norske Videnskaps-Akademi i Oslo*, n.s. 2.

Ebbesen, S. (1981) *Commentators and Commentaries on Aristotle's Sophistici Elenchi*, 4 vols, Leiden: Brill.

Ebner, P. (1966) 'Nuove epigrafe di Velia', *La Parola del Passato*, 108–10: 336–41.

Edel, E. (1976) *Ägyptische Ärzte und ägyptische Medizin am hethischen Königshof*, Opladen: Westdeutscher Verlag.

Edelstein, E. J. and Edelstein, L. (1945) *Asclepius: Collection and Interpretation of the Testimonies*, 2 vols, Baltimore: Johns Hopkins University Press; repr. 1998. (Cited as Edelstein 1945.)

Edelstein, L. (1967) *Ancient Medicine: Select Papers of Ludwig Edelstein*, Baltimore: Johns Hopkins University Press.

Edlow, R. B. (1977) *Galen on Language and Ambiguity*, Leiden: Brill.

Edwards, C. and Woolf, G. (eds) (2003) *Rome the Cosmopolis*, Cambridge: Cambridge University Press.

Edwards, M. (1997) 'Simon Magus, the bad Samaritan', in M. J. Edwards and S. Swain (eds) *Portraits: Biographical Representation in the Greek and Latin Literature of the Roman Empire*, Oxford: Clarendon Press: 69–91.

Effe, B. (1974) 'Der Aufbau von Nikanders Theriaka und Alexipharmaka', *Rheinisches Museum*, 117: 53–66.

Ehrhardt, N. (1989) 'Apollon Ietros: ein verschollener Gott Ioniens', *Istanbuler Mitteilungen*, 39: 115–22.

Ehrhardt, P. (1974) *Satirische Epigramme auf Ärzte: Eine medizinhistorische Studie auf der Grundlage des XI. Buches der Anthologia Palatina*, MD thesis, University of Erlangen.

Eisinger, J. (1982) 'Lead and wine: Eberhard Gockel and the *Colica Pictonum*', *Medical History*, 26: 279–302.

Eitrem, S. (1950) *Some Notes on Demonology in the New Testament*, Oslo: A. W. Brøgger.

el-Abbadi, M. (1992) *The Life and Fate of the Library of Alexandria*, Paris: Unesco.

el-Saghir, M. (1986) *Le Camp romain Lougsor*, Cairo: Institut français.

Engelmann, H. (1990) 'Ephesische Inschriften', *Zeitschrift für Papyrologie und Epigraphik*, 84: 89–94.

Erbse, H. (1974) *Scholia Graeca in Homeri Iliadem*, vol. 3, Berlin: De Gruyter.

Eschebach, H. (1984) *Die Ärztehäuser in Pompeii*, *Antike Welt, Suppl.*, 15.

Evershed, R. P., Berstan, R., Grew, F., Copley, M. S., Charmant, A. J. H., Barham, E., Mottram, H. R. and Brown, G. (2004) 'Archaeology: formulation of a Roman Cosmetic', *Nature*, 432: 35–6.

Eyben, E. (1980–1) 'Family planning in Graeco-Roman Antiquity', *Ancient Society*, 11/12: 5–82.

Eyers, J. (2011) *Yewden Roman Villa*, Hambleden, Lane End: Chiltern Archaeology.

Fabbri, M. and Trotta, A. (1989) *Una Scuola-collegio di Età Augustea*, Rome: L'Erma di Bretschneider.

Fabricius, C. (1972) *Galens Exzerpte aus älteren Pharmakologen*, Berlin: De Gruyter.

Fagan, G. G. (1999) *Bathing in Public in the Roman World*, Ann Arbor: University of Michigan Press.

—— (2006) 'Bathing for health with Celsus and the Elder Pliny', *Classical Quarterly*, 56: 190–207.

Faraone, C. A. and Obbink, D. (eds) (1991) *Magika Hiera: Ancient Greek Magic and Religion*, Oxford: Clarendon Press.

Fausti, D. (2005) 'Modelli espositivi relativi all prognosi nel Corpus Hippocraticum', in van der Eijk 2005a: 101–20.

Fazzo, S. (2002) 'Alexandre l'aphrodise contre Galien: la naissance d'une légende', *Philosophie antique: Problèmes, Renaissances, Usages*, 2: 109–44.

Feissel, D. (1999) 'Le Roufinion de Pergame au 6e siècle d'après un sceau nouvellement publié', *Revue des Études byzantines*, 57: 263–70.

Feissel, D., Gascou, J. and Teixidor, J. (1997) 'Documents d'archives romains inédits du Moyen Euphrate', *Journal des Savants*, 3–57.

Ferngren, G. (1992) 'Early Christianity as a religion of healing', *Bulletin of the History of Medicine*, 66: 1–15.

—— (2000) 'Early Christian views on the demonic etiology of disease', in Kottek and Horstmanshoff 2000: 183–202.

—— (2009) *Medicine and Health Care in Early Christianity*, Baltimore: Johns Hopkins University Press.

Ferraces Rodríguez, A. (ed.) (2009) *Fito-zooterapia antigua y altomedieval: Textos y Doctrina*, Corunna: Universidade da Coruña.

Festugière, A. J. (1939) 'L'expérience réligieuse du médecin Thessalos', *Revue biblique*, 48: 45–77.

—— (1975) *Études d'Histoire et de Philologie*, Paris: J. Vrin.

Feugère, M., Künzl, E. and Weisser, U. (1985) 'Les aiguilles à cataracte de Montbellet (Saône et Loire)', *Jahrbuch des Römisch-germanischen Zentralmuseums*, 32: 436–508.

Fichtner, G. (1984) *Corpus Hippocraticum*, Tübingen: Institut für Geschichte der Medizin.

—— (1990) *Corpus Galenicum: Verzeichnis der galenischen und pseudogalenischen Schriften*, ed. 2, Tübingen: Institut für Geschichte der Medizin.

Finch, J. (2011) 'The ancient origins of prosthetic medicine', *The Lancet*, 377: 548–9.

Finkel, I. L. (2000) 'On late Babylonian medical training', in A. R. George and I. L. Finkel (eds) *Wisdom, Gods and Literature: Studies in Assyriology in Honour of W. G. Lambert*, Winona Lake: Eisenbrauns: 137–223.

Fischer, K.-D. (1979) 'Kritisches zu den "Urkunden zur Hochschulpolitik der römischen Kaiser"', *Medizinhistorisches Journal*, 14: 312–21.

—— (1980) *Pelagonii Ars Veterinaria*, Leipzig: Teubner.

—— (2000a) 'Dr. Monk's Medical Digest', *Social History of Medicine*, 13: 247–51.

—— (2000b) *Premier Supplément à la Bibliographie des Textes médicaux latins: Antiquité et Haut Moyen Âge, 1986–1999*, St Etienne: Université de St Etienne.

—— (2000c) 'The *Isagoge* of Pseudo-Soranus', *Medizinhistorisches Journal*, 35: 3–30.

—— (2001) 'Wer lest, der findet. Versprengte kleinere Stücke medizinischer Werke in mittelalterlichen Handschriften', in Debru and Palmieri 2001: 69–90.

—— (2003) 'Galeni qui fertur ad Glauconem Liber tertius', in Garofalo and Roselli 2003: 101–32, 283–346.

—— (2012) *Ex occidente lux*. Greek medical works as represented in pre-Salernitan Latin translations', in Perilli *et al.* 2012: 29–56.

—— (ed.) (forthcoming) *Officina Hippocratica*.

Fischer, K.-D., Nickel, D. and Potter, P. (eds) (1998) *Text and Tradition: Studies in Ancient Medicine and its Transmission Presented to Jutta Kollesch*, Leiden: Brill.

Fitzgerald, W. A. (1948) 'Medical men, canonized saints', *Bulletin of the History of Medicine*, 22: 635–46.

Flashar, H. (1962) *Aristoteles: Problemata Physica*, Berlin: Akademie Verlag.

—— (1966) *Melancholie und Melancholiker in den medizinischen Theorien der Antike*, Berlin: De Gruyter.

Flashar, H. and Jouanna, J. (eds) (1997) *Médecine et Morale dans l'Antiquité*, Vandoeuvres: Fondation Hardt.

Flemming, R. (2000) *Medicine and the Making of Roman Women*, Oxford: Oxford University Press.

—— (2003) 'Empires of knowledge: medicine and health in the Hellenistic world', in A. Erskine (ed.) *A Companion to the Hellenistic World*, Oxford: Blackwell.

—— (2007a) 'Galen's imperial order of knowledge', in König and Whitmarsh 2007: 241–77.

—— (2007b) 'Women, writing, and medicine in the classical world', *Classical Quarterly*, 57: 257–79.

—— (2008) 'Commentary', in Hankinson 2008: 323–54.

—— (2009) 'Demiurge and emperor in Galen's world of knowledge', in Gill *et al.* 2009: 59–84.

Flint, V. I. J. (1991) *The Rise of Magic in Early Medieval Europe*, Oxford: Clarendon Press.

Floridi, L. (2002) *Sextus Empiricus: The Transmission and Recovery of Pyrrhonism*, Oxford: Oxford University Press.

Föllinger, S. (1996) *Differenz und Gleichheit: Das Geschlechterverhältnis in der Sicht griechischer Philosophen des 4. bis 1. Jahrhunderts v. Chr.*, Stuttgart: Steiner.

Forbes, H. and Foxhall, L. (1995) 'Ethnoarcheology and storage in the Ancient Mediterranean: beyond risk and survival', in Wilkins *et al.* 1995: 69–86.

Forrest, G. (1972) 'The inscriptions', in J. N. Coldstream and G. E. Huxley (eds) *Kythera*, London: Faber and Faber.

Forster, E. S. (1928) 'The pseudo-Aristotelian *Problems*', *Classical Quarterly*, 22: 162–5.

Fortenbaugh, W. W. and Gutas, D. (eds) (2002) *Theophrastus of Eresos: His Psychological, Doxographical and Scientific Writings, V*, New Brunswick: Transaction Publishers.

Fortenbaugh, W. W., Sharples, R. W. and Sollenberger, M. G. (2003) *Theophrastus of Eresos: On Sweat, On Dizziness and On Fatigue*, Leiden and Boston: Brill.

Fortuna, S., Garofalo, I., Lami, A. and Roselli, A. (eds) (2012) *Sulla tradizione indiretta dei testi medici greci: i commenti. Atti del quarto seminario internazionale, Siena, Certosa di Pontignano, 3–4 giugno 2011*, Pisa: F. Serra.

Fowden, E. K. (1999) *The Barbarian Plain: Saint Sergius between Rome and Iran*, Berkeley and London: University of California Press.

Fraisse, A. (2002) *Cassius Felix, De Medicina*, Paris: Les Belles Lettres.

Fraser, P. M. (1969) 'The career of Erasistratus of Ceos', *Rendiconti dell Istituto Lombardo, Classe di Lettere e Scienze Morali e Storiche*, 103: 518–37.

—— (1972) *Ptolemaic Alexandria*, 3 vols, Oxford: Clarendon Press.

Frede, M. (1981) 'On Galen's epistemology', in Nutton 1981a: 65–86; repr. in Frede 1987.

—— (1982) 'The method of the so-called Methodical school of medicine', in J. Barnes, J. Brunschwig, M. Burnyeat and M. Schofield (eds) *Science and Speculation*, Cambridge: Cambridge University Press: 1–23.

—— (1987) *Essays in Ancient Philosophy*, Oxford: Clarendon Press.

French, R. K. (1994) *Ancient Natural History*, London: Routledge.

—— (1997) *William Harvey's Natural Philosophy*, Cambridge: Cambridge University Press.

—— (1999) *Dissection and Vivisection in the European Renaissance*, Aldershot: Ashgate.

French, R. K. and Greenaway, F. (eds) (1986) *Science in the Early Roman Empire: Pliny the Elder, his Sources and Influence*, London: Croom Helm.

Frend, W. H. C. (2005) 'The place of miracles in the conversion of the ancient world to Christianity', in K. Cooper and J. Gregory (eds) *Signs, Wonders, Miracles: Representations of Divine Power in the Church. Studies in Church History, 41*, Woodbridge: The Boydell Press: 11–21.

Friedrich, H. V. (1968) *Thessalos von Tralles: Griechisch und Lateinisch, Beiträge zur klassischen Philologie, 28*, Meisenheim am Glan: Hain.

Frier, B. W. (2000) 'Demography', in A. K. Bowman, P. Garnsey and D. Rathbone, *The Cambridge Ancient History*, ed. 2, vol. XII, Cambridge: Cambridge University Press.

Frings, H. J. (1959) *Medizin und Arzt bei den griechischen Kirchenvätern bis Chrysostomos*, DD thesis, University of Bonn.

Frölich, H. (1879) *Die Militärmedicin Homers*, Stuttgart: F. Enke.

Furley, D. J. and Wilkie, J. S. (1984) *Galen on Respiration and the Arteries*, Princeton: Princeton University Press.

Gager, J. M. (1972) *Moses in Greco-Roman Paganism*, Nashville: Abingdon Press.

Gaillard-Seux, P. (2003) 'Sympathie et antipathie dans l'histoire naturelle de Pline l'Ancien', in Palmieri 2003: 113–28.

Galvao-Sobrino, C. R. (1996) 'Hippocratic ideals, medical ethics and the practice of medicine in the Early Middle Ages', *Journal of the History of Medicine and Allied Sciences*, 51: 438–55.

Garcia-Ballester, L. (1982) 'Arnau de Vilanova (c. 1240–1311) y la reforma de los estudios médicos en Montpellier (1309): el Hipócrates latino y la introduccíon del nuevo Galeno', *Dynamis*, 2: 97–158.

—— (1993) 'On the origin of the "six non-natural things" in Galen', in Kollesch and Nickel 1993: 105–15.

—— (1994) 'Introduction', in L. Garcia-Ballester, R. French, J. Arrizabalaga and A. Cunningham (eds) *Practical Medicine from Salerno to the Black Death*, Cambridge: Cambridge University Press.

Garland, R. (1987) *The Piraeus: From the Fifth to the First Century B.C.*, London: Duckworth.

—— (1992) *Introducing New Gods*, Ithaca: Cornell University Press.

—— (1995) *Deformity and Disability in the Graeco-Roman World*, London: Duckworth.

Garnsey, P. D. A. (1988) *Famine and Food Supply in the Graeco-Roman World: Responses to Risk and Crisis*, Cambridge: Cambridge University Press.

—— (1999) *Food and Society in Classical Antiquity*, Cambridge: Cambridge University Press.

Garnsey, P. D. A. and Whittaker, C. R. (eds) (1983) *Trade and Famine in Classical Antiquity, Proceedings of the Cambridge Philological Society, Suppl.*, 8.

Garofalo, I. (1988) *Erasistrati Fragmenta*, Pisa: Giardini.

—— (1994) 'La traduzione araba dei compendi alessandrini delle opere del canone di Galeno. Il compendio dell'Ad Glauconem', *Medicina nei Secoli*, 6: 329–48.

—— (1997) *Anonymi Medici de Morbis acutis et chroniis*, Leiden: Brill.

—— (1999) 'Una nuova opera di Galeno in traduzione araba', *Studi classici e orientali*, 47: 9–19.

Garofalo, I. and Debru, A. (2005) *Galien, Tome VII. Les Os pour les Debutants. L'Anatomie des muscles*, Paris: Les Belles Lettres.

—— (2008) *Galien, Tome VIII. L'Anatomie des Nerfs. L'Anatomie des Artères*. Paris: Les Belles Lettres.

Garofalo, I. and Roselli, A. (eds) (2003) *Galenismo e Medicina tardoantica. Fonti greche, latine e arabe. Atti del Seminario internazionale di Siena, Certosa di Pontignano – 9 e 10 Settembre 2002*, Naples: Istituto universitario orientale.

Garofalo, I., Lami, A., Manetti, D. and Roselli, A. (eds) (1999) *Aspetti della Terapia nel Corpus Hippocraticum*, Florence: Olschki.

Gärtner, H. (1962) *Rufi Quaestiones medicinales*, CMG Suppl., 4, Berlin: Akademie Verlag.

—— (1970) *Rufi Quaestiones medicinales*, Leipzig: Teubner.

Garzya, A. (ed.) (1996) *Storia e Ecdotica dei Testi medici greci*, Naples: M. D'Auria.

Garzya, A. and Jouanna, J. (eds) (1999) *I Testi medici greci: Tradizione e Ecdotica*, Naples: M. D'Auria.

Gauckler, P. (1895) *Le Musée de Cherchel*, Paris: E. Leroux.

Geller, M. J. (2001–2) 'West meets East: Early Greek and Babylonian diagnosis', *Archiv für Orientforschung*, 48/49: 50–75.

—— (2007) 'Phlegm and breath: Babylonian contributions to Hippocratic medicine', in I. L. Finkel and M. J. Geller (eds) *Disease in Babylonia*, Leiden: Brill: 187–99.

—— (2009) 'Introduction: Oeil malade et mauvais oeil', in Attia and Buisson 2009: 1–12.

—— (2010) *Ancient Babylonian Medicine: Theory and Practice*, Chichester: Wiley-Blackwell.

Geller, M. J. and Finkel, I. L. (eds) (2002) *Aspects of Disease in Ancient Mesopotamia*, Leiden: Brill.

Germanà, F. and Fornaciari, G. (1993) *Trapanazioni, Craniotomie, Traumi cranici in Italia: dalla Preistoria all'Età moderna*, Pisa: Giardini.

Gero, S. (1990) 'Galen on Jews and Christians: a reappraisal of the Arabic evidence', *Orientalia Christiana et Patristica*, 56: 371–411.

Geroulanos, S. and Bridler, R. (1994) *Trauma*, Mainz: P. von Zabern.

Gerstinger, H. (1970) *Dioskurides: Codex Vindobonensis med. gr. 1 der Österreichischen Nationalbibliothek*, Graz: Akademische Druck- und Verlagsanstalt.

Gil, L. and Rodriguez Alfageme, I. (1972) 'La figura del médico en la Comedia Atica', *Cuadernos de Filologia clásica*, 3: 81–91.

Gill, C. (2010) *Naturalistic Psychology in Galen and Stoicism*, Oxford: Oxford University Press.

Gill, C., Whitmarsh, T. and Wilkins, J. (eds) (2009) *Galen and the World of Knowledge*, Cambridge: Cambridge University Press.

Gilliam, J. F. (1961) 'The Plague under Marcus Aurelius', *American Journal of Philology*, 82: 225–51.

Ginouvès, R. (1994) 'L'eau dans les sanctuaires médicaux', in R. Ginouvès, A.-M. Guimier-Sorbets, J. Jouanna and L. Villard (eds) *L'Eau, la Santé et la Maladie dans le Monde grec*, Paris: École française d'Athènes: 237–46.

Girard, M. C. (1988) *Connaissance et Méconnaissance de l'Hellébore dans l'Antiquité*, Quebec: Université Laval.

—— (1990) 'L'hellébore: panacée ou placébo?', in Potter *et al.* 1990: 393–405.

Girone, M. (1998) Ἰάματα *Guarigioni miracolose di Asclepio in testi epigrafici*, Bari: Levante.

Gläser, P. P. (1986) 'Der Lepra-Begriff in der Bibel', in Wolf 1986: 63–8.

Gleason, M. (2009) 'Shock and awe: the performance dimension of Galen's anatomical demonstrations', in Gill *et al.* 2009: 85–114.

Golder, W. (2007) *Hippokrates und das Corpus Hippocraticum*, Würzburg: Königshausen und Neumann.

Goltz, D. (1974) *Studien zur alt-orientalischen und griechischen Heilkunde: Therapie, Arzneibereitung, Rezeptstruktur*, Wiesbaden: Steiner.

—— (1976) *Mittelalterliche Pharmazie und Medizin*, Stuttgart: Enke.

Good, B. J. (1994) *Medicine, Rationality, and Experience: An Anthropological Perspective*, Cambridge: Cambridge University Press.

Gordon, R. L., Beard, M., Reynolds, J. and Rouché, C. (1993) 'Roman inscriptions, 1986–1990', *Journal of Roman Studies*, 83: 131–58.

Gorrini, M. E. (2005) 'The Hippocratic impact on healing cults: the archeological evidence in Attica', in van der Eijk 2005a: 135–56.

Gorrini, M. E. and Melfi, M. (2002) 'L'archéologie des cultes guérisseurs: quelques observations', *Kernos*, 15: 247–65.

Goss, C. M. (1961) 'On anatomy of veins and arteries by Galen of Pergamos', *Anatomical Record*, 141: 355–66.

—— (1963) 'On the anatomy of muscles for beginners by Galen of Pergamon', *Anatomical Record*, 145: 477–501.

—— (1966) 'On anatomy of nerves by Galen of Pergamon', *American Journal of Anatomy*, 118: 327–36.

Gotthelf, A. (ed.) (1985) *Aristotle on Nature and Living Beings*, Pittsburgh: Mathesis Publications Inc.; Bristol: Bristol Classical Press.

Gotthelf, A. and Lennox, J. (eds) (1987) *Philosophical Issues in Aristotle's Biology*, Cambridge: Cambridge University Press.

Gourevitch, D. (1984a) *Le Mal d'être Femme*, Paris: Les Belles Lettres.

—— (1984b) *Le Triangle hippocratique*, Paris: École française de Rome.

—— (1987) 'Asclépiade de Bithynie dans Pline: problèmes de chronologie', in Pigeaud 1987b: 67–81.

—— (1991) 'Le pratique méthodique', in Mudry and Pigeaud 1991: 51–81.

—— (1999a) 'Fumigation et fomentation gynécologique', in Garofalo *et al.* 1999: 203–18.

—— (1999b) 'Le *Paul d'Égine* de Francis Adams: bonne ou mauvaise affaire?', in Garzya and Jouanna 1999: 227–40.

—— (2000) 'Hicesius' fish and chips: a plea for an edition of the Περὶ Ὕλης', in Braund and Wilkins 2000: 483–91.

—— (2001a) 'Un éléphant peut en cacher une autre, ou comment sauter du coq à l'âne peut mettre la puce à l'oreille', in Debru and Palmieri 2001: 157–76.

—— (2001b) *I iovani Pazienti di Galeno: per una Patocenosi dell'impero Romano*, Rome: Laterza.

—— (2004) 'Chirurgie obstétricale dans le monde romain: césarienne et embryotomie', in Dasen 2004: 239–64.

Gow, A. S. F. and Page, D. L. (1968) *The Greek Anthology: The Garland of Philip and Some Contemporary Epigrams*, Cambridge: Cambridge University Press.

Gow, A. S. F. and Scholfield, A. F. (1953) *Nicander of Colophon: Poems and Poetical Fragments*, Cambridge: Cambridge University Press.

Graf, F. (1985) *Nordionische Kulte*, Rome: Istituto Svizzero.

—— (1992) 'Heiligtum und ritual', in Reverdin and Grange 1992: 159–203.

—— (1996) 'Asclepius', in A. Spawforth and S. Hornblower (eds) *The Oxford Classical Dictionary*, ed. 3, Oxford: Clarendon Press: 188.

—— (1997) *Magic in the Ancient World*, Cambridge, MA: Harvard University Press.

Grant, M. (1996) *Anthimus: On the Observance of Foods*, Totnes: Prospect Books.

—— (2000) *Galen on Food and Diet*, London: Routledge.

Grant, R. L. (1960) 'Antyllus and his medical works', *Bulletin of the History of Medicine*, 34: 154–74.

Grant, R. M. (1983) 'Paul, Galen and Origen', *Journal of Theological Studies*, 34: 533–6.

Graumann, L. A. (2000) *Die Krankengeschichten der Epidemienbücher des Corpus Hippocraticum: Medizinhistorische Bedeutung und Möglichkeit der retrospektiven Diagnose*, Aachen: Shaker Verlag.

Green, M. H. (1989) 'Women's medical practice and medical care in medieval Europe', *Signs*, 14: 434–73.

—— (2008) *Making Women's Medicine Masculine: The Rise of Male Authority in Pre-modern Gynaecology*, Oxford: Oxford University Press.

Green, R. M. (1951) *A Translation of Galen's Hygiene (De Sanitate tuenda)*, Springfield, IL: C. C. Thomas.

—— (1955) *Asclepiades: His Life and Writings*, New Haven: E. Licht.

Greer, R. A. (1986) *Broken Lights and Mended Lives*, University Park and London: Pennsylvania State University Press.

Grensemann, H. (1968) *Die hippokratische Schrift 'Über die heilige Krankheit'*, Berlin: De Gruyter.

—— (1975) *Knidische Medizin. Teil I. Die Testimonien zur ältesten Lehre und Analysen knidischer Schriften im Corpus Hippocraticum*, Berlin: De Gruyter.

—— (1982) *Hippokratische Gynäkologie*, Wiesbaden: Steiner.

—— (1987) *Knidische Medizin, Teil III*, Stuttgart: Steiner.

Griffin, M. (1997) 'The Senate's story', *Journal of Roman Studies*, 87: 249–63.

Griffiths, A. (1987) 'Democedes of Croton: a Greek doctor at Darius' court', in H. Sancisi-Weerdenburg and A. Kuhrt (eds) *Achaemenid History II: The Greek Sources*, Leiden: Nederlands Instituut voor het Nahije Oosten: 37–51.

Grigorova, V. (2000) 'Médicaments et thermalisme à Pautalia, Thrace', *Gesnerus*, 57: 238–49.

Grimaudo, S. (2008) *Difendere la salute. Igiene e disciplina del soggetto nel De sanitate tuenda di Galeno*, Naples: Bibliopolis.

Griswold, C. L. (1986) *Self-knowledge in Plato's Phaedrus*, New Haven: Yale University Press.

Grmek, M. D. (1979) 'Les ruses de guerre biologiques dans l'antiquité', *Revue des Études grecques*, 92: 150–60.

—— (1989) *Diseases in the Ancient Greek World*, Baltimore: Johns Hopkins University Press.

—— (1990) *History of Aids*, Princeton: Princeton University Press.

—— (1991) 'La dénomination latine des maladies considérées comme nouvelles par les auteurs antiques', in Sabbah 1991: 195–214.

—— (1996) *Il Calderone di Medea: La sperimentazione sul vivente nell'Antichità*, Rome, Bari: Laterza.

—— (ed.) (1998) *Western Medical Thought from Antiquity to the Middle Ages*, Cambridge, MA: Harvard University Press.

Grmek, M. D. and Gourevitch, D. (1988) 'L'école médicale de Quintus et de Numisianus', *Mémoires du Centre Jean Palerne*, 8: 43–60.

—— (1994) 'Aux sources de la doctrine médicale de Galien: l'enseignement de Marinus, Quintus et Numisianus', *ANRW*, II, 37(2): 1491–528.

—— (1998) *Les Maladies dans l'Art antique*, Paris: Fayard.

Gruen, E. (1992) *Culture and National Identity in Republican Rome*, Ithaca: Cornell University Press.

Guardasole, A. (1997) *Eraclide di Taranto, Frammenti*, Naples: M. D'Auria.

—— (2000) *Tragedia e Medicina nell'Atene del V secolo a.C.*, Naples: M. D'Auria.

Guarducci, M. (1978) *Epigrafia Greca*, vol. 4, Rome: Istituto Poligrafico.

Gummerus, H. (1932) *Der Ärztestand im römischen Reiche. Societas Scientiarum Fennica, Commentationes Historiae et Litteraturae*, 3: 6.

Gundel, W. and Gundel, H. G. (1966) *Astrologoumena*, Wiesbaden: Steiner Verlag.

Gundert, B. (1998) 'Die Tabulae Vindobonenses als Zeugnis alexandrinischer Lehrtätigkeit um 600 n. Chr.', in Fischer *et al.* 1998: 91–144.

Habicht, C. (1969) *Die Inschriften des Asklepieions: Altertümer von Pergamon VIII. 3*, Berlin: De Gruyter.

—— (1985) *Pausanias' Guide to Ancient Greece*, Berkeley: University of California Press.

Hadot, P. (1984) 'Marc Aurèle, était-il opiomane?', in E. Lucchesi and H. D. Saffrey (eds) *Mémorial André-Jean Festugière: Antiquité païenne et chrétienne*, Geneva: P. Cramer: 33–50.

Hahn, J. (1991) 'Plinius und die griechischen Ärzte in Rom: Naturkonzeption und Medizinkritik in der *Naturalis Historia*', *Sudhoffs Archiv*, 75: 209–39.

Halfmann, H. (1986) *Itinera Principum*, Stuttgart: Steiner.

Hallof, L., Hallof, K. and Habicht, C. (1998) 'Aus der Arbeit der Inscriptiones Graecae II: Ehrendekrete von Kos', *Chiron*, 28: 101–42.

Hamilton, J. S. (1986) 'Scribonius Largus on the medical profession', *Bulletin of the History of Medicine*, 60: 209–16.

Hankinson, R. J. (1988) 'Galen explains the elephant', in M. Matthen and B. Linsky (eds) *Philosophy and Biology, Canadian Journal of Philosophy, Suppl.*, 14: 135–57.

—— (1989) 'Galen and the best of all possible worlds', *Classical Quarterly*, 39: 206–27.

—— (1990) 'Saving the phenomena', *Phronesis*, 35: 195–215.

—— (1991) *Galen on the Therapeutic Method, Books I and II*, Oxford: Clarendon Press.

—— (1992a) 'Doing without hypotheses: the nature of *Ancient Medicine*', in Lopez Ferez 1992: 55–68.

—— (1992b) 'Galen's philosophical eclecticism', *ANRW*, II, 36(5): 3505–22.

—— (1995) 'The growth of medical empiricism', in Bates 1995: 41–59.

—— (1998a) *Cause and Explanation in Ancient Greek Thought*, Oxford: Clarendon Press.

—— (ed.) (1998b) *Galen: On Antecedent Causes*, Cambridge: Cambridge University Press.

—— (ed.) (2008) *The Cambridge Companion to Galen*, Cambridge: Cambridge University Press.

Hanson, A. E. (1985) 'Papyri of medical content', *Yale Classical Studies*, 28: 25–47.

—— (1994) 'A division of labour: roles for men in Greek and Roman births', *Thamyris*, 1: 157–202.

—— (1996) 'Phaenarete: mother and *Maia*', in Wittern and Pellegrin 1996: 159–81.

—— (1997) 'Fragmentation and the Greek medical writers', in G. W. Most (ed.) *Collecting Fragments: Fragmente sammeln*, Göttingen: Vandenhoeck & Ruprecht: 289–314.

—— (2005) 'Greek medical papyri from the Fayum village of Tebtunis: patient involvement in a local health-care system?', in van der Eijk 2005a: 387–402.

—— (2006) 'Roman medicine', in D. S. Potter (ed.) *A Companion to the Roman World*, Oxford: Blackwell: 492–523.

—— (2010) 'Doctors' literacy and papyri of medical content', in Horstmanshoff 2010: 187–204.

Hanson, A. E. and Green, M. H. (1996) 'Methodicorum princeps: Soranus of Ephesus', *ANRW*, II, 37(2): 1834–55.

Harig, G. (1971) 'Zum Problem "Krankenhaus" in der Antike', *Klio*, 53: 179–95.

—— (1974) *Bestimmung der Intensität im medizinischen System Galens*, Berlin: Akademie Verlag.

—— (1987–8) 'Zur Datierung der Reisen Galens: ein Nachtrag', *Beiträge zur Hochschul- und Wissenschaftsgeschichte Erfurts*, 21: 13–20.

Harnack, A. (1892) 'Medicinisches aus der ältesten Kirchengeschichte', *Texte und Untersuchungen zur Geschichte der altchristlichen Literatur*, VIII: 4.

Harrauer, H. (1987) *Corpus Papyrorum Archiducis Raineri*, vol. 13, Vienna: Österreichische Nationalbibliothek.

Harris, C. R. S. (1973) *The Heart and the Vascular System in Ancient Greek Medicine*, Oxford: Clarendon Press.

Harris, J. R. (1971) *The Legacy of Egypt*, ed. 2, Oxford: Clarendon Press.

Harris, W. V. (1994) 'Child-exposure in the Roman Empire', *Journal of Roman Studies*, 84: 1–22.

—— (ed.) (forthcoming) *Madness in the Ancient World*, Oxford: Oxford University Press.

Harrison, S. J. (2000) *Apuleius: A Latin Sophist*, Oxford: Oxford University Press.

Harvey, S. A. (1984) 'Physicians and ascetics in John of Ephesus', *Dumbarton Oaks Papers*, 38: 87–94.

Harvey, W. (1628) *Exercitatio Anatomica de Motu Cordis et Anguinis in Animalibus*, Frankfurt: W. Fitzer.

Hasluck, F. W. (1929) *Christianity and Islam under the Sultans*, Oxford: Clarendon Press.

Havrda, M. (2011) 'Galenus Christianus? The doctrine of demonstration in Stromata VIII and the question of its source', *Vigiliae Christianae*, 65: 343–75.

Heeg, J. (1913) 'Pseudo-democritische Studien', *Abhandlungen der königlichen preussischen Akademie der Wissenschaften*, 4.

Heiberg, J. L. (1927) 'Geisteskrankheiten im klassischen Altertum', *Allgemeine Zeitschrift für Psychiatrie*, 86: 1–44.

Heitsch, E. (1963) 'Überlieferungsgeschichtliche Untersuchungen zu Andromachos, Markellos von Side und zum Carmen de viribus herbarum', *Nachrichten der Akademie der Wissenschaften zu Göttingen, phil.-hist. Kl.*, 2.

—— (1964) 'Die griechische Dichterfragmente der römischen Kaiserzeit', *Abhandlungen der Akademie der Wissenschaft zu Göttingen, phil.-hist. Kl.*, 58.

Helm, J. (2000) 'Sickness in early Christian healing narratives: medical, religious, and social aspects', in Kottek and Horstmanshoff 2000: 241–58.

Helman, C. G. (1978) 'Feed a cold, starve a fever', *Culture, Medicine, and Psychiatry*, 2: 107–37.

Hennecke, E., Schneemelcher, W. and Wilson, R. M. (1963) *New Testament Apocrypha*, 2 vols, London: Lutterworth Press.

Herbst, W. (1911) *Galeni de Studiis Atticissantium Testimonia*, PhD thesis, University of Leipzig.

Hermann, P. (1960) 'Inschriften aus dem Heraion von Samos', *Mitteilungen des deutschen archäologischen Instituts in Athen*, 75: 100–53.

Hershkowitz, D. (1998) *The Madness of Epic: Reading Insanity from Homer to Statius*, Oxford: Clarendon Press.

Herval, R. (1968) *Origines chrétiennes de la IIe Lyonnaise gallo-romaine à la Normandie ducale*, Rouen: Maugard.

Herzog, R. (1931) *Wunderheilungen: die Wunderheilungen von Epidauros, Philologus, Suppl.*, 22: 3.

—— (1939) 'Der Kampf um die Kult von Menuthis', in T. Klauser and A. Rücker (eds) *Pisciculi: Studien zur Religion und Kultur des Altertums. Festschrift F. J. Dölger*, Münster: Aschendorff: 117–24.

Herzog, R. and Schatzmann, P. (1932) *Kos I*, Berlin: Keller.

Hiller von Gärtringen, F. (1906) *Die Inschriften von Priene*, Berlin: Weidmann.

Hillert, A. (1990) *Antike Ärztedarstellungen*, Frankfurt: Peter Lang.

Hillgruber, M. (2010) 'Liebe, Weisheit und Verzichte. Zu Herkunft und Entwicklung der Geschchte von Antiochos und Stratonike', in T. Brüggemann, B. Meissner, C. Mileta, A. Pabst and O. Schmitt (eds) *Studia Hellenistica et Historiographica. Festschrift für Andreas Mehl*, Gutenberg: Comouter Druck Satz und Verlag: 73–102.

Hirschberg, J. (1982) *The History of Ophthalmology, vol. 1, Antiquity*, Bonn: Wayenborgh.

Hirschfeld, Y. (1992) *The Judaean Desert Monasteries in the Byzantine Period*, New Haven: Yale University Press.

Hirt, M. (1996) *Médecins et Malades de l'Égypte romaine*, PhD thesis, University of Geneva.

Hobson, B. (2009) *Latrinae et Foricae: Toilets in the Roman World*, London: Duckworth.

Hoessly, F. (2001) *Katharsis. Reinigung als Heilverfahren. Studien zur Ritual der archäischen und klassichen Zeit. Sowie zum Corpus Hippocraticum*, Göttingen: Vandenhoeck & Ruprecht.

Hoffmann, A. (1998) 'The Roman remodelling of the Asklepieion', in Koester 1998: 41–62.

Hoffmann, F. (forthcoming) 'Zur Neuedition des hieratisch-demotischen Papyrus Wien D 6257 aus römischer Zeit', in T. Pommerening and A. Imhausen (eds) *Writings of Early Scholars in the Ancient Near East, Egypt, Rome, and Greece*, Berlin: De Gruyter: 201–19.

Hoffmann-Axthelm, W. (1981) *A History of Dentistry*, Chicago: Quintessence.

—— (1985) *Geschichte der Zahnheilkunde*, Berlin, Chicago and London: Quintessenz, ed. 2.

Holcomb, R. C. (1941) 'The antiquity of congenital syphilis', *Bulletin of the History of Medicine*, 10: 148–72.

Holman, S. R. (2001) *The Hungry are Dying: Beggars and Bishops in Roman Cappadocia*, Oxford: Oxford University Press.

Holmes, B. (2006) 'Aelius Aristeides' illegible body', in W. V. Harris and B. Holmes (eds) *Aelius Aristeides between Greece, Rome and the East*, Leiden and Boston: Brill: 81–113.

—— (2009) 'Medicine', in G. Boys-Stones, B. Graziosi and P. Vasunia (eds) *The Oxford Handbook of Hellenic Studies*, Oxford: Oxford University Press: 552–68.

—— (2010) *The Symptom and the Subject: The Emergence of the Physical Body in Ancient Greece*, Princeton: Princeton University Press.

Holzmann, B. (1984) 'Asklepios', in J. C. Balty and J. Boardman (eds) *Lexikon Iconographicum Mythologiae Classicae*, Zurich and Munich: Artemis Verlag, vol. 2: 863–97, pl. 631–68.

Hommel, H. (1957) 'Euripides in Ostia', *Epigraphica*, 19: 109–64.

—— (1970) 'Das Datum der Munatier Grabstätte in Portus Trajani', *Zeitschrift für Papyrologie und Epigraphik*, 5: 293–303.

Hong, S., Candelone, J. P., Paterson, C. C. and Boutron, C. F. (1994) 'Greenland ice evidence of hemispheric lead pollution two millennia ago by Greek and Roman civilizations', *Science*, 265: 1841–3.

—— (1996) 'History of ancient copper-smelting pollution during Roman and medieval times recorded in Greenland ice', *Science*, 272: 246–9.

Honigmann, E. (1944) 'A trial for sorcery', *Isis*, 35: 281–4.

Hood, J. (2010) 'Galen's Aristotelian definitions', in D. Charles (ed.) *Definition in Greek Philosophy*, Oxford: Oxford University Press: 450–66.

Hope, V. M. and Marshall, E. (eds) (2000) *Death and Disease in the Ancient City*, London: Routledge.

Horden, P. (1982) 'Saints and doctors in the early Byzantine empire: the case of Theodore of Sykeon', *Studies in Church History*, 19: 1–13.

—— (1992) 'Disease, dragons, and saints: the management of epidemics in the Dark Ages', in Ranger and Slack 1992: 45–76.

—— (2000) 'Ritual and public health in the early medieval city', in S. Sheard and H. Power (eds) *Body and City: Histories of Urban Public Health*, Aldershot: Ashgate: 17–40.

—— (2008) *Hospitals and Healing from Antiquity to the Later Middle Ages*, Aldershot and Burlington: Ashgate.

Horden, P. and Purcell, N. (2000) *The Corrupting Sea: A Study of Mediterranean History*, Oxford: Blackwell.

Horstmanshoff, H. F. J. (1976) 'The ancient physician: craftsman or scientist?', *Bulletin of the History of Medicine*, 31: 448–59.

—— (1995) 'Galen and his patients', in van der Eijk *et al.* 1995: 83–99.

—— (ed.) (2010) *Hippocrates and Medical Education. Selected Papers Presented at the XIIth International Hippocrates Colloquium, Universiteit Leiden, 24–26 August 2005*, Leiden and Boston: Brill.

Howard-Johnston, J. and Hayward, P. A. (eds) (1999) *The Cult of Saints in Late Antiquity and the Early Middle Ages*, Oxford: Oxford University Press.

Hugonnard-Roche, H. (1989) 'Aux origines de l'exégèse orientale de la logique d'Aristote: Sergius de Res'aina (+536), médecin et philosophe', *Journal Asiatique*, 277: 1–17.

—— (1997) 'Note sur Sergius de Res'aina, traducteur du grec en syriaque et commentateur d'Aristote', in G. Endress and R. Kruk (eds) *The Ancient Tradition in Christian and Islamic Hellenism: Studies on the Transmission of Greek Philosophy and Science Dedicated to H. J. Drossaert Lulofs*, Leiden: Brill: 121–43.

Hull, J. M. (1974) *Hellenistic Magic and the Synoptic Tradition*, London: SCM Press.

Ideler, J. L. (1841) *Medici graeci minores*, 2 vols, Berlin: Reimer.

Ilberg, J. (1890) 'Die Hippokratesausgaben des Artemidoros Kapiton und Dioskurides', *Rheinisches Museum*, 45: 111–37.

—— (1893) 'Das Hippokratesglossar des Erotianos', *Abhandlungen der sächsischen Akademie der Wissenschaften*, 14: 101–47.

—— (1927) *Sorani Gynaeciorum Libri IV, De Signis Fracturarum, De Fasciis, Vita Hippocratis secundum Soranum, CMG* IV, Leipzig and Berlin: Teubner.

—— (1930) 'Rufus von Ephesos: ein griechischer Arzt in Traianischer Zeit', *Abhandlungen der sächsichen Akademie der Wissenschaften*, 41.

Inwood, B. (2001) *The Poems of Empedocles: A Text and Translation with an Introduction*, ed. 2, Toronto: University of Toronto Press.

Irigoin, J. (1997) *Tradition et critique des textes grecs*, Paris: Les Belles Lettres.

Iskandar, A. Z. (1976) 'An attempted reconstruction of the Late Alexandrian Medical Curriculum', *Medical History*, 20: 235–58.

Israelowich, I. (2012) *Society, Medicine and Religion in the Sacred Tales of Aelius Aristides*, Leiden and Boston: Brill.

Jackson, R. (1988) *Doctors and Diseases in the Roman Empire*, London: British Museum Publications.

—— (1990a) 'Roman doctors and their instruments: recent research into ancient practice', *Journal of Roman Archaeology*, 3: 5–27.

—— (1990b) 'Waters and spas in the classical world', in R. Porter (ed.) *The Medical History of Waters and Spas, Medical History Suppl.*, 10: 1–13.

—— (1992) 'Spas, waters, and hydrotherapy in the Roman world', in DeLaine and Johnston 1992: 107–16.

—— (1994) 'The surgical instruments, appliances and equipment in Celsus' De medicina', in Sabbah and Mudry 1994: 167–210.

—— (1996) 'Eye medicine in the Roman Empire', *ANRW*, II, 37(3): 2228–51.

—— (1997) 'An ancient British medical kit from Stanway, Essex', *The Lancet*, 350: 1471–3.

—— (2002a) 'A Roman doctor's house in Rimini', *British Museum Magazine*, 44: 20–3.

—— (2002b) 'Roman surgery: the evidence of the instruments', in R. Arnott (ed.) *The Archaeology of Medicine, BAR International Series*, 1046: 87–104.

Jackson, S. W. (1969) 'Galen: on mental disorders', *Journal of the History of the Behavioral Sciences*, 5: 365–84.

—— (1986) *Melancholia and Depression from Hippocratic Times to Modern Times*, New Haven: Yale University Press.

Jacobs, S. and Rütten, T. (1998) '*Democritus ridens* – ein weinender Philosoph? Zur Tradition des *Democritus melancholicus* in der Bildenden Kunst', *Wolfenbütteler Beiträge*, 11: 73–143.

Jacquart, D. and Thomasset, C. (1985) *Sexuality and Medicine in the Middle Ages*, London: Polity Press.

Jacques, J. M. (1979) 'Nicandre de Colophon poète et médecin', *Ktèma*, 4: 133–49.

—— (1997) 'La Méthode de Galien pharmacologue', in Debru 1997: 103–32.

—— (2002) *Nicandre, Oeuvres, Tome II: Les Thériaques*, Paris: Les Belles Lettres.

—— (2007) *Nicandre, Oeuvres, Tome III: Les Alexipharmaques*, Paris: Les Belles Lettres.

Jaeger, W. (1913) 'Das Pneuma im Lykeion', *Hermes*, 48: 29–74.

—— (1954) 'Aristotle's use of medicine as a model in his ethics', *Journal of Hellenic Studies*, 77: 54–66.

Janowitz, N. (2001) *Magic in the Roman World: Pagans, Jews, and Christians*, London: Routledge.

Jarcho, S. (1975–6) 'Medical and non-medical comments on Cato and Varro, with historical observations on the concept of infection', *Transactions and Studies of the College of Physicians of Philadelphia*, 43: 372–8.

Jarry, J. (1985) 'Nouveaux documents grecs et latins de Syrie', *Zeitschrift für Papyrologie und Epigraphik*, 60: 110–16.

Jebb, R. C. (1898) *Sophocles, Philoctetes*, Cambridge: Cambridge University Press.

John, J. (2001) *The Meaning in the Miracles*, Norwich: Canterbury Press.

Johnson, A. (1983) *Roman Forts of the First and Second Centuries AD in Britain and the German Provinces*, London: Batsford.

Johnson, W. A. and Parker, H. N. (eds) (2009) *Ancient Literacies: The Culture of Reading in Greece and Rome*, Oxford: Oxford University Press.

Johnston, I. (2006) *Galen: On Diseases and Symptoms*, Cambridge: Cambridge University Press.

Joly, R. (1961) 'Le question hippocratique et le témoinage de Phèdre', *Revue des Études grecques*, 74: 194–223.

—— (1969) 'Esclaves et médecins dans la Grèce antique', *Sudhoffs Archiv*, 53: 1–14.

—— (1984) *Hippocratis De Diaeta, CMG*, I, 2, 4, Berlin: Akademie Verlag.

Jones, C. P. (1998) 'Aelius Aristides and the Asclepieion', in Koester 1998: 63–76.

Jones, W. H. S. (1907) *Malaria: A Neglected Factor in Greek History*, Cambridge: Cambridge University Press.

—— (1923–31) *Hippocrates*, 4 vols, London: Heinemann.

—— (1928) *The Doctor's Oath*, Cambridge: Cambridge University Press.

—— (1947) *The Medical Writings of Anonymus Londinensis*, Cambridge; Cambridge University Press.

—— (1957) 'Ancient Roman folk medicine', *Journal of the History of Medicine*, 12: 459–72.

Jori, A. (1993) 'Platone e la "svolta dietetica" della medicina greca. Erodico di Selimbria e le insidie della techne', *Studi Italiani di Filologia Classica*, 11: 157–95.

—— (1996) *Medicina e Medici nell'Antica Grecia. Saggio sul PERÌ TÉCHNES Ippocratico*, Naples: Il Mulino.

Jost, M. (1985) *Sanctuaires et Cultes d'Arcadie*, Paris: J. Vrin.

Jouanna, J. (1961) 'Présence d'Empédocle dans la collection hippocratique', *Lettres d'Humanité*, 20: 452–63.

—— (1974) *Hippocrate et l'École de Cnide*, Paris: Les Belles Lettres.

—— (1988) *Hippocrate, Les Vents, De l'Art*, Paris: Les Belles Lettres.

—— (1991) 'Remarques sur la tradition arabe du commentaire de Galien aux traités hippocratiques des Airs, eaux, lieux et du serment', in J. A. López Férez (ed.) *Galeno: Obra, Pensamiento e Influencia*, Madrid: UNID: 235–52.

—— (1996a) *Hippocrate, Airs, Eaux, Lieux*, Paris: Les Belles Lettres.

—— (1996b) 'Hippocrate et les *Problemata* d'Aristote', in Wittern and Pellegrin 1996: 273–94.

—— (1996c) 'Un témoin méconnu de la tradition Hippocratique: l'Ambrosianus gr. 134 (B 113 sup.), fol. 1–2 (avec une nouvelle édition du *Serment* et de la *Loi*)', in Garzya 1996: 253–72.

—— (1997) 'La lecture de l'éthique hippocratique chez Galien', in Flashar and Jouanna 1997: 211–44. Trans. in Jouanna (2012).

—— (1999) *Hippocrates*, Baltimore: Johns Hopkins University Press.

—— (2000) *Hippocrate: Épidemies V et VII*, Paris: Les Belles Lettres.

—— (2003) *Hippocrate: La Maladie Secrète*, Paris: Les Belles Lettres.

—— (2005) 'Cause and crisis in historians and medical writers of the classical period', in van der Eijk 2005a: 3–28.

—— (2006) 'La posterité du traité hippocratique de la *Nature de l'homme*: la théorie des quatre humeurs', in Müller *et al.* 2006: 117–41. Trans. in Jouanna (2012).

—— (2007) 'Un pseudo-Galien inédit: le *Pronostic sur l'homme*. Contribution à l'histoire de la théorie quaternaire dans la médecine grecque tardive: l'insertion des quatre vents', in S. David and D. Geny (eds) *Troïka: Mélanges offerts à Michel Woronoff*, Besançon: Presses universitaires de Franche-Comté: I, 303–22.

—— (2010) 'Hippocrates as Galen's teacher', in Horstmanshoff 2010: 1–21.

—— (2011) 'Médecine rationelle et magie: le statut des amulettes et des incantations chez Galien', *Revue des Études grecques*, 124: 47–78.

—— (2012) *Greek Medicine from Hippocrates to Galen. Selected Papers*, Leiden and Boston: Brill.

Jouanna, J. and Magdelaine, C. (1999) *Hippocrate: L'Art de la Médecine*, Paris: GF Flammarion.

Judeich, W. (1898) *Altertümer von Hierapolis*, Berlin: Weidmann.

Jurina, K. (1985) *Vom Quacksalber zum Doctor Medicinae*, Cologne: Böhlau Verlag.

Kagan, J. (1994) *Galen's Prophecy: Temperament in Human Nature*, London: Free Association Books.

Kahn, J. (1975) *Job's Illness: Loss, Grief and Integration*, Oxford: Oxford University Press.

Kaimakis, D. (1976) *Die Kyraniden*, Meisenheim am Glan: Hain.

Kalbfleisch, K. (1895) *Die neuplatonische, fälschlich dem Galen zugeschriebene Schrift Πρὸς Γαῦρον περὶ τοῦ πῶς ἐμψυχοῦται τὰ ἔμβρυα, Abhandlungen der Berliner Akademie der Wissenschaften*, Anhang.

—— (1896) *Galeni Institutio logica*, Leipzig: Teubner.

Kaplan, M. S. (1978) 'Greeks and the Imperial Court from Tiberius to Nero', *Harvard Studies in Classical Philology*, 82: 353–5.

Karenberg, A. and Leitz, C. (eds) (2002) *Heilkunde und Hochkultur, II, 'Magie und Medizin' und 'Der alte Mensch' in den antiken Zivilisationen des Mittelmeerraumes*, Münster: Lit.

Karidas, P. (1968) *Das Amphiareion von Oropos in Medizingeschichtlicher Sicht*, MD thesis, University of Erlangen.

Kazhdan, A. P. and Sherry, L. F. (1998) 'Anonymous miracles of St. Artemios', in I. Sevcenko and I. Hutter (eds) Ἀετός. *Studies in Honour of Cyril Mango*, Stuttgart: Teubner.

Kearns, E. (1989) *The Heroes of Attica: Bulletin of the Institute of Classical Studies, Suppl.*, 57.

Kee, H. C. (1983) *Miracle in the Early Christian World*, New Haven: Yale University Press.

—— (1986) *Medicine, Miracle and Magic in New Testament Times*, Cambridge: Cambridge University Press.

Keller, A. (1988) *Die Abortiva in der römischen Kaiserzeit*, Stuttgart: Deutscher Apotheker Verlag.

Kelly, J. N. D. (1995) *Golden Mouth: The Story of John Chrysostom, Ascetic, Preacher, Bishop*, Ithaca: Cornell University Press.

Keyser, P. T. (1997) 'Science and magic in Galen's recipes (sympathy and efficacy)', in Debru 1997: 175–98.

Kibre, P. (1985) *Hippocrates Latinus*, New York: Fordham University Press.

Kieffer, J. S. (1964) *Galen's Institutio Logica*, Baltimore: Johns Hopkins University Press.

King, H. (1998) *Hippocrates' Woman*, London: Routledge.

—— (2001) *Greek and Roman Medicine*, Bristol: Bristol Classical Press.

—— (2002) 'The power of paternity: the Father of Medicine meets the Prince of Physicians', in Cantor 2002: 21–36.

—— (ed.) (2005) *Health in Antiquity*, London and New York: Routledge.

Kingsley, P. (1995) *Ancient Philosophy, Mystery and Magic: Empedocles and Pythagorean Tradition*, Oxford: Clarendon Press.

Kinneir Wilson, J. V. and Reynolds, E. H. (1990) 'Translation and analysis of a cuneiform text forming part of a Babylonian text on epilepsy', *Medical History*, 34: 185–98.

Kiple, K. (ed.) (1993) *The Cambridge World History of Human Disease*, Cambridge: Cambridge University Press.

Kislinger, E. (1984) 'Kaiser Julian und die (christlichen) xenodokeia', in W. Hörandner, J. Koder, O. Kresten and E. Trapp (eds) *Byzantios: Festschrift für Herbert Hunger*, Vienna: Ernst Becvar: 171–84.

Klibansky, R., Panowsky, E. and Saxl, F. (1964) *Saturn and Melancholy*, London: Nelson.

Klitsch, H. D. (1976) *Eine inschriftliche Krankengeschichte des 3. Jht. n. Chr.*, MD Diss., University of Erlangen.

Knibbe, K. (1981–2) 'Neue Inschriften aus Ephesos VIII', *Jahreshefte der österreichischen archäologischen Instituts*, 53: 136–40.

Knörzer, K.-H. (1970) *Römerzeitliche Pflanzenfunde aus Neuss*, Berlin: Deutsches Archäologisches Institut.

Koelbing, H. (1977) *Arzt und Patient*, Zurich: Artemis Verlag.

Koenen, L. (1996) 'The carbonized archive from Petra', *Journal of Roman Archaeology*, 9: 177–88.

Koester, H. (ed.) (1998) *Pergamon, Citadel of the Gods: Archaeological Record, Literary Description, and Religious Development*, Harrisburg: Trinity Press International.

Kolb, F. (1984) *Die Stadt in Altertum*, Munich: Beck.

Kolde, A. (2003) *Politique et Religion chez Isyllos d'Épidaure*, Basle: Schwabe.

Kollesch, J. (1973) *Untersuchungen zu den pseudogalenischen Definitiones medicae*, Berlin: Akademie Verlag.

—— (1981) 'Galen und die Zweite Sophistik', in Nutton 1981a: 1–11.

—— (1997) 'Die anatomischen Untersuchungen des Aristoteles und ihr Stellenwert als Forschungsmethode in der aristotelischen Biologie', in Kullmann and Föllinger 1997: 367–74.

Kollesch, J. and Kudlien, F. (1965) *Apollonius Citiensis In Hippocratis De articulis Commentarii*, *CMG* XI 1, 1, Berlin: Teubner.

Kollesch, J. and Nickel, D. (eds) (1993) *Galen und das Hellenistische Erbe*, Stuttgart: Steiner.

Kolta, K. S. and Schwazmann-Schafhauser, D. (2000) *Die Heilkunst im alten Ägypten: Magie und Ratio in der Krankheitsvorstellung und therapeutischen Praxis*, Stuttgart: Steiner.

König, J. (2005) *Athletics and Literature in the Roman Empire*, Cambridge: Cambridge University Press.

König, J. and Whitmarsh T. (eds) (2007) *Ordering Knowledge in the Roman Empire*, Cambridge: Cambridge University Press.

Korpela, J. (1987) *Das Medizinalpersonal im antiken Rom*, Helsinki: Finnish Academy of Sciences.

—— (1995) '*Aromatarii, pharmacopolae, thurarii et ceteri*. Zur Sozialgeschichte Roma', in van der Eijk *et al.* 1995: 101–11.

Kosak, J. C. (2000) '*Polis nosousa*: Greek ideas about the city and disease in the fifth century BC', in Hope and Marshall 2000: 35–54.

—— (2004) *Heroic Measures: Hippocratic Medicine in the Making of Euripidean Tragedy*, Leiden and Boston: Brill.

Kotansky, R. (1994) *Greek Magical Amulets, Papyrologica Coloniensia*, 22, 1, Opladen: Westdeutscher Verlag.

Kottek, S. and Horstmanshoff, M. (eds) (2000) *From Athens to Jerusalem*, Rotterdam: Erasmus Publishing.

Kötting, B. (1950) *Peregrinatio religiosa: Wahlfahrten in der Antike und das Pilgerwesen in der alten Kirche*, Münster: Aschendorff.

Kovačič, F. (2001) *Der Begriff der Physis bei Galen vor dem Hintergrund seiner Vorgänger*, Stuttgart: Steiner.

Kowalski, G. (1960) *Rufi De Corporis humani Appellationibus*, PhD thesis, University of Göttingen.

Kraus, P. and Walzer, R. (1951) *Galeni Compendium Timaei Platonis*, London: Oxford University Press.

Krug, A. (1985) *Heilkunst und Heilkult: Medizin in der Antike*, Munich: C. H. Beck.

—— (2008) *Das Berliner Arztrelief*, Berlin: De Gruyter.

Kudlien, F. (1962) 'Poseidonios und die Ärzteschule der Pneumatiker', *Hermes*, 90: 419–29.

—— (1963) 'Untersuchungen zu Aretaeus von Kappadokien', *Abhandlungen der Akademie der Wissenschaften in Mainz*, 11: 1151–230.

—— (1965) 'Zum Thema Homer und die Medizin', *Rheinisches Museum*, 108: 293–9.

—— (1967) *Der Beginn des medizinischen Denkens bei den Griechen*, Zurich: Artemis Verlag.

—— (1968a) *Die Sklaven in der griechischen Medizin*, Wiesbaden: Steiner.

—— (1968b) 'Pneumatische Ärzte', *RE, Suppl.*, 11: 1097–108.

—— (1968c) 'The third century A.D.: a blank spot in the history of medicine', in L. G. Stevenson and R. P. Multhauf (eds) *Medicine, Science, and Culture: Historical Essays in Honor of Owsei Temkin*, Baltimore: Johns Hopkins University Press: 25–34.

—— (1969) 'Antike Anatomie und menschlicher Leichnam', *Hermes*, 96: 78–94.

—— (1970a) 'Aretaeus', in C. C. Gillispie (ed.) *Dictionary of Scientific Biography*, vol. 1, New York: Scribner's: 234–5.

—— (1970b) 'Zu Arats Ὀστολογία und Aischylos' Ὀστολόγοι', *Rheinisches Museum*, 113: 297–304.

—— (1971) 'Galens Urteil über die Thukydideische Pestbeschreibung', *Episteme*, 5: 132–3.

—— (1975) 'Rufus of Ephesus', in C. C. Gillispie (ed.) *Dictionary of Scientific Biography*, 11: 603–5.

441

—— (1977) 'Das Göttliche und die Natur im hippokratischen *Prognostikon*', *Hermes*, 105: 268–74.

—— (1978) 'Beichte und Heilung', *Medizinhistorisches Journal*, 13: 1–14.

—— (1979) *Der griechische Arzt im Zeitalter des Hellenismus: Seine Stellung in Staat und Gesellschaft*, Wiesbaden: Steiner.

—— (1981) 'Galen's religious belief', in Nutton 1981a: 117–30.

—— (1983) 'Schaustellerei und Heilmittelvertrieb in der Antike', *Gesnerus*, 40: 91–8.

—— (1986a) *Die Stellung des Arztes in der römischen Gesellschaft*, Stuttgart: Steiner.

—— (1986b) 'Lepra in der Antike', in Wolf 1986: 39–44.

—— (1989) 'Hippokrates-Rezeption im Hellenismus', in Baader and Winau 1989: 355–76.

Kudlien, F. and Durling, R. J. (eds) (1991) *Galen's Method of Healing*, Leiden: Brill.

Kühn, K. G. (1821–33) *Claudii Galeni Opera Omnia*, 20 vols in 22, Leipzig: C. Cnobloch.

—— (1827–8) *Opuscula academica medica et philologica*, 2 vols, Leipzig: L. Voss.

Kullmann, W. and Föllinger, S. (eds) (1997) *Aristotelische Biologie*, Stuttgart: Steiner Verlag.

Künzl, E. (1982) *Medizinische Instrumente aus Sepulkralfunden der römischen Kaiserzeit*, Bonn: Rheinlandverlag.

—— (1986) 'Operationsräume in römischen Thermen', *Bonner Jahrbücher*, 186: 491–501.

—— (1995) 'Ein archäologisches Problem: Gräber römischer Chirurginnen', in van der Eijk *et al.* 1995: 309–19.

—— (1996) 'Forschungsbericht zu den antiken medizinischen Instrumenten', *ANRW*, II, 37(3): 2434–639.

—— (2002) *Medizinische Instrumenten der römischen Zentralmuseum, Mainz*, Bonn: Habelt.

Kutsche, F. (1913) *Attische Heilgötter und Heilheroen*, Giessen: Topelman.

Laes, C. (2011) 'Midwives in Greek inscriptions in Hellenistic and Roman Antiquity', *Zeitschrift für Papyrologie und Epigraphik*, 176: 154–62.

Laharie, M. (1991) *La Folie au Moyen Âge*, Paris: Le Léopard d'Or.

Lanata, G. (1969) *Medicina magica e Religione popolare in Grecia fino all'Ippocrate*, Rome: Edizioni dell'Ateneo.

Lane Fox, R. (1986) *Pagans and Christians in the Mediterranean World*, Harmondsworth: Penguin.

Lang, P. (2009) 'Goats and the sacred disease in Callimachus' Acontius and Cydippe', *Classical Philology*, 104: 85–90.

—— (forthcoming) *A Dream of Healing: Medicine in Ptolemaic Egypt*, Leiden and Boston: Brill.

Langholf, V. (1986) 'Kallimachos, Komödie und hippokratische Frage', *Medizinhistorisches Journal*, 21: 3–30.

—— (1990) *Medical Theories in Hippocrates*, Berlin: De Gruyter.

Langslow, D. R. (1994) 'Celsus and the makings of Latin medical terminology', in Sabbah and Mudry 1994: 297–318.

—— (1999) 'The language of poetry and the language of science: the Latin poets and medical Latin', in J. N. Adams and R. G. Mayer (eds) *Aspects of the Language of Latin Poetry*, *Proceedings of the British Academy*, 93: 183–226.

—— (2000) *Medical Latin in the Roman Empire*, Oxford: Oxford University Press.

Langslow, D. R. and Maire, B. (eds) (2010) *Body, Disease and Treatment in a Changing World: Latin Texts and Contexts in Ancient and Medieval Medicine*, Lausanne: Éditions BHMS.

Lanternari, V. (1994) *Medicina, Magia, Religione, Valori*, Naples: Liguori.

Laser, S. (1983) *Medizin und Körperpflege: Archaeologia Homerica*, fascicle S, Göttingen: Vandenhoeck & Ruprecht.

Laskaris, J. (1999) 'Ancient healing cults as a source for Hippocratic pharmacology', in Garofalo *et al.* 1999: 1–12.

—— (2002) *The Art is Long: On the Sacred Disease and the Scientific Tradition*, Leiden: Brill.

Latte, K. (1960) *Römische Religionsgeschichte*, Munich: Beck.

Lederer, S. E. (2002) 'Hippocrates American style: representing professional morality in early twentieth-century America', in Cantor 2002: 239–56.

Lefkowitz, M. (1981) *The Lives of the Greek Poets*, London: Duckworth.

Leith, D. (2006) 'The Antinoopolis illustrated herbal (PJohnson + PAntin. 3.214 = MP3 2095)', *Zeitschrift für Papyrologie und Epigraphik*, 156: 141–56.

—— (2008) 'The *diatritus* and therapy in Graeco-Roman medicine', *Classical Quarterly*, 58: 581–600.

—— (2012) 'Pores and void in Asclepiades' physical theory', *Phronesis*, 57: 164–91.

Lennox, J. (1994) 'The disappearance of Aristotle's biology: a Hellenistic mystery', in T. D. Barnes (ed.) *The Sciences in Greco-Roman Society*, Edmonton: Academic Printing and Publishing: 7–24.

Lenz, F. W. (1959) *The Aristeides Prolegomena*, Leiden: Brill.

Leven, K.-H. (1993) 'Miasma und Metadosis – antike Vorstellungen von Ansteckung', *Medizin, Gesellschaft und Geschichte*, 11: 44–73.

—— (1994) 'Hippokrates im 20. Jahrhundert: ärztliches Selbstbild, Idealbild und Zerrbild', in K.-H. Leven and C.-R. Prüll (eds) *Selbstbilder des Arztes im 20. Jahrhundert*, Freiburg im Breisgau: Hans Ferdinand Schulz Verlag: 39–96.

—— (1998) 'Krankheiten: historische Deutung versus retrospektive Diagnose', in N. Paul and T. Schlich (eds) *Medizingeschichte: Aufgaben, Probleme, Perspektiven*, Frankfurt: Campus Verlag: 153–85.

Lewis, Naphtali (1963) 'The non-scholar members of the Alexandrian Museum', *Mnemosyne*, ser. 4, 16: 257–60.

Lewis, Norman (1989) 'Snakes of San Domenico', *Independent Magazine*, 59, 21 October: 74–80.

Lichtenthaeler, C. (1984) *Der Eid des Hippokrates*, Cologne: Deutscher Ärzte-Verlag.

LiDonnici, L. R. (1995) *The Epidaurian Miracle Inscriptions*, Atlanta: Scholars Press.

Lieber, E. (1981) 'Galen in Hebrew: the transmission of Galen's works in the medieval Islamic world', in Nutton 1981a: 167–86.

—— (1996) 'The Hippocratic "Airs, Waters, Places" on cross-dressing eunuchs: "natural" yet also "divine"', in Wittern and Pellegrin 1996: 45–76.

—— (2000) 'Old Testament "leprosy", contagion and sin', in L. I. Conrad and D. Wujastyk (eds) *Contagion: Perspectives from Pre-modern Societies*, Aldershot: Ashgate: 99–136.

Lindemann, M. (1999) *Medicine and Society in Early Modern Europe*, Cambridge: Cambridge University Press.

Little, L. K. (ed.) (2007) *Plague and the End of Antiquity: The Pandemic of 541–750*, Cambridge: Cambridge University Press.

—— (2011) 'Plague historians in lab coats', *Past and Present*, 213: 267–90.

Littmann, R. J. and Littmann, M. L. (1973) 'Galen and the Antonine plague', *American Journal of Philology*, 94: 243–55.

Littré, E. (1839–61) *Oeuvres complètes d'Hippocrate*, 10 vols, Paris: J. B. Baillière.

Lloyd, G. E. R. (1968) 'Plato as a natural scientist', *Journal of Hellenic Studies*, 88: 68–92.

—— (1971) *Polarity and Analogy: Two Types of Argumentation in Early Greek Thought*, Cambridge: Cambridge University Press.

—— (1975) 'A note on Erasistratus of Ceos', *Journal of Hellenic Studies*, 95: 172–5.

—— (1978) *Hippocratic Writings*, Harmondsworth: Penguin.

—— (1979) *Magic, Reason and Experience*, Cambridge: Cambridge University Press.

—— (1983) *Science, Folklore, and Ideology*, Cambridge: Cambridge University Press.

—— (1987) *The Revolutions of Wisdom*, Berkeley and London: University of California Press.

—— (1990) *Demystifying Mentalities*, Cambridge: Cambridge University Press.

—— (1991) *Methods and Problems in Greek Science*, Cambridge: Cambridge University Press.

—— (1996) 'Theories and practices of demonstration in Galen', in M. Frede and G. Striker (eds) *Rationality in Greek Thought*, Oxford: Clarendon Press: 255–77.

—— (2001) 'Is there a future for ancient science?', *Proceedings of the Cambridge Philological Society*, 47: 196–210.

—— (2003) *In the Grip of Disease: Studies in the Greek Imagination*, Oxford: Oxford University Press.

—— (2009) 'Galen's un-Hippocratic case histories', in Gill *et al.* 2009: 115–31.

Lo Presti, R. (2008) *In forma di senso: l'encefalocentrismo del trattato ippocratico Sulla malattia sacra nel suo contesto epistemologico*, Rome: Carocci.

Long, A. A. and Sedley, D. N. (1987) *The Hellenistic Philosophers*, Cambridge: Cambridge University Press.

Longfield-Jones, G. M. (1986) 'A Graeco-Roman speculum in the Wellcome Museum', *Medical History*, 30: 81–9.

Longrigg, J. N. (1980) 'The great plague of Athens', *History of Science*, 18: 209–25.

—— (1981) 'Superlative achievement and comparative neglect: Alexandrian medical science and modern historical research', *History of Science*, 19: 155–200.

—— (1985) 'A seminal "debate" in the fifth century B.C.?', in A. Gotthelf (ed.) *Aristotle on Nature and Living Things: Philosophical and Historical Studies Presented to D. M. Balme*, Pittsburgh and Bristol: Bristol Classical Press.

—— (1988) 'Anatomy in Alexandria in the third century B.C.', *British Journal for the History of Science*, 21: 455–88.

—— (1992) 'Epidemics, ideas, and classical Athenian society', in Ranger and Slack 1992: 21–44.

—— (1993a) *Greek Rational Medicine: Philosophy and Medicine from Alcmaeon to the Alexandrians*, London: Routledge.

—— (1993b) 'Empedocles and the plague of Selinus: a cock and bull story?', *Tria Lustra: A Festschrift in Honour of John Pinsent*, Liverpool: Liverpool University Press.

—— (1997) 'Medicine in the classical world', in I. Loudon (ed.) *Western Medicine: An Illustrated History*, Oxford: Oxford University Press.

—— (1998) *Greek Medicine from the Heroic to the Hellenistic Age: A Source Book*, London: Duckworth.

Lonie, I. M. (1965) 'The Cnidian treatises of the Corpus Hippocraticum', *Classical Quarterly*, n.s. 15: 1–6.

—— (1975) 'The paradoxical text *On the Heart*', *Medical History*, 17: 1–15, 136–53.

—— (1977) 'A structural pattern in Greek dietetics', *Medical History*, 21: 235–69.

—— (1978) 'Cos versus Cnidus and the historians', *History of Science*, 16: 42–75, 77–92.

—— (1981) *The Hippocratic Treatises 'On Generation', 'On the Nature of the Child', 'Diseases IV'*, Berlin: De Gruyter.

Lopez Ferez, J. A. (ed.) (1992) *Tratados Hipocráticos: Estudios acerca de su Contenido, Forma e Influencia*, Madrid: UNED.

—— (2010) 'Some remarks by Galen about the teaching and studying of medicine', in Horstmanshoff 2010: 361–99.

Lorenz, R. (1976) *Beiträge zur Hygiene bei Homer*, Munich: Technical University.

Louis, P. (1991) *Aristote, Problèmes*, Paris: Les Belles Lettres.

Luck, G. (1985) *Arcana Mundi*, Baltimore and London: Johns Hopkins University Press.

McCann, A. M. (1978) *Roman Sarcophagi in the Metropolitan Museum of Art*, New York: Metropolitan Museum.

MacKinney, L. C. (1952) 'Medical ethics and etiquette in the early Middle Ages: the persistence of Hippocratic ideals', *Bulletin of the History of Medicine*, 26: 1–31.

—— (1965) *Medical Illustrations in Medieval Manuscripts*, London: Wellcome Historical Medical Library.

Macleod, R. M. (ed.) (2000) *The Library of Alexandria*, London: I. B. Tauris.

MacMullen, R. (1981) *Paganism in the Roman Empire*, New Haven: Yale University Press.

—— (1985) *Christianizing the Roman Empire (A.D. 100–400)*, New Haven and London: Yale University Press.

—— (1991) 'Hellenizing the Romans (2nd Century B.C.)', *Historia*, 40: 419–38.

—— (1997) *Christianity and Paganism in the Fourth to Eighth Centuries*, New Haven: Yale University Press.

Macridy, T. (1912) 'Inscriptions de Notion', *Jahreshefte der österreichischen archäologischen Instituts*, 15.

Magdelaine, C. (2007) 'Du char à la pratique routinière: à propos de l'ἐπιδίφριος ἰατρός', in Boudon-Millot *et al.* 2007: 295–306.

Magoulias, H. J. (1954) 'The lives of saints as sources of data for the history of Byzantine medicine in the sixth and seventh centuries', *Byzantinische Zeitschrift*, 57: 127–50.

Maire, B. (2002) *Gargilius Martialis, De Pomis et oleribus*, Paris: Les Belles Lettres.

Majno, G. (1975) *The Healing Hand: Man and Wound in the Ancient World*, Cambridge, MA: Harvard University Press.

Maloney, G. and Savoie, R. (1982) *Cinq cents ans de bibliographie hippocratique, 1473–1982*, St-Jean Chrystostome: Editions du Sphinx.

Manchester, K. (1992) 'Leprosy: the origin and development of the disease in antiquity', in D. Gourevitch (ed.) *Maladie et Maladies: Histoire et Conceptualisation*, Geneva: Droz: 31–50.

Manetti, D. (1994) 'Autografi e incompiuti: il caso dell'Anonimo Londinese P. Lit. Lond. 165', *Zeitschrift für Papyrologie und Epigraphik*, 100: 47–58.

—— (1996) 'Ὡς δ'αὐτὸς Ἱπποκράτης λέγει. Teoria causale e ippocratismo nell'Anonimo Londinese (VI 43ss.)', in Wittern and Pellegrin 1996: 296–310.

—— (1999a) 'Aristotle and the role of doxography in the Anonymus Londinensis (PBrLibr inv. 137)', in van der Eijk 1999a: 95–141.

—— (1999b) 'Il proemio di Erotiano e l'oscurità intenzionale di Ippocrate', in Garzya and Jouanna 1999: 363–78.

—— (2005) 'Medici contemporanei di Ippocrate: problemi d'identificazione', in van der Eijk 2005a: 295–314.

—— (2009a) 'The role of doxography in the Anonymus Londinensis', in T. Rütten (ed.) *Geschichte der Medizingeschichtsschreibung: Historiographie unter dem Diktat literarischer Gattungen von der Antike bis zur Aufklärung*, Remscheid: Gardez! Verlag: 87–110.

—— (2009b) 'Galen and Hippocratic medicine: language and practice', in Gill *et al.* 2009: 157–74.

—— (2011) *Anonymus Londiniensis, De medicina*, Berlin: De Gruyter.

Manetti, D. and Roselli, A. (1994) 'Galeno commentatore di Ippocrate', *ANRW*, II, 37(2): 1527–634.

Mani, N. (1959) *Die historischen Grundlagen der Leberforschung*, 2 vols, Basle: Juris.

—— (1991) 'Die wissenschaftlichen Grundlage der Chirurgie bei Galen', in Kudlien and Durling 1991: 26–49.

Mann, J. E. (2012) *Hippocrates: On the Art of Medicine*, Leiden and Boston: Brill.

Mansfeld, J. (1971) *The Pseudo-Hippocratic Tract ΠΕΡΙ ʽΕΒΔΟΜΑΔΩΝ*, Assen: Van Gorcum.

—— (1994) *Prolegomena: Questions to be Settled Before the Study of an Author, or a Book*, Leiden: Brill.

Mansfeld, J. and Runia, D. (1996) *Aetiana: The Method and Intellectual Context of a Doxographer*, Leiden: Brill.

Manuli, P. (1980) 'Claudio Tolomeo: il criterio e il principio', *Rivista critica di Storia della Filosofia*, 4: 2–26.

Manuli, P. and Vegetti, M. (1977) *Cuore, Sangue e Cervello: Biologia e Antropologia nel Pensiero antico*, Milan: Episteme Editrice.

—— (eds) (1988) *Le Opere psicologiche di Galeno*, Naples: Bibliopolis.

Manzoni, T. (2001) *Il Cervello secondo Galeno*, Ancona: Il Lavoro editoriale.

Marasco, G. (1995a) 'L'Introduction de la médecine grecque à Rome', in van der Eijk *et al.* 1995: 35–48.

—— (1995b) 'Cleopatra e gli esperimenti su cavie umane', *Historia*, 44: 317–25.

—— (1996) 'Les médecins de cour à l'époque hellénistique', *Revue des Études grecques*, 109: 435–66.

—— (2010) 'The curriculum of studies in the Roman Empire and the cultural role of physicians', in Horstmanshoff 2010: 205–22.

Marcos, N. F. (1975) *Los Thaumata de Sofronio: Contribucíon al Estudio de la Incubatio cristiana*, Madrid: Instituto Antonhio de Nebrija.

Marenghi, G. (1964) *Aristotele, Problemi di Medicina*, Milan: Istituto editoriale italiano.

Marganne, M. H. (1981) *Inventaire analytique des Papyrus grecs de Médecine*, Geneva: Droz.

—— (1993) 'Links between Egyptian and Greek medicine', *Forum*, 3(5): 35–43.

—— (1998) *La Chirurgie dans l'Egypte gréco-romaine d'après les Papyrus littéraires grecs*, Leiden: Brill.

—— (2001) 'Hippocrate et la médecine de l'Égypte gréco-romaine', *Revue de Philosophie ancienne*, 19: 39–62.

Marichal, R. (1994) Les Ostraca de Bu Njem, Tripoli, 1992; cited in *Journal of Roman Studies*, 84: 262.

Markus, R. A. (1990) *The End of Ancient Christianity*, Cambridge: Cambridge University Press.

Martin, A. (1984) 'À propos d'une inscription bilingue d'Apulie', *Epigraphica*, 46: 194–8.

Martin, A. and Primavesi, O. (1999) *L'Empédocle de Strasbourg*, Berlin: De Gruyter.

Martin, G. S. (1922) 'Miner's hookworm at the Centenillo Mines, Spain', *Transactions of the Institute of Mining and Metallurgy*, 13: 558.

Marx, K. F. H. (1877) 'Uebersichtliche Anordnung der die Medizin betreffenden Aussprueche des Philosopher Lucius Annaeus Seneca', *Abhandlungen der königlichen Gesellschaft der Wissenschaften zu Göttingen*, 22.

Massar, N. (2001) 'Un savoir-faire à l'honneur: "médecins" et "discours civique" en Grèce hellénistique', *Revue belge de Philologie et de l'Histoire*, 9: 175–201.

—— (2005) *Soigner et Servir: Histoire sociale et culturelle de la Médecine grecque à l'époque hellénistique*, Paris: De Boccard.

Mastrocinque, A. (1995) 'Les médecins des Séleucides', in van der Eijk *et al.* 1995: 143–51.

Masullo, R. (1999) *Filagrio. Frammenti*, Naples: Bibliopolis.

Mattern, S. P. (2008) *Galen and the Rhetoric of Healing*, Baltimore: Johns Hopkins University Press.

Matthaei, C. F. (1808) *XXI Medicorum veterum et clarorum graecorum varia Opuscula*, Moscow: Royal University.

Mattingly, D. J. (2011) *Imperialism, Power and Identity*, Princeton and Oxford: Princeton University Press.

Mavroudis, A. D. (2000) *Archigenes Philippou Apameus*, Athens: University of Athens.

May, M. T. (1968) *Galen on the Usefulness of Parts of the Body*, 2 vols, Ithaca: Cornell University Press.

Mazzini, I. (1997) *La Medicina dei Greci e dei Romani: Letteratura, Lingua, Scienza*, 2 vols, Rome: Jouvence.

—— (1999) *A. Cornelio Celso, la Chirurgia*, Pisa and Rome: Istituti editoriali.

Mazzini, I. and Fusco, F. (eds) (1985) *I Testi di Medicina latini antichi: Problemi filologici e storici*, Rome: G. Bretschneider.

Meier, L. (2009) 'Unveröffentlichte Inschriften aus dem Asklepieion und der Roten Halle von Pergamon', *Chiron*, 39: 395–404.

Meiggs, R. (1973) *Roman Ostia*, ed. 2, Oxford: Clarendon Press.

Meiggs, R. and Lewis, D. M. (1969) *A Selection of Greek Historical Inscriptions to the End of the Fifth Century B.C.*, Oxford: Clarendon Press.

Meinecke, B. (1927) 'Consumption (tuberculosis) in classical history', *Annals of Medical History*, 9: 379–402.

Meisami, J. S. (1989) 'Mas'udi on love and the fall of the Barmakids', *Journal of the Royal Asiatic Society*, 121: 252–77.

Melfi, M. (2007) *I santuari di Asclepio in Grecia*, Rome: L'Erma di Bretschneider.

Mentzou-Meimari, K. (1982) Ἐπαρχιακὰ εὐαγῆ ἱδρύματα μεχρὶ τοῦ τέλους τῆς εἰκονομαχίας', *Byzantina*, 11: 253–308.

Merkelbach, R. (1972) 'ΣΩΤΗΡ "Arzt"', *Zeitschrift für Papyrologie und Epigraphik*, 9: 133.

—— (1994) 'ΕΙΑΤΗΡΙΟΝ', *Zeitschrift für Papyrologie und Epigraphik*, 102: 296.

Mesk, J. (1913) 'Antiochos und Stratonike', *Rheinisches Museum*, 68: 366–94.

Metraux, A. G. (1995) *Sculptors and Physicians in Fifth-century Greece: A Preliminary Study*, Montreal: McGill-Queen's University Press.

Metzger, N. (2011) *Wolfsmenschen und nächtliche Heimsuchungen: zur kulturhistorischen Verortung vormoderner Konzepte von Lykanthropie und Ephialtes*, Remscheid: Gardez! Verlag.

Meyer (-Steineg), T. (1909) *Theodorus Priscianus und die römische Medizin*, Jena: Gustav Fischer.

Meyerhof, M. (1929) 'Autobiographische Bruchstücke Galens aus arabischen Quellen', *Sudhoffs Archiv*, 22: 72–86.

Meyerhof, M. and Schacht, J. (1930–1) 'Galen, über die medizinischen Namen', *Abhandlungen der Preussischen Akademie der Wissenschaften, philologisch-historische Klasse*, 3.

Michaelides, D. (1984) 'A Roman surgeon's tomb from Nea Paphos, I', *Report of the Department of Antiquities of Cyprus*, 19: 315–32.

—— (1988) 'A Roman surgeon's tomb from Nea Paphos, II', *Report of the Department of Antiquities of Cyprus*, 23: 229–34.

Michler, M. (1968) *Die hellenistische Chirurgie*, Wiesbaden: Steiner.

—— (1969) *Das Spezialisierungsproblem und die antike Chirurgie*, Berne, Stuttgart and Vienna: H. Huber.

—— (1975) 'Soranus', in C. C. Gillispie (ed.) *Dictionary of Scientific Biography*, vol. 12, New York: Scribner's: 538–42.

—— (1993) 'Principis medicus: Antonius Musa', *ANRW*, II, 2, 37, 1: 757–85.

—— (2003) *Westgriechische Heilkunde*, Pattensen: H. Wellm.

Migliorini, P. (1997) *Scienza e Terminologia medica nella Letteratura latina dell'Età Neroniana, Seneca, Lucano, Persio, Petronio*, Frankfurt: Peter Lang.

Miller, H. W. (1953) 'The concept of the divine in De Morbo Sacro', *Transactions of the American Philological Society*, 84: 1–15.

—— (1962) 'The aetiology of disease in Plato's *Timaeus*', *Transactions of the American Philological Association*, 86: 184–97.

Miller, T. S. (1990) 'The Sampson hospital of Constantinople', *Byzantinische Forschungen*, 15: 101–35.

—— (1997) *The Birth of the Hospital in the Byzantine Empire*, ed. 2, Baltimore: Johns Hopkins University Press.

Mitchell, L. G. (2001) 'Euboean Io', *Classical Quarterly*, 51: 339–52.

Mitchell, S. (1993) *Anatolia: Land, Men, and Gods in Asia Minor*, 2 vols, Oxford: Clarendon Press.

—— (1999) 'The cult of *theos hypsistos* between pagans, Jews, and Christians', in P. Athanassiadi and M. Frede (eds) *Pagan Monotheism in Late Antiquity*, Oxford: Oxford University Press: 81–146.

Möhler, R. (1990) *Epistula de vulture: Untersuchungen zu einer organotherapeutischen Drogenmonographie des Frühmittelalters*, Pattensen: H. Wellm.

Molland, E. (1970) *Opuscula patristica*, Oslo: Universitetsforlaget.

Moog, F. P. (1995) *Die Fragmente des Themison von Laodikeia*, MD thesis, University of Giessen.

—— (2002) 'Gladiatorenblut dei Epilepsie als etruskische Therapie – und der Bischof Marinos von Thrakien', in Karenberg and Leitz 2002: 153–82.

Moraux, P. (1984) *Der Aristotelismus bei den Griechen*, vol. 2, Berlin: De Gruyter.

Moreau, A. and Turpin, J. C. (eds) (2000) *La Magie*, Montpellier: Université Paul Valéry.

Mørland, H. (1933) *Rufi De Podagra, Symbolae Osloenses, Suppl.*, 6.

Morley, N. (2001) 'The transformation of Italy, 225–28 B.C.', *Journal of Roman Studies*, 91: 50–62.

Morton, A. G. (1986) 'Pliny on plants: his place in the history of botany', in French and Greenaway 1986: 86–96.

Most, G. W. (1981) 'Callimachus and Herophilus', *Hermes*, 109: 188–96.

—— (1993) 'A cock for Asclepius', *Classical Quarterly*, 43: 97–111.

Moule, C. F. D. (1965) *Miracles*, London: SCM Press.

Mudry, P. (1997) 'Ethique et médecine à Rome: la préface de Scribonius Largus ou l'affirmation d'une singularité', in Flashar and Jouanna 1997: 297–322.

—— (ed.) (1999) *Le Traité des Maladies aigües et des Maladies chroniques de Caelius Aurelianus*, Nantes: Université de Nantes.

Mudry, P. and Pigeaud, J. (eds) (1991) *Les Écoles médicales à Rome*, Geneva: Droz.

Müller, C. W., Brockmann, C. and Brunschön, C. W. (eds) (2006) *Ärzte und ihre Interpreten: Medizinische Fachtexte der Antike als Forschungsgegenstand der klassischen Philologie*, Munich and Leipzig: K. G. Saur.

Müller, H. (1987) 'Ein Heilungsbericht aus dem Asklepieion von Pergamon', *Chiron*, 17: 193–233.

Müller, I. W. (1993) *Humoralmedizin: physiologische, pathologische und therapeutische Grundlagen der galenistischen Heilkunst*, Heidelberg: Haug.

Müntzer, F. (1897) *Quellenkritik der Naturgeschichte des Plinius*, Berlin: Weidmann.

Müri, W. (1953) 'Melancholie und schwarze Galle', *Museum Helveticum*, 10: 21–38; repr. in *Griechische Studien*, Basle: F. Reinhardt, 1976: 139–64.

Nachmanson, E. (1917) *Erotianstudien*, Uppsala: Akademiske Bokhandeln.

—— (1918) *Erotiani Vocum Hippocraticarum Collectio*, Uppsala: Appelbergs Boktryckerei.

Nash Williams, V. E. (1950) *The Early Christian Monuments of Wales*, Cardiff: University of Wales Press.

Nelson, E. D. (2005) 'Coan promotions and the authorship of the Presbeutikos', in van der Eijk 2005a: 209–36.

Netz, R. (2011) 'The bibliosphere of ancient science (outside of Alexandria): a preliminary survey', *NTM*, n.s. 19: 239–69.

Neuburger, M. (1910) *A History of Medicine*, vol. 1, London: Oxford University Press.

Nicholls, M. C. (2011) 'Galen and libraries in the *Peri Alupias*', *Journal of Roman Studies*, 101: 123–42.

Nickel, D. (1971) *Galeni De Uteri Dissectione*, CMG 5, 2, 1, Berlin: Akademie Verlag.

—— (2005) 'Hippokratisches bei Praxagoras von Kos?', in van der Eijk 2005a: 315–24.

Niebyl, P. H. (1971) 'Old age, fever, and the lamp metaphor', *Bulletin of the History of Medicine*, 26: 351–68.

Nissen, C. (2001) 'Un oracle médical de Sarpédon à Séleucie du Calycadnos', *Kernos*, 14: 93–110.

—— (2009) *Entre Asklépios et Hippocrate: Étude des Cultes guérisseurs et des Médecins en Carie*, Liège: Centre international d'étude de la religion grecque antique.

Nissen, T. (1939) 'De SS. Cyri et Iohannis vitae formis', *Analecta Bollandiana*, 57: 65–71.

Nock, A. D. (1972) *Essays on Religion and the Ancient World*, 2 vols, Oxford: Clarendon Press.

Nörenberg, H. W. (1968) *Das Göttliche und die Natur in der Schrift über die Heilige Krankheit*, Bonn: Habelt.

Noy, D. (2000) *Foreigners at Rome: Citizens and Strangers*, London: Duckworth.

Nriagu, J. O. (1983) *Lead and Lead Poisoning in Antiquity*, New York: Wiley.

Nunn, J. F. (1996) *Ancient Egyptian Medicine*, London: British Museum Publications.

Nutton, V. (1968) 'A Greek doctor from Chester', *Journal of the Chester Archaeological Society*, 55: 7–13.

—— (1969) 'The doctor and the oracle', *Revue belge de philologie*, 47: 37–48.

—— (1970) 'The doctors of the Roman navy', *Epigraphica*, 32: 66–71.

—— (1971a) 'L. Gellius Maximus, physician and procurator', *Classical Quarterly*, 21: 262–72.

—— (1971b) 'Two notes on immunities: *Digest* 27, 1, 6, 10 and 11', *Journal of Roman Studies*, 61: 52–63; repr. in Nutton 1988.

—— (1972) 'Ammianus and Alexandria', *Clio Medica*, 7: 165–76.

—— (1973) 'The chronology of Galen's earlier career', *Classical Quarterly*, 23: 158–71; repr. in Nutton 1988.

—— (1975) 'Museums and medical schools in Classical Antiquity', *History of Education*, 4: 3–15.

—— (1977) '*Archiatri* and the medical profession in Antiquity', *Papers of the British School at Rome*, 45: 191–226; repr. in Nutton 1988.

—— (1979) *Galen, On Prognosis*, CMG 5, 8, 1, Berlin: Akademie Verlag.

—— (ed.) (1981a) *Galen: Problems and Prospects*, London: The Wellcome Institute.

—— (1981b) 'Continuity or rediscovery? The city physician in classical antiquity and medieval Italy', in A. W. Russell (ed.) *The Town and State Physician in Europe*, Wolfenbüttel: Herzog August Bibliothek: 9–46; repr. in Nutton 1988.

—— (1983) 'The seeds of disease: an explanation of contagion and infection from the Greeks to the Renaissance', *Medical History*, 27: 1–24; repr. in Nutton 1988.

—— (1984a) 'From Galen to Alexander: aspects of medical practice in late antiquity', *Dumbarton Oaks Papers*, 38: 1–14; repr. in Nutton 1988.

—— (1984b) 'Galen in the eyes of his contemporaries', *Bulletin of the History of Medicine*, 58: 315–24; repr. in Nutton 1988.

—— (1985a) 'Murders and miracle cures: lay attitudes towards medicine in classical antiquity', in R. Porter (ed.) *Patients and Practitioners*, Cambridge: Cambridge University Press: 23–53; repr. in Nutton 1988.

—— (1985b) 'The drug trade in antiquity', *Journal of the Royal Society of Medicine*, 78: 138–45; repr. in Nutton 1988.

—— (1986) 'The perils of patriotism: Pliny and Roman medicine', in French and Greenaway 1986: 30–58; repr. in Nutton 1988.

—— (1987) 'Numisianus and Galen', *Sudhoffs Archiv*, 71: 236–9.

—— (1988) *From Democedes to Harvey*, London: Variorum Reprints.

—— (ed.) (1990a) *Medicine at the Royal Courts of Europe*, London: Routledge.

—— (1990b) 'The patient's choice: a new treatise by Galen', *Classical Quarterly*, 40: 235–57.

—— (1990c) 'Therapeutic methods and Methodist therapeutics in the Roman Empire', in Y. Kawakita, S. Sakai and Y. Otsuka (eds) *History of Therapeutics*, Tokyo: Ishiyaku EuropAmerica Inc.: 1–36.

—— (1991a) 'From medical certainty to medical amulets: three aspects of ancient therapeutics', in W. F. Bynum and V. Nutton (eds) *Essays in the History of Therapeutics*, Amsterdam: Rodopi: 13–22.

—— (1991b) 'Style and context in the Method of Healing', in Kudlien and Durling 1991: 1–25.

—— (1992) 'Healers in the medical market place: towards a social history of Graeco-Roman medicine', in A. Wear (ed.) *Medicine in Society*, Cambridge: Cambridge University Press: 1–58.

—— (1993a) 'Beyond the Hippocratic oath', in A. Wear, J. Geyer-Kordesch and R. French (eds) *Doctors and Ethics: The Earlier Historical Setting of Professional Ethics*, Amsterdam: Rodopi: 10–37.

—— (1993b) 'Galen and Egypt', in Kollesch and Nickel 1993: 11–31.

—— (1993c) 'Galen at the bedside: the methods of a medical detective', in W. F. Bynum and R. Porter (eds) *Medicine and the Five Senses*, Cambridge: Cambridge University Press: 7–16.

—— (1993d) 'Greek science in the sixteenth-century Renaissance', in J. V. Field and F. James (eds) *Renaissance and Revolution: Humanists, Scholars, Craftsmen and Natural Philosophers in Early Modern Europe*, Cambridge: Cambridge University Press: 15–28.

—— (1993e) 'Roman medicine: tradition, confrontation, assimilation', *ANRW*, II, 37(1): 49–78.

—— (1995a) 'Medicine in the Greek world, 800–50 B.C.'; 'Roman medicine, 250 B.C. to A.D. 200'; 'Medicine in late antiquity and the early middle ages', in Conrad *et al.* 1995: 11–88.

—— (1995b) 'Galen *ad multos annos*', *Dynamis*, 15: 25–40.

—— (1995c) 'The changing language of medicine, 1450–1550', in O. Weijers (ed.) *Vocabulary of Teaching and Research between Middle Ages and Renaissance*, Turnhout: Brepols: 184–98.

—— (1995d) 'The medical meeting place', in van der Eijk *et al.* 1995: 3–25.

—— (1995e) 'What's in an oath?', *Journal of the Royal College of Physicians of London*, 29: 518–24.

—— (1996) 'Apollophanes [2]', *DNP*, 1: 891.

—— (1997a) 'Galen on theriac: problems of authenticity', in Debru 1997: 133–51.

—— (1997b) 'The rise of medical humanism: Ferrara, 1464–1555', *Renaissance Studies*, 11: 3–19.

—— (1998) 'To kill or not to kill? Caelius Aurelianus on contagion', in Fischer *et al.* 1998: 233–42.

—— (1999) *Galen, On My Own Opinions*, CMG V, 3, 2, Berlin: Akademie Verlag.

—— (2000a) 'Did the Greeks have a word for it?', in L. I. Conrad and D. Wujastyk (eds) *Contagion: Perspectives from Pre-modern Societies*, London: Routledge: 137–62.

—— (2000b) 'Medical thoughts on urban pollution', in Hope and Marshall 2000: 65–73.

—— (2001) 'God, Galen, and the depaganisation of ancient medicine', in P. Biller and J. Ziegler (eds) *Religion and Medicine in the Middle Ages*, York: York Medieval Press: 15–32.

—— (ed.) (2002a) *The Unknown Galen: Bulletin of the Institute of Classical Studies, Suppl.*, 77, London: Institute of Classical Studies.

—— (2002b) 'In defence of Kühn', in Nutton 2002a: 1–7.

—— (2008a) 'Greek medical astrology and the boundaries of medicine', in A. Akasoy, C. Burnett and R. Yoeli-Tlalim (eds) *Astro-Medicine: Astrology and Medicine, East and West*, Florence: SISMEL – Edizioni del Galluzzo: 17–31.

—— (2008b) 'The medical world of Rufus of Ephesus', in Pormann 2008: 139–58.

—— (2009) 'Galen's library', in Gill *et al.* 2009: 19–34.

—— (2010a) 'Galen in context', in F. Cairns and M. Griffin (eds) *Papers of the Langford Latin Seminar*, 14: 1–18.

—— (2010b) '*De virtute centaureae*: a neglected Methodist text?', in Langslow and Maire 2010: 213–22.

—— (2011) *Galen: On Problematical Movements*, Cambridge: Cambridge University Press.

—— (tr.) (2012a) 'Galen: avoiding distress', in Singer 2012.

—— (2012b) 'From Noah to Galen: a medieval Latin history of medicine', in C. Burnett and I. Csepregi (eds) *Ritual Healing in Antiquity and the Middle Ages*, Florence: SISMEL – Edizioni del Galluzzo.

—— (2012c) 'The commentary on the Hippocratic Oath ascribed to Galen', in S. Fortuna *et al.* (eds) (2012) *Sulla tradizione indiretta dei testi medici greci: i commenti. Atti del quarto seminario internazionale, Siena, Certosa di Pontignano, 3–4 giugno 2011*, Pisa: F. Serra: 15–24.

Oberhelman, S. M. (1994) 'Aretaeus of Cappocia: the Pneumatic physician of the first century A.D.', *ANRW*, II, 37(2): 941–66.

Oliver, J. H. (1936) 'The Sarapion monument and the Paean of Sophocles', *Hesperia*, 5: 91–122.

Olson, S. D. and Sens, A. (2000) *Archestratos of Gela: Greek Culture and Cuisine in the Fourth Century*, Oxford: Oxford University Press.

Önnerfors, A. (1993) 'Magische Formeln im Dienste römischer Medizin', *ANRW*, II, 37(1): 157–224.

Opsomer, C. and Halleux, R. (1985) 'La lettre d'Hippocrate à Mécène et la lettre d'Hippocrate à Antiochus', in Mazzini and Fusco 1985: 339–64.

—— (1991) 'Marcellus ou le mythe empirique', in Mudry and Pigeaud 1991: 159–78.

Oriel, J. D. (1973a) 'Anal and scrotal warts in the ancient world', *Paleopathological Newsletter*, 3: 5–7.

—— (1973b) 'Gonorrhea in the ancient world', *Paleopathological Newsletter*, 4: 7.

Ormos, I. (1993) 'Bemerkungen zur editorischen Bearbeitung der Galenschrift "Über die Sektion toter Lebewesen"', in Kollesch and Nickel 1993: 165–72.

Orth, E. (1925) *Cicero und die Medizin*, Berne and Leipzig: n.p.

Osbaldeston, T. A. and Wood, R. P. A. (2000) *Dioscorides De materia medica*, Johannesburg: Ibidis Press.

Osborne, C. (1987) 'Empedocles recycled', *Classical Quarterly*, 37: 24–50.

Osborne, R. (2011) *The History Written on the Classical Greek Body*, Cambridge: Cambridge University Press.

Oser-Gröte, C. M. (2004) *Aristoteles und das Corpus Hippocraticum*, Stuttgart: Steiner.

Padel, R. (1995) *Whom Gods Destroy: Elements of Greek and Tragic Madness*, Princeton: Princeton University Press.

Palfi, G., Dutour, O., Bérato, J. and Brun, J. P. (2000) 'La syphilis en Europe dans l'antiquité: le foetus de Costebelle et les autres nouvelles données ostéo archéologiques', *Vesalius*, 6: 55–63.

Palmieri, N. (2001) 'Nouvelles remarques sur les commentaires à Galien de l'école médicale de Ravenne', in Debru and Palmieri 2001: 209–46.

—— (2002) 'La médecine alexandrine et son rayonnement occidental (VIe–VIIe s. ap. J.-Ch.)', *Lettre d'Informations du Centre Jean Palerne: Médecine antique et mediévale*, n.s. 1: 5–23.

—— (ed.) (2003) *Rationel et Irrationnel dans la Médecine Ancienne et Médiévale*, St Etienne: Université de St Etienne.

Papagrigorakis, M. J., Yapijakis, C., Synodinos, P. N. and Baziotopoulou-Valavani, E. (2006) 'DNA examination of dental pulp incriminates typhoid as a probable cause of the Plague of Athens', *International Journal of Infectious Diseases*, 10(3): 206–14.

Papathomas, A. (2000) 'Eine Abrechnung über Getreidenüberlieferungen eines Xenodocheions an hilfsbedürftigen Personen: zur Wohltätigkeit Aktivität der spätantiken Kirche', in H. Mellaerts (ed.) *Papyri in honorem Johannis Bingen octogenarii (P. Bingen)*, Louvain: Peters: 561–71.

Paribeni, R. and Romanelli, P. (1914) 'Studi e ricerche archeologiche', *Monumenti antichi*, 23: 5–72.

Parker, H. (1997) 'Women physicians in Greece, Rome, and the Byzantine Empire', in L. R. Furst (ed.) *Women Physicians and Healers*, Lexington: University of Kentucky Press: 131–50.

—— (2012) 'Galen and the girls: sources for women medical writers revisited', *Classical Quarterly*, 62: 359–86.

Parker, R. (1983) *Miasma: Pollution and Purification in Early Greek Religion*, Oxford: Clarendon Press.

—— (1996) *Athenian Religion: A History*, Oxford: Clarendon Press.

Parkin, T. G. (1992) *Demography and Roman Society*, Baltimore and London: Johns Hopkins University Press.

—— (2003) *Old Age in the Roman World*, Baltimore and London: Johns Hopkins University Press.

Parsons, P. (2007) *The City of the Sharp-nosed Fish*, London: Weidenfeld and Nicolson.

Patlagean, E. and Riché, P. (eds) (1981) *Hagiographie, Cultures et Sociétés, IVe–XIIe Siècles*, Paris: Etudes Augustiniennes.

Pecere, O. and Stramaglia, A. (eds) (1996) *La Letteratura di Consumo nel Mondo grecolatino*, Cassino: Università degli Studi di Cassino.

Peek, W. (1969a) 'Inschriften aus dem Asklepieion von Epidauros', *Abhandlungen der sächsischen Akademie der Wissenschaften*, 60: 2.

—— (1969b) 'Inschriften von den Dorischen Inseln', *Abhandlungen der sächsischen Akademie der Wissenschaften*, 62: 1.

Peeters, P. (1929) 'La passion de S. Julien d'Emèse', *Analecta Bollandiana*, 47: 44–76.

—— (1939) 'S. Dometios le martyr et S. Dometios le médecin', *Analecta Bollandiana*, 57: 72–104.

Pellegrino, E. D. and Pellegrino, A. E. (1988) 'Humanism and ethics in Roman medicine: translation and commentary on a text of Scribonius Largus', *Literature and Medicine*, 7: 22–38.

Pellicer, L. (2000) 'A propos d'"Hippocrate refusant les présents d'Artaxerxès", esquisse de Girodet (Montpellier, Musée Fabre)', in R. Andréani, H. Michel and E. Pélaquier (eds) *Hellénisme et Hippocratisme dans l'Europe méditeranéenne: Autour de D. Coray*, Montpellier: Université française de Montpellier: 197–212.

Perilli, L. (2007) 'Da medico a lessicografo: Galeno e il Glossario Ippocratico', in Müller *et al.* 2006: 165–202.

Perilli, L., Brockmann, C., Fischer, K. D. and Roselli, A. (eds) (2012) *Officina Hippocratica: Beiträge zu Ehren von Anargyros Anastassiou und Dieter Irmer*, Berlin: De Gruyter.

Petrakis, B. Ch. (1997) *ΟΙ ΕΠΙΓΡΑΦΕΣ ΤΟΥ ΩΡΩΠΟΥ*, Athens: Greek Archaeological Society.

Petsalis-Diomidis, A. (2010) *Truly Beyond Wonders: Aelius Aristides and the Cult of Asklepios*, Oxford: Oxford University Press.

Petzl, G. (1983) *Die Inschriften von Smyrna*, Bonn: R. Habelt.

—— (1994) 'Die Beichtinschriften Westkleinasiens', *Epigraphica Anatolica*, 22.

Pfaff, F. (1932a) 'Die Überlieferung des Corpus Hippocraticum in der nach alexandrinischen Zeit', *Wiener Studien*, 50: 67–82.

—— (1932b) 'Rufus aus Samaria, Hippokrateskommentator und Quelle Galens', *Hermes*, 67: 356–9.

Pfeiffer, R. (1968) *History of Classical Scholarship from the Beginnings to the End of the Hellenistic Age*, Oxford: Clarendon Press.

Phillips, E. D. (1973) *Greek Medicine*, London: Thames and Hudson.

Phillips, J. H. (1984) 'On Varro's *animalia quaedam minuta* and etiology of disease', *Transactions and Studies of the College of Physicians of Philadelphia*, ser. 5(4): 12–25.

Pigeaud, J. (1981) *La Maladie de l'Âme*, Paris: Les Belles Lettres.

—— (1982) 'Pro Caelio Aureliano', *Mémoires du Centre Jean Palerne*, 3: 105–18; repr. in Pigeaud 2008: 247–62.

—— (1987a) *Folie et Cures de la Folie chez les Médecins de l'Antiquité gréco-romaine*, Paris: Les Belles Lettres.

—— (ed.) (1987b) *Pline l'Ancien, Témoin de son Temps*, Salamanca: Universidad Pontificia.

—— (1988) *Aristote: L'Homme de Génie et la Mélancholie. Problème XXX, 1*, Paris: Editions Rivage.

—— (1991) 'Les fondements du méthodisme', in Mudry and Pigeaud 1991: 9–50; repr. in Pigeaud 2008: 199–245.

—— (1993) 'L'introduction du méthodisme à Rome', *ANRW*, II, 37(1): 1718–44.

—— (2008) *Poétiques du Corps: Aux Origines de la Médecine*, Paris: Les Belles Lettres.

Pigulewskaja, N. (1969) *Byzanz auf den Weg nach Indien*, Berlin: Akademie Verlag.

Pilch, J. J. (2000) *Healing in the New Testament: Insights from Medical and Mediterranean Anthropology*, Minneapolis: Fortress Press.

Pingree, D. (1976) 'Thessalus Astrologus', in F. E. Cranz (ed.) *Catalogus Translationum et Commentariorum*, vol. 3, Washington: Catholic University of America Press.

—— (1986) *Vetti Valentis Antiocheni Anthologiae*, Leipzig: Teubner.

Pithis, J. A. (1983) *Die Schriften ΠΕΡΙ ΣΦΥΓΜΩΝ des Philaretos*, Husum: Matthiesen Verlag.

Pitts, L. F. and St Joseph, J. K. (1985) *Inchtuthil*, London: The Roman Society.

Pleket, H. W. (1958) *Greek and Latin Inscriptions in the Rijksmuseum at Leyden*, Leiden: Brill.

—— (1995) 'The social status of physicians in the Graeco-Roman world', in van der Eijk *et al.* 1995: 27–34.

Podolak, P. (2010) *Soranos von Ephesos, Peri psyches: Sammlung der Testimonien, Kommentar und Einleitung*, Berlin and New York: De Gruyter.

Polito, R. (1994) 'I quattri libri sull'anima di Sorano e lo scritto *De anima* di Tertulliano', *Rivista di Storia della Filosofia*, 3: 423–68.

—— (1999) 'On the life of Asclepiades of Bithynia', *Journal of Hellenic Studies*, 119: 48–66.

Popović, M. (2007) *Reading the Human Body: Physiognomics and Astrology in the Dead Sea Scrolls and Hellenistic–Early Roman Period*, Leiden: Brill.

Pormann, P. (1999) *Paul of Aegina's Therapy of Children*, MPhil thesis, University of Oxford.

—— (ed.) (2008) *Rufus of Ephesus: On Melancholy*, Tübingen: Mohr Siebeck.

—— (2010) 'Medical education in antiquity: from Alexandria to Montpellier', in Horstmanshoff 2010: 419–42.

Porter, R. and Rousseau, G. S. (1998) *Gout: The Patrician Malady*, New Haven: Yale University Press.

Potter, P. (1976) 'Herophilus of Chalcedon: an assessment of his place in the history of anatomy', *Bulletin of the History of Medicine*, 50: 45–60.

—— (1988) *A Short Handbook of Hippocratic Medicine*, Sillery: Editions du Sphinx.

—— (1989) 'Epidemien I/III: Form und Absicht der zweiundvierzig Fallbeschreibungen', in Baader and Winau 1989: 9–19.

—— (1993) 'Apollonius and Galen on "Joints"', in Kollesch and Nickel 1993: 117–24.

Potter, P., Maloney, G. and Desautels, J. (eds) (1990) *La Maladie et les Maladies dans la Collection hippocratique*, Quebec: Editions du Sphinx.

Potter, T. W. (1985) 'A Republican healing sanctuary at Tor di Nona near Rome and the classical tradition of votive medicine', *Journal of the British Archaeological Association*, 138: 23–47.

Powell, O. (2003) *Galen on the Properties of Foodstuffs (De Alimentorum Facultatibus)*, Cambridge: Cambridge University Press.

Prêtre, C. and Charlier, P. (2009) *Maladies humaines, Thérapies divines: Analyse épigraphique et paléopathologique de Textes de Guérison grecs*, Paris: Presses universitaires du Septentrion.

Preuss, J. (1978) *Biblical and Talmudic Medicine*, New York: Sanhedrin Press.

Prioreschi, P. (1996a) *A History of Medicine*, Omaha: Horatius Press.

—— (1996b) 'Galenicae Quaestiones disputatae duae: rete mirabile and pulmonary circulation', *Vesalius*, 2: 67–78.

Pritchett, W. K. (1993) *The Liar School of Herodotus*, Amsterdam: J. C. Gieben.

Pugliese Carratelli, G. (1939–40) 'Per la storia delle associazioni in Rodi antica', *Annuario della Scuola archeologica in Atene*, n.s. 1–2: 147–200.

Puschmann, T. (1878–9) *Alexander von Tralles*, 2 vols, Vienna: W. Braumüller.

Radt, S. (1999) *Tragicorum Graecorum Fragmenta*, vol. 4, Sophocles, Göttingen: Vandenhoeck & Ruprecht.

Ramsay, W. M. (1919) 'A noble Anatolian family of the fourth century', *Classical Review*, 33: 2.

—— (1941) *The Social Basis of Roman Power in Asia Minor*, Aberdeen: Aberdeen University Press.

Ranger, T. and Slack, P. (eds) (1992) *Epidemics and Ideas: Essays on the Historical Perception of Pestilence*, Cambridge: Cambridge University Press.

Raschke, M. G. (1978) 'New studies in Roman commerce with the East', *ANRW*, II, 2: 604–1378.

Rathbone, D. (1990) 'Villages, land and population in Graeco-Roman Egypt', *Proceedings of the Cambridge Philological Society*, 36: 103–42.

Raven, J. E. (2000) *Plants and Plant Lore in Ancient Greece*, Oxford: The Leopard's Head Press.

Rawson, E. D. (1982) 'The life and death of Asclepiades of Bithynia', *Classical Quarterly*, 32: 358–70.

—— (1985) *Intellectual Life in the Late Roman Republic*, London: Duckworth.

Rechenauer, G. (1991) *Thukydides und die hippokratische Medizin*, Hildesheim: Olms.

Reeds, K. M. (1991) *Botany in Medieval and Renaissance Universities*, New York: Garland.

Reizenstein, R. (1904) *Poimandres*, Leipzig: Teubner.

Rémondon, R. (1964) 'Problèmes de bilinguisme dans l'Égypte lagide', *Chronique d'Égypte*, 39: 126–46.

Renehan, R. (1975) *Greek Lexicographical Notes*, Göttingen: Vandenhoeck & Ruprecht.

—— (1992) 'The staunching of Odysseus' blood: the healing powers of magic', *American Journal of Philology*, 113: 1–4.

—— (2000) 'A rare surgical procedure in Plutarch', *Classical Quarterly*, 50: 222–9.

Rescher, N. (1965) 'Galen and the fourth figure of the Syllogism', *Journal of the History of Philosophy*, 3: 27–41.

—— (1966) *Galen and the Syllogism*, Pittsburgh: Pittsburgh University Press.

Reverdin, O. and Grange, B. (eds) (1992) *Le Sanctuaire grec: Entretiens de la Fondation Hardt*, 37, Vandoeuvres: Fondation Hardt.

Reymond, E. A. E. (1976) *From the Contents of the Libraries of the Suchos Temples in the Fayyum. Pt. 1, A Medical Book from Crocodilopolis*, Vienna: Hollinek.

Rich, J. and Wallace-Hadrill, A. (eds) (1991) *City and Country in the Ancient World*, London: Routledge.

Richmond, I. A. (1968) *Hod Hill*, London: Batsford.

Riddle, J. (1980) 'Dioscorides', in F. E. Cranz (ed.) *Catalogus Translationum et Commentariorum*, vol. 4, Washington: Catholic University of America Press: 1–143.

—— (1981) 'Pseudo-Dioscorides' *Ex herbis femininis* and early medieval medical botany', *Journal of the History of Biology*, 14: 43–81.

—— (1984) 'Gargilius Martialis as a medical writer', *Journal of the History of Medicine and Allied Sciences*, 39: 408–29; repr. in Riddle 1992b.

—— (1985) *Dioscorides on Pharmacy and Medicine*, Austin: University of Texas Press.

—— (1992a) *Contraception and Abortion from the Ancient World to the Renaissance*, Cambridge, MA: Harvard University Press.

—— (1992b) *Quid pro quo: Studies in the History of Drugs*, Aldershot: Variorum.

Riethmüller, J. W. (2005) *Asklepios: Heiligtümer und Kulte*, Heidelberg: Verlag Archäologie und Geschichte.

Rihll, T. (2010) 'Alexandrian science and technology', in A. B. Lloyd (ed.) *A Companion to Ancient Egypt*, Oxford: Blackwell: 409–24.

Rinne, F. (1896) *Das Rezeptbuch des Scribonius Largus, zum ersten Male theilweise ins Deutsche übersetzt und mit pharmakologischem Commentar versehen: Historische Studien aus dem Pharmakologischen Institut der Universität Dorpat*, 5, Halle: Tansche and Grosse.

Rippere, V. (1981) 'The survival of traditional medicine in lay medical views', *Medical History*, 25: 411–14.

Ritner, R. K. (1989) 'Review of Von Staden 1989', *Newsletter of the Society for the History of Ancient Medicine and Pharmacy*, 17: 39–40.

Robert, F. (1989) 'Médecine d'équipe dans les épidémies V', in Baader and Winau 1989: 20–7.

Robert, L. (1932) 'Hellenica', *Revue de Philologie*, ser. 3(13): 166–73.

—— (1937) *Etude anatoliennes*, Paris: De Boccard.

—— (1940a) *Les Gladiateurs dans l'Orient grec*, Paris: E. Champion.

—— (1940b) *Hellenica, I*, Limoges: A. Bontemps.

—— (1948) *Hellenica, IV*, Paris: Les Belles Lettres.

—— (1960) *Hellenica 11/12*, Paris: Les Belles Lettres.

—— (1962) 'Bulletin épigraphique', *Revue des Études grecques*, 75: 220–1.

—— (1969) *Opera Minora Selecta, Epigraphie et Antiquités grecques*, 7 vols, Amsterdam: Hakkert.

—— (1973) 'De Cilicie à Messine et à Plymouth', *Journal des Savants*, 161–211.

—— (1980) *A travers l'Asie Mineure*, Paris: Ecole française d'Athènes.

Robert, L. and Robert, J. (1954) *La Carie: Le Plateau de Tabai et ses Environs*, Paris: A. Maisonneuve.

Roberts, C. and Cox, M. (2003) *Health and Disease in Britain from Prehistory to the Present Day*, Stroud: Sutton.

Roberts, C. and Manchester, K. (1998) *The Archeology of Disease*, Ithaca: Cornell University Press.

Roberts, C., Lewis, M. E. and Manchester, C. (eds) (2002) *The Past and Present of Leprosy: Archaeological, Historical, Palaeopathological and Clinical Approaches*, Oxford: Archaeopress.

Rocca, J. (2002) 'The brain beyond Kühn: reflections on *Anatomical Procedures*, Book IX', in Nutton 2002a: 87–100.

—— (2003) *Galen on the Brain*, Leiden: Brill.

—— (2008) 'Anatomy', in Hankinson 2008: 242–62.

Rodriguez Alfageme, I. (1995) 'La médecine technique dans la comédie attique', in van der Eijk *et al.* 1995: 579–86.

Roesch, P. (1984) 'Médecins publics dans les cités grecques', *Histoire des Sciences médicales*, 18: 279–93.

Rohland, J. P. (1977) *Der Erzengel Michael, Arzt und Feldherr: Zwei Aspekte des vor- und frühbyzantinische Michaelskult*, Leiden: Brill.

Röhr, J. (1923) *Der okkulte Kraftbegriff im Altertum, Philologus, Suppl.*, 17: 1.

Römer, C. (1990) 'Ehrung für den Arzt Themison', *Zeitschrift für Papyrologie und Epigraphik*, 84: 81–8.

Rose, V. (1882) *Sorani Gynaeciorum Vetus Translatio Latina*, Leipzig: Teubner.

Roselli, A. (1988) 'Citazioni ippocratiche in Demetrio Lacone (PHerc. 1012)', *Cronache Ercolanesi*, 18: 53–7.

—— (1991) 'Le responsiones medicinales di Caelius Aurelianus', *Mémoires du Centre Jean Palerne*, 10: 75–86.

—— (1998) 'L'Anonimo *De medicina* (II 244–245 Dietz): un prolegomenon alla lettura di testi medici?', *Filologia antica e moderna*, 15: 7–25.

—— (1999) 'Notes on the *Doxai* of doctors in Galen's *Commentaries* on Hippocrates', in van der Eijk 1999a: 359–81.

—— (2005) 'Areteo di Cappadocia lettore di Ippocrate', in van der Eijk 2005a: 413–32.

Rosen, R. (2010) 'Galen and the compulsion to instruct', in Horstmanshoff 2010: 325–42.

Rosenthal, F. (1956) 'An ancient commentary on the Hippocratic oath', *Bulletin of the History of Medicine*, 30: 52–87; repr. in F. Rosenthal (1990) *Science and Medicine in Islam*, Guildford: Variorum.

—— (1975) *The Classical Heritage in Islam*, London: Routledge.

Ross, Sir David (1971) *Aristotle*, London: Methuen.

Rothschild, B. M. and Rothschild, C. (1977) 'Congenital syphilis: the archeological record', *International Journal of Paleopathology*, 7: 39–40.

Rouché, M. (1999) 'Did medical students study philosophy in Alexandria?', *Bulletin of the Institute of Classical Studies*, 43: 153–69.

Rousselle, A. (1990) *Croire et Guérir: La Foi en Gaule dans l'Antiquité tardive*, Paris: Fayard.

Rubin Pinault, J. (1992) *Hippocratic Lives and Legends*, Leiden: Brill.

Rubinstein, G. (1985) *The Methodist Method*, PhD thesis, University of Cambridge.

Russu, I. (1972) 'Getica lui Statilius Crito', *Studii Clasice*, 14: 111–28.

Rütten, T. (1992) *Demokrit: lachender Philosoph und sanguinischer Melancholiker: eine pseudohippokratische Geschichte*, Leiden: Brill.

—— (1993) *Hippokrates im Gespräch*, Münster: Universitäts- und Landesbibliothek.

—— (1997) 'Medizinethische Themen in den deontologischen Schriften des Corpus Hippocraticum', in Flashar and Jouanna 1997: 65–111.

—— (2007) *Geschichten vom Hippokratischen Eid*, Wiesbaden: Harrassowitz.

Rydén, L. (1981) 'The holy fool', in S. Hackel (ed.) *The Byzantine Saint*, London: Fellowship of St Alban and St Sergius.

Sabbah, G. (ed.) (1991) *Le Latin médical: la Constitution d'un Langage scientifique*, St Etienne: Publications de l'Université de St Etienne.

Sabbah, G. and Mudry, P. (eds) (1994) *La Médecine de Celse: Mémoires du Centre Jean Palerne*, 13.

Sabbah, G., Corsetti, P.-P. and Fischer, K.-D. (1987) *Bibliographie des Textes médicaux latins: Antiquité et Haut Moyen Âge*, St Etienne: Université de St Etienne.

Sachs, M. and Varelis, G. (2001a) 'Der griechische Arzt und Chirurg Antyllos (2. Jh. n. Chr.) und seine Bedeutung für die Entwicklung der operativen Chirurgie', *Würzburger medizinhistorische Mitteilungen*, 20: 43–60.

—— (2001b) Ἀντύλλου Χειρουγούμενα. Die chirurgische Schriften des Antyllos (2. Jh. n. Chr.), *Würzburger medizinhistorische Mitteilungen*, 20: 61–86.

Salazar, C. F. (2000) *The Treatment of War Wounds in Graeco-Roman Antiquity*, Leiden: Brill.

Sallares, R. (1991) *The Ecology of the Ancient Greek World*, London: Duckworth.

—— (2002) *Malaria and Rome: A History of Malaria in Ancient Italy*, Oxford: Oxford University Press.

Sallares, R., Bouwman, A. and Anderung, C. (2004) 'The spread of malaria to Southern Europe in Antiquity: new approaches to old problems', *Medical History*, 48: 311–28.

Samama, E. (2003) *Les Médecins dans le Monde grec: Sources épigraphiques sur la Naissance d'un Corps médical*, Geneva: Droz.

Sanchis Llopis, J. A. (2000) 'La lengua de los médicos en la comedia griega post aristofánica', in J. A. Lopez Ferez (ed.) *La Lengua científica griega: Orígines, Desarollo e Influencia en las Lenguas modernas europeas*, 2 vols, Madrid: Ediciones Clásicas: 123–56.

Sarton, G. (1954) *Galen of Pergamum*, Lawrence: University of Kansas Press.

Saunders, K. B. (1999) 'The wounds in *Iliad* 13–16', *Classical Quarterly*, 49: 345–63.

Savage-Smith, E. (2002) 'Galen's lost ophthalmology and the *Summaria Alexandrinorum*', in Nutton 2002a: 121–38.

Scarborough, J. (1970) 'Diphilus of Siphnos and Hellenistic medical dietetics', *Journal of the History of Medicine and Allied Sciences*, 25: 194–201.

—— (1971) 'Galen and the gladiators', *Episteme*, 2: 98–111.

—— (1978) 'Theophrastus on herbals and herbal remedies', *Journal of the History of Biology*, 11: 353–85; repr. in Scarborough 2010.

—— (1985a) 'Criton, physician to Trajan: historian and pharmacist', in J. W. Eadie and J. Ober (eds) *The Craft of the Ancient Historian: Essays in Honor of Chester G. Starr*, Lanham: University Press of America: 387–405; repr. in Scarborough 2010.

—— (1985b) 'Erasistratus, student of Theophrastus?', *Bulletin of the History of Medicine*, 59: 515–17.

—— (1985c) 'Galen's dissection of the elephant', *Koroth*, 8: 123–34.

—— (1986) 'Pharmacy in Pliny's *Natural History*: some observations of substances and sources', in French and Greenaway 1986: 59–95.

—— (2010) *Pharmacy and Drug Lore in Antiquity: Greece, Rome, Byzantium*, Farnham and Burlington: Ashgate.

—— (2012) 'Pharmacology and toxicology at the court of Cleopatra VII: traces of three physicians', in A. van Arsdall and T. Graham (eds) *Herbs and Healers from the Ancient Mediterranean through the Medieval West*, Farnham and Burlington: Ashgate.

Scarborough, J. and Nutton, V. (1982) 'The preface of Dioscorides' *Materia Medica*: introduction, translation and commentary', *Transactions of the College of Physicians of Philadelphia*, ser. 5(4): 187–227.

Scheidel, W. (1994) 'Libitina's bitter gains: seasonal mortality and endemic disease in the city of Rome', *Ancient Society*, 25: 151–75.

—— (ed.) (2001a) *Debating Roman Demography*, Leiden: Brill.

—— (2001b) 'Roman age structure: evidence and models', *Journal of Roman Studies*, 91: 1–26.

—— (2002) *Death on the Nile: Disease and the Demography of Roman Egypt*, Leiden: Brill.

Schiefsky, M. (2005) *Hippocrates: Ancient Medicine*, Leiden: Brill.

Schlange-Schöningen, H. (2001) *Die römische Gesellschaft bei Galen: Biographie und Sozialgeschichte*, Habilitationschrift: Freie Universität Berlin.

Schmidt, A. (1924) *Drogen und Drogenhandel im Altertum*, Leipzig: Barth.

Schölkopf, V. (1968) *Zum Problem der Religiosität älterer griechische Ärzte*, MD thesis, University of Kiel.

Schonack, W. (1913) *Die Rezepte des Scribonius Largus zum ersten Male vollständig ins Deutsche übersetzt und mit ausführlichem Arzneimittelregister versehen*, Jena: Gustav Fischer.

Schöne, H. (1896) *Apollonius Citiensis in Hippocratis De articulis Commentarii*, Leipzig: Teubner.

—— (1907) 'Markellinos' Pulslehre: ein griechisches Anekdoton', *Festschrift zur 49. Versammlung deutschen Philologen und Schulmänner in Basel im J. 1907*: 448–72.

—— (1909) 'Aus der antiken Kriegschirurgie', *Bonner Jahrbücher*, 118: 1–11.

—— (1910) 'Echte Hippokratesschriften', *Deutsche medizinische Wochenschrift*, 36(9): 418–19, 466–7.

Schöner, E. (1964) *Das Viererschema in der antiken Humoralpathologie*, Wiesbaden: Steiner.

Schubert, C. (2005) *Der hippokratische Eid: Medizin und Ethik von der Antike bis heute*, Berlin: Wissenschaftliche Buchgesellschaft.

Schultze, C. F. (1999) *Aulus Cornelius Celsus: Arzt oder Laie? Autor, Konzept und Adressaten der De medicina libri octo*, Trier: Wissenschaftlicher Verlag.

Schultze, R. (1934) 'Die römische Legionslazarette in Vetera und anderen Legionslagern', *Bonner Jahrbücher*, 139: 54–63.

Schürer, E. (1987) *Storia del Popolo Giudaico al Tempo di Jesu Cristo*, 2 vols, Brescia: Paideia Editrice.

Schwartz, E. (ed.) (1922–74) *Acta Conciliorum Oecumenicorum*, 4 vols, Berlin and Leipzig: De Gruyter.

Sconocchia, S. (1983) *Scribonii Largi Compositiones*, Leipzig: Teubner.

—— (1993) 'L'opera di Scribonio Largo e la letteratura medica latina del 1 sec. d. C.', *ANRW*, II, 37(1): 845–922.

—— (2000) 'L'eredità della medicina romana dell'età tardoantica e medioevale', in C. Baffioni (ed.) *L'Eredità classica nell'Età tardoantica e medioevale: Filiologia, Storia, Dottrina*, Alessandria: Edizioni dell'Orso.

Scurlock, J. (2006) *Magico-medical Means of Treating Ghost-induced Illnesses in Ancient Mesopotamia*, Leiden: Brill.

Segal, J. B. (1970) *Edessa, the Blessed City*, Oxford: Clarendon Press.

Semeria, A. (1986) 'Per un censimento degli Asklepieia della Grecia continentale e delle isole', *Annuario della Scuola normale di Pisa*, 16: 931–58.

Shapiro, B., Rambaut, A. and Thomas, P. G. (2006) 'No proof that typhoid caused the Plague of Athens (a reply to Papagrigorakis *et al.* 2006)', *International Journal of Infectious Diseases*, 10(4): 334–5.

Sharpe, W. D. (1964) 'Isidore of Seville: the medical writings: an English translation with an introduction and commentary', *Transactions of the American Philosophical Society*, n.s. 54: 2.

Sharples, R. W. (1982) 'Alexander of Aphrodisias, on time', *Phronesis*, 27: 72–8.

Sharples, R. W. and van der Eijk, P. J. (2008) *Nemesius on the Nature of Man*, Liverpool: Liverpool University Press.

Shaw, B. D. (1996) 'Seasons of death: aspects of mortality in imperial Rome', *Journal of Roman Studies*, 86: 100–38.

Sheils, W. J. (ed.) (1982) *The Church and Healing*, Oxford: Blackwell.

Sherman, I. W. (2006) *The Power of Plagues*, Washington: ASM Press.

Sherwin-White, S. M. (1978) *Ancient Cos*, Göttingen: Vandenhoeck & Ruprecht.

Shilts, R. (1987) *And the Band Played On: Politics, People and the AIDS Epidemic*, New York: St Martin's Press.

Sideras, A. (1977) *Rufi De Renum et Vesicae Morbis*, CMG, 3(1), Berlin: Akademie Verlag.

—— (1994) 'Rufus von Ephesos und sein Werk im Rahmen der antiken Medizin', *ANRW*, II, 37(2): 1077–253, 2036–62.

Siegel, R. E. (1976) *Galen on the Affected Parts*, Basle: Karger.

Sigerist, H. E. (1951–61) *A History of Medicine*, 2 vols, London: Oxford University Press.

Sikes, S. K. (1971) *The Natural History of the African Elephant*, London: Weidenfeld and Nicolson.

Simon, B. (1978) *Mind and Madness in Classical Greece*, Ithaca: Cornell University Press.

Singer, C. (1952) 'Galen's elementary course on bones', *Proceedings of the Royal Society of Medicine*, 4: 767–76.

—— (1956) *Galen on Anatomical Procedures*, London, Oxford and New York: Oxford University Press.

Singer, P. N. (1997) *Galen: Selected Works*, Oxford: Oxford University Press.

—— (ed.) (2012) *Galen: Psychological Writings*, Cambridge: Cambridge University Press.

Siraisi, N. G. (1981) *Taddeo Alderotti and his Pupils*, Princeton: Princeton University Press.

Skoda, F. (1988) *Médecine ancienne et Métaphore: Le Vocabulaire de l'Anatomie et de la Pathologie en grec ancien*, Paris: Les Belles Lettres.

Smith, D. C. (1996) 'The Hippocratic Oath and modern medicine', *Journal of the History of Medicine and Allied Sciences*, 51: 484–500.

Smith, M. (1978) *Jesus the Magician*, New York: Harper and Row.

Smith, R. R. R. (1990) 'Late Roman philosopher portraits from Aphrodisias', *Journal of Roman Studies*, 80: 127–55.

Smith, W. D. (1973) 'Galen on Coans v. Cnidians', *Bulletin of the History of Medicine*, 47: 569–85.

—— (1979) *The Hippocratic Tradition*, Ithaca: Cornell University Press.

—— (1982) 'Erasistratus' dietetic medicine', *Bulletin of the History of Medicine*, 56: 399–409.

—— (1990) *Hippocrates: Pseudepigraphic Writings*, Leiden: Brill.

—— (1999) 'The genuine Hippocrates and his theory of therapy', in Garofalo *et al.* 1999: 107–7.

Solbakk, J. H. (1993) *Forms and Functions of Medical Knowledge in Plato*, PhD thesis, University of Oslo.

Solmsen, F. (1961) 'Greek philosophy and the discovery of the nerves', *Museum Helveticum*, 18: 150–67.

Speyer, W. (1971) *Die literarische Fälschung im heidnischen und christlichen Altertum: ein Versuch ihrer Deutung*, Munich: Beck.

Stahl, W. H. (1962) *Roman Science: Origins, Development and Influence in the Later Middle Ages*, Madison: University of Wisconsin Press.

Stakelum, J. (1940) *Galen and the Logic of Propositions*, Rome: Angelicum.

Stannard, J. (1961) 'Hippocratic pharmacology', *Bulletin of the History of Medicine*, 35: 497–518; repr. in J. Stannard (1999) *Pristina Medicamenta*, Aldershot: Ashgate.

—— (1965) 'Pliny and Roman botany', *Isis*, 56: 420–5.

Steckerl, F. (1958) *The Fragments of Praxagoras of Cos and his School*, Leiden: Brill.

Sternberg, T. (1991) *Orientalium more secutus*, Munster: Aschendorff.

Sterpellone, L. (2002) *La Medicina Etrusca: Demoiatria di un'Antica Civiltà*, Nocero: Essebiemme.

Steuer, R. O. and Saunders, J. B. de C. M. (1959) *Ancient Egyptian and Cnidian Medicine*, Berkeley: University of California Press.

Stilwell, R. (ed.) (1976) *The Princeton Encyclopedia of Classical Sites*, Princeton: Princeton University Press.

Stol, M. (1993) *Epilepsy in Babylonia*, Groningen: Styx Publications.

Storer, T. (2005) 'Form and function in *Prorrhetic 2*', in van der Eijk 2005a: 345–62.

Strohmaier, G. (1970) 'Asklepios und das Ei: zur Ikonographie in einem arabisch erhaltenen Kommentar zum hippokratischen Eid', in R. Altheim and H. U. Stier (eds) *Beiträge zur Alten Geschichte und deren Nachleben*, Berlin: De Gruyter: II, 143–53.

—— (1981) 'Galen in Arabic: prospects and projects', in Nutton 1981a: 187–96.

—— (1998) 'Bekannte und unbekannte Zitate in den *Zweifeln an Galen* des Rhazes', in Fischer *et al*. 1998: 263–88.

—— (2004) 'Asklepios und seine Sippe', in R. Arnzen and J. Thielmann (eds) *Words, Texts and Concepts cruising the Mediterranean Sea: Studies on the Sources, Contents and Influences of Islamic Civilization and Arabic Philosophy and Science dedicated to Gerhard Endress on his Sixty-fifth Birthday*, Louvain, Paris and Dudley: Peeters: 151–8.

—— (2007) 'La longévité de Galien et les deux places de son tombeau', in Boudon-Millot *et al*. 2007: 393–404.

Stückelberger, A. (1994) *Bild und Wort: Das illustrierte Fachbuch in der antiken Naturwissenschaft*, Mainz: von Zabern.

Suder, W. (1988) '*A partu, utraque filiam enixa decessit*: mortalité maternelle dans l'Empire romain', *Mémoires du Centre Jean Palerne*, 8: 161–6.

Sudhoff, K. (1915–16) 'Die pseudohippokratische Krankheitsprognostik nach den Auftreten von Hautausschlägen "Secreta Hippocratis" oder "Capsula Eburnea" genannt', *Sudhoffs Archiv*, 9: 79–116.

—— (1929) 'Ἐπαφή der Aussatz?', *Sudhoffs Archiv*, 21: 204–6.

Swain, S. (1996) *Hellenism and Empire*, Oxford: Clarendon Press.

—— (ed.) (2007) *Seeing the Face, Seeing the Soul: Polemon's Physiognomy from Classical Antiquity to Medieval Islam*, Oxford: Oxford University Press.

—— (2008) 'Social stress and political pressure: *On Melancholy* in context', in Pormann 2008: 113–38.

Syme, R. (1971) *Emperors and Biography*, Oxford: Clarendon Press.

Tassinari, P. (1994) 'Il trattato sulle febri dello ps. Alessandro d'Afrodisia', *ANRW*, II, 37(2): 2019–34.

Tecusan, M. M. (2004) *The Fragments of the Methodists*, 2 vols, Leiden: Brill.

Telfer, W. (1955) *Nemesius of Emesa: On the Nature of Man*, London: SCM Press.

Temkin, O. (1932) 'Geschichte des Hippokratismus im ausgehenden Altertum', *Kyklos*, 4: 1–80.

—— (1934) 'Galen's advice for an epileptic boy', *Bulletin of the History of Medicine*, 2: 179–89.

—— (1956) *Soranus' Gynaecology*, Baltimore: Johns Hopkins University Press.

—— (1971) *The Falling Sickness*, ed. 2, Baltimore: Johns Hopkins University Press.

—— (1973) *Galenism: Rise and Decline of a Medical Philosophy*, Ithaca and London: Cornell University Press.

—— (1977) *The Double Face of Janus*, Baltimore: Johns Hopkins University Press.

—— (1991) *Hippocrates in a World of Pagans and Christians*, Baltimore: Johns Hopkins University Press.

—— (2002) *'On Second Thought' and Other Essays in the History of Medicine and Science*, Baltimore and London: Johns Hopkins University Press.

Theoharides, T. C. (1971) 'Galen, on marasmus', *Journal of the History of Medicine*, 26: 369–90.

Thévenot, M. (1968) *Divinités et Sanctuaires de la Gaule*, Paris: Fayard.

Thivel, A. (1981) *Cnide et Cos? Essai sur les Doctrines médicales dans la Collection hippocratique*, Paris: Les Belles Lettres.

—— (1999) 'Quale scoperta ha reso celebre Ippocrate?', in Garofalo *et al.* 1999: 149–63.

Thivel, A. and Zucker, A. (eds) (2002) *Le Normal et le Pathologique dans la Collection hippocratique*, Nice: Université de Nice.

Thomas, J. P. (1987) *Private Religious Foundations in the Byzantine Empire*, Washington: Dumbarton Oaks Center.

Thomas, R. (2000) *Herodotus in Context: Ethnography, Science, and the Art of Persuasion*, Cambridge: Cambridge University Press.

Thomassen, H. and Probst, C. (1994) 'Die Medizin des Rufus von Ephesos', *ANRW*, II, 37(2): 1254–92.

Thompson, D. J. (1988) *Memphis under the Ptolemies*, Princeton: Princeton University Press.

Thorndike, L. (1923) *A History of Magic and Experimental Science*, vol. 1, New York: Columbia University Press.

—— (1946) 'Translations of the works of Galen from the Greek by Niccolò da Reggio (c.1308–1345)', *Byzantina Metabyzantina*, 1: 213–35.

—— (1960) 'The three Latin translations of the pseudo-Hippocratic Tract on Astrological Medicine', *Janus*, 49: 103–29.

—— (1963) 'The pseudo-Galen, *De Plantis*', *Ambix*, 11: 87–94.

Tibiletti, G. (1979) *Le Lettere private di Papiri greci del III e IV secolo d. C.*, Milan: Università Cattolica.

Tick, E. (2001) *The Practice of Dream Healing*, Wheaton: Quest Books.

Tieleman, T. (1997) 'The hunt for Galen's shadow: Alexander of Aphrodisias, *De anima* 94.7–100 Bruns reconsidered', in K. A. Algra (ed.) *Polyhistor: Studies in the History and Historiography of Ancient Philosophy Presented to J. Mansfeld*, Leiden: Brill: 256–83.

Till, W. C. (1951) *Die Arzneikunde der Kopten*, Berlin: Akademie Verlag.

Todd, R. B. (1976) 'Greek medical ideas in the Greek Aristotelian Commentators', *Symbolae Osloenses*, 52: 117–34.

Toledo-Pereyra, L. (1973) 'Galen's contribution to surgery', *Journal of the History of Medicine*, 28: 356–75.

Tomlinson, R. A. (1983) *Epidauros*, Austin: University of Texas Press.

Toomer, G. J. (1985) 'Galen on the astronomers and astrologers', *Archive for the History of Exact Science*, 32: 193–206.

Totelin, L. M. V. (2004) 'Mithridates' antidote: a pharmacological ghost', *Early Science and Medicine*, 9: 1–19.

—— (2009) *Hippocratic Recipes: Oral and Written Transmission of Pharmacological Knowledge in Fifth- and Fourth-century Greece*, Leiden and Boston: Brill.

Touwaide, A. (1994) 'Galien et la toxicologie', *ANRW*, II, 37(2): 1887–986.

—— (1997) 'La thérapeutique médicamenteuse de Dioscoride à Galien', in Debru 1997: 255–82.

—— (1999) 'Krankheit', *DNP*, 6: 793–803.

—— (2012) 'Research breakthrough: 200-year-old medicine revealed', published on-line at: http://medicaltraditions.org/institute/news/2-general/168-research-breakthrough-2000-year-old-medicine-revealed (accessed 1994).

Trease, G. E. and Evans, W. C. (1978) *Pharmacognosy*, ed. 11, London: Baillière Tindall.

Tuplin, C. J. (2004) 'Doctoring the Persians: Ctesias of Cnidus, physician and historian', *Klio*, 86: 305–47.

Ullmann, M. (1972a) 'Das Steinbuch des Xenokrates von Ephesos', *Medizinhistorisches Journal*, 7: 49–64.

—— (1972b) 'Kleopatra in einer arabischen alchemistischen Disputation', *Wiener Zeitschrift für die Kunde des Morgenlandes*, 63/64: 158–75.

—— (1973) 'Neues zum Steinbuch des Xenokrates', *Medizinhistorisches Journal*, 8: 59–76.

—— (1974) 'Neues zu den diätetischen Medizin des Rufus von Ephesos', *Medizinhistorisches Journal*, 9: 23–40.

—— (1975) 'Die Schrift des Rufus de infantium curatione', *Medizinhistorisches Journal*, 10: 165–90.

—— (1977) 'Galens Kommentar zu der Schrift *De aere aquis locis*', in R. Joly (ed.) *Actes du Colloque hippocratique de Mons*, Mons: Université de Mons: 353–65.

—— (1978a) *Die Medizin im Islam*, Leiden: Brill.

—— (1978b) *Islamic Medicine*, Edinburgh: Edinburgh University Press.

—— (1978c) *Rufus von Ephesos: Krankenjournale*, Wiesbaden: Harrassowitz.

—— (1983) 'Die Schrift des Rufus von Ephesos über die Gelbsucht in arabischer und lateinischer Übersetzung', *Abhandlungen der Akademie der Wissenschaften in Göttingen*, 138.

—— (1994) 'Die arabische Überlieferung der Schriften des Rufus von Ephesos', *ANRW*, II, 37(2): 1293–349.

Urso, A. M. (1997) *Dall'Autore al Traduttore: Studi sulle Passiones celeres et tardae di Celio Aureliano*, Messina: EDAS.

Vallance, J. T. (1990) *The Lost Theory of Asclepiades of Bithynia*, Oxford: Clarendon Press.

—— (1993) 'The medical system of Asclepiades of Bithynia', *ANRW*, II, 37(1): 693–727.

—— (2000) 'Doctors in the library: the strange tale of Apollonius the bookworm and other stories', in Macleod 2000: 95–114.

van der Eijk, P. J. (1996) 'Diocles and the Hippocratic writings on the method of dietetics and the limits of causal explanation', in Wittern and Pellegrin 1996: 239–57; repr. in van der Eijk 2005b.

—— (1997a) 'Galen's use of the concept of "qualified experience" in his dietetic and pharmacological works', in Debru 1997: 35–58; repr. in van der Eijk 2005b.

—— (1997b) 'Towards a rhetoric of scientific discourse: some formal characteristics of Greek medical and philosophical texts (Hippocratic Corpus, Aristotle)', in E. J. Bakker (ed.) *Grammar as Interpretation: Greek Literature in its Linguistic Context*, Leiden: Brill.

—— (1999a) *Ancient Histories of Medicine*, Leiden: Brill.

—— (1999b) 'The anonymus Parisinus and the doctrines of "the Ancients"', in van der Eijk 1999a: 295–332.

—— (1999c) 'Aristotle on "distinguished physicians" and on the medical significance of dreams', in van der Eijk 1999a: 447–59.

—— (1999d) 'Antiquarianism and criticism: forms and functions of medical doxography in methodism (Soranus and Caelius Aurelianus)', in van der Eijk 1999a: 397–452.

—— (1999e) *On Sterility* ("HA X"), a medical work by Aristotle', *Classical Quarterly*, 49: 490–502; repr. in van der Eijk 2005b.

—— (2000–1) *Diocles of Carystus: A Collection of the Fragments with Translation and Commentary*, 2 vols, Leiden: Brill.

—— (2005a) *Hippocrates in Context: Papers Read at the 11th International Hippocrates Colloquium, University of Newcastle upon Tyne, 27–31 August 2002*, Leiden and Boston: Brill.

—— (2005b) *Medicine and Philosophy in Classical Antiquity: Doctors and Philosophers on Nature, Soul, Health and Disease*, Cambridge: Cambridge University Press.

—— (2008) 'Therapeutics', in Hankinson 2008: 283–303.

—— (2010) 'Principles and practices of compilation and abbreviation in the medical "Encyclopaedias" of late antiquity', in M. Horster and C. Reitz (eds) *Condensing Texts: Condensed Texts*, Stuttgart: Steiner Verlag: 519–54.

—— (2011) 'Medicine and health in the Graeco-Roman world', in M. Jackson (ed.) *The Oxford Handbook of the History of Medicine*, Oxford: Oxford University Press: 21–39.

van der Eijk, P. J., Horstmanshoff, H. F. J. and Schrijvers, P. H. (eds) (1995) *Ancient Medicine in its Socio-cultural Context*, 2 vols, Amsterdam: Rodopi.

van der Meer, L. B. (1987) *The Bronze Liver of Piacenza*, Amsterdam: J. C. Gieben.

van der Toorn, K. (1985) *Sin and Sanction in Israel and Mesopotamia: A Comparative Study*, Assen: Van Gorcum.

van der Toorn, K., Becking, B. and van der Horst, P. W. (eds) (1995) *Dictionary of Deities and Demons in the Bible*, Leiden: Brill.

van Effenterre, H. and Ruze, F. (1994) *Receuil des Inscriptions politiques et juridiques de l'Archaisme grec*, vol. I, Rome: Ecole française de Rome.

van Esbroeck, M. (1981) 'La diffusion orientale de la légende orientale des saints Cosme et Damien', in Patlagean and Riché 1981: 61–77.

van Straten, F. T. (1981) 'Gifts for the gods', in H. S. Versnel (ed.) *Faith, Hope, and Worship*, Leiden: Brill: 65–151.

—— (1992) 'Votives and votaries in Greek sanctuaries', in Reverdin and Grange 1992: 247–84; repr. in R. Buxton (2000) *Oxford Readings in Greek Religion*, Oxford: Oxford University Press: 191–223.

van Uytfanghe, M. (1981) 'La controverse biblique et patristique autour du miracle, et ses répercussions sur l'hagiographie dans l'antiquité tardive et le haut moyen âge latin', in Patlagean and Riché 1981: 205–31.

Varinoglu, E. (1989) 'Eine Gruppe von Sühneinschriften aus dem Museum von Usak', *Epigraphica Anatolica*, 13: 37–50.

Vegetti, M. (1993) 'I nervi dell'anima', in Kollesch and Nickel 1993: 63–77.

—— (1996) 'Iatromantis: previsione e memoria nella Grecia antica', in M. Bettini (ed.) *I signori della memoria e dell'Oblio*, Florence: La Nuova Italia: 65–81.

—— (1998a) 'Empedocle medico e sophista: l'antica medicina 20', *Elenchos*, 19: 345–60.

—— (1998b) 'Between knowledge and practice: Hellenistic medicine', in Grmek 1998: 72–103.

Ventris, M. and Chadwick, J. (1973) *Documents in Mycenaean Greek*, ed. 2, Cambridge: Cambridge University Press.

Verbanck-Piérard, A. (ed.) (1998) *Au Temps d'Hippocrate: Médecine et Société en Grèce ancienne*, Mariemont: Musée royale de Mariemont.

—— (2000) 'Les héros guérisseurs des dieux comme les autres! A propos des cultes médicaux dans l'attique classique', in V. Pirenne-Delforge and E. Suárez de la Torre (eds) *Héros et Héroines dans les Mythes et les Cultes grecs, Kernos, Suppl.*, 10: 281–332.

Verbeke, G. (1945) *L'Evolution de la Doctrine du Pneuma du Stoïcisme à S. Augustin*, Paris and Louvain: Desclée de Brouwer.

Vermes, G. (1973) *Jesus the Jew*, London: Macmillan.

Viano, C. A. (1984) 'Perché non'c'era sangue delle arterie? La cecità epistemologica degli anatomisti antichi', in G. Giannatone and M. Vegetti (eds) *La Scienza Ellenistica*, Naples: Bibliopolis: 297–352.

Viellefond, J. R. (1970) *Les 'Cestes' de Julius Africanus: Étude sur l'Ensemble des Fragments avec Édition, Traduction et Commentaires*, Paris: Librairie Marcel Didier.

Vikan, G. (1984) 'Art, medicine, and magic in early Byzantium', *Dumbarton Oaks Papers*, 38: 65–86.

Vogt, S. (2008) 'Drugs and pharmacology', in Hankinson 2008: 242–62.

Voinot, J. (1999) *Les Cachets à Collyres dans le Monde romain*, Montagnac: Libraire archéologique Monique Mergoil.

—— (1999–2000) 'Bibliographie des cachets à collyres (cachets d'oculistes)', *Lettre d'Informations du Centre Jean Palerne*, 32: 2–29.

von Grot, R. (1899) 'Über die in der hippokratischen Schriftensammlung enthaltenen pharmakologischen Kentnisse', *Historische Studien aus dem Pharmakologischen Institute der Kaiserl. Universität Dorpat*, 1: 58–133.

von Müller, I. (1895) 'Über Galens Werk vom wissenschaftlichen Beweis', *Abhandlungen der kgl. bayerischen Akademie der Wissenschaften*, 20: 2.

von Staden, H. (1975) 'Experiment and experience in Hellenistic medicine', *Bulletin of the Institute of Classical Studies*, 22: 178–99.

—— (1982) 'Hairesis and heresy: the case of the "haireseis iatrikai"', in B. F. Meyer and E. P. Sanders (eds) *Jewish and Christian Self-definition in the Graeco-Roman World*, London: SCM: 76–100, 199–206.

—— (1989) *Herophilus: The Art of Medicine in Early Alexandria*, Cambridge: Cambridge University Press.

—— (1990) 'Incurability and hopelessness: the Hippocratic Corpus', in Potter *et al.* 1990: 75–112.

—— (1992a) 'The discovery of the body: human dissection and its cultural contexts in Ancient Greece', *Yale Journal of Biology and Medicine*, 65: 223–41.

—— (1992b) 'Jaeger's "Skandalon der historischen Vernunft": Diocles, Aristotle, and Theophrastus', in W. M. Calder, III (ed.) *Werner Jaeger Reconsidered*, Atlanta: Scholars' Press: 227–65.

—— (1992c) 'Women and dirt', *Helios*, 19: 7–30.

—— (1996a) 'In a pure and holy way: personal and professional conduct in the Hippocratic oath', *Journal of the History of Medicine and Allied Sciences*, 51: 404–37.

—— (1996b) 'Liminal perils: early Roman receptions of Greek medicine', in F. J. Ragep and S. Ragep (eds) *Tradition, Transmission, Transformation*, Leiden: Brill, 369–409.

—— (1997a) '"Hard Realism" and "A Few Romantic Moves": Henry Sigerist's versions of Ancient Greece', in E. Fee and T. M. Brown (eds) *Making Medical History: The Life and Times of Henry E. Sigerist*, Baltimore and London: Johns Hopkins University Press: 136–61.

464

—— (1997b) 'Inefficacy, error and failure: Galen on δόκιμα φάρμακα ἄπρακτα', in Debru 1997: 59–84.

—— (1997c) 'Teleology and mechanism: Aristotelian biology and early Hellenistic medicine', in Kullmann and Föllinger 1997: 183–208.

—— (1999) 'Caelius Aurelianus and the Hellenistic epoch: Erasistratus, the Empiricists, and Herophilus', in Mudry 1999: 85–119.

—— (2000) 'Body, soul, and nerves: Epicurus, Herophilus, Erasistratus, the Stoics, and Galen', in J. P. Wright and P. Potter (eds) *Psyche and Soma*, Oxford: Clarendon Press.

—— (2002a) 'Division, dissection and specialization: Galen's *On the Parts of the Medical Techne*', in Nutton 2002a: 19–48.

—— (2002b) Ὡς ἐπὶ τὸ πολύ. "Hippocrates" between generalization and individualization', in Thivel and Zucker 2002: 23–43.

—— (2003) 'Galen's daimon: reflections on "rational" and "irrational"', in Palmieri 2003: 15–44.

—— (2007) '"The *Oath*", the oaths and the Hippocratic Corpus', in Boudon-Millot *et al.* 2007: 425–66.

—— (2009a) 'The Hellenistic character of Celsus, *Artes X–XII* (*Medicina V–VI*): history, structure and system', in Ferraces Rodríguez 2009: 13–32.

—— (2009b) 'Staging the past, staging oneself: Galen on Hellenistic exegetical traditions', in Gill *et al.* 2009: 132–56.

—— (2010) 'How Greek was the Latin body? The parts and the whole in Celsus' *Medicina*', in Langslow and Maire 2010: 3–23.

von Wilamowitz-Moellendorff, U. (1928) *Marcellus von Side*, Sitzungsberichte der deutschen Akademie der Wissenschaften.

Vööbus, A. (1965) *History of the School of Nisibis*, SCO 266, subsid. 26, Louvain: CSCO.

—— (1967) *The Statutes of the School of Nisibis*, Stockholm: ETSE.

—— (1970) *Syrische Kanonessammlungen. 1 Westsyrische Originalurkunden*, Louvain: CSCO.

—— (1982) *The Canons of Maruta of Maipherqat and Related Sources*, Louvain: E. Peeters.

Waldron, H. A. and Wells, C. (1979) 'Exposure to lead in ancient populations', *Transactions and Studies of the College of Physicians of Philadelphia*, ser. 5(1): 102–15.

Walzer, R. (1935) 'Galeni De septimestri partu', *Rivista di Studi orientali*, 13: 346–8.

—— (1944) *Galen: On Medical Experience*, Oxford: Clarendon Press.

—— (1949) *Galen on Jews and Christians*, Oxford: Clarendon Press.

—— (1962) *From Greek into Arabic*, London: B. Cassirer.

Walzer, R. and Frede, M. (1985) *Galen: Three Treatises on the Nature of Science*, Indianapolis: Hackett.

Wasserstein, A. (1982) 'Galen's commentary on the Hippocratic treatise *Airs, Waters and Places* in the Hebrew translation of Solomon ha-Me'ati', *Proceedings of the Israel Academy of Sciences and Humanities*, 6: 3.

Watermann, R. (1974) *Medizinisches und Hygienisches aus Germania Inferior*, Neuss: R. Watermann.

Watson, G. (1966) *Theriac and Mithridatium: A Study in Therapeutics*, London: The Wellcome Historical Medical Library.

Waugh, W., Bernabò, M. and Grmek, M. D. (1984) 'La scena ortopedica', *Kos*, 1(5): 33–60.

Wear, A. (1983) 'William Harvey and "The Way of the Anatomists"', *History of Science*, 21: 223–49.

—— (2000) *Knowledge and Practice in English Medicine, 1550–1650*, Cambridge: Cambridge University Press.

Weeks, K. R. (1970) *The Anatomical Knowledge of the Ancient Egyptians and the Representation of the Human Figure in Egyptian Art*, PhD thesis, Yale University.

Weinreich, O. (1909) *Antike Heilungswunder*, Giessen: Topelmann.

Weinstock, S. (1948) 'The author of Ps. Galen's Prognostica de Decubitu', *Classical Quarterly*, 42: 41–3.

Weisser, U. (1989) 'Das Corpus Hippocraticum in der arabischen Medizin', in Baader and Winau 1989: 377–408.

Weisz, G. (2002) 'Hippocrates, holism and humanism in interwar France', in Cantor 2002: 257–79.

Wellmann, M. (1889) 'Sextius Niger', *Hermes*, 24: 530–69.

—— (1895) *Die pneumatische Schule bis auf Archigenes*, Berlin: Weidmann.

—— (1897) 'Krateuas', *Abhandlungen der königlichen Gesellschaft der Wissenschaften in Göttingen*.

—— (1901) *Die Fragmente der sikelischen Ärzte Akron: Philistion und des Diokles von Karystos*, Berlin: Weidmann.

—— (1906–14) *Pedanius Dioscorides, De Materia Medica*, 3 vols, Berlin: Weidmann.

—— (1907) 'Eine neue Schrift des Alexander von Tralles', *Hermes*, 42: 532–41.

—— (1908a) 'Aelius Promotus Ἰατρικὰ καὶ ἀντιπαθητικά', *Sitzungsberichte der preussischen Akademie der Wissenschaften*, 37.

—— (1908b) 'Asklepiades von Bithynien von einem herrschenden Vorurteil befreit', *Neue Jahrbücher für das Klassische Altertum*, 18: 684–703.

—— (1916) 'Pamphilos', *Hermes*, 51: 1–64.

—— (1921) 'Die Georgika des Demokritos', *Abhandlungen der preussischen Akademie der Wissenschaften, phil.-hist. Kl.*

—— (1929) 'Spuren Demokrits von Abdera im Corpus Hippocraticum', *Sudhoffs Archiv*, 22: 290–312.

—— (1934) *Marcellus von Side als Arzt und die Koiraniden des Hermes Trismegistos, Philologus, Suppl.*, 27(2).

Wendel, C. (1943) 'Pamphilos, 23', *RE*, 18: 336–49.

Wenkebach, E. (1932–3) 'Der hippokratische Arzt als das Ideal Galen', *Quellen und Studien zur Geschichte der Naturwissenschaften und Medizin*, 3: 155–75.

Wenskus, O. (1990) *Astronomische Zeitangaben von Homer bis Theophrast*, Stuttgart: Steiner.

West, M. L. (1971) 'The cosmology of "Hippocrates", De hebdomadibus', *Classical Quarterly*, 21: 365–88.

—— (1978) *Hesiod: Works and Days*, Oxford: Clarendon Press.

—— (1982) 'Magnus and Marcellinus: unnoticed acrostics in the *Cyranides*', *Classical Quarterly*, 32: 480–1.

—— (1997) *The East Face of Helicon*, Oxford: Clarendon Press.

Westendorf, W. (1999) *Handbuch der altägyptischen Medizin*, Leiden: Brill.

Westerink, L. G. (1964) 'Philosophy and medicine in late antiquity', *Janus*, 51: 169–77.

Weyh, W. (1911–12) *Die syrische Barbara-Legende, mit einem Anhang: Die syrische Kosmas und Damian-Legende in deutscher Übersetzung*, Programm des k. Humanistischen Gymnasiums, Schweinfurt: J. Reichardt.

Wickkiser, B. L. (2008) *Asklepios, Medicine, and the Politics of Healing in Fifth-century Greece*, Baltimore: Johns Hopkins University Press.

Wilberding, J. (2011) *Porphyry: To Gaurus on how Embryos are Ensouled and On What is in our Power*, London: Duckworth.

Wilkins, J. (2005) 'The social and intellectual context of *Regimen II*', in van der Eijk 2005a: 121–34.

466

—— (2007) 'Galen and Athenaeus in the Hellenistic Library', in König and Whitmarsh 2007: 69–87.

—— (2011) 'Galen the scholar', in P. Millett, S. P. Oakley and R. J. E. Thompson (eds) *Ratio et res ipsa: Classical Essays presented by Former Pupils to James Diggle on his Retirement*, Cambridge: Cambridge Philological Society: 45–60.

Wilkins, J. and Hill, S. (1994) *The Life of Luxury: Europe's Oldest Cookery Book*, Totnes: Prospect Books.

Wilkins, J., Harvey, D. and Dobson, M. (eds) (1995) *Food in Antiquity*, Exeter: Exeter University Press.

Williams, B. A. O. (1973) 'The analogy of city and soul in Plato's Republic', in A. N. Lee, A. P. D. Mourelatos and R. M. Rorty (eds) *Exegesis and Argument, Phronesis, Suppl.*, 1, Assen: Van Gorcum: 196–206.

Wilmanns, J. C. (1995) *Der Sanitätsdienst im römischen Reich*, Hildesheim: Olms Weidmann.

Winnington-Ingram, R. P. (1980) *Sophocles: An Interpretation*, Cambridge: Cambridge University Press.

Winter, F. E. (1980) 'Tradition and innovation in Doric design III: the work of Ictinus', *American Journal of Archeology*, 84: 399–416.

Wiseman, J. N. (1973) *Studies in the Antiquities of Stobi*, Belgrade: Tito Najowski.

Wissowa, G. (1909) 'Febris', *RE*, 6: 2095–6.

Witt, M. (2009) *Weichteil- und Viszeralchirurgie bei Hippokrate: Ein Rekonstruktionsversuch der verlorenen Schrift Perì trōmátou kaì belõu (De vulneribus et telis)*, Berlin: De Gruyter.

Wittern, R. and Pellegrin, P. (eds) (1996) *Hippokratische Medizin und antike Philosophie*, Hildesheim, Zurich and New York: Olms Weidmann.

Wohlers, M. (1999) *Heilige Krankheit: Epilepsie in antiker Medizin, Astrologie und Religion*, Marburg: N. Elwert.

Wöhrle, G. (1990) *Studien zur Theorie der antiken Gesundheitslehre*, Stuttgart: Steiner.

Wolf, J. H. (ed.) (1986) *Aussatz, Lepra, Hansen-Krankheit: Ein Menschheitsproblem im Wandel, Teil II. Aufsätze*, Würzburg: Deutsches Aussätzigen-Hilfswerk.

Wolska-Conus, W. (1989) 'Stéphanos d'Athènes et Stéphanos d'Alexandrie: Essai d'identification et de biographie', *Revue des Études Byzantines*, 47: 5–89.

Wolstenholme, G. (ed.) (1982) *Lives of the Fellows of the College of Physicians of London, Continued to 1975*, London: The Royal College of Physicians.

Worp, K. A. (1982) 'Der Arzt in P. Lips. 42', *Zeitschrift für Papyrologie und Epigraphik*, 45: 227–8.

Worthington, M. (2009) 'Medical information outside the medical corpora', in Attia and Buisson 2009: 47–77.

Wulf-Rheidt, U. (1998) 'The Hellenistic and Roman houses of Pergamum', in Koester 1998: 299–330.

Yegül, F. K. (1992) *Baths and Bathing in Classical Antiquity*, New York: Architectural Heritage Foundation.

—— (2010) *Bathing in the Roman World*, Cambridge: Cambridge University Press.

Youtie, H. C. and Winter, J. G. (1951) *Michigan Papyri*, vol. 8, Ann Arbor: University of Michigan Press.

Yunis, H. (ed.) (2003) *Written Texts and the Rise of Literate Culture in Ancient Greece*, Cambridge: Cambridge University Press.

Zaccagnini, C. (1983) 'Patterns of mobility among ancient Near Eastern craftsmen', *Journal of Near Eastern Studies*, 41: 245–64.

Ziegenaus, O. and De Luca, G. (1968–84) *Das Asklepieion von Pergamum, Altertümer von Pergamon*, XI, Berlin: De Gruyter.

Ziegler, R. (1994) 'Aegeai, das Asklepioskult, das Kaiserhaus der Decier und das Christentum', *Tyche*, 9: 187–212.

Zunino, M. L. (1997) *Hiera Messeniaka: La Storia religiosa della Messenia dall'Età micenea all'Età hellenistica*, Udine: Forum.

INDEX OF NAMES

INDEX OF TOPICS

body/soul relationship
  in Galenic medicine 240–1
  Platonic theory 118
botany, medical: development 143
breasts: cancer 35
bubo: lancing 54 *illus.*

camp fever (typhus) 25
cancers 23, 30 *see also* under affected part
  surgery 23
  treatments 35
carminatives 98
carphology 90
case histories 22, 89
  at healing shrines 110
  role 90–2
cataracts: surgery 31
cauterisation 93
chief doctor (archiatros) 153–4
chlamydia trachomatis 30
Christianity
  charity to the ill 295–302
  and healing 332 *n*104, 412 *n*142
  and healing cults 310–1
chronic conditions 34–5, 204, 334 *n*144,
  382 *n*29
circulators (travelling doctors) 162, 327 *n*39
  see also healers
climate
  role in disease 331 *n*63
climate: role in disease 25
clyster: administration of 95 *illus.*
Colles fracture 31 *see also*
  fractures/dislocations
constipation 34
contagion 26
critical days 123
  origin of doctrine 46
cult of Asclepius 109, 216, 286–9
  dedication 287 *illus.*
  devotion to 286–9
  expansion 109,111
  introduced in Rome 161–4
  and secular healers 112
  spread 105–8
  universality 282–3
cupping glass 93, 94 *illus.*
cure tablets 35, 109–10
cures *see* therapies/therapeutic practices
cystitis 30

deficiency diseases 21 *see also* disease/diseases;
  specific deficiency diseases
degenerative diseases 23 *see also* disease/
  diseases; specific disease e.g. arthritis
demography 19–20 *see also* pathocoenosis
  and malnutrition 21
diagnosis 353 *n*80
  Galenic 228 in Galenic medicine 244
  and humoral colour 339 *n*82
  and individual disposition 92
  methodology 121
diatritos 197
diet
  and disease 25, 26
  and healing 362 *n*77
  and health 33–4, 36
dietetics 124
  beginnings 102
  Dogmatic 126–7
  in Galenic medicine 246–8
  Hellenistic 143
  Hippocratic 96–7, 352 *n*74
  origin 352 *n*69
  pre-Hippocratic theories 49
digestion: pre-Hippocratic theories 47
digestive complaints 29
Dioclean spoon 122
Diocles: reduction of fractures 362 *n*76
disease/diseases 19 *see also* affected part;
  affected system; degenerative diseases;
  digestive omplaints; health; name;
  name e.g. leprosy; occupational diseases;
  parasitic infections; pathocoenosis;
  respiratory conditions; sexually
  transmitted diseases
  Ancient perception of 36 and bile 360
    *n*10
  causes/explanations 26, 330 *n*51, 366
    n84
    divine origin 113, 290–2
    elemental imbalance 45–6
    mechanical 137–9
    natural 39, 51, 114, 123–4
    rational 114–15
  classification and description 22, 397
    *n*86
  communicable 24
  concept 28
  contagion 26, 328 *n*17
  and degeneration of tissues 360*n*10
  equating to modern 28–9
  Hippocratic theories 58–9

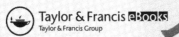